LEARNSMART® >

The market-leading **adaptive study tool** proven to strengthen memory recall, increase class retention, and boost grades.

> Moves students beyond memorizing

> Allows instructors to align content with their goals

> Allows instructors to spend more time teaching higher-level concepts

SMARTBOOK® >

The first—and only—adaptive reading experience designed to transform the way students read.

> Engages students with a personalized reading experience

> Ensures students retain knowledge

LEARNSMART
PREP®

An adaptive course preparation tool that quickly and efficiently helps students prepare for college-level work.

> Levels out student knowledge

> Keeps students on track

LEARNSMART
ACHIEVE®

A learning system that continually adapts and provides learning tools to teach students the concepts they don't know.

> Adaptively provides learning resources

> A time management feature ensures students master course material to complete their assignments by the due date

WWW.LEARNSMARTADVANTAGE.COM

Fourth Edition

Nutrition

FOR HEALTHY LIVING

Updated with *2015–2020 Dietary Guidelines for Americans*

Wendy J. Schiff, MS, RDN

McGraw Hill Education

NUTRITION FOR HEALTHY LIVING Updated with *2015–2020 Dietary Guidelines for Americans*, FOURTH EDITION

Published by McGraw–Hill Education, 2 Penn Plaza, New York, NY 10121. Copyright © 2016 by McGraw–Hill Education. All rights reserved. Printed in the United States of America. Previous editions © 2013, 2011, and 2009. No part of this publication may be reproduced or distributed in any form or by any means, or stored in a database or retrieval system, without the prior written consent of McGraw–Hill Education, including, but not limited to, in any network or other electronic storage or transmission, or broadcast for distance learning.

Some ancillaries, including electronic and print components, may not be available to customers outside the United States.

This book is printed on acid–free paper.

1 2 3 4 5 6 7 8 9 RMN 21 20 19 18 17 16

ISBN 978–1–259–89350–6
MHID 1–259–89350–2

Senior Vice President, Products & Markets: *Kurt L. Strand*
Vice President, General Manager, Products & Markets: *Marty Lange*
Vice President, Content Design & Delivery: *Kimberly Meriwether David*
Managing Director: *Michael S. Hackett*
Director of Digital Content: *Michael G. Koot, PhD*
Brand Managers: *Marija Magner/Amy Reed*
Director, Product Development: *Rose Koos*
Product Developer: *Darlene M. Schueller*
Marketing Manager: *Kristine Rellihan*
Digital Product Analyst: *Christine Carlson*
Director, Content Design & Delivery: *Linda Avenarius*
Program Manager: *Angela R. FitzPatrick*
Content Project Managers: *MaryJane Lampe/Brent Dela Cruz*
Buyer: *Jennifer Pickel*
Designers: *Michelle D. Whitaker/Matt Backhaus*
Content Licensing Specialists: *Lori Hancock (image)/Lorraine Buczek (text)*
Cover Image: *© Fred Hirschmann/Getty Images*
Compositor: *SPi Global*
Printer: *R. R. Donnelley*

All credits appearing on page or at the end of the book are considered to be an extension of the copyright page.

Library of Congress Cataloging–in–Publication Data

Names: Schiff, Wendy.
Title: Nutrition for healthy living / Wendy J. Schiff M.S., R.D.
Description: Fourth edition, updated with 2015–2020 dietary guidelines for
   Americans. | New York, NY: McGraw–Hill Education, [2016]
Identifiers: LCCN 2016008796 | ISBN 9781259893506 (alk. paper)
Subjects: LCSH: Human nutrition—Textbooks.
Classification: LCC QP141 .S3435 2016b | DDC 612.3—dc23
LC record available at https://lccn.loc.gov/2016008796

The Internet addresses listed in the text were accurate at the time of publication. The inclusion of a website or photo or mention of a specific product does not indicate an endorsement by the authors or McGraw–Hill Education, and McGraw–Hill Education does not guarantee the accuracy of the information presented at these sites.

www.mhhe.com

Brief Contents

1 The Basics of Nutrition   2

2 Evaluating Nutrition Information   32

3 Planning Nutritious Diets   60

4 Body Basics   98

5 Carbohydrates   128

6 Fats and Other Lipids   164

7 Proteins   214

8 Vitamins   256

9 Water and Minerals   314

10 Energy Balance and Weight Control   370

11 Nutrition for Physically Active Lifestyles   424

12 Food Safety Concerns   456

13 Nutrition for a Lifetime   492

Appendix A English-Metric Conversions and Metric-to-Household Units   A-1
Appendix B Daily Values Table   A-2
Appendix C Energy Metabolism   A-3
Appendix D Amino Acids   A-6
Appendix E Vitamins Involved in Energy Metabolism   A-7
Appendix F Body Mass Index-for-Age Percentiles   A-8
Appendix G Answers to Concept Checkpoint
Questions and Practice Test Questions   A-10
Appendix H References   A-24

Glossary   G-1

Photo Credits   C-1

Index   I-1

Dietary Reference Intakes (DRIs)

Meet the Author

Wendy J. Schiff MS, RDN received her BS in biological health/medical dietetics and MS in human nutrition from The Pennsylvania State University. She has taught introductory foods and nutrition courses at the University of Missouri–Columbia as well as nutrition, human biology, and personal health courses at St. Louis Community College–Meramec. She has worked as a public health nutritionist at the Allegheny County Health Department (Pittsburgh, Pennsylvania) and State Food and Nutrition Specialist for Missouri Extension at Lincoln University in Jefferson City, Missouri. In addition to authoring *Nutrition for Healthy Living and Nutrition Essentials: A Personal Approach,* Wendy has coauthored *Human Nutrition: Science for Healthy Living* and a college-level personal health textbook, and authored many other nutrition-related educational materials. She is a registered dietitian nutritionist and a member of the Academy of Nutrition and Dietetics.

To my mother and late father.

Welcome to the Fourth Edition of Nutrition for Healthy Living Updated with 2015-2020 Dietary Guidelines for Americans

We think of ourselves as consumers when we purchase homes, cars, computers, and food. We are also consumers of nutrition-related information. Nearly every day, we are literally bombarded with messages in media and from acquaintances concerning nutrition, foods, and health. Much of this information is unreliable, and often it is intended to promote sales of products or services. Unfortunately, many consumers lack the knowledge and skills needed to analyze such information critically and decide whether or not to apply it to their decision-making process.

Helping students become better-informed consumers, particularly as this relates to food and nutrition, is the foundation of Nutrition for Healthy Living. This major theme flows throughout the textbook by providing students with practical information, critical thinking skills, and the scientific foundation needed to make better-informed choices about their diet and health. By reading Nutrition for Healthy Living, not only will students learn basic principles of nutrition, they will also be able to evaluate various sources of nutrition information critically and to apply sound nutrition practices to improve their lives.

Wendy J. Schiff

Personalized, Adaptive Learning

Adaptive learning resources offer students a personalized learning experience.

"LearnSmart has helped me to understand exactly what concepts I do not yet understand. I feel like after I complete a module I have a deeper understanding of the material and a stronger base to then build on to apply the material to more challenging concepts."

Student

LEARNSMART®

McGraw—Hill LearnSmart® is one of the most effective and successful adaptive learning resources available on the market today. More than 2 million students have answered more than 1.3 billion questions in LearnSmart since 2009, making it the most widely used and intelligent adaptive study tool that's proven to strengthen memory recall, keep students in class, and boost grades. Students using LearnSmart are 13% more likely to pass their classes and 35% less likely to drop out.

LearnSmart continuously adapts to each student's needs by building an individual learning path so students study smarter and retain more knowledge. Turnkey reports provide valuable insight to instructors, so precious class time can be spent on higher—level concepts and discussion.

SMARTBOOK®

Fueled by LearnSmart—the most widely used and intelligent adaptive learning resource—**SmartBook®** is the first and only adaptive reading experience available today.

Distinguishing what a student knows from what they don't, and honing in on concepts they are most likely to forget, SmartBook personalizes content for each student in a continuously adapting reading experience. Reading is no longer a passive and linear experience, but an engaging and dynamic one where students are more likely to master and retain important concepts, coming to class better prepared. Valuable reports provide instructors insight as to how students are progressing through textbook content and are useful for shaping in—class time or assessment.

As a result of the adaptive reading experience found in SmartBook, students are more likely to retain knowledge, stay in class, and get better grades.

Digital efficacy study shows results!

Digital efficacy study final analysis shows students experience higher success rates when required to use LearnSmart.

- Passing rates increased by an average of **11.5%** across the schools and by a weighted average of **7%** across all students.
- Retention rates increased an average of **10%** across the schools and by a weighted average of **8%** across all students.

Study details:

- Included two state universities and four community colleges.
- Control sections assigned chapter assignments consisting of test bank questions and the experimental sections assigned LearnSmart, both through McGraw—Hill Connect®.
- Both types of assignments were counted as a portion of the grade, and all other course materials and assessments were consistent.
- 358 students opted into the LearnSmart sections and 332 into the sections where test bank questions were assigned.

> "After collecting data for five semesters, including two 8-week intensive courses, the trend was very clear: students who used LearnSmart scored higher on exams and tended to achieve a letter grade higher than those who did not."
>
> Gabriel Guzman
> Triton College

Personalized Teaching and Learning Environment

Saves students and instructors time while improving performance.

|NUTRITION

McGraw—Hill Connect® Nutrition is a digital teaching and learning environment that saves students and instructors time while improving performance over a variety of critical outcomes.

- *Auto—grade assessments and tutorials*

  Instructors can easily create customized assessments that will be automatically graded. All Connect content is created by nutrition instructors so it is pedagogical, instructional, and at the appropriate level. Interactive questions using high—quality art from the textbook and animations and videos from a variety of sources take students way beyond multiple choice.

- *Gather assessment information*

  All Connect questions are tagged to a learning outcome, specific section and topic, and Bloom's level for easy tracking of assessment data.

- *Access content anywhere, anytime*

  The **media—rich eBook** allows students to do full text searches, add notes and highlights, and access their instructor's shared notes and highlights.

- *Streamline lecture creation*

  Presentation tools, such as PowerPoint® lecture outlines including art, photos, tables, and animations, allow instructors to customize their lectures.

McGraw—Hill Connect® Insight is a powerful data analytics tool that allows instructors to leverage aggregated information about their courses and students to provide a more personalized teaching and learning experience.

LEARNSMART
PREP®

LearnSmart Prep® is designed to get students ready for a forthcoming course by quickly and effectively addressing prerequisite knowledge gaps that may cause problems down the road.

McGraw–Hill Tegrity® is a fully automated lecture capture solution used in traditional, hybrid, "flipped classes" and online courses to record lesson, lectures, and skills.

NutritionCalc Plus is a suite of powerful dietary self–assessment tools that help students track their food intake and activity and analyze their diet and health goals. Students and instructors can trust the reliability of the ESHA database while interacting with a robust selection of reports.

McGraw–Hill Campus® integrates all of your digital products from McGraw–Hill Education with your school's learning management system for quick and easy access to best–in–class content and learning tools.

Create what you've only imagined

Introducing **McGraw–Hill Create™**—a self–service website that allows you to create custom course materials—print and eBooks—by drawing upon McGraw–Hill Education's comprehensive, cross–disciplinary content. Add your own content quickly and easily. Tap into other rights–secured third–party sources as well. Then, arrange the content in a way that makes the most sense for your course.

Even personalize your book with your course name and information! Choose the best format for your course: color print, black–and–white print, or eBook. The eBook is now even viewable on an iPad®! And when you are done, you will receive a free PDF review copy in just minutes!

Visit McGraw–Hill Create—www.mcgrawhillcreate.com—today and begin building your perfect book.

The ABCs of Nutrition

Who Was *Nutrition for Healthy Living* Written for?

Writing a nutrition textbook is not an easy task. Throughout the process, I relied on my experience in teaching nutrition, foods, biology, and personal health classes at both the university and the community college level to develop a vision for a fresh approach to presenting basic information about nutrition. My teaching experiences also provided valuable insights into the diversity, as well as the needs, interests, and capabilities, of today's students. In addition, manuscript reviews by colleagues helped define the shared goals of those who teach the course, which in turn helped shape the content of this textbook.

Nutrition for Healthy Living is intended for students who are interested in learning about nutrition for personal reasons, as well as students considering majoring in nutrition, nursing, or other health– and science–related fields. Students from a wide variety of academic backgrounds often enroll in introductory nutrition courses, and in many instances, they have not taken college–level science courses prior to this nutrition course. With this in mind, I wrote the textbook with the understanding that an introductory textbook must appeal to students who represent a broad range of interests and academic backgrounds—English majors as well as nursing majors. My hope is that this introductory course, along with my textbook, can spark students' interest in adopting healthier dietary practices and possibly even inspire some students to consider nutrition as their major.

The *Nutrition for Healthy Living* Difference Is *ABC*

When I began to write this textbook, I felt strongly that I wanted to craft an alternative to established nutrition textbooks, while maintaining a focus on concepts that are fundamental to introductory nutrition courses. By building upon my experiences as coauthor of a college–level personal health textbook, I sought to develop a nutrition textbook that not only was scientifically up–to–date but also included consumer–oriented content and features. I wanted to create a textbook that would be visually appealing and fun to read, engage students' interest, be well organized, and have features that contribute to the pedagogy without being distracting. As my developmental editor gathered feedback from numerous instructors, the advantages that the new textbook would offer took shape—what my team at McGraw–Hill Education and I refer to as the **"ABCs of *Nutrition for Healthy Living.*"**

A = Accessible Science

Nutrition is an "offspring" science that requires a basic understanding of certain chemical and physiological concepts and terms. Ignorance about chemistry and physiology contributes to food faddism and health quackery. By providing a solid scientific foundation, nutrition educators can more easily dispel commonly held but inaccurate beliefs, such as "When you're inactive, muscle turns into fat," and "Cellulite is a special type of body fat."

Becoming knowledgeable about nutrition involves a certain level of understanding of basic scientific principles. *Nutrition for Healthy Living* recognizes the importance of introducing such principles in a manner that every college student can understand. As my primary goal for students who use this textbook, I want students to acquire a basic understanding of nutritional science so that they can make intelligent, practical choices that can result in improved nutrition and health.

Chapter 4 (Body Basics) presents basic principles of chemistry and human physiology as they apply to the study of nutrition, but at a level that students can easily understand. This chapter, for example, introduces and defines terms that relate to nutrition and foods, such as *acid*, *basic*, *enzyme*, and *solvent*. Because students and courses vary in the depth of scientific foundation required, this chapter features some flexibility. The chapter is divided into two main sections, chemistry and human physiology, so professors can choose to skip the chemistry section if they prefer.

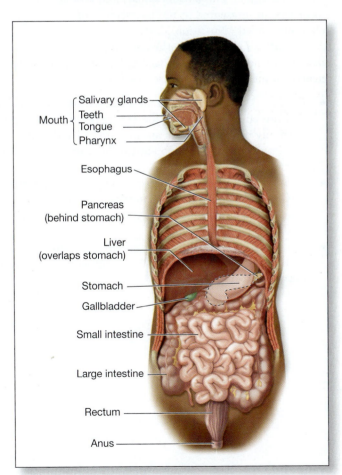

"I find the writing style good. It is engaging and clear. It gets the scientific facts across in an easy-to-understand way."

Sarah Brunnig
Seminole State College

B = Brief Organization

In developing the structure of this book, a new approach emerged; instructors often do not have the time to cover all the material in their textbooks. Based upon their feedback, I chose to organize the core content into 13 chapters. I believe this organization makes teaching introductory nutrition more manageable and fits the time frame of most courses better than textbooks that include 15 or more chapters. Furthermore, basic information concerning world nutrition, diet and cancer, and dietary supplements is incorporated where it is relevant throughout the book.

Although some topics were important to cover, they did not warrant using a full chapter. Thus, topics such as global nutrition concerns, alcohol and alcohol abuse, and eating disorders are presented in the last section of chapters, called "Nutrition Matters." *Nutrition for Healthy Living* covers the core material instructors need in a format that is logical and practical for nearly all introductory nutrition courses:

- Chapter 1 introduces students to nutrition and nutrients, and presents 10 key nutrition concepts, such as "Most naturally occurring foods are mixtures of nutrients" and "variety of foods can help ensure the nutritional adequacy of a diet."
- Chapter 2 presents basic information about scientific methodology as it relates to nutrition research and provides tips for becoming a more wary consumer of nutrition– and health–related information.
- Chapter 3 discusses dietary standards and guidelines, food groups and guides, and how to use information provided on nutrient labels.

- Chapter 4 introduces basic chemical and physiological concepts and key terms that relate to the science of nutrition. This chapter also provides basic information about human digestion and nutrient absorption.
- Chapters 5, 6, 7, 8, and 9 present basic and practical information about the nutrients, such as their major functions in the body, food sources, and roles in health.
- Chapters 10, 11, 12, and 13 focus on applying basic nutrition information for important concerns or different age groups. Chapter 10, for example, covers weight management; Chapter 11 presents information relating to physical fitness; Chapter 12 features information about food–borne illness; and Chapter 13 discusses nutrition during the life span.

Nutrition for Healthy Living follows a more traditional approach to the study of nutrition in that the textbook's organization focuses on nutrients rather than certain functions, tissues, or diseases. Additionally, the textbook integrates health information, particularly diet–related chronic diseases, within each chapter where it is appropriate, rather than relegate it to a single chapter near the end of the textbook. For example, the chapters that discuss nutrients provide fundamental information first and then present applications, including the nutrient–related health effects of certain lifestyle practices, particularly dietary choices. Additionally, the quantity and length of boxed features in the chapters are limited, as they tend to disrupt the flow of content and students often skip reading them.

Nutrition Matters

Chapter 1 The Basics of Nutrition	**Malnutrition: A Worldwide Concern** Includes information about undernutrition, federal food assistance programs, biotechnology, sustainable agriculture, and the world food crisis.
Chapter 2 Evaluating Nutrition Information	**What Are Dietary Supplements?** Discusses complementary and alternative medicine, and regulations regarding dietary supplements, along with a table with information about some of the more popular dietary supplements.
Chapter 3 Planning Nutritious Diets	**The Melting Pot** Examines the influences that various cultures and ancestral groups have had on the American diet and the possible effects that these practices have on health.
Chapter 4 Body Basics	**Gut Reaction** Includes information concerning common digestion and intestinal problems, such as constipation, vomiting, heartburn, peptic ulcer, and irritable bowel syndrome.
Chapter 5 Carbohydrates	**Glycemic Index and Glycemic Load** Provides information about the glycemic index and glycemic load and their usefulness as standards for menu planning.
Chapter 6 Fats and Other Lipids	**Drink to Your Health?** Includes information about alcohol and its health effects.
Chapter 7 Proteins	**Stretching Your Food Dollars** Provides practical tips for saving money on food.
Chapter 8 Vitamins	**Diet and Cancer** Discusses cancer, including factors that may cause cancer and the role of diet in cancer development.
Chapter 9 Water and Minerals	**Bottled Water Versus Tap Water** Provides information about the safety of the American water supply as well as the pros and cons of drinking bottled water.
Chapter 10 Energy Balance and Weight Control	**Eating Disorders: Over the Deep Edge** Discusses major eating disorders, including risk factors and treatments.
Chapter 11 Nutrition for Physically Active Lifestyles	**Developing a Personal Physical Fitness Plan** Provides practical advice for designing a personal fitness plan that can be followed for a lifetime.
Chapter 12 Food Safety Concerns	**Avoiding "The Revenge"** Includes information about travelers' diarrhea, including risky food-related practices and high-risk parts of the world.
Chapter 13 Nutrition for a Lifetime	**In Search of the Fountain** Includes information concerning the possibility of "defying" the aging process by manipulating one's diet.

C = Consumer Focus

Regardless of their backgrounds, students are consumers of nutrition information from a wide variety of sources, including popular magazines, friends, diet books, infomercials, and the Internet. Oftentimes these students arrive in class with many misconceptions about their diet and health. As nutrition educators, we seek to identify these beliefs and to impart sound, reliable nutrition and health information. We also strive to equip our students with the tools they need to make intelligent, informed food– and nutrition–related decisions beyond the classroom. Chapter 2 (Evaluating Nutrition Information) presents a practical introduction to becoming an informed consumer of nutrition and nutrition–related information. This book is unique among nutrition textbooks in its inclusion of this chapter, which provides basic information concerning scientific research and a thorough discussion of how to evaluate nutrition– and health–related sources and messages.

In addition to devoting an entire chapter to the topic of evaluating nutrition–related information and ways of becoming a more wary consumer of nutrition information, the consumer emphasis is integrated throughout the book.

Food & Nutrition tip

Often, the only difference between a creamy salad dressing, such as ranch or blue cheese, and the "light" version of the dressing is the amount of water they contain. Instead of paying more for calorie-reduced bottled salad dressings, make your own light salad dressing by adding about ¼ cup water to a jar of regular creamy salad dressing, then stir or shake the mixture.

- **Food & Nutrition Tips** present practical suggestions that apply material discussed in a section. These tips provide information students can use every day—and for the rest of their lives. Such features include tips for selecting fresh foods, managing energy intake, and keeping foods safe to eat.

REAL PEOPLE | REAL STORIES

Katie Adams

When Katie Adams was an American college student, she had the opportunity to attend England's renowned Cambridge University during her junior year. Within a few months after Katie began her studies in England, she began to experience frequent bouts of abdominal pain not long after eating. Making matters even worse, she suffered from nearly constant diarrhea. Although her weight was at a healthy level when she first went to England, she began to lose pounds despite eating adequate amounts of food.

Eventually, Katie reached the point at which she could no longer ignore her health problems. While at Cambridge, she was examined by a physician who thought her signs and symptoms were the result of celiac disease. Although Katie was unfamiliar with the disease, she decided to forgo being tested for the condition until she returned to the United States.

After coming home from England, Katie underwent specialized testing by a physician who diagnoses and treats conditions affecting the intestinal tract. This testing detected the presence of antibodies to proteins in gluten. She also underwent an endoscopic examination of her upper gastrointestinal tract. This exam enabled the gastroenterologist to see the condition of her small intestine and remove a small part of the damaged tissue to view under a microscope. As a result of these definitive tests, Katie was diagnosed with celiac disease. The only treatment for celiac disease is complete avoidance of gluten-containing foods.

Eating out is especially difficult for people with celiac disease, because of restaurants' widespread inclusion of breads, rolls, pasta, and desserts made from wheat flour in menus. Katie learned how to locate the few restaurants in her community that cater to people with celiac disease by having kitchens that are dedicated to gluten-free food preparation.

Today, Katie maintains her good health by continuing to avoid gluten. Although her diet is very restrictive, she knows from experience that if she "cheats" by eating even a small amount of food that contains gluten, she'll get sick again. After such occasions, she returns to following a gluten-free diet, and within several days, her intestinal tract heals itself.

According to Katie, people who are unfamiliar with celiac disease should take the condition seriously and accommodate the special dietary needs of people who have the disease. For example, if you invite someone with celiac disease to share a meal or snack with you, wash your hands after you prepare foods that contain gluten and don't offer those foods to the person. Additionally, prepare some gluten-free foods for your guest who has celiac disease to eat safely. She says, "It's discouraging when people think I'm simply a 'picky eater' and just making life hard for them. The more people who understand celiac disease, the easier my life becomes!"

- **Real People, Real Stories** feature information about people who actually have recovered from or are currently living with nutrition–related conditions such as celiac disease, type 1 diabetes, eating disorders, and hypertension. This feature is designed to help students recognize the daily challenges people with such conditions face and the role diet and physical activity play in managing health.

- **Recipe for Healthy Living** is a practical application of nutrition and food information that will appeal to most college students. Each chapter features an easy−to−make, kitchen−tested recipe that helps bring the chapter's content to life (e.g., "Nutty Energy Bars"). In addition to the pie graph for macronutrient content and a bar chart to illustrate % Daily Value for energy and key nutrients in a serving of the food, this feature also indicates which MyPlate food groups the major ingredients in the dish represent. This feature demonstrates that preparing nutritious foods can be fun and economical. By trying the recipes, students can develop basic food preparation skills and may be inspired to cook more foods "from scratch." As a result, they may rely less on vending machines and fast−food outlets.

- **My Diverse Plate.** To attract consumers who seek to maintain their traditional diets, major supermarkets offer foods that have been imported from around the world. Additionally, many people travel to distant countries, where unfamiliar foods are dietary mainstays. The My Diverse Plate feature introduces students to foods and dietary practices that are ethnically and culturally diverse.

Recipe for Healthy Living

Mango Lassi

Lassi (*luh-see*) is a simple yogurt-based beverage that originated in India. Lassi is usually made and served before a meal, but the drink can also be a refreshing, nutritious snack. This recipe makes about four ½-cup servings. Each serving supplies approximately 97 kcal, 4 g protein, 9 g digestible carbohydrate, 0.5 g fat, 1 g fiber, 122 mg calcium, and 30 mg vitamin C.

INGREDIENTS:

1 ripe mango
1 cup plain, fat-free yogurt
1 Tbsp sugar
6 ice cubes

PREPARATION STEPS:

1. Wash and peel mango. Remove fruit pulp from mango and discard large seed and peel.
2. Dice mango pulp and place in blender.
3. Add yogurt, sugar, and ice cubes to the blender.
4. Blend ingredients until smooth.
5. Serve immediately or refrigerate for up to 24 hours.

Choose **MyPlate**.gov

- Fat 5%
- Protein 16%
- Carbohydrate 79%

	% of DV/serving
Calories*	5
Protein	8
Carbohydrate**	6
Fiber	4
Calcium	12
Vitamin A	4
Vitamin C	50
Sodium	2
Potassium	33

*2000 daily total kcal
**Digestible forms

connect | NUTRITION   Further analyze this and other recipes through activities on Connect at www.mcgrawhillconnect.com.

- **Did You Know?** This margin feature notes interesting nutrition−related tidbits that relate to information presented in that section of the chapter. Some of these features dispel commonly held beliefs about food and nutrition that are inaccurate.

MY DIVERSE PLATE

Ghee (Indian Clarified Butter)

Ghee is a solid fat that is used for cooking, primarily in India. Traditionally, ghee was made from the milk of a type of buffalo that was native to India and Pakistan, but milk from other animals can be used. To make ghee, butter is heated until its water content evaporates completely and the solids (primarily lactose and some proteins) brown and sink to the bottom. After heating, the fat is strained to remove the solids. Scientists are exploring whether certain lipids in ghee have antioxidant activity in cells.

Did You Know?

Have you heard of the "Freshman 15," the popular belief that college students gain 15 pounds during their freshman year? Results of scientific studies confirm that freshmen are likely to gain weight, but the increase is much less than 15 pounds—only 3 to 5 pounds on average.[19]

Assessment and Evaluation of Learning

One of our primary goals as nutrition educators is to ensure that our students leave the introductory nutrition course with a better understanding of the nutrition principles and concepts needed to improve their diet and health. To assess how well faculty are achieving that goal, many colleges and universities are implementing Student Learning Outcomes as a way to measure what students have learned upon completing an introductory nutrition course. Student Learning Outcomes can also be used to help instructors identify content areas that need more refined teaching methods. *Nutrition for Healthy Living* has been developed around the following coursewide outcomes.

Coursewide Student Learning Outcomes

1. Identify functions and sources of nutrients.
2. Demonstrate basic knowledge of digestion, absorption, and metabolism.
3. Apply current dietary guidelines and nutrition recommendations.
4. Analyze and evaluate nutrition information scientifically.
5. Relate roles of nutrients in good health, optimal fitness, and chronic diseases.
6. Summarize basic concepts of nutrition throughout the life span.
7. Evaluate a personal diet record using a computer database.

Additionally, each major section of a chapter opens with a list of section–specific learning outcomes that build upon the broader coursewide outcomes. The "Learning Outcomes" help students prepare for reading the section and clarify major concepts they are expected to learn. These measurable outcomes are further supported by assessment methods and study aids found within the chapters and in Connect.

Quiz Yourself

This pretest, comprised of five true–or–false questions, appears at the beginning of each chapter; answers to the quiz are provided at the end of the chapter. The purpose of "Quiz Yourself" is to stimulate interest in reading the chapter. By taking the quiz, students may be surprised to learn how little or how much they know about the chapter's contents.

Practice Test

Each chapter ends with a series of 10 or more multiple–choice questions that test students' comprehension and recall of information presented in the chapter. Answers to the test questions are in Appendix G. The multiple–choice questions prepare students for classroom exams, because they are similar in type and format to those in the test bank. In many instances, the test questions are correlated to the Coursewide Student Learning Outcomes and Learning Outcomes.

Learning Outcomes

1 List the primary function of proteins in the body.

2 Identify the basic structural unit of proteins and its components.

3 Classify an amino acid as essential or nonessential.

Quiz Yourself

Before reading Chapter 2, test your knowledge of scientific methods and reliable sources of nutrition information by taking the following quiz. The answers are on page 59.

1. Scientists use anecdotes as scientific evidence to support their findings. _____ T _____ F

2. Popular health-related magazines typically publish articles that have been peer reviewed. _____ T _____ F

3. By conducting a prospective epidemiological study, medical researchers can determine risk factors that may influence health. _____ T _____ F

4. Dietary supplements include vitamin pills as well as products that contain echinacea, ginseng, and garlic. _____ T _____ F

5. In general, registered dietitians are reliable sources of food and nutrition information. _____ T _____ F

Practice Test

Select the best answer.

1. The first step of the scientific method usually involves
   a. gathering data.
   b. developing a hypothesis.
   c. identifying relationships between variables.
   d. making observations.

2. A group of scientists observe a group of college students over 4 years to determine which of their characteristics leads to weight gain. This study is an example of
   a. a case–control study.
   b. a prospective study.
   c. a retrospective study.
   d. an experimental study.

3. An aspect of _____ involves studying causes of health problems in a population.
   a. epidemiology
   b. technobiology
   c. diseasiology
   d. censusology

4. Comparing individuals with iron–deficiency anemia to individuals who have very similar characteristics but are healthy would be an example of
   a. a prospective study.
   b. an anecdotal study.
   c. a retrospective study.
   d. a case–control study.

5. Generally, epidemiological studies
   a. establish causation.

Critical Thinking

The "Critical Thinking" feature involves higher–level cognitive skills, including applying, analyzing, synthesizing, and evaluating information. This assessment features a series of thought–provoking questions at the end of the chapter. The questions can help students develop higher–level cognitive skills using nutrition–related content. Acquiring and/or sharpening these skills can help students become better consumers of nutrition–related information.

Concept Checkpoint

The "Concept Checkpoint" feature includes review questions, many of which involve critical thinking skills, posed at the end of major headings. Such questions enable students to test their acquisition of information presented in the section. Answers to the questions in each "Concept Checkpoint" are located in Appendix G.

End-of-Chapter Summary

This feature provides a brief review of the main points of each major section of the chapter. Sometimes students have difficulty determining the key points in a chapter; the chapter summary helps them focus on these points.

References

Nutrition for Healthy Living includes in–text citations and extensive lists of references in Appendix H. References provide readers with access to sources of information for more in–depth understanding or for topics that hold particular interest.

Key Terms and Pronunciation Guide

Key terms and definitions are provided in the margins on the same two–page spread where the terms first appear in the chapter. Many unfamiliar terms have pronunciations provided within the text. A glossary of these key terms is at the end of the textbook. These tools facilitate students' recall and understanding of important, and possibly unfamiliar, terminology.

Personal Dietary Analysis

Many chapters include an end–of–chapter activity for analyzing personal eating habits. Most of these activities require the use of a dietary analysis software program, such as NutritionCalc Plus. Students can gain insight into their eating behaviors by completing this activity.

What's New in This Edition?

The first edition of this textbook included beautiful, pedagogically based illustrations and creative page layouts that were designed to facilitate learning. The updated fourth edition maintains this energetic and visually appealing design. We retained the engaging photos that draw students' attention to the written information and relate content to the "real world." It is important to note that the use of products in photos is for example representation only and does not constitute an endorsement.

The updated fourth edition of *Nutrition for Healthy Living* incorporates the *2015−2020 Dietary Guidelines for Americans*. In addition, the content has been updated extensively and many of the diagrams and illustrations have been modified to increase their clarity. The following list describes updates to specific chapters:

Chapter 2: Evaluating Nutrition Information

- Content has been streamlined to facilitate reading.

Chapter 3: Planning Nutritious Diets

Information from the *2015–2020 Dietary Guidelines for Americans* has been used to update Section 3.3.

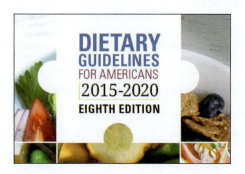

- Section 3.3 ("Dietary Guidelines"):
  - Highlights the five "overarching guidelines" that recommend basic food− and nutrition−related practices for consumers such as "Focus on variety, nutrient density, and amount of food" and "Shift to healthier food and beverage choices."
  - Presents the components of a "healthy eating pattern," according to the new dietary guidelines.
  - Describes specific recommendations concerning the new guidelines, including "Choose foods that provide potassium, dietary fiber, calcium, and vitamin D, which are nutrients of public health concern..." and, for pregnant women: "Do not consume alcohol."
  - Identifies "nutrients of public health concern," according to the 2015–2020 edition of the dietary guidelines.
  - Includes revised Tables 3.3, 3.4, and 3.5 to help support the updated narrative.
  - Has a new "Did You Know?" box, which briefly explains the process that led to the publication of the 8th edition of the dietary guidelines.
- Section 3.4 ("Food Guides"):
  - Includes the leading sources of empty calories and explains how to minimize intake of empty calories.
  - Has information about changes the USDA made to ChooseMyPlate.gov that reflect the new dietary guidelines.
  - The proposed Nutrition Facts panel is presented and compared to the original panel.

Chapter 4: Body Basics

- New "Real People, Real Stories" feature about a person with ulcerative colitis.

Chapter 5: Carbohydrates

- Updated with information from the *2015–2020 Dietary Guidelines for Americans* concerning the importance of consuming foods that supply dietary fiber (a nutrient of "public health concern") and the need to limit intakes of foods and beverages that contain added sugars.
- A new "Real People, Real Stories" feature about a young woman with type 1 diabetes.

Chapter 6: Fats and Other Lipids

- Updated with information from the *2015–2020 Dietary Guidelines for Americans* that focuses on limiting saturated fat. Although the guidelines suggest keeping cholesterol intake "as low as possible," the author explains why most people can consume some cholesterol.
- Updated Table 6.2, Comparing Fats and Oils: Saturated, Monounsaturated, and Polyunsaturated Fatty Acids.
- New figure (6.9) that illustrates fat digestion and absorption.
- New figure (6.12) that illustrates enterohepatic circulation.
- New figure (6.20) that illustrates what can happen to certain lipoproteins in the bloodstream.

Chapter 7: Proteins

- New figure (7.16) on complementary combinations.
- New subsection about nutritional genomics.

Chapter 8: Vitamins

- Updated with information from the *2015–2020 Dietary Guidelines for Americans* that identifies vitamin D as a nutrient of public health concern.
- New sections about biotin and pantothenic acid.
- New "Real People, Real Stories" about a young woman whose body lacked vitamin D.
- Updated information about cancer and diet in the "Nutrition Matters" section of the chapter.

Chapter 9: Water and Minerals

- Updated with information from the *2015–2020 Dietary Guidelines for Americans* that indicates the maximum daily limit for sodium intake and identifies calcium, potassium, and iron (for pregnant women or those who can become pregnant) as mineral nutrients of public health concern.

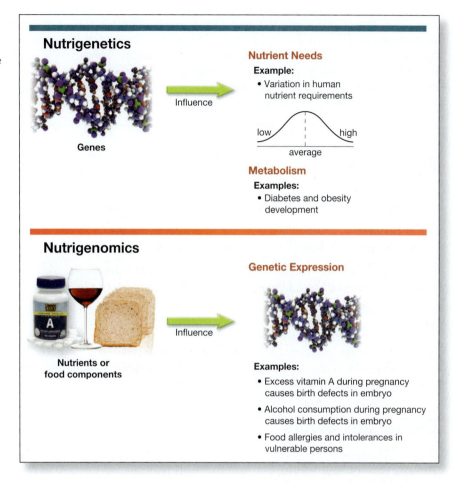

- New sections on sulfur, chloride, fluoride, copper, manganese, and molybdenum.

Chapter 10: Energy Balance and Weight Control

- This chapter has been reorganized to improve readability.
- Information about the usefulness of the "3500 kcal rule-of-thumb" is provided.
- "Nutrition Matters" section on eating disorders has been completely updated and rewritten.
- New "Real People, Real Stories" feature about a young woman with a history of eating disorders.

Chapter 11: Nutrition for Physically Active Lifestyles

- Table 11.9, which focuses on popular ergogenic supplements and aids, has been updated.

Chapter 13: Nutrition for a Lifetime

- The latest information about childhood obesity has been included.

Acknowledgments

The development of an accurate and current manuscript for *Nutrition for Healthy Living*, Fourth Edition, was facilitated by the input of numerous college instructors and emeriti. These individuals reviewed chapters and contributed encouraging comments and constructive suggestions concerning content and pedagogy. Moreover, certain reviewers contributed additional input on specific sections of the manuscript. Their willingness to provide suggestions for developing content was gratifying.

I offer my sincere thanks to the following colleagues who provided a wide range of valuable input, including reviewing manuscript, class–testing chapters, serving on our Advisory Board blog, and preparing supplemental materials:

Reviewers

Stephanie F. Beplay
Colorado Community Colleges

Sarah Brunnig
Seminole State College

Mary Dean Coleman–Kelly
The Pennsylvania State University

Janet Colson
Middle Tennessee State University

Jessica Coppola
Sacramento City College

June Gnass
Butte College

Betty Joynes
Camden County College

Tonia Marchena
Daytona State College

Anne Marietta
Southeast Missouri State University

Cheryl Neudauer
Minneapolis Community and Technical College

Wanda Ragland
Macomb Community College

Jennifer Ravia
The University of Arizona

Carole Sloan
Henry Ford Community College

Tammy Stephenson
University of Kentucky

Sonya J. Williams
Oklahoma City Community College

Digital Reviewers

Natalia Abramova
Husson University

Linda Armstrong
Normandale Community College

Denise Boutwell
Wiregrass Georgia Technical College

Cheryl Davis
Diablo Valley College

Iveta D. Dinbergs
Middlesex Community College

April Engel
Valencia College

Purti Gadkari
Wharton County Junior College

Elaine Higgins
Camden County College

Jean Jackson
Bluegrass Community and Technical College

Phyllis Kennedy
Wiregrass Georgia Technical College

Betty J. Klein
Ivy Tech Community College

Kathryn Link
Alfred State College

Tonia Marchena
Daytona State College

Liza Mohanty
Olive–Harvey College

Gloria C. Payne
Middle Tennessee State University

Eimear Towler
Miami University Ohio

Allisha Weeden
Idaho State University

Najat Yahia
Central Michigan University

I would also like to thank Kelly Webber for updating the PowerPoint lecture outlines and Robin Polokoff for updating the LearnSmart questions.

Additionally, Kevin D. Hall (National Institutes of Health) deserves my gratitude for reviewing some new material in Chapter 10.

My very special thanks is necessary to Matthew Lang; Stephanie Patton; Anne Buchanan, the mother of the late Jason Reinhardt; Dallas Clasen; Amanda Croker; Justin Steinbruegge; Katie Adams; Sarah Marie; and Jan Haapala. These individuals helped make *Nutrition for Healthy Living* more real and interesting by contributing their stories to

"Nutrition Matters" and "Real People, Real Stories" features. I also appreciate the assistance of Deborah McEnery for graciously providing her grandfather's baby photo that appears in Chapter 13 and Trip Straub of Straub's Markets for allowing me to take photographs in his stores.

Many McGraw–Hill Education employees invested a great deal of time and effort into the development and production of this updated edition of *Nutrition for Healthy Living*. My sincerest thanks is extended to all the members of the McGraw–Hill Education editorial, design, production, and marketing team for their enthusiastic support and encouragement. While I was writing this textbook, the team consulted me when making important decisions that directly affected the textbook's features, layout, design, and pedagogy. It was a pleasure to work with people who were willing to listen to my concerns and incorporate many of my suggestions.

A few members of the team deserve special recognition. Amy Reed and Marija Magner served as my brand managers. Under their very capable direction, I was able to focus my attention on the preparation of this edition. I am also grateful to Kristine Rellihan, Marketing Manager, for her work in promoting this edition. Thanks as well to Matt Backhaus, Designer; Brent Dela Cruz, Assessment Content Project Manager; and Content Licensing Specialists, Lorraine Buczek and Lori Hancock. When the first edition was in development,

Michelle Whitaker managed the production of the unique and visually stimulating design. The first edition's design won a first place award at the Chicago Book Clinic in 2008. Michelle along with Matt Backhaus provided their creative talents to the development of the fourth edition. MaryJane Lampe had the difficult task of managing my chapters as they progressed through production, and she helped convey my wishes concerning the art and layout to the compositor. MaryJane's efforts were instrumental in the production of a superior textbook.

I also want to thank Marty Lange, Vice President, General Manager, Products & Markets, and Michael Hackett, Managing Director, for being instrumental in making certain that McGraw–Hill Education provided ample financial support for the production of a superior textbook. Last, but not least, my Product Developers, Angie FitzPatrick and Darlene Schueller, deserve my heartfelt gratitude for the hard work, long hours, and extraordinary dedication they invested in the production of *Nutrition for Healthy Living*.

Wendy J. Schiff

Contents

1 **The Basics of Nutrition 2**

Quiz Yourself   2

1.1 **Nutrition: The Basics**   3
Why Learn about Nutrition   3
Introduction to Nutrition   4
Dietary Supplements   7

1.2 **Factors That Influence Americans' Health**   9

1.3 **Metrics for Nutrition**   11

1.4 **Key Nutrition Concepts**   13

1.5 **Nutrition Matters: Undernutrition—A Worldwide Concern**   20

Summary   24
Recipe for Healthy Living   27
Personal Dietary Analysis   29
Critical Thinking   30
Practice Test   30

2 **Evaluating Nutrition Information 32**

Quiz Yourself   32

2.1 **Nutrition: Science for Consumers**   33
Understanding the Scientific Method   33
Confusion and Conflict   42

2.2 **Nutrition Information: Fact or Fiction**   43
Become a Critical Consumer of Nutrition Information   43
Ask Questions   45
Look for Red Flags   46
Using the Internet Wisely   47

2.3 **Reliable Nutrition Experts**   49
Becoming a Registered Dietitian Nutritionist   49

2.4 **Nutrition Matters: What Are Dietary Supplements?**   50

Summary   55
Recipe for Healthy Living   57
Critical Thinking   58
Practice Test   58

3 **Planning Nutritious Diets 60**

Quiz Yourself   60

3.1 **From Requirements to Standards**   61
What Is a Nutrient Requirement?   61
Dietary Reference Intakes   62
Applying Nutrient Standards   64

3.2 **Major Food Groups**   65
Other Foods   66

3.3 **Dietary Guidelines**   68
Follow a Healthy Eating Pattern Across the Lifespan   68
Focus on Variety, Nutrient Density, and Amount of Food   68
Limit Calories from Added Sugars and Saturated Fats and Reduce Sodium Intake   69
Shift to Healthier Food and Beverage Choices   69
Support Healthy Eating Patterns for All   69
Applying the Dietary Guidelines   69

3.4 **Food Guides**   71
MyPlate   71
Other Food Guides   74

Do Americans Follow Dietary
    Recommendations? 74
What Is the Exchange System? 75

3.5 Food and Dietary Supplement Labels 76
Nutrition Facts Panel 76
Daily Values 78
Health- and Nutrition-Related Claims 80
Structure/Function Claims 81
Nutrient Content Claims 81
Dietary Supplement Labels 82
Organic Food 83

3.6 Using Dietary Analysis Software 85
Government-Sponsored Dietary Analysis
    Websites 86

3.7 Nutrition Matters: The Melting Pot 87

Summary 91
Recipe for Healthy Living 93
Personal Dietary Analysis 94
Critical Thinking 95
Practice Test 96

4 Body Basics 98

Quiz Yourself 98

4.1 Nutrition: Chemistry Foundations 99
Basic Chemistry Concepts 99
What Is a Chemical Reaction? 102

4.2 Basic Physiology Concepts 104
The Cell 105
From Cells to Systems 106

Cardiovascular System 107
Respiratory System 107
Lymphatic System 108
Urinary System 108
Muscular System 108
Skeletal System 109
Nervous System 109
Endocrine System 109
Integumentary System 110
Reproductive System 110
Digestive System 111

**4.3 Digestion, Absorption, Transport, and
    Elimination 111**
Mouth 111
Esophagus 112
Stomach 113
Small Intestine 114
The Liver, Gallbladder, and Pancreas 115
Absorbing and Transporting Nutrients 115
Large Intestine 117
The Adaptable Digestive Tract 118

Real People, Real Stories: Matthew Lang 119

4.4 Nutrition Matters: Gut Reaction 120

Summary 123
Recipe for Healthy Living 125
Critical Thinking 126
Practice Test 126

5 Carbohydrates 128

Quiz Yourself 128

5.1 Introducing Carbohydrates 129

5.2 Simple Carbohydrates: Sugars 130
Monosaccharides 130
Disaccharides 131
Sucrose 131
Nutritive and Nonnutritive Sweeteners 132

5.3 **Complex Carbohydrates** 136
Starch and Glycogen 136
Fiber 136

5.4 **What Happens to Carbohydrates in the Body?** 138
Maintaining Blood Glucose Levels 140
Glucose for Energy 141

5.5 **Carbohydrate Consumption Patterns** 142
Reducing Your Intake of Refined Carbohydrates 143

5.6 **Understanding Nutrient Labeling: Carbohydrates and Fiber** 143

5.7 **Carbohydrates and Health** 144
Are Carbohydrates Fattening? 144
What Is Diabetes? 146

Real People, Real Stories: Stephanie Patton 150
What Is Hypoglycemia? 150
Metabolic Syndrome 151
Lactose Intolerance 152
Does Sugar Cause Hyperactivity? 153
Fiber and Health 153

5.8 **Nutrition Matters: Glycemic Index and Glycemic Load** 156

Summary 158
Recipe for Healthy Living 159
Personal Dietary Analysis 160
Critical Thinking 162
Practice Test 162

6 Fats and Other Lipids 164

Quiz Yourself 164

6.1 **Introducing Lipids** 165

6.2 **Fatty Acids, Triglycerides, Phospholipids, and Sterols** 166
Fatty Acids 166
Triglycerides 169
Phospholipids 171
Sterols 172

6.3 **What Happens to Lipids in the Body?** 174
Bile 174
What Are Lipoproteins? 174
Using Triglycerides for Energy 178

6.4 **Lipid Consumption Patterns** 179

6.5 **Understanding Nutritional Labeling: Lipids** 180

6.6 **Lipids and Health: Cardiovascular Disease (CVD)** 181
From Atherosclerosis to Cardiovascular Disease 181
Lipoproteins and Atherosclerosis 183
Risk Factors for Atherosclerosis 184
Assessing the Risk of Atherosclerosis 186
Reducing the Risk of Atherosclerosis: Dietary Changes 188
What If Lifestyle Changes Do Not Work? 194

6.7 **Nutrition Matters: Drink to Your Health?** 195

Summary 204
Recipe for Healthy Living 207
Personal Dietary Analysis 208
Critical Thinking 212
Practice Test 212

7 Proteins 214

Quiz Yourself 214

7.1 **What Are Proteins?** 215
Proteins in the Body 215
Amino Acids 216

7.2 Proteins in Foods 218
Protein Quality 219

7.3 What Happens to Proteins in the Body? 220
How the Body Uses Amino Acids to Synthesize
    Proteins 220
Protein Denaturation 222
Protein Digestion and Absorption 222
Protein Turnover 223
Nitrogen Balance 224
How Much Protein Do You Need? 225

7.4 Protein Consumption Patterns 226
MyPlate: Recommendations for Protein
    Intake 226

7.5 Understanding Nutritional Labeling 228

7.6 Proteins: Economical Considerations 228
Combining Complementary Proteins 229

7.7 Vegetarianism 232
Is Vegetarianism a Healthy Lifestyle? 233
Meatless Menu Planning 234

7.8 Protein Adequacy 235
Excessive Protein Intake 235
What About High-Protein Weight-Loss
    Diets? 236
Protein Deficiency 236

7.9 Food Allergies, Celiac Disease, and PKU 238
What Is a Food Allergy? 238
What Is Celiac Disease? 240

Real People, Real Stories: Katie Adams 241
What Is PKU? 242
What Is Nutritional Genomics? 242

Real People, Real Stories: Dallas Clasen 243

**7.10 Nutrition Matters: Stretching Your Food
    Dollars 245**

Summary 249
Recipe for Healthy Living 251
Personal Dietary Analysis 252
Critical Thinking 254
Practice Test 254

8 Vitamins 256

Quiz Yourself 256

8.1 Vitamins: Basic Concepts 257
What Is a Vitamin? 258
Classifying Vitamins 259
Roles of Vitamins 259
Sources of Vitamins 260
Vitamin Absorption 262
Vitamin Deficiency and Toxicity Disorders 263
Preserving the Vitamin Content of Foods 264

8.2 Fat-Soluble Vitamins 266
Vitamin A 267
Food Sources of Vitamin A 269
Dietary Adequacy 270
Vitamin D 272

Real People, Real Stories: Amanda Croker 273
Why Is Vitamin D Necessary? 273
Sources of Vitamin D 274
Dietary Adequacy 276
Vitamin E 277
Food Sources of Vitamin E 277
Dietary Adequacy 277
Vitamin K 278
Why Is Vitamin K Necessary? 279
Food Sources of Vitamin K 279
Dietary Adequacy 280

8.3 Water-Soluble Vitamins 281
Thiamin 281
Riboflavin 284
Niacin 285
Vitamin B-6 286
Folate 287
Vitamin B-12 290
Pantothenic Acid 294
Biotin 294
Vitamin C 294
Choline 297

8.4 Vitamins as Medicines 297
Niacin as Medicine? 298
Vitamin B-6 as Medicine? 298
Folic Acid, B-6, and B-12 as Medicine? 298
Vitamin C as Medicine? 298
Vitamin E as Medicine? 299
Vitamin A and Carotenoids as Medicine? 300
Dietary Supplements and AMD 300
Some Final Thoughts 301

8.5 Nutrition Matters: Diet and Cancer 302

Summary 306
Recipe for Healthy Living 309
Personal Dietary Analysis 310
Critical Thinking 311
Practice Test 312

9 Water and Minerals 314

Quiz Yourself 314

9.1 Introducing Water and Minerals 315

9.2 Water 316
Membrane Transport 317

Body Water Distribution 318
Sources of Water 320
The Essential Balancing Act 320

9.3 Minerals: Basic Concepts 324
Why Are Minerals Necessary? 325
Sources of Minerals 326

9.4 Major Minerals 327
Calcium (Ca) 329
Sodium (Na) 335
Potassium (K) 340

Real People, Real Stories: Justin Steinbruegge 340
Magnesium (Mg) 342
Chloride 344
Sulfur 345

9.5 Trace Minerals 345
Iron (Fe) 347
Zinc (Zn) 352
Copper 354
Iodine (Iodide) 354
Fluoride 356
Selenium (Se) 357
Chromium (Cr) 358
Manganese 359
Molybdenum 359

9.6 Minerals with Possible Physiological Roles 360

9.7 Nutrition Matters: Bottled Water Versus Tap Water 361

Summary 363
Recipe for Healthy Living 366
Personal Dietary Analysis 367
Critical Thinking 368
Practice Test 368

10 Energy Balance and Weight Control 370

Quiz Yourself 370

10.1 The Obesity Epidemic 371
Prevalence of Overweight and Obesity 371

10.2 Body Composition   372
Adipose Tissue   373
Subcutaneous Fat and Visceral Fat   373
Measuring Body Fat   374
How Much Body Fat Is Too Much?   376

10.3 Energy for Living   377
Energy Intake   377
Energy Output   378
Basal and Resting Metabolism   378
Energy for Physical Activity   381
Putting It All Together   382

10.4 Energy Balance   383

10.5 Classifying Overweight and Obesity   385
How Can I Calculate My BMI?   386
Excess Body Fat: Effects on Health   386
Body Fat Distribution: Effects on Health   387

10.6 What Causes Overweight and Obesity?   388
Physiological Factors   388
Environmental Influences   391
Genes and Environment: Interactions   392
Other Factors That Influence Weight   393

10.7 Weight Loss and Its Maintenance   393
Features of Medically Sound Weight-Loss
Plans   395
Key Factors   395
Community-Based Weight-Loss
Programs   399

Real People, Real Stories: Jan Haapala   400
Successful Losers: How Do They Manage Their
Weight?   401

10.8 Medical Treatments for Obesity   401
Weight-Loss Medication   401
Bariatric Surgical Procedures   402
What Is Liposuction?   403

10.9 Unreliable Weight-Loss Methods   404
Fad Diets   404
Dietary Supplements for Weight
Loss   406

10.10 Gaining Weight   409

**10.11 Nutrition Matters: Eating Disorders and
Disordered Eating   410**

Real People, Real Stories: Sarah Marie   415

Summary   416
Recipe for Healthy Living   419
Personal Dietary Analysis   421
Critical Thinking   422
Practice Test   422

11 Nutrition for Physically Active Lifestyles 424

Quiz Yourself   424

**11.1   Introduction to Nutrition for Fitness and
Sport   425**

11.2 Benefits of Regular Exercise   426
Determining the Intensity of Physical
Activity   426
Physical Activity Pyramid   428

11.3 Energy for Muscular Work   429
Energy Metabolism   429
How Do Cells Use ATP?   432
Energy Systems for Exercising Muscles   432
PCr-ATP Energy System   432
Lactic Acid Energy System   433
Oxygen Energy System   434
Fat or Carbohydrate for Fueling Exercise?   436

11.4 General Dietary Advice for Athletes   437
Energy for Athletic Performance   438
Focusing on Carbohydrate Intake   438
What About Protein?   441
Raising the Bar?   442
Focusing on Fluids   443
Antioxidant Vitamins   445
Iron   445
Calcium   446

**11.5 Ergogenic Aids: Separating Fact from
Fiction   446**
Caffeine   447

**11.6 Nutrition Matters: Developing a Personal Fitness
Plan   449**

Summary   452
Recipe for Healthy Living   453
Critical Thinking   454
Practice Test   454

12 **Food Safety Concerns 456**

Quiz Yourself   456

12.1 Introduction to Food Safety   457
Pathogens   457

12.2 Protecting Our Food   458

12.3 Microbes in Food   459
Sources of Pathogens   460
High-Risk Foods   461

12.4 Food-Borne Illness   462

12.5 Common Food-Borne Pathogens   463
Bacteria   463
Viruses   463
Protozoans and Parasitic Worms   465
Fungi   465

12.6 Preventing Food-Borne Illness   467
Purchasing Food   467
Setting the Stage for Food Preparation   468

Preparing Food   469
Storing and Reheating Food   471

12.7 Food Preservation   474
Home-Canned Foods   475
Irradiation   476

12.8 Preparing for Disasters   476
Emergency Food Supply   477

12.9 Food Additives   478
Food Safety Legislation: Food Additives   479
Other Substances in Foods   480

**12.10 Nutrition Matters: Avoiding "The
Revenge"   483**

Summary   486
Recipe for Healthy Living   488
Critical Thinking   489
Practice Test   489

13 **Nutrition for a Lifetime 492**

Quiz Yourself   492

13.1 Introduction to Nutrition for a Lifetime   493

13.2 Pregnancy   494
Low-Birth-Weight and Preterm
Newborns   495
Nutrition-Related Signs of Pregnancy   496
Pregnancy: General Dietary
Recommendations   497
Weight Gain During Pregnancy   499
The Importance of Prenatal Care   500

13.3 Infant Nutrition   503
Breast Milk Is Best Milk   503
The Milk Production Process: Lactation   504
Dietary Planning for Lactating Women   506
Quitting Too Soon   507
Infant Formula Feeding   507
Introducing Solid Foods   509
What Not to Feed an Infant   510

13.4 The Preschool Years   512
Snacks   513
Fostering Positive Eating Behaviors   513
Common Food-Related Concerns   514

13.5 School-Age Children   515

13.6 Adolescence   517
Nutrition-Related Concerns of Adolescents   517

13.7 Childhood Obesity   519
Defining Obesity in Children   519
Health Problems Associated with Childhood
   Obesity   519
Childhood Obesity: Contributing Factors   519
Preventing Childhood Obesity   521
Treating Childhood Obesity   521

13.8 Nutrition for Older Adults   522
The Aging Process   523
Common Nutrition-Related Concerns   524
Dietary Planning in Older Adulthood   527
Community Nutrition Services for Older
   Adults   528

13.9 Nutrition Matters: In Search of the Fountain   529

Summary   530

Recipe for Healthy Living   533
Critical Thinking   534
Practice Test   534

**Appendix A English-Metric Conversions and Metric-to-
   Household Units   A-1**

Appendix B Daily Values Table   A-2

Appendix C Energy Metabolism   A-3

Appendix D Amino Acids   A-6

**Appendix E Vitamins Involved in Energy
   Metabolism   A-7**

**Appendix F Body Mass Index-for-Age
   Percentiles   A-8**

**Appendix G Answers to Concept Checkpoint
   Questions and Practice Test Questions   A-10**

Appendix H References   A-24

Glossary   G-1

Photo Credits   C-1

Index   I-1

Dietary Reference Intakes (DRIs)

CHAPTER 1

The Basics of Nutrition

Quiz Yourself

Take the following quiz to test your basic nutrition knowledge; the answers are on page 31.

1. There are four classes of nutrients: proteins, lipids, sugars, and vitamins. _____ T _____ F

2. Proteins are the most essential class of nutrients. _____ T _____ F

3. All nutrients must be supplied by the diet, because they cannot be made by the body. _____ T _____ F

4. Vitamins are a source of energy. _____ T _____ F

5. Milk, carrots, and bananas are examples of "perfect" foods that contain all nutrients. _____ T _____ F

Mc Graw Hill Education **connect** | NUTRITION   **www.mcgrawhillconnect.com**

A wealth of proven resources are available on Connect® Nutrition including McGraw-Hill LearnSmart®, SmartBook®, NutritionCalc Plus, and many other dynamic learning tools. Ask your instructor about Connect!

1.1 Nutrition: The Basics

Learning Outcomes

1 Explain why it is important to learn about foods and nutrition.

2 Identify factors that influence personal food choices.

3 Identify lifestyle factors that contribute to some of the leading causes of death in the United States.

4 List the six classes of nutrients, and identify a major role of each class of nutrient in the body.

5 Explain how to determine whether a substance is a phytochemical or an essential nutrient.

When you were an infant and a young child, your parents or other adult caregivers were the "gatekeepers" of your food; they chose what you ate and prepared it, and you probably ate most of it. If you balked at eating steamed broccoli or baked salmon, they may have told you, "Eat your vegetables if you expect to get dessert," or "Finish that fish. People in Africa are starving!" As you grew older, your **diet,** your usual pattern of food choices, came increasingly under your control. Today, your diet is more likely to be composed of foods that you enjoy as well as can afford and probably those you can prepare easily or obtain quickly. Your family's ethnic and cultural background may also play a role in determining what you eat regularly. For example, do you eat tamales, tripe, goat, or kim chee because you ate these foods as a child? Numerous other factors influence your food choices, including friends and food advertising, as well as your beliefs and moods (Fig. 1.1).

Food is a basic human need for survival. You become hungry and search for something to eat when your body needs **nutrients,** the life-sustaining substances in food. Nutrients are necessary for the growth, maintenance, and repair of your body's cells. However, you have no instinctual drive that enables you to select the appropriate mix of nutrients your body requires for proper functioning. To eat well, you need to learn about the nutritional value of foods and the effects that your diet can have on your health.

Simply having information about nutrients and foods and their effects on health may not be enough for people to change ingrained food-related behaviors; a person must be motivated to make such changes. Some people become motivated to improve their diets because they want to lose or gain weight. Others are so concerned about their health, they are motivated to change their eating habits in specific ways, such as by eating fewer salty or fatty foods. Many people, however, do not care if the food they eat is beneficial or harmful to their health.

diet usual pattern of food choices

nutrients chemicals necessary for proper body functioning

- Family
- Childhood experiences
- Peers • Ethnic background
- Education • Occupation • Income
- Rural vs. urban residence
- Food composition, convenience, and availability • Food flavor, texture, and appearance • Religious beliefs
- Nutritional beliefs • Health beliefs
- Current health status • Habits
- Advertising and media
- Moods

Figure 1.1 What influences your eating practices? Numerous factors influence food choices, including food advertising, peers, income, moods, and personal beliefs.

Why Learn about Nutrition

Why should you care about your diet? In the United States, poor eating habits contribute to several leading causes of death, including heart disease, some types of cancer, stroke, and type 2 diabetes (Fig. 1.2). Results of a national study that followed over 350,000 older adult Americans for 10 years indicated the likelihood of dying was 20 to 25% lower for subjects who followed nationally recommended dietary guidelines.[1] According to the *2015–2020 Dietary Guidelines for Americans*, people can reduce their chances of developing serious diseases that contribute to premature deaths by consuming more fruits, vegetables, unsalted nuts, fat–free or low–fat dairy products, and whole–grain cereals, as well as exercising regularly.[2]

Are you concerned about the nutritional quality of your diet? The fact that you are taking this course indicates you have a strong interest in nutrition and a desire to learn more about the topic. A major objective of this textbook is to provide you with the basic information you need to better understand how your diet can influence your health. Managing your diet is your responsibility. We will not tell you what to eat to guarantee optimal health: No one can make that promise. After reading this textbook and learning about foods and the nutrients they contain, you can use the information to make informed decisions concerning the foods you eat. Furthermore, you will be able to evaluate your diet and decide if it needs to be changed.

Each chapter of this textbook begins with "Quiz Yourself," a brief true–or–false quiz to test your knowledge of the material covered in the chapter. Each major section of a chapter ends with "Concept Checkpoints," a series of multiple–choice questions that can help you determine whether you understood the major concepts in the section. Answers to the "Concept Checkpoints" are given in Appendix G. At the end of each chapter, you will find the answers to the opener quiz, as well as a group of multiple–choice questions that test your understanding of the material in the chapter. The answers to those questions are also provided in Appendix G. References for information cited in chapters are in Appendix H.

Introduction to Nutrition

nutrition scientific study of nutrients and how the body uses these substances

chemistry study of the composition and characteristics of matter and changes that can occur to it

Nutrition is the scientific study of nutrients, chemicals necessary for proper body functioning, and how the body uses them. Understanding nutrition requires learning about chemistry. **Chemistry** is the study of the composition and characteristics of matter, and changes that can occur to it. Matter is anything that takes up space and has mass or weight (on Earth). The air you breathe, this textbook, and even your body consist of chemicals and are forms of matter.

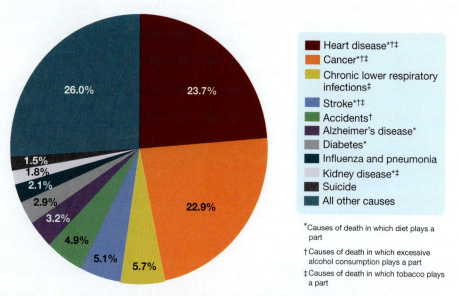

- Heart disease*†‡
- Cancer*†‡
- Chronic lower respiratory infections‡
- Stroke*†‡
- Accidents†
- Alzheimer's disease*
- Diabetes*
- Influenza and pneumonia
- Kidney disease*‡
- Suicide
- All other causes

*Causes of death in which diet plays a part

†Causes of death in which excessive alcohol consumption plays a part

‡Causes of death in which tobacco plays a part

Source: Hoyert DL, Jiaquan X: Deaths: Preliminary data for 2011. *National Vital Statistics Reports* 61[6], 2012.

Figure 1.2 Ten leading causes of U.S. deaths (preliminary data, 2011). Lifestyle factors contribute to many of the 10 leading causes of death in the United States.

"There are chemicals in our food!" This statement may sound frightening, but it is true. Food is matter; therefore, it contains chemicals, some of which are nutrients.

There are six classes of nutrients: carbohydrates, fats and other lipids, proteins, vitamins, minerals, and water. Your body is comprised of these nutrients (Fig. 1.3). Although an average healthy young man and woman have similar amounts of vitamins, minerals, and carbohydrates in their bodies, the young woman has less water and protein, and considerably more fat.

Table 1.1 presents major roles of nutrients in your body. In general, your body uses certain nutrients for energy, growth and development, and regulation of processes, including the repair and maintenance of cells. A **cell** is the smallest living functional unit in an organism, such as a human being. There are hundreds of different types of cells in your body. Cells do not need food to survive, but they need the nutrients in food to carry out their metabolic activities. **Metabolism** is the total of all chemical processes that occur in living cells, including chemical reactions (changes) involved in generating energy, making proteins, and eliminating waste products.

Understanding nutrition also involves learning about human *physiology*, the study of how the body functions. Chapter 4 (Body Basics) prepares you for

Figure 1.3 **Comparing composition.** These illustrations present the approximate percentages of nutrients that comprise the bodies of a healthy young man and woman. Note that the amount of vitamins in the human body is so small, it is not shown.

TABLE 1.1   Major Functions of Nutrients in the Body

Nutrient	Major Functions
Carbohydrates	Energy (most forms)
Lipids	Energy (fat)
	Cellular development, physical growth and development
	Regulation of body processes (certain chemical messengers, for example)
	Absorption of certain vitamins
Proteins	Production of structural components, such as cell membranes, and functional components, such as enzymes
	Cellular development, growth, and maintenance
	Regulation of body processes (certain chemical messengers, for example)
	Immune function and fluid balance
	Energy
Vitamins	Regulation of body processes, including cell metabolism
	Maintenance of immune function, production and maintenance of tissues, and protection against agents that can damage cellular components
Minerals	Regulation of body processes, including fluid balance and metabolism; formation of certain chemical messengers; structural and functional components of various substances and tissues; physical growth, maintenance, and development
Water	Maintenance of fluid balance, regulation of body temperature, elimination of wastes, and transportation of substances
	Participant in many chemical reactions

cell smallest living functional unit in an organism

metabolism total of all chemical processes that take place in living cells

essential nutrient nutrient that must be supplied by food

deficiency disease state of health that occurs when a nutrient is missing from the diet

phytochemicals compounds made by plants that are not nutrients

the study of nutrition by presenting basic information about chemistry and human physiology. Chapters 5 (Carbohydrates), 6 (Fats and Other Lipids), 7 (Proteins), 8 (Vitamins), and 9 (Water and Minerals) provide information about the functions of nutrients in the body.

What Is an Essential Nutrient?

The body can synthesize (make) many nutrients, such as the lipids cholesterol and fat, but about 50 nutrients are dietary essentials. An **essential nutrient** must be supplied by food, because the body does not synthesize the nutrient or make enough to meet its needs. Water is the most essential nutrient.

There are three key features that help identify an essential nutrient:

- If the nutrient is missing from the diet, a **deficiency disease** occurs as a result. The deficiency disease is a state of health characterized by certain abnormal physiological changes. (*Physiological* refers to the functioning of the body.) Visible or measurable changes are referred to as *signs* of disease. Disease signs include rashes, failure to grow properly, and elevated blood pressure. *Symptoms* are subjective complaints of ill health that are difficult to observe and measure, such as dizziness, fatigue, and headache.

- When the missing nutrient is added to the diet, the abnormal physiological changes are corrected. As a result, signs and symptoms of the deficiency disorder resolve as normal functioning is restored and the condition is cured.

- After scientists identify the nutrient's specific roles in the body, they can explain why the abnormalities occurred when the substance was missing from the diet.

If you wanted to test your body's need for vitamin C, for example, you could avoid consuming foods or vitamin supplements that contain the vitamin. When the amount of vitamin C in your cells became too low for them to function normally, you would develop physical signs of *scurvy*, the vitamin C deficiency disease. Early in the course of the deficiency, tiny red spots that are actually signs of bleeding under the skin (tiny bruises) would appear where the elastic bands of your clothing applied pressure. When you brushed your teeth, your gums would bleed from the pressure of the toothbrush. If you cut yourself, the wound would heal slowly or not at all. If you started consuming vitamin C–containing foods again, the deficiency signs and symptoms would disappear within a few days as your body recovered. By reading about vitamin C in Chapter 8, you will learn that one of the physiological roles of vitamin C is maintaining a substance in your body that literally holds cells together. This substance is also needed to produce scar tissue for wound healing. Thus, vitamin C meets all the required features of an essential nutrient.

Table 1.2 lists nutrients that are generally considered to be essential. Fortunately, the human body is designed to obtain these substances from a wide variety of foods. Chapter 3 provides information about ways to plan nutritious diets.

What Are Nonnutrients? Some foods contain nonnutrients—substances that are not nutrients, yet they may have healthful benefits. Plants make hundreds of nonnutrients called **phytochemicals** (*phyto* = plant). Caffeine, for example, is a phytochemical naturally made by coffee plants that has a stimulating effect on the body. Many phytochemicals are antioxidants that may reduce risks of heart disease and certain cancers. An **antioxidant** protects cells and their components from being damaged or destroyed by exposure to certain harmful environmental and internal factors. Not all phytochemicals, however, have beneficial effects on the body; some are *toxic* (poisonous) or can interfere with the absorption of nutri‐ ents. Scientific research that explores the effects of phy‐ tochemicals on the body is ongoing. Table 1.3 lists several phytochemicals that are currently under scientific inves‐ tigation, identifies rich food sources of these compounds, and indicates their biological effects on the body, including possible health benefits.

Dietary Supplements

Many Americans purchase dietary supplements such as vitamin pills and herbal extracts to improve their health. The Dietary Supplement and Health Education Act of 1994 (DSHEA) allows manufacturers to classify nutrient supplements and certain herbal products as foods.[3] The DSHEA defines a **dietary supplement** as a product (excluding tobacco) that contains a vitamin, a mineral, an herb or other plant product, an amino acid, or a dietary substance that supplements the diet by increasing total intake. According to scientific evidence, some dietary supplements, such as vitamins and certain herbs, can have beneficial effects on health. However, results of scientific testing also indicate that many popular dietary supplements are not helpful and may even be harmful. The "Nutrition Matters" feature in Chapter 2 ("What Are Dietary Supplements?") discusses dietary supplements. Informa‐ tion about specific dietary supplements is also woven into chapters where it is appropriate.

TABLE 1.2 Essential Nutrients for Humans

Water	Glucose[†]	Fats that contain linoleic and alpha-linolenic acids
Vitamins:	**Minerals:**	
A	Calcium	
B vitamins	Chloride	
Thiamin	Chromium	**The following amino acids are generally recognized as essential:**
Riboflavin	Copper	
Niacin	Iodine	
Pantothenic acid	Iron	
Biotin	Magnesium	Histidine
Folic acid (folate)	Manganese	Leucine
B-6	Molybdenum	Isoleucine
B-12	Phosphorus	Lysine
Choline*	Potassium	Methionine
C	Selenium	Phenylalanine
D**	Sodium	Threonine
E	Sulfur	Tryptophan
K	Zinc	Valine

*The body makes choline but may not make enough to meet needs. Often classified as a *vitamin-like* compound.

**The body makes vitamin D after exposure to sunlight, but a dietary source of the nutri‐ ent is often necessary.

[†]A source of glucose is needed to supply the nervous system with energy and spare pro‐ tein from being used for energy.

antioxidant substance that protects other compounds from being damaged or destroyed by certain factors

dietary supplements nutrient preparations, certain hormones, and herbal products

---

Concept **Checkpoint 1.1**

1. Identify at least two of the 10 leading causes of death that are diet related.
2. Identify at least four factors that influence your eating habits.
3. List the six major classes of nutrients.
4. What is the smallest living functional unit in the body?
5. What are three key factors that determine whether a substance is an essential nutrient?
6. What is a phytochemical?
7. Define "dietary supplement."

TABLE 1.3   Phytochemicals of Scientific Interest

Classification and Examples	Rich Food Sources	Biological Effects/Possible Health Benefits
Carotenoids		May reduce risk of certain cancers, may reduce risk of macular degeneration (a major cause of blindness)
Alpha-carotene, beta-carotene, lutein, lycopene, zeaxanthin	Orange, red, yellow fruits and vegetables; egg yolks	
Phenolics		Antioxidant activity; may inhibit cancer growth, may reduce risk of heart disease
Quercetin	Apples, tea, red wine, onions, olives, raspberries, cocoa	
Catechins	Green and black tea, chocolate, plums, apples, berries, pecans	
Naringenin, hesperitin	Citrus fruits	
Anthocyanins	Red, blue, or purple fruits and vegetables	
Resveratrol	Red wine, purple grapes and grape juice, dark chocolate, cocoa	
Isoflavonoids	Soybeans and other legumes	
Lignans	Flaxseed, berries, whole grains, bran, nuts	
Tannins	Tea, coffee, chocolate, blueberries, grapes, persimmons	
Ellagic acid	Raspberries, strawberries, cranberries, walnuts, pecans, pomegranates	
Monterpenes	Oranges, lemons, grapefruit, cherries	
Organosulfides		Antioxidant effects; may improve immune system functioning and reduce the risk of heart disease
Isothiocyanates, indoles, allylic sulfur compounds	Garlic, onions, leeks, cruciferous vegetables (broccoli, cauliflower, cabbage, kale, bok choy, collard and mustard greens)	
Alkaloids		Stimulant effects
Caffeine	Coffee, tea, kola nuts, cocoa	
Glycosides		May kill certain microbes, inhibit certain cancers, and reduce risk of heart disease
Saponins	Chickpeas, beans, oats, grapes, olives, spinach, garlic, quinoa	
Capsaicinoids		May provide some pain relief
Capsaicin	Chili peppers	
Fructooligosaccharides		May stimulate the growth of beneficial bacteria in the human intestinal tract
	Onions, bananas, asparagus, wheat	

1.2 Factors That Influence Americans' Health

Learning Outcomes

1 Explain why people should be concerned about their lifestyle and risk factors for chronic diseases.

2 Compare Americans' current typical eating habits to the population's typical eating habits in 1970.

3 Describe the general goals of *Healthy People 2020.*

As mentioned in the opener of this chapter, poor eating habits contribute to several of the leading causes of death in the United States. Note in Figure 1.2 that heart disease is the leading cause of death for all Americans, and cancer is the second leading cause of death. In 2011, these two diseases accounted for almost 50% of all deaths.[4]

Conditions such as heart disease and cancer are *chronic* diseases. Chronic diseases usually take many years to develop and have complex causes. A **risk factor** is a personal characteristic that increases your chances of developing a chronic disease. For example, genetic background or family history is an important risk factor for heart disease. If your father's father had a heart attack before he was 55 years old and your mother is being treated for having a high blood cholesterol level (a risk factor for heart disease), your family history indicates you have a higher-than-average risk of having a heart attack. For many people, however, having a family history of a chronic disease does not mean that they definitely will develop the condition. Other risk factors that contribute to health are age, environmental conditions, psychological factors, access to health care, and lifestyle practices.

Lifestyle is a person's usual way of living that includes dietary practices, physical activity habits, use of drugs such as tobacco and alcohol, and other typical patterns of behavior. Your lifestyle may increase or reduce your chances of developing a chronic disease or delay its occurrence for years, even decades. Poor diet, cigarette smoking, and excess alcohol consumption, for example, are risk factors that increase the likelihood of heart disease, stroke, and many forms of cancer. Cigarette smoking is the primary cause of preventable cancer deaths, but dietary habits and physical activity patterns also contribute to the development of certain cancers.[5,6] Additionally, poor diet and lack of physical activity can result in obesity, a condition characterized by the accumulation of too much body fat. Obesity is a risk factor for numerous health problems, including heart disease, certain cancers, type 2 diabetes, and *hypertension* (chronic high blood pressure).

Chapter 5 discusses diabetes, and Chapter 6 explains the role of diet and other lifestyle factors in the development of heart disease and hypertension. The Chapter 8 "Nutrition Matters" feature takes a closer look at the diet and cancer connection. Chapter 10 (Energy Balance and Weight Control) provides information about obesity.

risk factor personal characteristic that increases a person's chances of developing a disease

lifestyle usual way of living, including dietary practices and physical activity habits

Our Changing Eating Habits

Americans' diets have changed significantly over the past 40 years.[7] According to U.S. Department of Agriculture (USDA) estimates, we eat less red meat, eggs, and milk, and more fish, poultry, and cheese than in 1970. Our diet also supplies more food energy from flour and cereal products than in 1970, but *refined* grain foods, such as white bread and pasta, make up the majority of these products. In general, the more refined a food is, the more processing it has undergone before it reaches your plate, and as a result, the food has lost vitamins, minerals, and

Smoking is the leading cause of preventable death in the United States.

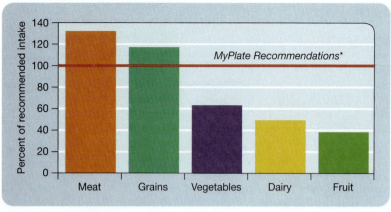

*Data based on a 2000-calorie diet.

Source: Calculated by ERS/USDA based on data from various sources (see Loss-Adjusted Food Availability Documentation). U.S. Department of Agriculture, Agricultural Research Service: *Food availability (per capita) data system*. Data as of February 2013.

Figure 1.4 Americans' diets generally do not meet dietary recommendations.

Did You Know?

Overall, the health status of minorities lags behind that of the rest of the U.S. population. Efforts to improve the health of minorities is a major focus of *Healthy People 2020* nutrition-related programs.

other beneficial naturally occurring substances. Compared to past years, Americans are eating more fruits and vegetables, but many people do not consume enough to meet recommended amounts (Fig. 1.4).

In 2010, the typical American diet provided more added fat, added sugar, and total food energy than in 1970 (Table 1.4).[7] If a person's energy intake is more than needed, especially for physical activity, his or her body fat increases. Nationwide surveys indicate that Americans are fatter than in previous decades. Dietary practices, however, should not receive all the blame for this unhealthy finding; during the same period, we have become increasingly dependent on various labor-saving gadgets and machines that make our lives easier but also reduce the amount of energy we need to expend. Chapter 10 examines weight management in detail.

Healthy People

Since the late 1970s, health promotion and disease prevention have been the focus of public health efforts in the United States. A primary focus of such efforts is developing educational programs that can help people prevent chronic and infectious diseases, birth defects, and other serious health problems. In many instances, it is more practical and less expensive to prevent a serious health condition than to treat it.

Healthy People 2010, a report issued in 2000 by the U.S. Department of Health and Human Services (DHHS), included 467 specific national health promotion and disease prevention objectives that were to be met by 2010. The main goals of *Healthy People 2010* were to promote healthful lifestyles and reduce preventable death and disability among Americans.

In early 2011, DHHS issued *Healthy People 2020*, a report that includes national health promotion and disease prevention objectives to be met by 2020. The "vision" of *Healthy People 2020* is "A society in which all people live long, healthy lives."[8] *Healthy People 2020* goals encourage Americans to:

- attain higher-quality, longer lives that are free of preventable disease, disability, injury, and premature death;

- achieve health equity by eliminating disparities to improve the health of all groups;

- create social and physical environments that promote good health for all;

- promote quality of life, healthy development, and healthy behaviors across all life stages.

TABLE 1.4   Changing Dietary Patterns: Energy Intakes and Added Fats and Sugars (per Person)

Dietary Component (per day)	1970	2010
Food energy	2064 Calories	2538 Calories
Added fats	1.6 oz	2.8 oz
Added sugars (equivalent to teaspoons of sugar)	20.8 teaspoons	23.0 teaspoons

Source: USDA, Economic Research Service: *Food availability (per capita) data system*.
http://www.ers.usda.gov/data-products/food-availability-%28per-capita%29-data-system/.aspx#.Ue8s-G0qmSo

Accessed: February 21, 2014

TABLE 1.5 Some *Healthy People 2020* Objectives: Nutrition and Weight Status (NWS)

Goal: Promote health and reduce chronic disease associated with diet and weight.

Goal Number	Objective's Short Title
NWS 8	Healthy weight in adults
NWS 9	Obesity in adults
NWS 10	Obesity in children and adolescents
NWS 14	Fruit intake
NWS 15	Vegetable intake
NWS 16	Whole grain intake
NWS 17	Solid fat and added sugar intake
NWS 18	Saturated fat intake
NWS 19	Sodium intake
NWS 20	Calcium intake
NWS 21	Iron deficiency in young children and in females of childbearing age

Healthy People 2020 has several major nutrition–related objectives, some of which are listed in Table 1.5. You can access more information about these objectives at the government's website (http://www.healthypeople.gov/2020/topicsobjectives2020/default.aspx).

Concept **Checkpoint 1.2**

8. What is a risk factor?
9. Explain how your lifestyle can affect your health.
10. Discuss how Americans' eating habits have changed since 1970.
11. Identify at least one main diet-related objective of *Healthy People 2020*.

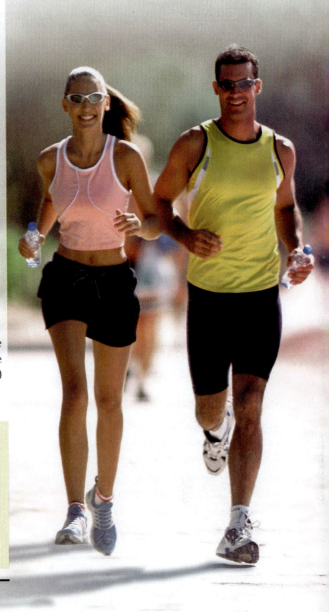

1.3 Metrics for Nutrition

Learning Outcomes

1 Identify basic units of the metric system often used in nutrition.

2 Use the caloric values of macronutrients and alcohol to estimate the amount of energy (kcal) in a food.

Scientists classify specific nutrients according to their chemical composition and major functions in the body. Nutrients can also be classified based on how much of them are in food. Americans usually refer to length in terms of inches and feet, weight in pounds, and amounts of food in familiar household measures (e.g., teaspoons, tablespoons, cups). Scientists, however, generally use metric values to report length (**meter**), weight (**gram**), and volume (**liter**). The following sec–tion provides a basic review of the metric system. Appendix A provides common English–to–metric and metric–to–household unit conversions.

TABLE 1.6   Common Metric Prefixes in Nutrition

kilo- (k) = one thousand
deci- (d) = one-tenth (0.1)
centi- (c) = one-hundredth (0.01)
milli- (m) = one-thousandth (0.001)
micro- (mc or μ) = one-millionth

kilocalorie or **Calorie** heat energy needed to raise the temperature of 1 liter of water 1° Celsius; measure of food energy

macronutrients nutrients needed in gram amounts daily and that provide energy; carbohydrates, proteins, and fats

micronutrients vitamins and minerals

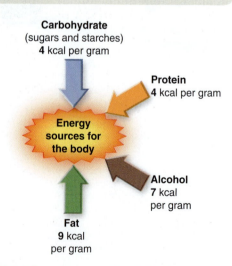

Carbohydrate
(sugars and starches)
4 kcal per gram

Protein
4 kcal per gram

Energy sources for the body

Alcohol
7 kcal per gram

Fat
9 kcal per gram

Figure 1.5 Energy sources for the body. Most forms of carbohydrate supply 4 kcal/g; protein also provides 4 kcal/g. Fat supplies 9 kcal/g, and alcohol (a nonnutrient) provides 7 kcal/g.

Metric Basics

The metric prefixes **micro–, milli–, centi–, deci–,** and **kilo–** indicate whether a measurement is a fraction or a multiple of a meter (m), gram (g), or liter (l or L) (Table 1.6).

There are approximately 2.54 centimeters (cm) per inch. To obtain your approximate height in centimeters, multiply your height in inches by 2.54. For example, a person who is 5′5″ in height (65″) measures about 165 cm (65 × 2.54) in length. There are approximately 28 g in an ounce and 454 g in a pound. A kilo–gram (**kilo** = 1000) equals 1000 g or about 2.2 pounds. To determine your weight in kilograms (kg), divide your weight in pounds by 2.2. A person who weighs 130 pounds, for example, weighs about 59 kg.

Assume that a small raisin weighs 1 gram. If you cut this raisin into 1000 equal pieces, then each piece weighs 1 milligram (**milli** = 1000). Thus, 1000 milligrams (mg) equal 1 gram (g). Imagine cutting a small raisin into 1 million equal pieces. Each piece of raisin would weigh 1–millionth of a gram, or a microgram (mcg or μg). Amounts of nutrients in blood are often reported as the number of milligrams or micrograms of the substance per deciliter of blood. For example, a normal blood glucose level for a healthy fasting person is 90 milligrams/deciliter (90 mg/dl).

What's a Calorie?   Running, sitting, studying—your body uses energy even while sleeping. Every cell in your body needs energy to carry out its various activities. As long as you are alive, you are constantly using energy. You are probably familiar with the term *calorie,* the unit that describes the energy con–tent of food. A calorie is the heat energy necessary to raise the temperature of 1 g (1 ml) of water 1° Celsius (C). A calorie is such a small unit of measurement, the amount of energy in food is reported in 1000–calorie units called kilocalories or Calories. Thus, a **kilocalorie** (kcal) or **Calorie** is the heat energy needed to raise the temperature of 1000 g (a liter) of water 1° Celsius (C). A small apple, for example, supplies 40,000 calories or 40 kcal or 40 Calories. If no number of kilocalories is specified, it is appropriate to use "calories." In this textbook, the term *kilocalories* (kcal) is interchangeable with *food energy* or simply *energy.*

A gram of carbohydrate and a gram of protein each supply about 4 kcal; a gram of fat provides about 9 kcal (Fig. 1.5). Although alcohol is not a nutrient, it does provide energy; a gram of pure alcohol furnishes 7 kcal. If you know how many grams of carbohydrate, protein, fat, and/or alcohol are in a food, you can estimate the number of kilocalories it provides. For example, if a serving of food contains 10 g of carbohydrate and 5 g of fat, multiply 10 by 4 (the number of kcal each gram of carbohydrate supplies). Then multiply 5 by 9 (the number of kcal each gram of fat supplies). By adding the two values (40 kcal from carbohydrate and 45 kcal from fat), you will determine that this food provides 85 kcal/serving.

Macronutrients and Micronutrients

Carbohydrates, fats, and proteins are referred to as **macronutrients** because the body needs relatively large amounts (grams) of these nutrients daily. Vitamins and minerals are **micronutrients,** because the body needs very small amounts (milligrams or micrograms) of them to function properly. In general, a serving of food supplies grams of carbohydrate, fat, and protein, and milligram or micro–gram quantities of vitamins and minerals. It is important to understand that macronutrients supply energy for cells, whereas micronutrients do not. Although the body requires large amounts of water, this nutrient provides no energy and is not usually classified as a macronutrient.

Amounts of nutrients present in different foods vary widely, and even the same food from the same source can contain different amounts of nutrients. Therefore, food composition tables and nutrient analysis software generally indicate average amounts of nutrients in foods. By using these tools, however, you can obtain approximate values for each nutrient measured and estimate your nutrient intake.

Concept **Checkpoint 1.3**

12. Scientists generally use which metric values to report volume, weight, and length?
13. A person weighs 154 pounds. How many kilograms does this person weigh?
14. A slice of whole-wheat bread supplies approximately 13 g of carbohydrate, 1 g of fat, 3 g of protein, and 11 g of water. Based on this information, estimate the number of kilocalories this food provides.
15. Which nutrients are classified as macronutrients? Which are classified as micronutrients?

1.4 Key Nutrition Concepts

Learning Outcomes

1 Give examples of empty-calorie, energy-dense, and nutrient-dense foods.

2 Discuss key basic nutrition concepts, such as the importance of eating a variety of foods and why food is the best source of nutrients.

Before learning about the nutrients and their roles in health, it is important to grasp some key basic nutrition concepts (Table 1.7). The content in the chapters that follow will build upon these key concepts and can help you make more informed choices concerning your dietary practices.

Concept 1: Most Naturally Occurring Foods Are Mixtures of Nutrients

Which foods do you think of when you hear the words *protein* or *carbohydrate?* You probably identify meat, milk, and eggs as sources of protein; and potatoes, bread, and candy as sources of carbohydrate. Most naturally occurring foods, however, are mixtures of nutrients. In many instances, water is the major nutrient in foods. For example, an 8–fluid–ounce serving of fat–free milk is about 91% water by weight, but it is an excellent source of protein and supplies carbohydrate, very little fat, and several vitamins and minerals. A 6–ounce plain white potato baked in its skin is 75% water and only about 23% carbohydrate by weight. The baked potato also supplies iron and potassium (minerals) and vitamins C and niacin.

Many sweet snacks are sources of nutrients other than sugar, a carbohydrate. Although sugar comprises about 44% of the weight of a chocolate with almonds candy bar, over one–third of the sweet snack's energy is from fat. The candy bar also contains small amounts of protein, iron, calcium, vitamin A, and the B–vitamin riboflavin. Figure 1.6 compares the energy, water, protein, carbohydrate, fat, and calcium contents of a 6–ounce baked potato, a slice of whole–wheat bread, 8 ounces of fat–free milk, and a chocolate–glazed doughnut (4–inch diameter) You can find information about the energy and nutrient contents of foods by using "What's in the Foods You Eat *Search Tool*" at the U.S. Department of Agriculture's website: www.ars.usda.gov/Services/docs.htm?docid=17032.

TABLE 1.7   Key Basic Nutrition Concepts

- Most naturally occurring foods are mixtures of nutrients.
- Variety can help ensure the nutritional adequacy of a diet.
- There are no "good" or "bad" foods.
- Enjoy eating all foods in moderation.
- For each nutrient, there is a range of safe intake.
- Food is the best source of nutrients and phytochemicals.
- There is no "one size fits all" approach to planning a nutritionally adequate diet.
- Foods and the nutrients they contain are not cure-alls.
- Malnutrition includes *under*nutrition as well as *over*nutrition.
- Nutrition is a dynamic science.

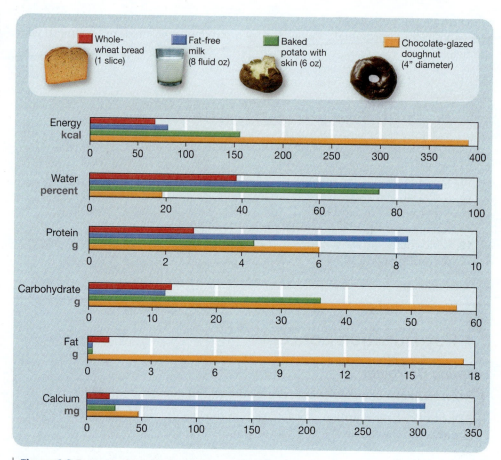

Figure 1.6 Energy and nutrient comparison. These foods contribute very different amounts of energy, water, protein, carbohydrate, fat, and calcium to diets.

Concept 2: Variety Can Help Ensure the Nutritional Adequacy of a Diet

No natural food is "perfect" in that it contains all nutrients in amounts that are needed by the body. To help ensure the nutritional adequacy of your diet, choose a diet that contains a variety of foods from each food group that is shown in Figure 1.7, including fruits, low–fat or fat–free dairy products, and whole grains. To make menu planning more interesting and dishes more appealing, try unfa– miliar foods and new recipes for preparing your usual fare. Chapter 3 (Planning Nutritious Diets) provides information about the food groups and practical menu planning tools, such as the MyPlate plan. MyPlate is a personalized approach to menu planning that can help you incorporate a variety of foods from all food groups into your daily diet.

Concept 3: There Are No "Good" or "Bad" Foods

Are some foods "good" and others "bad" for your body? If you think there are such foods, which ones are good and which are bad? Do you sometimes feel guilty about eating "junk foods"? What is a junk food? Should pizza, chips, candy, doughnuts, ice cream, and sugar–sweetened soft drinks be classified as junk food?

No food deserves the label of "bad" or "junk," because all foods have nutritional value. For example, many people think pumpkin pie is a junk food. Pumpkin pie, however, is a good source of protein, the mineral iron, and the phytochemical beta–carotene that the body can convert to vitamin A. Even

| Figure 1.7 MyPlate.

Pumpkin pie is a good source of beta-carotene, a substance the body can convert to vitamin A. Because the pie is made with eggs and milk, this holiday favorite is also a good source of protein.

sugar–sweetened soft drinks provide water and the carbohydrate sugar, a source of energy. Although pies, doughnuts, and ice cream contain a lot of fat and sugar, these foods also supply small amounts of protein, vitamins, and minerals to diets. Healthy diets, however, generally contain limited amounts of such foods.

Empty-Calorie Foods

Some foods and beverages, such as bacon, candy, pastries, snack chips, and alcoholic or sugar–sweetened drinks, are described as sources of "empty calories." An **empty–calorie** food contributes a large portion of its energy from unhealthy solid fat, added sugar, and/or alcohol.[9] Therefore, people should limit their intake of empty–calorie foods. Consuming too much food energy in relation to one's needs can result in depositing excess body fat. Furthermore, eating too many empty–calorie foods may displace more nutritious foods from the diet. Chapter 3 provides more information about empty–calorie foods.

Nutrient Density

Certain foods are more nutritious than others. A **nutrient–dense** food contains more vitamins and minerals in relation to its unhealthy fat, added sugar, and/or alcohol contents. Broccoli, leafy greens, fat–free milk, orange juice, lean meats, and whole–grain cereals are examples of nutrient–dense foods. Figure 1.8 compares the nutritional values of 8–fluid–ounce servings of a sugar–sweetened soft drink and fat–free milk. Note that milk supplies water, protein, and certain vitamins and minerals, whereas the soft drink supplies water and carbohydrate but is a poor source of protein and micronutrients. A nutritious diet contains a variety of nutrient–dense foods.

Energy Density

Energy density describes the energy value of a food in relation to the food's weight. For example, a chocolate, cake–type frosted doughnut that weighs about 2 ounces provides 242 kcal; 5 medium strawberries also weigh about 2 ounces, but they provide only 19 kcal. You would have to eat nearly 64 of the strawberries to obtain the same amount of food energy that is in the chocolate doughnut. Therefore, the doughnut is an energy–dense food in comparison to the berries. In general, high–fat foods such as doughnuts are energy dense because they are concentrated sources of energy. Most fruits are not energy dense, because they contain far more water than fat.

Figure 1.9 compares a group of foods that each weigh about the same but differ in their energy densities. Not all energy–dense foods are empty–calorie foods. Nuts, for example, are high in fat and, therefore, energy dense. However, nuts are also nutrient dense because they contribute protein, vitamins, minerals, and fiber to diets. Most forms of fiber are classified as carbohydrates.

A food *is* bad for you if it contains toxic substances or is contaminated with bacteria, viruses, or microscopic animals that cause food–borne illness. Chapter 12 (Food Safety Concerns) focuses on food safety concerns, including major types of food–borne illnesses and how to prevent them.

Concept 4: Enjoy Eating All Foods in Moderation

Dietary **moderation** involves obtaining enough nutrients from food to meet one's needs while avoiding excessive amounts and balancing calorie intake with calorie expenditure, primarily by physical activity. This can be accomplished by choosing nutrient–dense foods, limiting serving sizes, and incorporating moderate– to

83 kcal
8.26 g protein
299 mg calcium
247 mg phosphorus
0.446 mg riboflavin
149 µg vitamin A

91 kcal
0.17 g protein
5 mg calcium
25 mg phosphorus
0 mg riboflavin
0 µg vitamin A

8 fluid ounces   8 fluid ounces

Figure 1.8 Comparing nutrient densities. Although the milk and soft drink have similar caloric contents, milk is a much better source of proteins and micronutrients.

empty calorie describes food or beverage that supplies excessive amounts of unhealthy solid fat, added sugars, and/or alcohol

nutrient-dense describes food or beverage that has more vitamins and minerals in relation to its unhealthy fat, added sugar, and/or alcohol contents

energy density energy value of a food in relation to the food's weight

moderation obtaining adequate amounts of nutrients while balancing calorie intake with calorie expenditure

When a diet meets nutritional needs, including some empty-calorie items such as these brownies adds enjoyment when such foods are consumed in moderation.

physiological dose amount of a nutrient that is within the range of safe intake and enables the body to function optimally

megadose generally defined as 10 times the recommended amount of a vitamin or mineral

Figure 1.9 Energy density. Although each of these portions of food weigh about the same, they differ in their energy densities. For example, you would need to eat over 4 cups of whole strawberries to consume the same amount of energy in a 3-ounce, broiled hamburger patty (10% fat).

vigorous—intensity physical activities into your daily routine. Although mod—eration requires planning meals and setting aside time for physical activity daily, it can help you achieve your health and fitness goals. If, for example, you overeat during a meal or snack, you can regain dietary moderation and balance by eating less food and exercising more intensely during the next 24 hours.

Eliminating all empty—calorie foods from your diet is not generally recommended or necessary. If your core diet is comprised primarily of nutrient—dense foods and meets your nutritional needs, including some empty—calorie items adds enjoyment to living when they are consumed in moderation. Physically active individuals, such as athletes in training programs, often find it difficult to consume enough energy from foods to sustain healthy body weights, unless they include some empty—calorie items in their diets.

Concept 5: For Each Nutrient, There Is a Range of Safe Intake

By eating a variety of nutrient—dense foods, you are likely to obtain adequate and safe amounts of each nutrient. The **physiological dose** of a nutrient is the amount that is within the range of safe intake and enables the body to func—tion optimally. Consuming less than the physiological dose can result in mar—ginal nutritional status. In other words, the person's body has just enough of the nutrient to function adequately, but that amount is not sufficient to overcome the added stress of infection or injury. If a person's nutrient intake falls below the marginal level, the individual is at risk of developing the nutrient's deficiency disease. For example, the recommended amounts of the B—vitamin niacin are 16 mg for men and 14 mg for women. People whose diets contain little or no nia—cin are at risk of developing *pellagra*, the vitamin's deficiency disease.

Most people require physiological amounts of micronutrients. A **megadose** is generally defined as an amount of a vitamin or mineral that is at least 10 times the recommended amount of the nutrient.[10] When taken in high amounts, many vitamins behave like drugs and can produce unpleasant and even toxic side effects. For example, physicians sometimes use megadoses of the B—vitamin niacin to treat high blood cholesterol levels, but such amounts may cause painful facial flushing and liver damage. Minerals have very narrow ranges of safe intakes.

Many consumers take megadoses of vitamin and/or mineral supplements without consulting physicians, because they think the micronutrients will prevent or treat ailments such as the common cold or heart disease. For most people, consuming amounts of nutrients that exceed what is necessary for good health is economically wasteful and could be harmful to the body. "More is not always better," when it relates to optimal nutrition.

In their natural states, most commonly eaten foods do not contain toxic levels of vitamins and minerals. You probably do not need to worry about consuming toxic levels of micronutrients, unless you are taking megadoses of vitamin/mineral supplements or eating large amounts of foods that are fortified with these nutrients regularly. The diagram shown in Figure 1.10 illustrates the general concept of deficient, safe, and toxic intake ranges for nutrients such as vitamins and minerals. Chapters 8 and 9 provide more information about micronutrients, including deficiencies and toxicities.

Concept 6: Food Is the Best Source of Nutrients and Phytochemicals

The most natural, reliable, and economical way to obtain nutrients and beneficial phytochemicals is to base your diet on a variety of "whole" and minimally processed foods. Plant foods naturally contain a variety of nutrients and phytochemicals, but processing the foods often removes some of the most healthful parts. For example, a wheat kernel is stripped of its germ and outer hull (bran) during refinement into white flour (Fig. 1.11). Wheat germ is a rich source of vitamin E and beneficial lipids. Wheat bran contains fiber and certain phytochemicals, and it is a concentrated source of micronutrients. The endosperm that remains is primarily starch (a form of carbohydrate) with some protein and very small amounts of micronutrients and fiber. By replacing refined grain products, such as white bread, with whole-grain products, you can increase the likelihood of obtaining a wide variety of nutrients and phytochemicals.

In addition to eating food, many people take nutrient supplements in the form of pills, powders, bars, wafers, or beverages. The human body, however, is designed to obtain nutrients from foods, not supplements. In some instances, nutrients from food are more available, that is, more easily digested and absorbed, than those in supplements.

It is important to understand that nutrient supplements do not contain everything one needs for optimal nutrition. For example, they do not contain the wide variety of phytochemicals found in plant foods. Although supplements that contain phytochemicals are available, they may not provide the same healthful benefits as consuming the plants that contain these compounds. Why? Nutrients and phytochemicals may need to be consumed together to provide the desirable effects in the body. Food naturally contains combinations of these chemicals in very small amounts and certain proportions. There is nothing "natural" about gulping down handfuls of supplements.

Some individuals have increased needs for certain nutrients, particularly micronutrients. People who have chronic illnesses, digestive disorders that interfere with nutrient absorption, and certain inherited disorders may require supplemental nutrients. Additionally, many older adults may need higher amounts of vitamins and other nutrients than those found in food. Because it is often difficult

Figure 1.10 Intake continuum. For each nutrient, there is a range of safe intake.

Death

Toxic

Upper limit of safe intake

Safe physiologic doses (range of safe intake for optimal body function)

Marginal

Deficient

Death

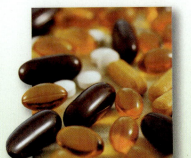

Dietary supplements should not be considered substitutes for nutrient-dense food.

This product is a functional food because it was manufactured with ingredients that may reduce the body's cholesterol level.

to plan and eat nutritious menus each day, taking a supplement that contains a variety of vitamins may be advisable, even for healthy adults.[11] In general, there appears to be little danger in taking a dietary supplement that provides 100% of recommended amounts of the micronutrients daily.[12] However, healthy adults should consider taking such supplements as an "insurance policy" and not a sub-stitute for eating a variety of nutrient-dense foods.

Concept 7: There Is No "One Size Fits All" Approach to Planning a Nutritionally Adequate Diet

By using food guides presented in Chapter 3, you can individualize your diet so that it is nutritionally adequate and suits your food likes and dislikes, budget, and lifestyle. Individualizing a diet does not mean only eating foods that "match" your blood type, hair color, personality, or shoe size. If someone promotes a diet based on such personal traits, steer clear of the diet and the promoter. Consider this: Human beings would not have survived as a species for thousands of years if their diets had to be matched to physical characteristics or personalities.

Physicians often prescribe special diets, sometimes referred to as *medical nutrition therapies*, for people with chronic health conditions such as diabe-tes. Even the nutritional needs of healthy people vary during different stages of their lives. Chapter 13 (Nutrition for a Lifetime) provides information about the importance of diet during pregnancy, childhood, and other stages of the life cycle.

Concept 8: Foods and the Nutrients They Contain Are Not Cure-Alls

Although specific nutrient deficiency diseases, such as scurvy, can be cured by eating foods that contain the nutrient that is missing or in short supply, nutrients do not "cure" other ailments. Diet is only one aspect of a person that influences his or her health. By making certain dietary changes, however, a person may be able to prevent or forestall the development of certain diseases, or possibly lessen their severity if they occur.

Although there is no legal definition for "functional foods," such prod-ucts have health-related purposes.[13] Functional foods are often manufactured to boost nutrient intakes or help manage specific health problems. For example, consumers who want to increase their calcium intake can purchase orange juice

Figure 1.11 **What is white flour?** During refinement, a wheat kernel is stripped of its nutrient-rich germ and bran. The endosperm (white flour) that remains is mostly starch.

Bran

Endosperm

Germ

White Flour

NET WT 4LB

that has the mineral added to it. Certain margarine substitutes contain phyto–chemicals that interfere with the body's ability to absorb cholesterol from food and, as a result, may lower the risk of heart disease. Although some functional foods can help Americans improve their health, more research is needed to determine their benefits as well as possible harmful effects.

Concept 9: Malnutrition Includes *Under*nutrition as Well as *Over*nutrition

Malnutrition is a state of health that occurs when the body is improperly nour–ished. Everyone must consume food and water to stay alive, yet despite the abundance and variety of nutritious foods, many Americans consume nutrition–ally poor diets and suffer from malnutrition as a result. Some people select nutri–tionally inadequate diets because they lack knowledge about nutritious foods or the importance of nutrition to health. Low–income people, however, are at risk for malnutrition because they have limited financial resources for making wise food purchases. Other people who are at risk of malnutrition include those who have severe eating disorders, are addicted to drugs such as alcohol, or have cer–tain serious medical problems. This chapter's "Nutrition Matters" feature dis–cusses the international problem of *under*nutrition.

Although many people associate malnutrition with undernutrition and starvation, *over*nutrition, the long–term excess of energy or nutrient intake, is also a form of malnutrition. Overnutrition is often characterized by obesity. You may be surprised to learn that overnutrition is more common in the United States than undernutrition (Fig. 1.12). Obesity is widespread in countries where most people have the financial means to buy food, have an ample food supply, and obtain little exercise. Chapter 10 provides information about obesity.

Concept 10: Nutrition Is a Dynamic Science

As researchers continue to explore the complex relationships between diets and health, nutrition information constantly evolves. As a result, dietary practices and recommendations undergo revision as new scientific evidence becomes avail–able and is reviewed and accepted by nutrition experts. Unfortunately such changes can be confusing to the general public, who expect medical researchers to provide definite answers to their nutrition–related questions and rigid advice concerning optimal dietary practices.

Even nutrition educators find it difficult to keep up with the vast num–ber of research articles published in scientific journals. Chapter 2 explains how nutrition research is conducted using scientific methods. Furthermore, Chapter 2 provides information to help you become a better consumer of nutrition and health information that appears in popular sources such as magazines, infomercials, and the Internet.

Figure 1.12 Obesity. Obesity is a prevalent nutrition-related health problem in many nations.

malnutrition state of health that occurs when the body is improperly nourished

MY DIVERSE PLATE

Locusts

In parts of Africa, Cambodia, and the Philippines, many people eat locusts, especially when the insects are plentiful. Popular ways to cook locusts include removing the wings and legs before frying with seasonings or placing locusts on skewers and roasting them over hot embers. The legs and wings are removed from the grilled insects before they are cooked or eaten. Over 60% of the dry weight of a locust is protein, so the insect is an excellent source of the macronutrient.

Source: Food and Agricultural Organization, http://www.fao.org/ag/locusts/en/info/info/faq/

Concept **Checkpoint 1.4**

16. Identify at least five of the key nutrition-related concepts presented in this section.

17. What is the difference between an empty-calorie and a nutrient-dense food?

18. What is the difference between a physiological dose and a megadose of a nutrient?

1.5 Nutrition Matters: Undernutrition—A Worldwide Concern

Learning Outcomes

1 Discuss factors that contribute to undernutrition in the world.

2 Describe how undernutrition during pregnancy and childhood can affect a child's physical and intellectual development.

3 Identify major federal food assistance programs and the populations served by each program.

4 Discuss how sustainable agriculture can improve the environment.

Over 6.5 billion people inhabit the Earth. In 2009, an estimated 1 billion of these persons were chronically undernourished and on the brink of starvation.[14] Chronic undernutrition is a condition that occurs when a person's long−term energy and nutrient intakes are insufficient to meet his or her needs.

Many factors contribute to undernutrition (Fig. 1.13). Poverty and lack of access to nutritious food are serious problems, particularly in sub−Saharan Africa and certain regions of Asia, where decades of civil unrest, wars, and the AIDS epidemic have left millions of people impover−ished and living in uncertainty. Furthermore, unfavorable weather conditions and crop failures can cause regional food shortages. In many developing countries, impoverished people lack supplies of clean cooking and drinking water. Throughout the world, lack of access to clean water causes the majority of all diseases and more than one−third of all deaths (Fig. 1.14).

Undernutrition During Periods of Growth

When undernutrition occurs during periods of rapid growth, such as pregnancy, infancy, and childhood, the long−term effects can be devastating. Each year, maternal and child undernutrition contributes to 3.5 million deaths; nutrition−related factors such as under−nutrition and vitamin A deficiency are responsible for 35% of deaths in children under 5 years of age.[15] The vast majority of childhood deaths associated with under−nutrition occur among poor populations in developing countries, particularly in Africa and Southeast Asia.[16]

Figure 1.13 Factors that contribute to undernutrition. Many factors, including war, disease, and overpopulation, contribute to undernutrition in developing countries.

Figure diagram labels: Parasites; Overpopulation; Depleted farmland and other natural resources; Cultural traditions; UNDERNUTRITION; Disease; Lack of sanitary water supplies; War and political / civil unrest; Food distribution problems (such as lack of good roads)

Undernutrition During Pregnancy. Women who are undernourished during pregnancy are more likely to die while giving birth than pregnant women who are adequately nourished. Furthermore, malnourished pregnant women have a high risk of giving birth to infants that are born too soon. These babies often suffer from breathing problems and have low birth weights—conditions that increase their risk of dying during their first year of life. Each year, an estimated 18 million low−birth−weight infants are born in the world.[17] The vast majority of low−birth−weight infants are born in developing countries. Chapter 13 provides more information about the importance of adequate nutrition during pregnancy.

Undernutrition During Infancy. As explained in Chapter 13, breast milk is the best food for young infants because it is sanitary, is nutritionally adequate, and provides babies with immu−nity to some infectious diseases. In developing countries, many new mothers do not exclusively breastfeed their babies for more than a few weeks.[15] Although infant formulas are nutritious substitutes for breast milk, they do not provide immunity to diseases, and they are generally more expensive.

Figure 1.14 Unsafe water source. In developing countries, lack of clean cooking and drinking water contribute to the spread of infectious diseases.

To increase the volume of infant formula that they can afford to give their children, poor parents in developing countries often add excessive amounts of water. This practice dilutes the nutritional value of the formula and increases the likelihood of contaminating it with disease-causing microbes. Infants who drink formula that has been mixed with unsanitary water can develop diarrhea that causes loss of body water (*dehydration*) and death.

Ideally, babies should be exclusively breast fed for their first six months and then consume breast milk in addition to solid foods well into their second year.

Undernutrition During the Preschool Years. In undernourished children, nutrient deficiencies are responsible for stunted physical growth, delayed physical development, blindness, impaired intellectual development, and premature death (Fig. 1.15). In the United States and other developed countries, children are usually well nourished and vaccinated against common childhood diseases such as measles. In poorer nations, however, many children are malnourished and not protected against infectious agents, such as the virus that causes measles. Measles can be a life-threatening illness in undernourished children, because their immune systems do not function normally.

Undernutrition in the United States Undernutrition also occurs in wealthy, developed nations such as the United States. In some instances, undernutrition is not due to poverty in these countries. For example, many people suffering from anorexia nervosa and chronic alcoholism are undernourished despite having enough money to purchase food. Nevertheless, Americans with low incomes have a higher risk of malnutrition than members of the population who are in higher income categories. Between 2008–2012, 14.9% of the population were living at or below the U.S. Department of Health and Human Services *poverty guideline*.[18] In 2011, the poverty guideline was $22,350 for a family of four.[19] In 2014, this guideline was $23,850 for a family of four. Most American households are *food secure*, which means the people in those households have access to and can purchase sufficient food to lead healthy, active lives. In 2011, **food insecurity** was reported in almost 15% of all households in the United States.[20] Food insecurity describes individuals or families who are concerned about running out of food or not having enough money to buy more food. People who are unemployed, work in low-paying jobs, or have excessive medical and housing expenses often experience food insecurity. Food insecurity may also affect elderly Americans who live on fixed incomes, especially if they are forced to choose between purchasing nutritious food and buying life-extending medications.

Charities and churches in many cities operate food pantries and "soup kitchens" to feed food-insecure people (Fig. 1.16). In addition to the help provided by the private sector, low-income individuals can obtain food aid from federal food assistance programs. Table 1.8 summarizes information about major federally subsidized food programs in the United States. Although not every eligible food-insecure person has access to or takes advantage of the aid, federal food assistance programs protect most American children from hunger and undernutrition. For more information

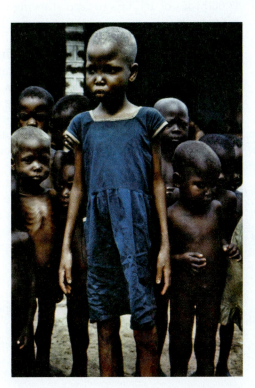

Figure 1.15 Chronic undernutrition. This photograph shows a group of undernourished children outside a Nigerian orphanage during the late 1960**s.**

food insecurity situation in which individuals or families are concerned about running out of food or not having enough money to buy more food

Figure 1.16 Feeding the hungry. In many cities, charities and churches operate food pantries and "soup kitchens" to feed food-insecure people.

TABLE 1.8   Major Federally Subsidized Food Programs in the United States

Program	General Eligibility Requirements	Description
Supplemental Nutrition Assistance Program (SNAP)	Low-income individuals and families	Participants use an electronic benefit transfer (debit) card to purchase allowable food items.
Commodity Distribution Program	Certain low-income groups, including pregnant women, preschool-age children, and the elderly	In some states, state agencies distribute USDA surplus foods to eligible people.
Women, Infants, and Children (WIC)	Low-income pregnant or breastfeeding women, infants, and children under 5 years of age who are at nutritional risk	Participants receive checks or vouchers to purchase milk, cheese, fruit juice, certain cereals, infant formula, and other specific food items at grocery stores. Nutrition education is also provided.
School Lunch and School Breakfast Programs	Low-income children of school age	Certain schools receive subsidies from the government to provide free or reduced-price nutritionally balanced lunches and breakfasts.
Elderly Nutrition Program	Age 60 or older (no income guidelines)	Provides grants for sites to provide nutritious congregate and home-delivered meals
Child and Adult Care Food Program	Children enrolled in organized childcare programs and seniors in adult care programs	Site receives reimbursement for nutritious meals and snacks supplied to participants.
Food Distribution Program on Indian Reservations	Low-income American Indian or non-Indian households on reservations; members of federally recognized Native American tribes	Distribution of monthly food packages. This program is an alternative to SNAP and includes a nutrition education component.

about the federal government's nutrition assistance pro-grams, visit www.nutrition.gov/food-assistance-programs.

World Food Crisis: Finding Solutions   Reducing hunger through food aid programs is a major goal of the United Nations. The World Food Program and United Nations Children's Fund (UNICEF) are agencies within the United Nations that provide high-quality food for undernourished populations. UNICEF also supports the development and distribution of ready-to-use therapeutic food (RUTF) to treat severe undernutrition among young children in developing countries. *Plumpy'Nut*, for example, is

Any child who attends a school that participates in the School Lunch Program can purchase a nutritious lunch. After selecting from the menu, the child enters his or her personal identification number (PIN) into the device shown in the photo. The device records the purchase and debits the child's school lunch account. By using this system, the program protects the identity of children who receive free or reduced-price lunches.

an energy- and nutrient-dense paste made from a mixture of peanuts, powdered milk, oil, sugar, vitamins, and minerals. During processing, the paste is placed in foil packets to keep the food clean and make it easy to transport to remote places without refrigeration. In 2013, UNICEF supplied over 37,000 tons of RUTFs to feed starving children in developing nations.[21]

The Promise of Biotechnology.   **Biotechnology** involves the use of living things—plants, animals, microbes—to manufacture new products. Biotechnology in agriculture has led to the development of crops that supply higher yields, resist pests, or are tolerant of drought conditions. By increasing food production or modifying the nutritional content of foods, biotechnology offers another way of alleviating the world food crisis.

Genetic modification methods, such as *genetic engineering*, involve scientific methods that alter an animal or plant's hereditary material (**genes** or DNA). For example, genes that produce a desirable trait are transferred from

biotechnology using living things to manufacture new products

genetic modification techniques that alter an organism's DNA

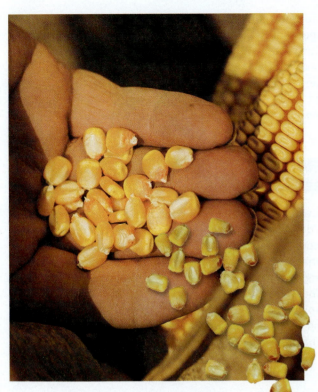

Figure 1.17 Genetically modified corn. This seed corn is the result of genetic engineering.

one organism into the DNA of a second organism, altering its genes. Most of the cotton, corn, and soybeans grown in the United States are the result of genetic engineering (Fig. 1.17).[22] These crops have been genetically altered to resist pests and tolerate chemicals that farmers use to kill pests (pesticides). In the future, genetic engineering of food crops will provide the opportunity to enhance the plants' nutritional qualities.

According to Dr. J. Craig Venter, geneticist and founder of the Institute for Genomic Research, the safety of genetically engineered crops destined for human consumption has been tested extensively.[23] Some scientists, however, have raised concerns that *genetically modified organisms (GMOs)* introduce new proteins into the food chain, creating the potential for environmental harm. The U.S. Food and Drug Administration (FDA) regulates the safety of genetically engineered foods. Nevertheless, researchers continue to examine the long-term safety of GMOs.

Feeding the World, Protecting Natural Resources. Our current system of food production relies primarily on conventional agricultural methods. In general, conventional farming requires considerable amounts of water and pesticides that can harm the environment. Irrigation systems often remove fresh water from rivers and other natural sources at a faster rate than it is restored. This activity

reduces water flow to many communities. The water that runs off conventional farms can carry with it precious topsoil and pesticides that pollute waterways. Such farming methods also release greenhouse gases, especially carbon dioxide and methane, which contribute to global warming. Furthermore, the need for new farmland often requires cutting down trees so that forests can be converted to croplands. The loss of forests eliminates native animal and plant habitats. About 40% of the Earth's land (excluding Greenland and Antarctica) is used for food production; very little suitable land remains to be farmed.[24] What can be done to feed the world's population without destroying the Earth's natural resources?

What's Sustainable Agriculture? **Sustainable agriculture** involves farming methods that meet the demand for more food without depleting natural resources and harming the environment. The challenge is finding ways for farmers and ranchers to make the conversion from primarily conventional farming techniques to sustainable agriculture. Farming needs to be profitable for farmers and ranchers, so any switch from conventional to sustainable agricultural methods must not reduce their profit margins.

To solve the problems created by conventional agricultural methods, an international team developed the following points for establishing a universal policy:[24]

- Stop expanding agricultural activity, especially into tropical forests and grasslands.
- Find ways to improve crop yields on existing farms. Biotechnology in agriculture has led to the development of crops that supply higher yields, resist pests, or are tolerant of drought conditions. By increasing food production or modifying the nutritional content of foods, biotechnology offers a way of reducing the world food crisis.
- Find ways to use natural resources and pesticides more efficiently. Use irrigation systems that apply water directly to a plant's base instead of spraying it into the air, where much of the water evaporates.
- Rely more on nonchemical methods of pest management (see Chapter 12).
- Eat less meat. Sixty percent of the world's crops (primarily grains) are grown for human consumption. Most of the remaining crops are used to feed cattle and other farm animals. It takes about 30 pounds of grains to produce 1 pound of hamburger. By reducing the consumption of meat, especially beef, more grains could be produced to feed people. Grass-fed beef also spares grains for human consumption, because grass is not eaten by people.

sustainable agriculture farming methods that do not deplete natural resources or harm the environment while meeting the demand for food

- Reduce food waste—about 30% of food is wasted. In many instances, the food spoils before it is eaten or it is thrown out as garbage. Smaller portion sizes and better menu planning can reduce the amount of food that people waste each day.

Taking Action. Poverty and hunger have always plagued humankind; the causes of poverty and hunger are complex and, therefore, difficult to eliminate. Nevertheless, certain social, political, economic, and agricultural changes can reduce the number of people who are chronically hungry. In the short run, wealthy countries can provide food aid to keep impoverished people from starving to death. Families and small farmers in underdeveloped nations need to learn new and more efficient methods of growing, processing, preserving, and distributing nutritious regional food products. Additionally, governments can support programs that encourage breastfeeding and fortify locally grown or commonly consumed foods with vitamins and minerals that are often deficient in local diets.

In the long run, population control is critical for preserving the Earth's resources for future generations. Impoverished parents in poor countries often have many children because they expect only a few to survive to adulthood. When people are financially secure, adequately nourished, and well educated, they tend to have fewer, healthier children. Thus, long-term ways to slow population growth include providing well-paying jobs, improving public education, and increasing access to health care services.

Concept **Checkpoint 1.5**

19. How do unfavorable environmental and political factors in developing countries affect the health status of people living in those nations?
20. What effects can undernutrition have on the health of pregnant women and young children?
21. What is the "WIC program"?
22. Explain the difference between conventional and sustainable agricultural methods.
23. What is a genetically modified organism?

Chapter References

See Appendix H.

Summary

1.1 Nutrition: The Basics

- Lifestyle choices, including poor eating habits and lack of physical activity, contribute to the development of many of the leading causes of premature deaths for American adults, including heart disease, cancer, stroke, and diabetes. However, you may be able to extend your life span and improve your quality of life by applying what you learn about nutrition and the role of diet and health.

- There are six classes of nutrients: carbohydrates, lipids, proteins, vitamins, minerals, and water. The body needs certain nutrients for energy, growth and development, and regulation of processes, including the repair and maintenance of cells. The human body can synthesize many nutrients, but about 50 nutrients are dietary essentials that must be supplied by food.

- Nonnutrients, which include phytochemicals, are substances in food that may have healthful benefits. Many phytochemicals are antioxidants that protect cells from being damaged or destroyed by exposure to certain environmental factors. However, some phytochemicals are toxic. The Dietary Supplement Health and Education Act of 1994 (DSHEA) allows manufacturers to classify herbal products and nutrient supplements as dietary supplements.

1.2 Factors That Influence Americans' Health

- Heart disease is the leading cause of death for all Americans. Chronic diseases, such as heart disease, are complex conditions that have multiple risk factors. A risk factor is a personal characteristic that increases a person's chances of developing diseases. In many instances, people can live longer and healthier by modifying their diets, increasing their physical activity, and altering other aspects of their lifestyles. Objectives to improve the status of Americans' health, including nutrition-related programs, are an important focus of *Healthy People 2020*.

1.3 Metrics for Nutrition

- Scientists generally use metric values when measuring volume, weight, and length. The metric prefixes *micro-, milli-, deci-, centi-,* and *kilo-* indicate whether a measurement is a fraction or a multiple of a meter, gram, or liter. Approximately 28 g are in an ounce and 454 g are in a pound; a kilogram equals 1000 grams or about 2.2 pounds. Each gram equals 1000 milligrams or 1 million micrograms.

- Every cell needs energy. A Calorie is the heat energy needed to raise the temperature of 1 liter of water 1° Celsius (C). Calories or kilocalories (kcal) are used to indicate the energy value in food. If no number of kilocalories is specified, it is appropriate to use "calories." A gram of carbohydrate and a gram of protein each supply about 4 kcal; a gram of fat provides about 9 kcal. Although alcohol is not a nutrient, a gram of pure alcohol furnishes 7 kcal.

- Carbohydrates, fats, and proteins are referred to as macronutrients because the body needs relatively large amounts of these nutrients daily. Vitamins and minerals are micronutrients, because the body needs very small amounts. Although the body requires large amounts of water, this nutrient provides no energy and is not usually classified as a macronutrient.

1.4 Key Nutrition Concepts

- There are several key points to understanding nutrition. Most naturally occurring foods are mixtures of nutrients, but no food contains all the nutrients needed for optimal health. Thus, nutritionally adequate diets include a variety of foods from all food groups. Instead of classifying foods as "good" or "bad," people can focus on eating all foods in moderation and limiting empty-calorie foods. For each nutrient, there is a range of safe intake. Healthy people should rely on eating a variety of foods to meet their nutrient needs instead of taking dietary supplements. Foods and the nutrients they contain are not cure-alls. There is no "one size fits all" approach to planning a nutritionally adequate diet. Malnutrition includes overnutrition as well as undernutrition. Finally, nutrition is a dynamic science; new scientific information about nutrients and their roles in health is constantly emerging. Therefore, ways the science of nutrition is applied, such as dietary recommendations, also change.

1.5 Nutrition Matters: Undernutrition—A Worldwide Concern

- Poverty and undernutrition are commonplace in many developing countries. Impoverished people must often cope with infectious diseases and polluted water supplies. In developing countries, poor sanitation practices and lack of clean cooking and drinking water contribute to diseases and deaths. In undernourished children, nutrient deficiencies are responsible for stunted physical growth, delayed physical development, blindness, impaired intellectual development, and premature death. Chronic undernutrition depresses the body's immune functioning, increasing the risk of death from infectious diseases, such as measles, especially in childhood. The vast majority of childhood deaths associated with undernutrition occur among poor populations in developing countries, particularly in sub-Saharan Africa and Southeast Asia. When undernutrition occurs during the first 5 years of life, the effects can be devastating to the child's brain and result in permanent learning disabilities. Additionally, chronically undernourished children do not grow normally and tend to be shorter if they survive to adulthood.

- Reducing hunger through food aid programs is a major goal of the United Nations. Biotechnological advances in agriculture have led to the development of crops that supply higher yields, resist pests, or are tolerant of drought conditions. Conventional farming methods can cause soil loss and add pesticides to water supplies. Sustainable agriculture refers to farming methods that do not deplete natural resources or harm the environment while meeting the demand for food.

Recipe for Healthy Living

Food Preparation Basics (Yes, You *Can* Cook!)

By learning how to prepare dishes, experiment with recipe ingredients, and use a variety of spices and herbs as seasonings, you can make home-cooked meals that are more tasty, more appealing, and lower in fat, sugar, salt, and calories than the usual choices at fast-food restaurants. Additionally, you can save money by making your meals and snacks instead of purchasing them from restaurants and vending machines.

At the end of each chapter, you will find the "Recipe for Healthy Living," a nutritious, easy-to-prepare recipe. Each recipe includes a list of ingredients, instructions, and some information concerning the energy and selected nutrient contents in a serving of the product. The "MyPlate" icon indicates which of the USDA's food groups are primarily represented in the recipe (see Fig.1.7). The circle graph shows approximate percentages of total calories for each macronutrient in the food. The bar graph indicates approximate percentages of Daily Values (DVs) for energy and some key nutrients. Daily Values are a set of nutrient standards used for food labeling purposes (see Chapter 3).

Even if you've had little or no cooking experience, you can learn the basics of preparing foods. Some cooks don't measure ingredients; they know from experience how to estimate amounts of foods and seasonings to add when preparing dishes. Until you feel confident with your food preparation skills, it is best to follow recipes and measure ingredients carefully.

You'll need some basic food preparation equipment to get started. You don't have to spend a lot of money, but buy well-made stainless steel (rustproof) cooking utensils and mixing bowls that will last for decades. Baking pans should also be stainless steel. A square or rectangular tempered-glass baking dish can be used for a variety of cooking needs, including heating foods in a toaster oven or microwave oven.

Understanding how to use household measurements is a good place to begin when learning how to cook. Purchase a set of metal measuring spoons that includes ⅛ teaspoon (tsp), ¼ tsp, ½ tsp, 1 tsp, and 1 tablespoon (Tbsp) measures. You'll also need a set of plastic or metal measuring cups that includes the following measures: ¼ cup, ⅓ cup, ½ cup, and 1 cup. These cups are used to measure dry ingredients such as flour or sugar. Finally, purchase a 2-cup glass or clear plastic measuring pitcher that is marked to indicate fluid ounces. This pitcher is used for measuring liquid ingredients such as water, milk, and oil.

To measure dry ingredients, fill the appropriate measuring cup or spoon to the top, and skim off the excess with the straight edge of a knife. To measure liquid ingredients, use a liquid measuring pitcher. Fill the pitcher to the desired amount, and place it on a level surface. Crouch down so you are at eye level with the fluid's level, and then carefully add more or remove some fluid as needed.

HOUSEHOLD UNITS

Common household units often used for measuring food ingredients and their commonly used abbreviations are listed below. Ounces (oz) are a measure of weight; *fluid* ounces are a measure of volume. Appendix A provides information about English-to-metric and metric-to-household unit conversions.

COMMON HOUSEHOLD UNITS FOR MEASURING FOOD INGREDIENTS

3 tsp = 1 Tbsp	1 cup = 8 fluid ounces (oz)
4 Tbsp = ¼ cup	1 cup = ½ pint
5 Tbsp + 1 tsp = ⅓ cup	2 cups = 1 pint
8 Tbsp = ½ cup	4 cups or 2 pints = 1 quart
16 Tbsp = 1 cup	4 quarts = 1 gallon

Low-Fat Applesauce Oatmeal Muffins

The following muffin recipe is simple and will give you an opportunity to practice measuring dry and liquid ingredients. This recipe makes 12 small muffins, so you'll need a muffin tin with 12 muffin cups. Each muffin supplies about 168 kcal, 4.6 g fat, 27.0 g digestible carbohydrate, 4.5 g protein, 1.5 g fiber, and 5.7 mg iron.

INGREDIENTS:

1 ½ cups quick oats, enriched, uncooked
1 ¼ cups all-purpose enriched flour
1 tsp baking powder
¾ tsp baking soda
1 tsp ground cinnamon
¼ tsp ground nutmeg
1 cup unsweetened applesauce
½ cup fat-free milk
½ cup brown sugar
3 Tbsp vegetable oil
1 medium egg
vegetable oil cooking spray

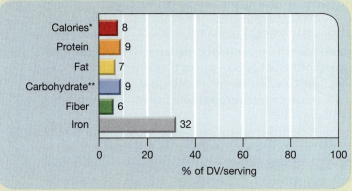

PREPARATION STEPS:

1. Preheat oven to 400° F. Spray vegetable oil spray lightly on the bottom of each cup of the muffin tin.

2. Combine oats, flour, baking powder, baking soda, and spices in a large bowl. Stir until well mixed. By using a large spoon, form a depressed area (a "well") in the center of the dry ingredients.

3. In another bowl, break the egg and use a fork to beat the egg to blend the white and yolk into a yellow mixture.

4. Add applesauce, milk, brown sugar, and oil to the beaten egg, and stir with a large spoon until ingredients are well mixed.

5. Pour the applesauce-containing mixture into the "well" of dry ingredients in the first bowl. Stir gently and just until the dry ingredients have been moistened by the applesauce mixture. Do not be concerned if small lumps of dry ingredients are in the batter. Do not beat or overmix the ingredients; otherwise, the muffins will form air tunnels and have peaked rather than rounded tops.

6. Spoon batter into muffin cups until the cup is half full of batter.

7. Bake 20 minutes or until muffins are golden brown. Use pot holders to protect your hands when taking the muffin tin out of the oven. Cool muffins for about 5 minutes before removing them from the tin. Muffins can be stored in a closed container in the refrigerator for up to a week. Before eating, warm each muffin in a microwave oven for about 15 seconds.

Tip: For easier cleanup, soak the bowl that contained the batter in cold, soapy water.

Further analyze this and other recipes through activities on Connect at www.mcgrawhillconnect.com.

Personal Dietary Analysis

1. For 1 week, keep grocery and convenience store receipts.

    a. How much money did you spend on foods purchased at these markets?

    b. Which foods were the most expensive items purchased?

    c. How much money did you spend on empty-calorie foods and beverages such as salty snacks, cookies, soft drinks, and candy? _____

    d. What percentage of your food dollars were spent on empty-calorie foods? _____ (Divide the amount of money spent on empty-calorie foods by the total cost of food for the week. Move the decimal point over 2 places to the right and place a percent sign after the number.)

    e. How much money did you spend on nutrient-dense foods such as whole-grain products, fruits, and vegetables? _____

    f. What percentage of your food dollars were spent on nutrient-dense foods? _____ (Divide the amount of money spent on nutrient-dense foods by the total cost of food for the week. Move the decimal point over 2 places to the right and place a percent sign after the number.)

2. For 1 week, keep a detailed log of your usual vending machine purchases, including the item(s) purchased and amount of money spent for each purchase.

    a. What types of foods and beverages did you buy from the machines?

    b. How many soft drinks did you consume each day? _____

    c. How much money did you spend on vending machine foods and beverages? _____

    d. Based on this week's vending machine expenditures, estimate how much money you spend on such purchases in a year. _____

3. For 1 week, keep a detailed log of your usual fast-food consumption practices, including fast-food purchases at convenience stores. List the types of food and beverages you purchased and amount of money you spent.

    a. According to your weekly record, how often do you buy food from fast-food places and convenience stores? _____

    b. What types of foods did you usually buy?

    c. How much money did you spend on fast foods? _____

    d. Based on this week's expenditures, estimate how much money you spend on fast-food purchases in a year. _____

Complete this Personal Dietary Analysis activity online at www.mcgrawhillconnect.com.

Critical Thinking

1. Identify at least six factors that influence your food and beverage selections. Which of these factors is the most important? Explain why.

2. Consider your current eating habits. Explain why you think your diet is or is not nutritionally adequate.

3. "Everything in moderation." Explain what this state‐ment means in terms of your diet.

4. If you were at risk of developing a chronic health con‐dition that could be prevented by changing your diet,

would you make the necessary changes? Explain why or why not.

5. Have you ever used certain foods or dietary supplements, such as vitamins, to treat or prevent illnesses? If you have, describe the situations and discuss which foods or supplements were used.

6. What actions have you taken or can you take to help hun‐gry or food‐insecure people obtain adequate nutrition?

Practice Test

Select the best answer.

1. Diet is a

  a. practice of restricting energy intake.
  b. pattern of food choices.
  c. method of reducing portion sizes.
  d. technique to reduce carbohydrate intake.

2. Which of the following conditions is not one of the 10 leading causes of death in the United States?

  a. tuberculosis
  b. cancer
  c. heart disease
  d. stroke

3. The nutrients that provide energy are

  a. carbohydrates, vitamins, and lipids.
  b. lipids, proteins, and minerals.
  c. vitamins, minerals, and proteins.
  d. proteins, fats, and carbohydrates.

4. _____ refers to all chemical processes that occur in living cells.

  a. Physiology   b. Catabolism
  c. Anatomy   d. Metabolism

5. Phytochemicals

  a. are essential nutrients.
  b. may have healthful benefits.
  c. should be avoided.
  d. are in animal sources of food.

6. Which of the following foods is energy and nutrient dense?

  a. peanut butter
  b. sugar‐sweetened soft drink
  c. fat‐free milk
  d. iceberg lettuce

7. Which of the following foods is a rich source of phytochemicals?

  a. hamburger
  b. fish
  c. peaches
  d. chicken

8. An antioxidant is a(an)

  a. essential nutrient found only in animal foods.
  b. dietary supplement that is available without prescription.
  c. substance that protects cell components from being damaged or destroyed.
  d. nonnutrient produced by plants that provides health benefits.

9. In the United States, the primary cause of preventable cancer deaths is

  a. physical inactivity.
  b. tobacco use.
  c. high‐fat diet.
  d. excessive alcohol intake.

10. Lena weighs 165 pounds. What is her weight in kilograms?

  a. 75 kg
  b. 7.5 kg
  c. 82 kg
  d. 8.2 kg

11. A serving of food contains 10 g carbohydrate, 2 g pro‐tein, and 4 g fat. Based on this information, a serving of this food supplies _____ kcal.

  a. 64
  b. 74
  c. 84
  d. 94

12. A serving of food supplies 20 g carbohydrate, 4 g protein, 10 g fat, and 50 g water. Which of the following statements is true about a serving of the food?

a. Fat provides the most food energy.
b. Carbohydrate provides the most food energy.
c. Water provides the most food energy.
d. Fat provides about 25% of total calories.

13. Which of the following foods is the most nutrient dense?

a. potato chips
b. broccoli
c. butter
d. chocolate chip cookie

14. Which of the following statements is false?

a. A megadose is 10 times the recommended amount of a nutrient.
b. Megadoses of nutrients may behave like drugs in the body.
c. In general, megadoses of nutrients are safe to consume.
d. A physiological dose of a vitamin is less than a megadose of the vitamin.

15. The _____ Program enables eligible low-income participants to use a special debit card to purchase food at authorized stores.

a. Nutritious Food Purchase
b. Supplemental Nutrition Assistance
c. Healthy Diets for All
d. Eat Better for Less

LEARNSMART®
ADVANTAGE

Get the most out of your study of nutrition with McGraw-Hill's innovative suite of adaptive learning products including McGraw-Hill LearnSmart®, SmartBook®, LearnSmart Achieve®, and LearnSmart Prep®. Visit www.learnsmartadvantage.com.

Answers to **Quiz Yourself**

1. There are four classes of nutrients: proteins, lipids, sugars, and vitamins. **False** (p. 5)

2. Proteins are the most essential class of nutrients. **False** (p. 6)

3. All nutrients must be supplied by the diet, because they cannot be made by the body. **False** (p. 6)

4. Vitamins are a source of energy. **False** (p. 12)

5. Milk, carrots, and bananas are examples of "perfect" foods that contain all nutrients. **False** (p. 14)

CHAPTER 2

Evaluating Nutrition Information

Quiz Yourself

Before reading Chapter 2, test your knowledge of scientific methods and reliable sources of nutrition information by taking the following quiz. The answers are on page 59.

1. Scientists use anecdotes as scientific evidence to support their findings.
   _____ T _____ F

2. Popular health-related magazines typically publish articles that have been peer reviewed. _____ T _____ F

3. By conducting a prospective epidemiological study, medical researchers can determine risk factors that may influence health.
   _____ T _____ F

4. Dietary supplements include vitamin pills as well as products that contain echinacea, ginseng, and garlic.
   _____ T _____ F

5. In general, registered dietitians are reliable sources of food and nutrition information. _____ T _____ F

Mc Graw Hill Education **connect** **www.mcgrawhillconnect.com**
| NUTRITION

A wealth of proven resources are available on Connect® Nutrition including McGraw-Hill LearnSmart®, SmartBook®, NutritionCalc Plus, and many other dynamic learning tools. Ask your instructor about Connect!

2.1 Nutrition: Science for Consumers

Learning Outcomes

1 Explain the basic steps of the scientific method.

2 Explain the importance of having controls when performing experiments.

3 Design a nutrition-related study that involves human subjects.

4 Explain why nutrition information derived from anecdotes is not evidence based.

5 Discuss why similar scientific studies often have different results.

We consume food, and we consume nutrition information. There seems to be no way to avoid nutrition information: If you browse shelves of books and magazine at a bookstore, watch television, listen to the radio, or shop for groceries, you will encounter information about the subject. Even family members and friends contribute to the flood of nutrition information. Much of the information from such popular sources is not **evidence based,** that is, it is not supported by scientific evidence. The challenge for you and other consumers is to understand how scientists collect evidence about nutrition and health, and how to analyze this information to determine whether it is factual and based on solid evidence (reliable) or misinformation that is unsupported by the facts.

How do nutrition scientists determine facts about foods, nutrients, and diets? Why do nutrition scientists seem to contradict themselves so much? How can you evaluate the reliability of nutrition information? Where can you obtain up—to—date, accurate nutrition information? This chapter will provide answers to these questions and help you become a more critical and careful consumer.

evidence based information that is based on results of scientific studies

anecdotes reports of personal experiences

Understanding the Scientific Method

In the past, nutrition facts and dietary practices were often based on intuition, common sense, "conventional wisdom" (tradition), or **anecdotes** (reports of personal experiences). Today, *registered dietitians* and other nutrition experts discard conventional beliefs, explanations, and practices when the results of current scientific research no longer support them.

Scientists ask questions about the natural world, such as: "How do cells make proteins?" and "What causes stomach ulcers?" To obtain answers for their questions, researchers design studies that follow generally accepted methods. Figure 2.1 presents the general steps nutrition researchers take when conducting scientific investigations. The following sections take a closer look at some common methods that scientists use to collect nutrition information and establish nutrition facts.

Laboratory Experiments

An experiment is a systematic way of testing a hypothesis (question). Because of safety and ethical concerns, nutrition scientists often conduct experiments on small mammals before performing similar research on humans. Certain kinds of mice and rats are raised for experimentation purposes (Fig. 2.2). These rodents are inexpensive to house in laboratories, and their food and other living conditions can be carefully controlled. An experiment that uses whole living organisms,

1. Make observations that generate questions

2. Formulate hypotheses to explain events

3. Review current scientific literature (published studies) that relate to the questions

4. Design studies, perform tests, and collect data

5. Analyze data and draw conclusions based on the results

6. Share results with peers (report findings)

7. Conduct more research, the results of which may confirm or refute previous findings

SCIENTIFIC METHOD

Figure 2.1 **Nutrition science: Scientific method.** Nutrition scientists generally follow these steps when conducting research.

treatment group group being studied that receives a treatment

control group group being studied that does not receive a treatment

variable personal characteristic or other factor that changes and can influence an outcome

Figure 2.2 **Rodents for research.** Nutrition scientists often conduct *in vivo* experiments on small rodents that are raised for experimentation purposes.

such as mice, is called an *in vivo* experiment. Nutrition researchers also perform controlled laboratory experiments on cells or other components derived from living organisms. These studies are *in vitro* or "test tube" experiments.

Experiments generally involve the basic steps shown in Figure 2.1. A team of nutrition scientists, for example, makes observations and generates questions that result in the development of a hypothesis. According to their hypothesis, consuming "chemical X" in charcoal–grilled meat is harmful. To test this hypothesis, the scientists divide 100 genetically similar 3–week old mice into two groups of 50 mice. One group **(treatment group)** is fed a certain amount of chemical X daily for 52 weeks; the second group **(control group)** does not receive the treatment during the period (Fig. 2.3).

Why is a control group necessary? Having a control group enables scientists to compare results between the two study groups to determine whether the treatment had any effect. A **variable** is a characteristic or other factor that can change and influence an outcome. Many variables can influence the outcome of an experimental study. Therefore, scientists who want to determine the effect or effects of a single variable, such as chemical X intake, need to control the influence of other variables. Therefore, all other conditions, including timing of feedings and amount of handling by caregivers must be the same for both groups of mice. If researchers design an experiment in which they fail to control variables that are not being tested, their findings are likely to be unclear or inaccurate.

For the duration of this study, the scientists examine the mice regularly for signs of health problems and record their results (data). If the mice in the treatment group are as healthy as the mice in the control group at the end of this experiment, the researchers may conclude that mice can safely consume the amount of chemical X used in the study on a daily basis for a year.

Researchers are cautious when drawing conclusions from results of *in vitro* experiments, because components removed from a living thing may not function the same way they do when they are in the entire life form.

Figure 2.3 **An experiment.** Based on the findings shown in the graph, is it safe for mice to consume chemical X daily for a year?

Medical researchers must also be careful when applying the results of *in vivo* animal studies to people, because of the physiological differences between humans and other animals. Nevertheless, scientists are often able to determine the safety and effectiveness of treatments by conducting research on laboratory animals before engaging in similar testing on humans. Two types of research that involve human subjects are *experimental* (intervention) studies and *observational* studies. Such investigations can provide clues about the causes, progression, and prevention of diet—related diseases.

Human Research: Experimental (Intervention) Studies

Nutrition scientists often conduct experimental studies to obtain information about health conditions (*outcomes*) that may result from specific dietary practices. When conducting an experimental study involving human subjects, researchers usually randomly divide a large group of people into treatment and control groups.

For example, every other person who enrolls in a study is placed in the treatment group. The remaining subjects become control group members. Random assignment helps ensure that the members of the treatment and control groups have similar variables, such as age and other characteristics. All subjects will be instructed to maintain their usual lifestyle during the duration of the study, except for the activities required by their participation in the research.

Then the scientists provide all study participants with the same instructions and a form of intervention, such as a dietary supplement or experimental food. However, only members of the treatment group actually receive the treatment. Subjects in the control group are given a **placebo.** Placebos are not simply "sugar pills"; they are a fake treatment, such as a sham pill, injection, or medical procedure. The placebo mimics the treatment. For example, a placebo dietary supplement pill looks, tastes, and smells like the supplement pill with an active ingredient that is given subjects in the treatment group. The placebo pill,

placebo fake treatment, such as a sham pill, injection, or medical procedure

Did You Know?

| Man with pellagra

Today, the idea that something missing in diets can cause a nutrient deficiency disease is widely accepted. A hundred years ago, however, it was a novel idea that most medical experts dismissed because they thought only "germs" caused disease. In the early 1900s, the disease *pellagra* was widespread in the United States, especially in southern states. Each year, thousands of Americans died from this dreaded illness. Most medical experts thought pellagra was an infectious disease, because it often occurred where people lived in close quarters, such as prisons, orphanages, and mental health institutions.

Joseph Goldberger, a physician who worked in a federal government laboratory, observed that not everyone who was exposed to people suffering from pellagra developed the condition. Dr. Goldberger also noted that prisoners ate a diet that was typically eaten by other people with pellagra. The diet emphasized corn bread, hominy grits (a corn product), molasses, potatoes, cabbage, and rice. At the time, this monotonous, low-protein diet was associated with poverty throughout the southern United States. He also observed that people who did not develop pellagra had higher incomes and ate more meat, milk, and fresh vegetables. Based on his observations, Goldberger rejected the medical establishment's notion that pellagra was an infectious disease. He proposed the idea that pellagra resulted from the lack of something in poor people's diet and the missing dietary factor was in meat, milk, and other foods eaten regularly by people with high incomes. To test his dietary hypothesis, Goldberger gave these foods to children in two Mississippi orphanages and patients in a Georgia mental institution who were suffering from pellagra, and they were cured of the disease. Many members of the medical establishment, however, rejected his finding that a poor diet was the cause of pellagra.

To satisfy his critics, Goldberger enrolled a group of healthy Mississippi prison inmates in an experiment that involved consuming the corn- and molasses-based diet commonly eaten in the southern states at the time. After a few months, more than half of the inmates developed pellagra. Once again, however, many of Goldberger's critics rejected his finding that poor diet was the cause of pellagra.

In 1916, Dr. Goldberger experimented on himself and some volunteers during what they called a "filth party." The group applied secretions taken from inside the nose and throat of a patient with pellagra into their noses and throats; they also swallowed pills made with flakes of skin scraped from the rashes of people with the disease. Additionally, Goldberger and one of his colleagues gave each other an injection of blood from a person who had pellagra. If pellagra were infectious, filth-party participants should have contracted the disease—but none of them did. Despite the results of Dr. Goldberger's extraordinary experiment, a few physicians still resisted the idea that pellagra was associated with diet.[1]

Dr. Goldberger died in 1929—8 years before Dr. Conrad Elvehjem and his team of scientists at the University of Wisconsin isolated a form of the vitamin niacin from liver extracts. Elvehjem and his colleagues discovered niacin cured "black tongue," a condition affecting dogs that was similar to pellagra.[2] Soon after Elvehjem's discovery, other scientists determined that niacin was effective in treating pellagra, and the medical establishment finally accepted the fact that the disease was the result of a dietary deficiency.

| *Dr. Joseph Goldberger*

however, has *inert* ingredients; that is, the pill contains substances that do not produce any measurable physical changes. Providing placebos to members of the control group enables scientists to compare the extent of the treatment's response with that of the placebo.

What Is the Placebo Effect? People may report positive or negative reactions to a treatment even though they received the placebo. If a patient believes a medical treatment will improve his or her health, the patient is more likely to report positive results for the therapy. Such wishful thinking is called the **placebo effect.**

People who take certain herbal products or use other unconventional medical therapies to prevent or treat diseases are often convinced the products and treatments are effective, despite the general lack of scientific evidence to support their beliefs. Such personal findings may be examples of the placebo effect. However, placebos can produce beneficial physiological and psychological changes, particularly in conditions that involve pain.[3] Because subjects in the control group believe they are receiving a real treatment, their faith in the "treatment" can stimulate the release of chemicals in the brain that alter pain perception, reducing their discomfort. Therefore, when people report that a treatment was beneficial, they may not have been imagining the positive response, even when they were taking a placebo.

placebo effect response to a placebo

double-blind study experimental design in which neither the participants nor the researchers are aware of each participant's group assignment

epidemiology study of the occurrence, distribution, and causes of health problems in populations

Double-Blind Studies

Human experimental studies are usually **double–blind studies;** that is, neither the investigators nor the subjects are aware of the subjects' group assignments. Codes are used to identify a subject's group membership, and this information is not revealed until the end of the study. Maintaining such secrecy is important during the course of a human study involving placebos, because researchers and subjects may try to predict group assignments based on their expectations. If the investigators who interview the participants are aware of their individual group assignments during the study (a single–blind study), they may unwittingly convey clues to each subject, perhaps in the form of body language, that could influence the subject's belief about being in the experimental or control group. Subjects who suspect they are in the control group and taking a placebo may report no changes in their condition, because they expect a placebo should have no effect on them. On the other hand, subjects who think they are in the treatment group could insist that they feel better or have more energy as a result of the treatment, even though the treatment may not have produced any measurable changes in their bodies. Ideally, subjects should not be able to figure out their group assignment while researchers are collecting information from them.

Human Research: Epidemiological Studies

For decades, medical researchers have noted differences in rates of chronic diseases and causes of death among various populations. The most common type of diabetes, for example, occurs more frequently among Native American, Hispanic, and non–Hispanic African–American adults than among non–Hispanic, white American adults.[4] To understand why this difference exists, medical researchers rely on the findings of epidemiological studies.

Epidemiology (*ehp–e–dee–me–all'–uh–jee*) is the study of the occurrence, distribution, and causes of health problems in populations. Epidemiologists often use physical examinations of people to obtain health data, such as height and weight. Additionally, they may collect other kinds of information by conducting surveys. Such surveys question people about their personal and family medical histories, environmental exposures, health practices, and attitudes. Since 1999, National Nutrition and Health Examination Survey (NHANES) researchers have used interviews and physical examinations to assess the health and nutritional status of a nationally representative sample of Americans. Data collected from NHANES help epidemiologists determine the prevalence of major diseases, risk factors for such diseases, and national standards for measurements that are associated with health status, including height, weight, and blood pressure.

In cases involving chronic diseases such as heart disease and cancer, it is often difficult to determine a single variable that is responsible for the development of the condition. Multiple factors, including a person's *genetic susceptibility* (inherited proneness), exposure to certain environmental conditions, and diet as well as other lifestyle practices can influence his or her likelihood of developing a disease.

By conducting studies that explore differences in dietary practices and disease occurrences among populations, nutrition epidemiologists may learn much about the influence of diet on health. If one group of people is more likely to develop a certain health disorder than another group and the two populations consume very different diets, scientists can speculate about the role diet plays in this difference.

Observational Epidemiological Studies   Most epidemiological research is observational and involves either case–control study or cohort study designs (Fig. 2.4). In a **case–control study,** individuals with a health condition (cases) such as heart disease or breast cancer are matched to persons with similar characteristics who do not have the condition (controls). Information such as personal and family medical histories, eating habits, and other lifestyle behaviors are collected from each participant in the study. By analyzing the results of case–control studies, researchers identify factors that may have been responsible for the illness. Scientists, for example, may be able to identify dietary practices that differ between the two groups, such as long–term fruit and vegetable intakes.

In a **cohort study,** epidemiologists collect and analyze various kinds of information about a large group of people over time. The scientists are generally interested in making associations between exposure to a specific factor and the subsequent development of health conditions. Cohort studies can be *retrospective* or *prospective*. Retrospective means "to look back" and prospective means "to look forward" in time. (See Figure 2.4.) In a retrospective cohort study, researchers collect information about a group's past exposures and identify current health outcomes. For example, nutritional epidemiologists might examine whether a group of people who have stomach cancer consumed more charcoal–broiled meat (the exposure) in the past than a group of people with similar characteristics who do not have stomach cancer. In a prospective cohort study, a group of healthy people are followed over a time period and any diseases that eventually develop are recorded. Scientists then try to identify links between exposures and diseases that occurred between the beginning and end of the study period.

The Framingham Heart Study that began in 1949 in Framingham, Massachusetts, is one of the most well–known prospective studies. At the beginning of the study, the over 5200 healthy participants (men and women) underwent extensive physical examinations and questioning about their family and personal medical histories as well as their lifestyle practices. Over the following years, a group of medical researchers periodically collected data concerning each participant's health and, if the person died, cause of death. The scientists analyzed this information and found relationships between a variety of personal characteristics and health outcomes. Findings from the Framingham Heart Study identified numerous risk factors for heart disease, including elevated

case-control study study in which individuals who have a health condition are compared with individuals with similar characteristics who do not have the condition

cohort study study that measures variables of a group of people over time

EPIDEMIOLOGICAL STUDIES

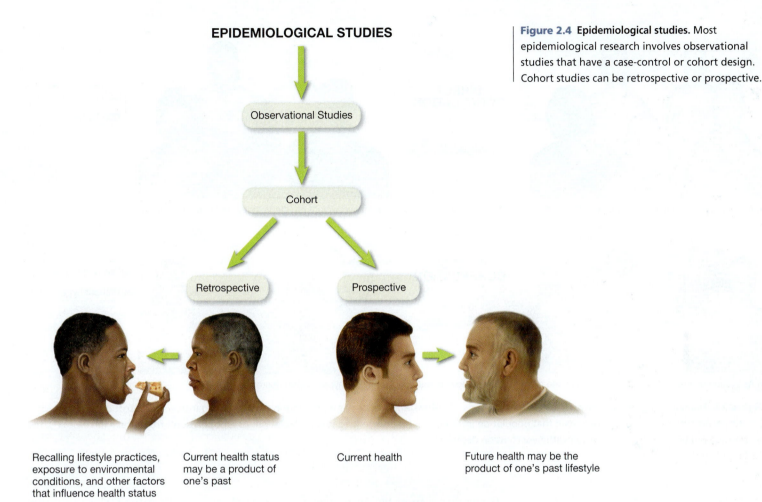

Figure 2.4 **Epidemiological studies.** Most epidemiological research involves observational studies that have a case-control or cohort design. Cohort studies can be retrospective or prospective.

Recalling lifestyle practices, exposure to environmental conditions, and other factors that influence health status

Current health status may be a product of one's past

Current health

Future health may be the product of one's past lifestyle

blood cholesterol levels, cigarette smoking, and hypertension. Today, medical researchers are still collecting information from the original Framingham Heart Study participants as well as their descendants.

Limitations of Epidemiological Studies Epidemiological studies cannot establish *causation*, that is, whether a practice is responsible for an effect. When two different natural events occur simultaneously within a population, it does not necessarily mean they are correlated. A **correlation** is a relationship between variables. A correlation occurs when two variables change over the same period; for example, when a population's intake of sugar—sweetened soft drinks increases, the percentage of overweight people in the population also increases (Fig. 2.5a). In this case, the correlation is *direct* or *positive* because the two variables—body weight and regular soft drink consumption—are changing in the same direction; they are both increasing. An *inverse* or *negative* correlation occurs when one variable increases and the other one decreases (the variables change in opposite directions). An example of an inverse correlation is the relationship between fruit intake and hypertension; as a population's fruit consumption increases, the per—centage of people with hypertension in that population decreases (Fig. 2.5b).

What appears to be a correlation between a behavior and an outcome could be a coincidence, that is, a chance happening, and not an indication of a *cause—and—effect* relationship between the two variables. For example, in a survey of lemonade consumption in Colorado over a 10—year period, we might observe that fewer people drank lemonade during the winter than during

correlation relationship between two variables

DIRECT CORRELATION

10 years →

Healthy weight
Overweight

(a) As a population's intake of sugar-sweetened soft drinks increases (↑), the percentage of overweight people in that population increases (↑).

INVERSE CORRELATION

10 years →

With hypertension
Without hypertension

(b) As a population's fruit intake increases (↑), the percentage of people in that population with hypertension decreases (↓).

Figure 2.5 Examples of direct and inverse correlations. (a) Direct (positive) correlation: As a population's intake of sugar-sweetened soft drinks increases (↑), the percentage of overweight people in that population increases (↑). (b) Inverse (negative) correlation: As a population's fruit intake increases (↑), the percentage of people in that population with hypertension declines (↓).

the summer months. In a survey of snow skiing accidents in Colorado during the same 10—year period, we might also find that snow skiing accidents were more likely to occur during the winter than in the summer. Thus, as lemonade consumption declined, snow skiing accidents increased. Does this mean lem—onade consumption is inversely correlated to skiing accidents and people who do not drink lemonade have a greater risk of having a skiing accident at this time of year? It is more likely that the relationship between snow skiing and lemonade drinking is coincidental, because both activities are associated with seasonal weather conditions. Although this example is obviously far—fetched, it illustrates the problems scientists can have when analyzing results of epide—miological studies.

Analyzing Data, Drawing Conclusions, and Reporting Findings

Nutrition researchers use a variety of statistical methods to analyze data collected from observations and experiments. These methods may enable the researchers to find relationships between the variables and health outcomes that were studied. As a result, scientists can determine whether their hypotheses are supported by the data.

When an experiment or study is completed and the results analyzed, researchers summarize the findings and seek to publish articles with informa—tion about their investigation in scientific journals. Before articles are accepted for publication, they undergo **peer review,** a critical analysis conducted by a group of "peers." Peers are investigators who were not part of the study but are experts involved in related research. If peers agree that a study was well conducted, its results are fairly represented, and the research is of interest to

peer review expert critical analysis of a research article before it is published the journal's readers, these scientists are likely to recommend that the journal's editors publish the article. Examples of peer–reviewed medical and nutrition journals include the *The New England Journal of Medicine*, *Journal of the American Medical Association*, and the *Journal of the American College of Nutrition*.

Research Bias Scientists expect other researchers to avoid relying on their per–sonal attitudes and biases ("points of view") when collecting and analyzing data, and to evaluate and report their results objectively and honestly. This process is important because much of the scientific research that is conducted in the United States is supported financially by the federal government, nonprofit foundations, and drug companies and other private industries. Some funding sources can have certain expectations or biases about research outcomes, and as a result, they are likely to finance studies of scientists whose research efforts support their inter–ests. The beef industry, for example, might not fund scientific investigations to find connections between high intakes of beef and the risk of certain cancers. On the other hand, the beef industry might be interested in supporting a team of scientists whose research indicates that a high–protein diet that contains plenty of beef is useful for people who are trying to lose weight.

Peer–reviewed journals usually require authors of articles to disclose their affiliations and sources of financial support. Such disclosures may appear on the first page or at the end of the article. By having this information, readers can decide on the reliability of the findings. Although peer review helps ensure that the scientists are as ethical and objective as possible, it is impossible to eliminate all research bias.

Spreading the News After the results of a study are published in a nutrition–related journal or reported to health professionals attending a meeting of a nutrition or medical society, the media (e.g., newspapers, magazines, Internet news sources) may receive notice of the findings. If the information is simplistic and sensational, such as a finding that drinking green tea can result in weight loss, it is more likely to be reported in the popular press. In many instances, you learn about the study's results when they are reported in a television or radio news broadcast as a 15– or 30–second "sound bite." Such sources generally provide very little information concerning the way the study was conducted or how the data were collected and analyzed.

Popular sources of nutrition information, such as magazines and the Internet, generally do not sub–ject articles or blogs to peer review or other scientific scrutiny, and as a result, they may feature faulty, biased information. For example, a health news column in a popular magazine may report findings from a few nutrition journal articles that support the use of garlic supplements for reducing blood cholesterol levels. However, you may conclude that the column is biased if it excludes results of other studies that do not indicate such benefits. You can often distinguish a peer–reviewed scientific journal from a popular magazine simply by looking at their covers and skimming their pages. Compared to scientific journals, magazines typically have more colorful, attractive covers and photographs, and their articles are shorter and easier for the average person to read (Fig. 2.6).

| Examples of peer-reviewed medical and nutrition journals.

Figure 2.6 Judging by the cover. Consumers can be trained to look for features, such as "busy," brightly colored covers, that distinguish peer-reviewed scientific journals from popular magazines. Also, popular sources of nutrition information, such as these magazines, are readily available at supermarkets and convenience stores.

It is important to keep in mind that sensational media coverage of a medical "breakthrough" is not necessarily an indication of the value or quality of research that resulted in the news story or magazine article. The results of one study are rarely enough to gain widespread acceptance for new or unusual findings or to provide a basis for nutritional recommendations. Thus, the findings obtained by one research team must be supported by those generated in other studies. If the results of several scientific investigations conducted under similar conditions confirm the original researchers' conclusions, then these findings are more likely to be accepted by other nutrition scientists.

Confusion and Conflict

One day, the news highlights dramatic health benefits from eating garlic, dark chocolate, brown rice, or cherries. A few weeks later, the news includes reports of more recent scientific investigations that do not support the earlier find—ings. When consumers become aware of conflicting results generated by nutrition studies, they often become confused and disappointed. As a result, some people may mistrust the scientific community and think nutrition scientists do not know what they are doing.

Consumers need to recognize that conflicting findings often result from dif—ferences in the ways various studies are designed. Even when investigating the same question, different groups of scientists often conduct their studies and analyze the results differently. For example, the numbers, ages, and physical conditions of subjects; the type and length of the study; the amount of the treatment provided; and the statistical tests used to analyze results typically vary among studies. Additionally, individual genetic differences often contribute to a person's response to a treatment. Not only are people genetically different, they also have different lifestyles, and they typically recall dietary information and follow instructions con—cerning health care practices differently. These and other factors can influence the results of nutrition research involving human subjects.

The science of nutrition is constantly evolving; old beliefs and practices are discarded when they are not supported by more recent scientific evidence, and new principles and practices emerge from the new findings. By now you should understand that science involves asking questions, developing and testing hypotheses, gathering and analyzing data, drawing conclusions from data, and, sometimes, accepting change.

Concept **Checkpoint 2.1**

1. What is epidemiology?
2. Explain the importance of having a control group when conducting experimental research.
3. What is the major difference between a prospective study and a retrospective study?
4. What is a "placebo"? Why are placebos often used in studies involving human subjects?
5. What is a "double-blind study"?
6. What is a "peer-reviewed" article?
7. Explain why results of similar studies may provide different findings.

2.2 Nutrition Information: Fact or Fiction

Learning Outcomes

1 Explain why there is so much nutrition misinformation.

2 Discuss how people can become more critical and careful consumers of nutrition information.

3 Identify common "red flags" that are signs of nutrition misinformation.

While "channel surfing" one afternoon, you stop and watch the host of a televised home shopping program promote FatMegaMelter, his company's brand of a dietary supplement for losing weight. According to the host, the supplement contains a chemical derived from a plant that grows naturally in South Africa. This amazing chemical reduces the appetite for fattening foods, enabling an overweight person taking FatMegaMelter to lose up to 30 pounds in 30 days, without the need to exercise more or eat less. The host interviews an attractive young actress who claims to have lost a lot of weight after she started taking FatMegaMelter pills. A few days later, a friend mentions that she has lost 3 pounds since she began taking this product a week ago. You would like to lose a few pounds without resorting to restricting your food intake or exercising. Should you take FatMegaMelter? The supplement helped the actress and your friend; will it help you?

Although the actress's health history appears to be compelling evidence that the weight−loss supplement is effective, her information is a **testimonial,** a personal endorsement of a product. People are usually paid to provide their testimonials for advertisements; therefore, their remarks may be biased in favor of the product. Your friend's experience with taking the same weight−loss product is intriguing, but it is an anecdote and not *proof* that FatMegaMelter promotes weight loss. When your source of nutrition information is a testimonial, anecdote, or advertisement, you cannot be sure that the information is based on scientific facts and, therefore, reliable.

testimonial personal endorsement of a product

Become a Critical Consumer of Nutrition Information

People may think they have learned facts about nutrition by reading popular magazine articles or best−selling books; visiting Internet websites; or watching television news, infomercials, or home shopping programs. In many instances, however, they have been misinformed. To be a careful consumer, do not assume that all nutrition information presented in the popular media is reliable. The First Amendment to the U.S. Constitution guarantees freedom of the press and freedom of speech, so people can provide nutrition information that is not true. Thus, the First Amendment does not protect consumers with freedom from nutrition misinformation or false nutrition claims.

The U.S. Food and Drug Administration (FDA) can regulate nutrition− and health−related claims on product labels, but the agency cannot prevent the spread of health and nutrition misinformation published in books or pamphlets or presented in television or radio programs. As a consumer, you are responsible for questioning and

Be wary of ads for nutrition-related products that rely on testimonials and anecdotes.

researching the accuracy of nutrition information as well as the credentials of the people making nutrition–related claims.

Promoters of worthless nutrition products and services often use sophis–ticated marketing methods to lure consumers. For example, some promoters of dietary supplements claim their products are "scientifically tested," or they include citations to what appear to be scientific journal articles in their ads or articles. Consumers, however, cannot be certain the information is true. Few dietary supplements have been thoroughly evaluated by reputable scientists. In some instances, these products have been scientifically tested, but the bulk of the research has shown that most dietary supplements, other than vitamins and minerals, provide little or no measurable health benefits. Nevertheless, promoters of nonnutrient dietary supplements usually ignore the scientific evidence and continue to sell their goods to an unsuspecting, trusting public. The "Nutrition Matters" feature at the end of this chapter focuses on dietary supplements.

Consumers also need to be alert for promoters' use of **pseudoscience,** the presentation of information masquerading as factual and obtained by scientific methods. In many instances, pseudoscientific nutrition or physiology information is presented with complex scientific–sounding terms, such as "enzymatic therapy" or "colloidal extract." Such terms are designed to convince people without science backgrounds that the nutrition–related information is true. Often, promoters of nutrition misinformation try to confuse people by weaving false information with facts into their claims, making the untrue material seem credible too.

Although people's lives have improved as a result of scientific advancements in medicine, the general public tends to mistrust scientists, medical professionals, and the pharmaceutical industry. Promoters of nutrition misinformation exploit this mistrust to sell their products and services. For example, they may tell consumers that physicians rely on costly diagnostic methods and treatments for serious diseases because they are more interested in making money than doing what is best for their patients, such as rec–ommending a dietary supplement. Are physicians driven by the desire to make money from their patients' illnesses, and do they hide information about natural cures from them?

Over the past 100 years, people's lives have been greatly improved by contributions of medical researchers. As a group, physicians are dedicated to improving their patients' health and saving lives. Physicians have nothing to gain from concealing a cure from the public. They strive to diagnose and treat diseases using scientifically tested and approved techniques. Moreover, a physician may face a malpractice lawsuit if he or she fails to diagnose and treat a condition effectively. Additionally, physicians have much to gain from treating their patients kindly and effectively. Consider this: If you follow a physician's advice and have positive results, are you likely to be that doctor's patient for a long time and recommend the practitioner to others?

If your car is not functioning properly, you probably would want people who have the best training, tools, and equipment to determine the problem and repair it. If you think something is wrong with your body, it is prudent to seek information and opin–ions from medical professionals who have the best training and experience to diagnose and treat health disorders.

pseudoscience presentation of information masquerading as factual and obtained by scientific methods

Ask Questions

If you are like most people, you do not want to waste your money on things you do not need or that are useless or potentially harmful. How can you become a more careful, critical consumer of nutrition–related information or products? The following questions should help you evaluate various sources of nutrition information:

- *What motivates the authors, promoters, or sponsors to provide the information? Do you think they are more interested in your health and well–being or in selling their products?* Salespeople often have favorable biases toward the things they sell, and therefore, they may not be reliable sources of information about these products. A clerk in a dietary supplements outlet store, for example, may wear a white lab coat to look as though he or she has a science or medical educational background, but you should keep in mind that the clerk was hired to sell dietary supplements and may have little or no scientific training. Furthermore, salespeople who work in such outlets may be unwilling to inform customers about the potential health hazards of taking certain products, particularly when they earn a commission from each sale.

- *Is the source scientific, such as an article from a peer–reviewed nutrition journal?* In general, popular sources of nutrition information, such as best–selling books and articles in magazines, are not peer–reviewed by scientists. Additionally, radio or TV programs that promote nutrition information may actually be sophisticated advertisements for nutrition–related products.

- *If a study is cited, how was the research conducted? Did the study involve humans or animals? If people participated in the study, how many subjects were involved in the research? Who sponsored the study?* As mentioned earlier in this chapter, epidemiological studies are not useful for finding cause–and–effect relationships. Additionally, the results of studies involving large numbers of human subjects are more reliable than studies of animals. Sponsors may influence the outcomes of the studies they fund.

- *To provide scientific support for claims, does the source cite respected nutrition or medical journals or mention reliable experts?* Be careful if you see citations in popular nutrition or health books and magazines. Promoters of nutrition misinformation may refer to scientific–appearing citations from phony medical journals to convince people that their information is reliable. Furthermore, be wary of nutrition experts introduced or identified as "Doctor" because they may not be physicians or scientists. Furthermore, a so–called nutrition expert who is referred to as "Doctor" may not have a doctorate degree (Ph.D.) in human nutrition from an accredited university. Such experts may have obtained their degrees simply by purchasing them on the Internet or through a mail–order outlet, without having taken appropriate coursework or graduated from an accredited university or college.

If this person appeared on a television show or in a magazine advertisement, would you consider him to be a reliable source of nutrition information? Explain why you would or would not trust his nutrition-related advice.

quackery promotion of useless medical treatments

Practicing medicine without the proper training and licensing is illegal. How—ever, providing nutrition information and advice without the proper training and licensing is legal. **Quackery** involves promoting useless medical treatments, such as copper bracelets to treat arthritis.

To obtain information about a nutrition expert's credentials, enter the person's name at an Internet search engine and evaluate the results. For example, is the person associated with an accredited school of higher education or a government agency such as the U.S. Department of Agriculture? You can also visit www.quackwatch.org and submit an "Ask a Question" e—mail requesting information about a person's credentials from the site's sponsors.

Look for Red Flags

To become a critical consumer of nutrition information, you need to be aware of "red flags," clues that indicate a source of information is unreliable. Common red flags include the following:

1. **Promises of quick and easy remedies for complex health—related problems:** "Our product helps you lose weight *without* exercising or dieting," or "Garlic cures heart disease."

2. **Claims that sound too good to be true:** "Our all—natural product blocks fat and calories from being absorbed, so you can eat everything you like and still lose weight." Such claims are rarely true. Remember, if the claim sounds too good to be true, it probably is not true.

3. **Scare tactics that include sensational, frightening, false, or misleading statements about a food, dietary practice, or health condition:** "Dairy products cause cancer," or "Eating sugar causes hyperactivity."

4. **Personal attacks on the motives and ethical standards of registered dietitians or conventional scientists:** "Dietitians and medical researchers don't want you to know the facts about natural cures for cancer, diabetes, and heart disease because it will dry up their funding." Such statements indicate unsubstantiated biases against bona fide nutrition experts and the scientific community.

5. **Statements about the superiority of certain dietary supplements or unconventional medical practices:** "Russian scientists have discovered the countless health benefits of taking Siberian ginseng," or "Colon cleansing with herbs is the only cure for intestinal cancer."

6. **Testimonials and anecdotes as evidence of effectiveness:** "I lost 50 pounds in 30 days using this product," or "I rubbed this vitamin E—containing lotion on my scar and it disappeared in days." As mentioned earlier, these sources of information are unreliable. Reliable nutrition information is based on scientific evidence.

7. **Information that promotes a product's benefits while overlooking its risks:** "Our all—natural supplement boosts your metabolism naturally so it won't harm your system." Anything you consume, even water, can be toxic in high doses. Beware of any source of information that fails to mention the possible side effects of using a dietary supplement or nutrition—related treatment.

8. **Vague, meaningless, or scientific—sounding terms to impress or confuse consumers:** "Our *all—natural, clinically tested, patented, chelated* dietary supplement works best."

9. **Sensational statements with incomplete references of sources:** "Clinical research performed at a major university and published in a distinguished medical journal indicates food manufacturers have added ingredients to products that make you hungry and fat," or "Millions of Americans suffer from various nutritional deficiencies." Which "major university" and "distinguished medical journal"? What study reported that "millions of Americans" are deficient in nutrients?

10. **Recommendations based on a single study:** "Research conducted at our private health facility proves coffee enemas can cure cancer."

11. **Information concerning nutrients or human physiology that is not supported by reliable scientific evidence:** "This book explains how to combine certain foods based on your blood type," or "Most diseases are caused by undigested food that gets stuck in your guts," or "People with alkaline bodies don't develop cancer."

12. **Results disclaimers, usually in small or difficult–to–read print:** "Results may vary," or "Results not typical" (Fig. 2.7). Disclaimers are clues that the product may not live up to your expectations or the manufacturer's claims.

Using the Internet Wisely

You can find abundant sources of information about nutrition and the benefits of dietary supplements on the Internet. However, you must be careful and consider the sources. Who or what organization sponsors the site? Is the information intended to promote sales? Be wary if the site discusses benefits of dietary supplements and enables you to purchase these products online. Furthermore, a site is likely to be unreliable if it includes comprehensive disclaimers such as "The manufacturer is not responsible or obligated to verify statements," or "The FDA has not evaluated this website. This product is not intended to diagnose, cure, or prevent any disease." Also avoid sites that publish disclaimers such as "The nutrition and health information at this site is provided for educational purposes only and not

Figure 2.7 Results disclaimer. This disclaimer may be a red flag indicating the product has limited effectiveness, despite its promoter's claims.

Food & Nutrition tips

If you are looking for a recipe for guacamole, cranberry chutney, or sweet and sour cabbage, simply use the Internet—it is like having a cookbook at your fingertips. Recipes for nearly every food and from various countries and ethnic groups are available on the Internet, and you can also find menu planning and cooking tips from this vast resource.

When searching the Web for recipes, you need to recognize that many food manufacturers use the sites to promote their products in recipes. If the brand name of a product is mentioned in the recipe, you can usually substitute another company's product. Additionally, recipes do not always provide accurate information about the nutrients and calories in a serving of food, and you cannot be certain that the recipes have been tested for quality. Therefore, it is a good idea to check more than one site for a recipe and compare the information.

TABLE 2.1 Tips for Searching Nutrition Information on the Internet

To be a Careful Consumer of Internet Sources of Information:

1. Use multiple sites, especially government sites such as the Centers for Disease Control and Prevention (www.cdc.gov) and the Food and Drug Administration (www.fda.gov), as well as the sites of nationally recognized nutrition- or health-related associations such as the Academy of Nutrition and Dietetics (www.eatright.org) and the American Heart Association (www.americanheart.org).

2. Be wary of sites that have surveys for you to complete, advertisements for diet-related products, and promotions in pop-up windows.

3. Rely primarily on sites that are managed or reviewed by a group of qualified health professionals. Blogs might be fun and interesting to read, but they are not necessarily reliable.

4. Look for the Health on the Net symbol at the bottom of the main page of the website. The Health on the Net Foundation is a nonprofit, international organization that promotes the HONcode, a set of principles for standardizing the reliability of health information on the Internet. Currently, website sponsors are not required to follow HONcode standards. For more information about HONcode, you can visit the organization's website (www.hon.ch/).

5. Do not trust information at a site that does not indicate valid sources, such as well-respected peer-reviewed scientific journals or nationally recognized universities or medical centers. Contributing authors and their credentials should be identified; when they are, perform an online search of the scientific journals, as well as the authors' names and credentials to determine their validity.

6. Do not trust a site that includes attacks on the trustworthiness of the medical or scientific establishment.

7. Avoid sites that provide online diagnoses and treatments.

8. Be wary of commercial sites (*.com) with links to government sites or the sites of well-known medical, nutrition, or scientific associations. An unreliable *.com site can be linked to reliable sites without having received their endorsements.

9. Avoid providing your personal information at the site because its confidentiality may not be protected.

Be wary of nutrition information provided at websites that sell diet-related products.

For more tips, visit: http://ods.od.nih.gov/Health_Information/How_To_Evaluate_Health_Information_on_the_Internet_Questions_and_Answers.aspx.

as a substitute for the advice of a physician or dietitian. The author and owner of this site are not liable for personal actions taken as a result of the site's contents."

Be wary of websites that are authored or sponsored by one person, or sites that promote or sell products for profit (*.com), because such sources of information may be biased. In general, websites sponsored by nationally recognized health associations such as the Academy of Nutrition and Dietetics, (www.eatright.org) and nonprofit organizations such as the National Osteoporosis Foundation (www.nof.org) are reliable sources of nutrition information. Government agencies (*.gov) and nationally accredited colleges and universities (*.edu) are also excellent sources of credible nutrition information. Table 2.1 presents some tips for using the Internet to obtain reliable nutrition information.

The Federal Trade Commission (FTC) enforces consumer protection laws and investigates complaints about false or misleading health claims that appear on the Internet. For information to help you evaluate nutrition and health–related claims, visit the agency's website (www.ftc.gov/bcp/edu/pubs/consumer /health/hea07.shtm). To complain about a product, you can complete and submit the FTC's complaint form at the website or call the agency's toll–free line (1−877−382−4357).

Concept **Checkpoint 2.2**

8. What is the difference between a testimonial and an anecdote?

9. List at least three "red flags" that may indicate a questionable source of nutrition information.

10. List at least three tips for using the Internet as a reliable source of nutrition information.

2.3 Reliable Nutrition Experts

Learning Outcome

1 Explain how to identify reliable nutrition experts.

registered dietitian (RD), registered dietitian nutritionist (RDN), or licensed dietitian nutritionist (LDN) college-trained health care professional who has extensive knowledge of foods, nutrition, and dietetics

If you have questions about food or nutrition, where do you find factual answers? Although many states regulate and license people who call themselves nutritionists, you cannot always rely on someone who refers to him— or herself as a "nutritionist" or "nutritionalist" for reliable nutrition information, because there are no standard legal definitions for these descriptors. Should you ask a physician for nutrition advice? Physicians are not necessarily the best sources of nutrition information, because most doctors do not have extensive college coursework in the subject.

If your university or college has a nutrition or dietetics department, you are likely to find nutrition experts, including professors, registered dietitians, and registered dietitian nutritionists, who are faculty members. A **registered dietitian (RD), registered dietitian nutritionist (RDN), or licensed dietitian nutritionist (LDN)** is a college—trained health care professional who has extensive knowledge of foods, nutrition, and *dietetics*, the application of nutrition and food information to treat many health—related conditions. The titles "registered dietitian (RD)" and "registered dietitian nutritionist (RDN)" are legally protected.

You can also locate registered dietitians by consulting the phone directories, contacting your local dietetic association or dietary department of a local hospital, or visiting the Academy of Nutrition and Dietetics website (www.eatright.org) or the Dietitians of Canada's website (www.dietitians.ca).

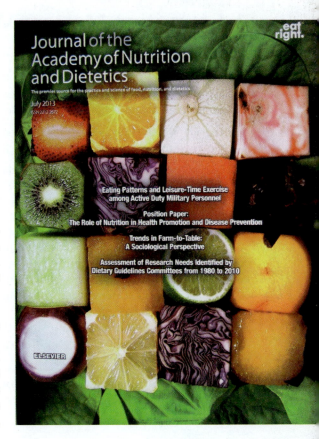

Becoming a Registered Dietitian Nutritionist

There are three major professional divisions for RDs, RDNs, and LDNs: clinical dietetics, community nutrition, and food service systems management. Clinical dietitians can work as members of medical teams in hospitals or clinics. Clinical dietitians can also work as community nutritionists in public health settings or as dietary counselors in private practice or with wellness programs. Food service systems management dietitians direct food systems in hospitals, schools, or other settings. Although most registered dietitians work in health care settings, some are educators or researchers.

An RD/RDN/LDN has completed a baccalaureate degree program approved by the Accreditation Council for Education in Nutrition and Dietetics of the Academy of Nutrition and Dietetics, the largest organization of dietitians in the United States. As undergraduate students, dietetics majors are required to take a wide variety of college—level courses, including food and nutrition sciences, organic chemistry, biochemistry, biology, physiology, microbiology, food service systems management, business, and communications classes. If you are attending a major university, you can check the course or program catalog at your school to determine whether an accredited dietetics program is offered.

In addition to taking the required college coursework, the student dietitian must complete a *supervised practice program (SPP)* that provides professional training in a health care facility such as a hospital, a food service company, or a community health care agency such as a state or local health department. Finally, this individual has to pass the national registration examination to become cer—tified as an RD. After becoming certified, RDs are also required to fulfill con—tinuing education requirements to maintain their certification. The Academy of Nutrition and Dietetics provides information about becoming an RD and roles these professionals play in health care settings.

Concept **Checkpoint 2.3**

11. What is the difference between a nutritionist and a registered dietitian nutritionist?

12. List three ways of locating reliable nutrition experts.

2.4 Nutrition Matters: What Are Dietary Supplements?

Learning Outcomes

① Explain the difference between conventional medicine and complementary and alternative medicine (CAM).

② Explain how the FDA regulates medicines differently than dietary supplements.

③ Discuss the risks and benefits of taking dietary supplements.

Do you take a daily vitamin or mineral pill because you are concerned about the nutritional quality of your diet? Do you use herbal pills or extracts to strengthen your immune system, boost your memory, or treat illnesses such as the common cold? If you follow any of these practices, you are not alone. According to results of national surveys, almost 50% of the American population takes one or more dietary supplements regularly.[6]

According to the Dietary Supplement and Health Edu—cation Act of 1994 (DSHEA), a dietary supplement is a product (other than tobacco) that

- adds to a person's dietary intake and contains one or more dietary ingredients, including nutrients or *botanicals* (herbs or other plant material)

- is taken by mouth
- is not promoted as a conventional food or the only item of a meal or diet[7]

Dietary supplements include nutrient pills, protein pow—ders, and herbal extracts, as well as energy bars and drinks. Many dietary supplements are often referred to as "nutraceuticals," but there is no legal definition for this term.

In the United States, the most commonly used dietary supplements are **multivitamin/mineral (MV/M)** prod—ucts.[8] There is no standard definition for the contents of a MV/M supplement, but such products may contain several vitamins and minerals.[6] Among American adults, the most popular nonvitamin, nonmineral dietary supplements are fish oil or "omega 3," glucosamine, echinacea, and flaxseed oil and pills. Some people use dietary supplements, particu—larly those containing nutrients, because the products are recommended by their physicians or dietitians. Physicians, for example, may prescribe a prenatal MV/M supplement for their pregnant patients. Most dietary supplements are available without the need for prescriptions, so people can take them without their doctors' knowledge and approval. When researchers asked a group of people why they used dietary supplements, subjects gave a variety of reasons, including to boost their nutrient intakes, to prevent certain diseases, to obtain more energy, to enhance good health, and to treat existing ailments.[9]

Table 2.2 provides information about some non-micronutrient dietary supplements that are popular among adult Americans. Benefits and risks of supplementing diets with micronutrients are discussed in Chapters 8 and 9.

What Is Complementary and Alternative Medicine?

The use of herbal products and other dietary supplements to treat disease or promote good health is an aspect of **complementary and alternative medicine (CAM).** CAM includes a variety of health care practices and products that are not accepted by the majority of physicians and other conventional health care providers. In 2007, approximately 38% of American adults and 12% of American children used CAM therapies, including chiropractic manipulations, homeopathy, naturopathy, and massage therapy.[10] Among American adults, taking nonvitamin, nonmineral natural products was the most popular form of CAM therapy. However, there is little scientific evidence that supports the usefulness as well as the safety of taking most nonnutrient dietary supplements, including botanicals.[10]

A few types of CAM are gaining acceptance among conventional medical practitioners, primarily because there is sufficient scientific support for the practices. For example, species of "unfriendly" bacteria can overpopulate the large intestine when a person takes an antibiotic for infection. The overgrowth of these bacteria can cause cramping and diarrhea. Some physicians recommend probiotics in yogurt or tablet form for patients who are taking antibiotics. Research has shown that certain probiotics can help prevent or limit diarrhea that results from antibiotic use.[11]

The practice of using CAM with conventional medicine is called *integrative medicine.* The National Center for Complementary and Integrative Health (NCCIH), an agency within the National Institutes of Health, funds research intended to increase scientific evidence about the usefulness and safety of CAM practices.

How Are Dietary Supplements Regulated?

The U.S. Food and Drug Administration (FDA) is the federal agency that is responsible for ensuring the safety and effectiveness of medications and other health–related products. The FDA strictly regulates the development, production, and marketing of new medications (drugs). A drug is a substance, natural or human–made, that alters body functions. As a result, drugs can produce beneficial as well as harmful effects on the body. Before marketing a new drug, the manufacturer must submit evidence to the FDA indicating that the product has been tested extensively and is safe and effective. If FDA experts have serious concerns about a medication's side effects or question its usefulness, the agency may reject the manufacturer's petition to sell the product.

When consumed, many dietary supplements act as drugs in the body. However, the FDA regulates dietary supplements as foods, not medications.[12] As a result, dietary supplement manufacturers can bypass most of the strict regulations that the FDA applies to the introduction of new medications into the marketplace. Supplement manufacturers, for example, generally do not need FDA approval before manufacturing or marketing their products. Additionally, the manufacturers are not required to provide the FDA with scientific evidence indicating their products provide measurable health benefits. Manufacturers, however, must notify the FDA and provide the agency with information about the safety of any supplement that contains dietary ingredients that were not marketed in dietary supplements prior to 1994, unless the substance had been used in foods.

The FDA regulates the labeling of dietary supplements, including the kinds of claims that are permitted on labels. The "Food and Dietary Supplement Labels" section of Chapter 3 provides information about supplement labeling.

The FDA's role in regulating dietary supplements generally begins after products enter the marketplace.[13] Supplement manufacturers are required to keep records concerning reports they receive about serious adverse (negative) health effects that may have been caused by their products. Furthermore, the manufacturers must also inform the FDA about such reports. Consumers and health care professionals can also report health problems that are possibly associated with supplement use directly to the FDA.

When the FDA determines that a particular supplement presents a significant or unreasonable risk of harm, the agency alerts consumers about the risk and seeks to recall the product, that is, initiates efforts to have it removed

multivitamin/mineral (MV/M) describes a dietary supplement that contains vitamins and minerals

complementary and alternative medicine (CAM) variety of health care practices that are not accepted by the majority of conventional medical practitioners

TABLE 2.2 Some Popular Dietary Supplements

Dietary Supplement	Major Claims	Known Health Effects	
		Benefits	Risks
Alfalfa	Treats kidney problems and improves urine flow Relieves arthritis symptoms	May be effective in lowering total cholesterol and "bad" cholesterol levels, but little scientific evidence that it has other benefits	Although alfalfa leaves may be safe to ingest, consuming alfalfa seeds may be hazardous to health; may lower blood sugar levels, which could be dangerous for people with diabetes
Bitter orange	Useful for causing weight loss and treating heartburn, upset stomach, and constipation	None	May increase heart rate and blood pressure, which could result in stroke
Chondroitin	Relieves joint damage associated with arthritis	Some scientific evidence supports health benefit claims, but more research is needed. Often combined with glucosamine	Some products may contain poisonous levels of the mineral manganese.
Coenzyme Q-10	Increases exercise tolerance, prevents heart disease and cancer, and reverses signs of aging	Antioxidant made by the body and involved in energy metabolism Insufficient scientific evidence to support most claims	May improve heart function Low toxicity but may interfere with certain blood thinners
Echinacea	Boosts immune system Prevents the common cold and reduces cold symptoms	May reduce cold symptoms if taken in the early stage of the infection process May reduce recurrence of vaginal yeast infections Not effective for treating recurrent genital herpes outbreaks	Generally safe for short-term use but may provoke allergic response or intestinal upset; some products may be contaminated with arsenic and lead
Evening primrose oil	Treats eczema (a common skin condition) Relieves arthritis and postmenopausal symptoms	Little scientific evidence to support health benefit claims	Long-term safety has not been established.
Fish oil	Prevents heart disease and stroke Cures rheumatoid arthritis Reduces depression and risk of Alzheimer's disease	Lowers elevated blood triglyceride (fat) levels, but consuming fatty fish may be more helpful in reducing heart disease risk than taking fish oil supplements Can slightly lower blood pressure May reduce pain and stiffness associated with rheumatoid arthritis More research is need to determine other health benefits.	Taking more than 3 g/day may interfere with blood clotting, increasing the risk of hemorrhagic stroke. Can reduce blood vitamin E concentration
Flaxseed and flaxseed oil	Acts as a laxative (flaxseed) Reduces blood cholesterol levels	Nonanimal source of omega-3 fatty acids Seeds have laxative effects. May benefit people with heart disease, but more research is needed	Generally safe but may cause diarrhea
Garlic	Lowers blood cholesterol levels	May slow the development of atherosclerosis that can result in heart attack and stroke May reduce the risk of stomach and colon cancers May reduce elevated blood pressure	Can cause allergic reaction, cause unpleasant body odor, and interfere with prescription blood thinners
Ginger	Treats "morning sickness" and other forms of nausea Relieves stomach upsets Relieves joint and muscle pain	Can safely treat morning sickness and may reduce other forms of nausea Lack of scientific evidence to support other health benefit claims	In general, few side effects when taken in small amounts; powdered ginger may cause intestinal upset

Sources: National Institutes of Health, National Center for Complementary and Alternative Medicine: Health topics A-Z *http://nccam.nih.gov/health/atoz.htm*
Accessed: July 31, 2014

TABLE 2.2 Some Popular Dietary Supplements *(Continued)*

Dietary Supplement	Major Claims	Known Health Effects	
		Benefits	**Risks**
Ginkgo biloba	Improves memory Reduces the risk of Alzheimer's disease and other forms of dementia	Taking ginkgo leaf extracts by mouth may produce mild improvements in cognitive (thinking) processes and reduce dizziness. Lack of scientific evidence to support many other health benefit claims	Reacts with several prescription medications May increase the risk of bleeding and cause allergic reactions, headaches, intestinal upsets, and nausea Ginkgo seeds are toxic.
Ginseng (Asian)	Boosts overall health Treats erectile dysfunction (male impotence)	May lower elevated blood glucose levels and benefit immune system Lack of scientific evidence to support other health benefit claims	May cause headaches, sleep disturbances, allergic responses, and gastrointestinal upsets Long-term use may increase risk of toxicity.
Glucosamine sulfate	Relieves joint damage associated with arthritis	Some scientific evidence supports health benefit claims, but more research is needed (frequently used with chondroitin).	Appears to be safe but may cause mild gastrointestinal side effects, including nausea and heartburn
Green tea	Prevents or treats cancer Promotes weight loss Reduces blood cholesterol levels	Results of some laboratory studies indicate green tea protects against cancer or reduces cancer cell growth, but results of human studies are not conclusive. Lack of reliable evidence to support other health benefit claims, including promoting weight loss	Green tea extracts may damage the liver. Caffeine content may cause sleep disturbances, irritability, and digestive upset.
Kava	Reduces stress	Potential harm of using kava outweighs any benefit.	Toxic—can damage the liver May cause abnormal muscle movements, yellowed skin, and sleepiness
L-arginine	Treats heart disease Improves male sexual functioning Improves mental functioning of older adults Lowers blood pressure Increases male fertility	Amino acid (component of proteins) Does not prevent heart attacks May reduce recovery time after surgery and improve erectile function More research is needed to support other health benefits.	Probably safe when taken for short term but may cause side effects, including abdominal pain, diarrhea, gout, breathing problems, and low blood pressure May worsen recurrent herpes outbreaks Should not be taken by people who are recovering from a heart attack, because the supplement may cause another heart attack
Melatonin	Treats some sleep disorders Prevents jet lag Treats cancer, headaches, and irritable bowel syndrome Delays the aging process	May be effective for treating certain sleep disorders and preventing jet lag May help relieve withdrawal symptoms in smokers who quit tobacco use Lack of evidence that the supplement is useful for other conditions	Probably safe for short-term use, but people should not drive or operate heavy machinery for 4–5 hours after taking the supplement Interacts with several prescription medications and other herbs that produce sedation (calming effects) May interfere with female fertility and worsen depression in people with the condition
St. John's wort	Reduces depression	At this time, most studies do not support using the supplement to treat depression.	May interact with other herbal products and many medications, including prescription antidepressants and oral contraceptives

from the market.[14] In most instances, the manufacturer voluntarily recalls the product after determining there is a problem with it or being notified by the FDA about the problem. In some cases, however, the FDA requests a recall. If the FDA determines that the manufacturer's response to the recall is inadequate, the agency can take enforcement steps, such as initiating legal action against the company to seize products or stop producing the items.

Using Dietary Supplements Wisely

When used properly, many dietary supplements, particularly micronutrient products, are generally safe. Herbal supplements, however, are made from plants that may have toxic parts. Comfrey, pennyroyal, sassafras, kava, lobelia, and ma huang are among the plants known to be highly toxic or cancer-causing. Products containing material from these plants should be avoided. The use of botanical products can also evoke allergic or inflammatory responses that often result in signs and symptoms of skin, sinus, or respiratory illnesses. Herbal teas may contain pollens and other parts of plants that can cause allergies, particularly in people who are sensitive to the herbs or their related species. Echinacea (purple cone flower) is related to ragweed, a plant that is often associated with seasonal respiratory allergies. When people who are allergic to ragweed pollen take supplements that contain echinacea, they may develop allergic responses that mimic symptoms of the common cold (watery eyes, runny nose, and sneezing). In some instances, inflammatory responses, such as asthma attacks, can occur after exposure to echinacea or other plants. Asthma can be a life-threatening condition. Therefore, people who have asthma or allergies should be very careful when using botanical supplements.

Consumers also need to be aware that medicinal herbs may contain substances that interact with prescription or over-the-counter medications as well as other herbs. Such responses can produce unwanted and even dangerous side effects (see Table 2.2). Ginkgo biloba, for example, can interact with aspirin, increasing the risk of bleeding. Garlic, ginseng, and vitamin E supplements can also increase bleeding. Kava and valerian act as sedatives (calming agents) and can amplify the effects of anesthetics and other medications used during surgery. Therefore, consult a physician or pharmacist before using any dietary supplement or giving such products to your children. Additionally, treat dietary supplements as drugs: store them away from children and provide your physicians and other health care professionals with a list of the ones you are taking.

If you use or are thinking about using one or more dietary supplements:

- Determine whether the supplement is necessary. Some people have medical reasons for taking dietary

supplements that contain one or more micronutrients, such as folic acid, calcium, or vitamin D. Discuss your need for the supplement with your physician or a registered dietitian before you purchase or use the product. This action is particularly important if you are pregnant, are breastfeeding a baby, or have a chronic medical condition such as diabetes or heart disease.

- Consult a physician as soon as you develop signs and symptoms of a serious illness. Using supplements to treat serious diseases instead of seeking conventional medical care that has proven effectiveness is a risky practice. In these instances, delaying or forgoing useful medical treatment may result in the worsening of the condition or even be life threatening.

- Be wary of claims made about a supplement's benefits and investigate the claims used to promote the product. The following government websites provide reliable information about dietary supplements:

U.S. National Library of Medicine http://www.nlm.nih.gov/medlineplus/herbalmedicine.html

Food and Drug Adminstration www.fda.gov/Food/DietarySupplements/default.htm

National Institutes of Health, National Center for Complementary and Integrative Health https://nccih.nih.gov/health/integrative-health

Office of Dietary Supplements http://ods.od.nih.gov/

- Determine hazards associated with taking the supplement. Information about the risks and benefits of various dietary supplements can be found at the **Office of Dietary Supplements'** website: http://ods.od.nih.gov/factsheets/dietarysupplements/.

- Avoid using dietary supplements as substitutes for nutritious foods. Plant foods provide a wide array of phytochemicals, many of which may have health benefits when taken in their natural forms—foods. When these substances are isolated from plants and manufactured into supplements, they may lose their beneficial properties.

If you experience negative side effects after using a particular dietary supplement, it is a good idea to be examined by a physician immediately. Furthermore, you as well as your physician should report the problem to the FDA's MedWatch program by calling (800) FDA-1088 or visiting the agency's website: http://www.fda.gov/Safety/MedWatch/HowToReport/default.htm.

It is important to recognize that the manufacturing of dietary supplements is a profitable industry in the

United States. In 2011, Americans spent $30 billion on such products.[15] In many instances, however, people do not need dietary supplements, and they are wasting their money by purchasing them—money that could be better spent on natural sources of nutrients and phyto—chemicals, particularly fruits, vegetables, and whole—grain cereals.[16]

Concept **Checkpoint 2.4**

13. List at least three examples of complementary and alternative medical practices.
14. Explain why a prescription medication that is used to treat the common cold is not a dietary supplement.
15. List at least two examples of dietary supplements.

Chapter References

See Appendix H.

Summary

2.1 Nutrition: Science for Consumers

• Scientists ask questions about the natural world and follow generally accepted methods to obtain answers to these questions. Nutrition research relies on scientific methods that may involve making observations, asking questions and developing possible explanations, performing tests, collecting and analyzing data, drawing conclusions from data, and reporting on the findings. Other scientists can test the findings to confirm or reject them.

• Epidemiology is the study of the occurrence, distribution, and causes of health problems in populations. By studying differences in dietary practices and disease occurrences among populations, epidemiologists can suggest nutrition-related hypotheses for the prevalence of certain diseases. Epidemiological studies cannot indicate whether two variables are correlated, because the relationship could be a coincidence.

• Researchers summarize the findings and seek to publish articles with information about their investigations in scientific journals. Before articles are accepted for publication, they undergo peer review. Scientists generally do not accept a hypothesis or the results of a study until they are supported by considerable research evidence. Media coverage of a medical breakthrough is not necessarily an indication of the value or quality of research that resulted in the news story. More research is often necessary for scientists to determine whether the results are valid and can be generalized.

• Consumers may think scientists do not know what they are doing when conflicting research findings are reported in the media. Conflicting findings often result because different teams of researchers use different study designs when investigating the same hypothesis. Furthermore, each team of scientists may analyze the results differently. Other factors, such as genetic and lifestyle differences, can also influence the results of nutrition research involving human subjects. The science of nutrition is constantly evolving.

2.2 Nutrition Information: Fact or Fiction

- Although testimonials and anecdotes are often used to promote nutrition-related products and services, consumers cannot be sure that this information is reliable or based on scientific facts. Personal observations are not evidence of a cause-and-effect relationship because many factors, such as lifestyle and environment, can influence outcomes.

- Popular magazine articles, best-selling trade books, Internet websites, television news reports, and other forms of media are often unreliable sources of nutrition information. Consumers need to be careful and question the reliability of such sources, because the First Amendment to the U.S. Constitution guarantees freedom of the press and freedom of speech.

- Consumers need to ask questions to determine the author's reasons for promoting the information. Consumers should also look for red flags, such as scare tactics and claims that sound too good to be true.

- Much of the nutrition information that is on the Internet is unreliable and intended to promote sales. Websites sponsored by nonprofit organizations, nationally recognized health associations, government agencies, and nationally accredited colleges and universities are generally reliable sources of information.

2.3 Reliable Nutrition Experts

- Although some states regulate and license nutritionists, there is no standard legal definition for "nutritionist" in the United States. For reliable food, nutrition, and dietary information, consumers can consult persons with degrees in human nutrition from accredited institutions of higher learning, such as nutrition instructors and registered dietitians, registered dietitian nutritionists, or licensed dietitian nutritionists.

2.4 Nutrition Matters: What Are Dietary Supplements?

- A dietary supplement is a product (other than tobacco) that adds to a person's dietary intake, contains one or more dietary ingredients, is taken by mouth in tablet or other forms, and is not promoted as a conventional food or the only item of a meal or diet.

- Dietary supplements include nutrient pills, protein powders, and herbal extracts, as well as energy bars and drinks. In many instances, people do not need dietary supplements. Healthy people should focus on obtaining nutrients and phytochemicals from foods, particularly fruits, vegetables, and whole-grain cereals. Before taking a dietary supplement, discuss the matter with your physician.

Recipe for Healthy Living

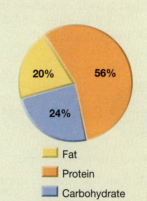

Grandma's Chicken Soup

Long before the advent of over-the-counter antihistamines and cough syrups, there was chicken soup. Sometimes referred to as "Jewish penicillin," chicken soup has been used as a cold remedy for over 1000 years. Chicken soup is not a cure for the common cold. However, results of a laboratory study indicated chicken soup contains substances that can subdue the body's inflammatory response to upper respiratory tract infections. This inflammatory response typically results in common cold symptoms such as cough and excess nasal discharge. Although the soup's specific actions on cold-causing microbes still need to be determined, consuming a soothing, warm bowl of chicken soup contributes to the sick person's fluid and other nutrient intake at a time when he or she may not feel like eating anything else. Even if you don't have a cold, the following chicken soup recipe is delicious and easy to make. You can freeze the soup in small, covered plastic containers for future meals.

Source: Rennard BO and others: Chicken soup inhibits neutrophil chemotaxis in vitro. *Chest* 118(4):1, 2000.

This recipe makes approximately 6 cups of soup. A 1-cup serving of the soup supplies approximately 135 kcal, 19 g of protein, 3 g fat, 323 mg sodium, 431 mg potassium, and 6.4 mg niacin.

INGREDIENTS:

    1 package of raw chicken wings, approx. 3 to 4 lbs
    1 large onion, cut in wedges
    4 large carrots, cleaned and cut into 3-inch lengths
    ⅛ tsp black pepper
    1 chicken bouillon cube
    3 large celery stalks, cleaned and cut into 3-inch lengths
    ⅛ tsp paprika
    ⅛ tsp thyme
    ⅛ tsp curry seasoning
    few parsley sprigs (optional)

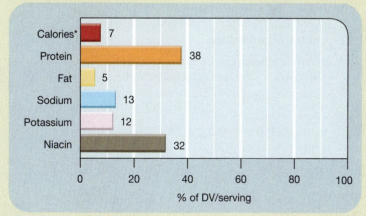

PREPARATION STEPS:

1. Place the raw chicken in a large cooking pot and add enough cold water to cover chicken, approximately 2 quarts of water.

2. Add onion, carrots, celery, pepper, bouillon cube, and spices to chicken and water; turn burner on high. When mixture comes to a boil, reduce heat to medium and cover the pot with a lid. Soup should boil for at least an hour.

3. Turn off the heat, remove chicken wings from the soup, and place them in a bowl. Cover and refrigerate.

4. Cover soup and refrigerate for 12 hours.

5. Skim chicken fat from top of soup. Remove skin from the wings and discard skin. Separate the meat from the bones, discard bones, and add the meat to the soup. Reheat soup before eating; sprinkle with parsley sprigs, if desired.

6. Cover and store leftover soup in refrigerator for up to 3 days, or freeze.

Note: When you reheat the soup, you can also add your favorite soup ingredients, such as frozen vegetables, broccoli florets, kale, whole-wheat noodles, or cooked brown rice.

 Further analyze this and other recipes through activities on Connect at www.mcgrawhillconnect.com.

Critical Thinking

1. A news broadcaster reports the results of a study in which people who took fish oil and vitamin E supplements daily did not reduce their risk of heart attack. Moreover, the researchers stopped the study when they determined the supplements increased the subjects' risk of stroke! Explain how you would determine whether this information is reliable.

2. Explain how you can verify the reliability of advice about dietary supplements provided at an Internet website.

3. Design a study that involves observing a nutrition–related practice of college students, such as vending machine choices or fast–food preferences, and share your idea with the class. Your study should be designed so that it is ethical and does not harm subjects physically or psychologically.

4. A group of scientists conduct a study to determine risk factors for breast cancer. According to their results, women who consume soy foods have a lower risk of breast cancer than women who do not eat soy foods. Think of two questions this finding is likely to generate that could be answered by further scientific investigation.

5. Browse through popular health–related magazines to find an article or advertisement that relates to nutrition, and make a copy of the article or advertisement. Analyze each sentence or line of the article or advertisement for signs of unreliability. Is the article or advertisement a reliable source of information? Explain why it is or why it is not.

Practice Test

Select the best answer.

1. The first step of the scientific method usually involves

   a. gathering data.
   b. developing a hypothesis.
   c. identifying relationships between variables.
   d. making observations.

2. A group of scientists observe a group of college students over 4 years to determine which of their characteristics leads to weight gain. This study is an example of

   a. a case–control study.
   b. a prospective study.
   c. a retrospective study.
   d. an experimental study.

3. An aspect of _____ involves studying causes of health problems in a population.

   a. epidemiology
   b. technobiology
   c. diseasiology
   d. censusology

4. Comparing individuals with iron–deficiency anemia to individuals who have very similar characteristics but are healthy would be an example of

   a. a prospective study.
   b. an anecdotal study.
   c. a retrospective study.
   d. a case–control study.

5. Generally, epidemiological studies

   a. establish causation.
   b. prove correlations.
   c. cannot determine cause–and–effect relationships.
   d. are experimental–based research efforts that examine two variables.

6. Which of the following journals does not have peer–reviewed articles?

   a. *Journal of the American Medical Association*
   b. *The New England Journal of Medicine*
   c. *Journal of the American College of Nutrition*
   d. *Men's Journal*

7. The government agency that enforces consumer protection laws by investigating false or misleading health–related claims is the

    a. Federal Trade Commission (FTC).
    b. Environmental Protection Agency (EPA).
    c. Agricultural Research Service (ARS).
    d. Centers for Disease Control and Prevention (CDC).

8. A testimonial is

    a. an unbiased report about a product's value.
    b. a scientifically valid claim.
    c. a personal endorsement of a product.
    d. a form of scientific evidence.

9. Which of the following websites is most likely to provide biased and unreliable nutrition information?

    a. the site of a nationally recognized health association (*.org)
    b. a site that promotes or sells dietary supplements (*.com)
    c. the site of a U.S. government agency (*.gov)
    d. an accredited college or university's site (*.edu)

10. A fake treatment is a(an)

    a. anecdote.
    b. double–blind study.
    c. pseudoscience experiment.
    d. placebo.

11. Which of the following substances would be classified as a dietary supplement according to the Dietary Supplement and Health Education Act of 1994?

    a. tobacco   c. ginseng
    b. aspirin   d. ibuprofen

12. The _____ is the federal agency that tries to ensure the safety and effectiveness of health–related products.

    a. FDA   c. EPA
    b. FTC   d. USGS

Answers to Quiz Yourself

1. Scientists use anecdotes as scientific evidence to support their findings. **False.** (p. 33)

2. Popular health-related magazines typically publish articles that have been peer-reviewed. **False.** (p. 45)

3. By conducting a prospective epidemiological study, medical researchers can determine risk factors that may influence health. **True.** (p. 38)

4. Dietary supplements include vitamin pills as well as products that contain echinacea, ginseng, and garlic. **True.** (p. 50)

5. In general, registered dietitians are reliable sources of food and nutrition information. **True.** (p. 49)

LEARNSMART ADVANTAGE

Get the most out of your study of nutrition with McGraw-Hill's innovative suite of adaptive learning products including McGraw-Hill LearnSmart®, SmartBook®, LearnSmart Achieve®, and LearnSmart Prep®. Visit www.learnsmartadvantage.com.

CHAPTER 3

Planning Nutritious Diets

Quiz Yourself

Before reading the rest of Chapter 3, test your knowledge of dietary standards, recommendations, and guides, as well as nutrient labels, by taking the following quiz. The answers are found on page 97.

1. According to the latest U.S. Department of Agriculture food guide, fruits and vegetables are combined into one food group. _____ T _____ F

2. According to the recommendations of the *2015–2020 Dietary Guidelines for Americans,* it is acceptable for certain adults to consume alcoholic beverages in moderation. _____ T _____ F

3. Last week, Colin didn't consume the recommended amount of vitamin C for a couple of days. Nevertheless, he is unlikely to develop scurvy, the vitamin C deficiency disease. _____ T _____ F

4. The Food and Drug Administration develops Dietary Guidelines for Americans. _____ T _____ F

5. The Nutrition Facts panel on a food label provides information concerning amounts of energy, fiber, and sodium that are in a serving of the food. _____ T _____ F

3.1 From Requirements to Standards

Learning Outcomes

1 Explain the difference between a dietary requirement and a dietary allowance.

2 Identify the various dietary standards and explain how they can be used.

When you shop for groceries, do you sometimes feel overwhelmed by the vast array of foods that are available? If your answer is "yes," your response is not surprising, considering the average supermarket offered nearly 44,000 items in 2013.[1] Every time you enter a supermarket, you are likely to find food items that were not on the shelves during your last visit to the store. In 2010, for example, over 21,500 new food and beverage products were introduced into the marketplace.[2]

Chapter 1 introduced some key nutrition concepts, including the need for dietary adequacy, moderation, balance, and a variety of foods. Chapter 2 described how you can become a more careful consumer of nutrition information. However, you are also a consumer of food. With so many grocery items from which to choose, what are the primary factors that influence your food purchases? Do you select foods simply because they taste good, are reasonably priced, or are easy to prepare? Do you ever consider the effects certain foods may have on your health before you purchase them?

Your lifestyle reflects your health–related behaviors, including your dietary practices and physical activity habits. Americans of all ages may reduce their risk of chronic disease by adopting nutritious diets and engaging in regular physical activity. However, consumers need practical advice to help them make decisions that can promote more healthy lifestyles.

Chapter 3 discusses dietary standards, including how the standards are established and used. The information in this chapter also presents practical ways to plan a nutritionally adequate, well–balanced diet using tools such as the Dietary Guidelines and MyPlate. Furthermore, Section 3.5 explains how to interpret and use nutrition–related information that appears on food and dietary supplement labels.

What Is a Nutrient Requirement?

By using research methods discussed in Chapter 2, scientists have been able to estimate the amount of many nutrients required by the body. A **requirement** can be defined as the smallest amount of a nutrient that maintains a defined level of nutritional health.[3] In general, this amount, when consumed daily, prevents the nutrient's deficiency disease. The requirement for a particular nutrient varies to some degree from person to person. A person's age, sex, general health status, physical activity level, and use of medications and drugs are among the factors that influence his or her nutrient requirements.

Many nutrients are stored in the body, including vitamin D and most minerals. Major storage sites include the liver, body fat, and bones. Other nutrients, such as vitamin C and most B vitamins, are not stored by the body. For optimal nutrition, you need to consume enough of those nutrients to maintain storage levels. Your body uses its nutrient stores much like you can

requirement smallest amount of a nutrient that maintains a defined level of nutritional health

61

use a savings account to help manage your money. When you have some extra cash, it is wise to place the money in a savings account, so you can withdraw some of the reserves to meet future needs without going into debt. When your consumption of certain nutrients is more than enough to meet your needs, the body stores the excess. When your intake of a stored nutrient is low or needs for this nutrient become increased, such as during recovery from illness, your body withdraws some from storage. As a result of having optimal levels of stored nutrients, you may recover more quickly and avoid or delay developing deficiencies of those nutrients.

Dietary Reference Intakes

Dietary Reference Intakes (DRIs) various energy and nutrient intake standards for Americans

Food and Nutrition Board (FNB) group of nutrition scientists who develop DRIs

Estimated Average Requirement (EAR) amount of a nutrient that meets the needs of 50% of healthy people in a life stage/sex group

Estimated Energy Requirement (EER) average daily energy intake that meets the needs of a healthy person maintaining his or her weight

Dietary Reference Intakes (DRIs) encompass a variety of daily energy and nutrient intake standards that nutrition experts in the United States use as references when making dietary recommendations. DRIs are intended to help people reduce their risk of nutrient deficiencies and excesses, prevent disease, and achieve optimal health.[4] The standards (Fig. 3.1) are the Estimated Average Requirement (EAR), which includes Estimated Energy Requirement (EER); Recommended Dietary Allowance (RDA), Adequate Intake (AI), and Tolerable Upper Intake Level (UL).

A group of nutrition scientists, the **Food and Nutrition Board (FNB)** of the Institute of Medicine, develop DRIs. Periodically, members of the board adjust DRIs as new information concerning human nutritional needs and dietary adequacy becomes available. You can find tables for the latest DRIs on the last pages of this book. The following sections provide basic information about the various DRI standards. It is important to become familiar with these terms, because we refer to them in this and other chapters.

Estimated Average Requirement

An **Estimated Average Requirement (EAR)** is the daily amount of the nutrient that meets the needs of 50% of healthy people who are in a particular *life stage/sex group*. Life stage/sex groups classify people according to age, sex, and whether females are pregnant or breastfeeding. A typical 20–year–old female college student, for example, would be classified as a female, between 19 and 30 years old, and not pregnant or breastfeeding.

To establish an EAR for a nutrient, the Food and Nutrition Board identifies a physiological marker, a substance in the body that reflects proper functioning and can be measured. This marker indicates whether the level of a nutrient in the body is adequate. A marker for vitamin C, for example, is the amount of the vitamin in certain blood cells. When these cells contain nearly all the vitamin C they can hold, the body has an optimal supply of the vitamin. Thus, a physician can diagnose whether a patient is vitamin C deficient by taking a blood sample from the person and measuring the vitamin C content of certain blood cells.

Figure 3.1 Dietary Reference Intakes. The Dietary Reference Intakes (DRIs) encompass a variety of terms that represent standards for energy and nutrient recommendations.

Estimated Energy Requirement The **Estimated Energy Requirement (EER)** is the average daily energy intake that meets the needs of a healthy person who is maintaining his or her weight. Dietitians can use EERs to evaluate an individual's energy intake. The EER takes into account the person's physical activity level, height, and weight, as well as sex and life stage. Because the EER is an average figure, some people have energy needs that are higher or lower. Chapter 10 provides formulas for calculating your EER.

Recommended Dietary Allowances

The **Recommended Dietary Allowances (RDAs)** are standards for recommending daily intakes of several nutrients. RDAs meet the nutrient needs of nearly all healthy individuals (97 to 98%) in a particular life stage/sex group. To establish an RDA for a nutrient, nutrition scientists first determine its EAR. Then scientists add a "margin of safety" amount to the EAR that allows for individual variations in nutrient needs and helps maintain tissue stores (Fig. 3.2). For example, the adult EAR for vitamin C is 60 mg for women who are not pregnant or breastfeeding and 75 mg for men.[3] However, the adult RDA for vitamin C is 15 mg higher than the EAR: 75 mg for women who are not pregnant or breastfeeding and 90 mg for men. Thus, the margin of safety for vitamin C is 15 mg. Because smoking cigarettes increases the need for vitamin C, smokers should add 35 mg to their RDA for the nutrient.

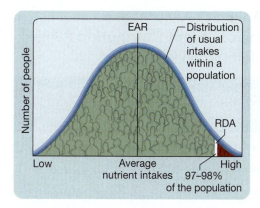

Figure 3.2 Establishing RDAs. A nutrient's RDA is high enough to meet or exceed the requirements of 97 to 98% of the population for the nutrient. In other words, about 98% of the population will have their needs for the nutrient met by just consuming the RDA amount.

Adequate Intakes

In some instances, nutrition scientists are unable to develop RDAs for nutrients because there is not enough information to determine human requirements. Until such information becomes available, scientists set **Adequate Intakes (AIs)** for these nutrients. To establish an AI, scientists record eating patterns of a group of healthy people and estimate the group's average daily intake of the nutrient. If the population under observation shows no evidence of the nutrient's deficiency disorder, the researchers conclude that the average level of intake must be adequate and use that value as the AI (Fig. 3.3). Vitamin K and the mineral potassium are among the nutrients that have AIs instead of RDAs.

Tolerable Upper Intake Level

Nutrition scientists also establish a **Tolerable Upper Intake Level (Upper Level or UL)** for many vitamins and minerals. The UL is the highest average amount of a nutrient that is unlikely to harm most people when the amount is consumed daily (see Fig. 3.3).[4] The risk of a toxicity disorder increases when a person regularly consumes amounts of a nutrient that exceed its UL. The UL for vitamin C, for example, is 2000 mg/day for adults.

Recommended Dietary Allowances (RDAs) standards for recommending daily intakes of several nutrients

Adequate Intakes (AIs) dietary recommendations that assume a population's average daily nutrient intakes are adequate because no deficiency diseases are present

Tolerable Upper Intake Level (Upper Level or UL) standard representing the highest average amount of a nutrient that is unlikely to be harmful when consumed daily

Acceptable Macronutrient Distribution Ranges (AMDRs) macronutrient intake ranges that are nutritionally adequate and may reduce the risk of diet-related chronic diseases

Acceptable Macronutrient Distribution Ranges

The results of scientific research suggest that food energy sources (macronutrients) are associated with risk of developing certain diet-related chronic diseases, such as heart disease. **Acceptable Macronutrient Distribution Ranges (AMDRs)** indicate ranges of carbohydrate, fat, and protein intakes that provide adequate amounts of vitamins and minerals and may reduce the risk of diet-related chronic diseases.[4] The AMDR for carbohydrates, for example, is 45 to 65% of total energy intake. If a person's total energy intake is 2300 kcal/day, then his or her recommended carbohydrate intake is 1035 to 1495 kcal/day. To obtain the range of energy from carbohydrate, multiply total kcal/day (in this case, 2300 kcal) by 0.45 (45%) and then

Figure 3.3 Adequate Intakes and Upper Limits. Consuming too much or not enough of a nutrient can cause health problems.

TABLE 3.1 Acceptable Macronutrient Distribution Ranges: Adults (2000 kcal/day)

Macronutrient	AMDR (% of total energy intake)	Calories
Carbohydrate	45–65	900–1300
Protein	10–35	200–700
*Fat**	20–35	400–700

* Fat intake should include essential fatty acids (see Chapter 6).

multiply 2300 kcal by 0.65 (65%). Table 3.1 lists adult AMDRs for a person who consumes 2000 kcal/day.

Applying Nutrient Standards

Table 3.2 summarizes information about the DRIs. Dietitians refer to DRIs as standards for planning nutritious diets for groups of people and evaluating the nutritional adequacy of a population's diet. Nevertheless, RDAs and AIs are often used to evaluate an individual's dietary practices.[4] Your diet is likely to be nutritionally adequate if your average daily intake for each nutrient meets the nutrient's RDA or AI value. If your diet consistently supplies less than the EAR for a nutrient, you may be at risk of eventually developing the nutrient's deficiency disorder (see Fig. 3.3). On the other hand, if your intake of a nutrient is consistently above its UL, you are at risk of developing that nutrient's toxicity disorder. Nutrient toxicity disorders are more likely to occur when people take high doses of individual nutrient supplements, particularly vitamins and minerals. If you do not take large doses of nutrient supplements and you eat reasonable amounts of food, your risk of developing a nutrient toxicity disorder is low.

Nutritional standards have a variety of commercial applications. Pharma— ceutical companies refer to DRIs when developing formulas that replace breast milk for infants and special formulas for people who cannot consume regular foods. As a result, babies can be nourished by consuming commercially prepared formulas, and adults who are unable to swallow can survive for years on formula feedings administered through tubes inserted into their bodies.

For nutrition labeling purposes, the Food and Drug Administration (FDA) uses RDAs to develop a set of standards called *Daily Values (DVs)*. Consumers may find DVs useful for comparing the nutritional contents of similar foods. The "Food and Dietary Supplement Labels" section of this chapter provides more information about nutritional labeling, including DVs.

TABLE 3.2 Summary of Dietary Reference Intakes

Standard	Definition	Example
Estimated Average Requirement (EAR)	Amount of a nutrient that meets the needs of 50% of healthy people who are in a particular life stage/sex group	**Vitamin C** 75 mg/day for males and 60 mg/day for females ages 19 through 50 years
Recommended Dietary Allowance (RDA)	Amount of a nutrient that meets the needs of nearly all healthy individuals (97.5%) in a particular life stage/sex group	**Vitamin C** 90 mg/day for males (nonsmokers) and 75 mg/day for females ages 19 through 50 years (nonsmokers)
Adequate Intake (AI)	Amount of a nutrient that is considered to be adequate based on the population's typical intakes, but there is not enough scientific information available to determine an RDA for the nutrient at this time	**Vitamin C** 40 mg/day for infants from birth through 6 months of age
Tolerable Upper Intake Level or Upper Limit (UL)	Highest average amount of a nutrient that is unlikely to harm most people when the amount is consumed daily	**Vitamin C** 2000 mg/day for adults
Acceptable Macronutrient Distribution Range (AMDR)	Ranges of carbohydrate, fat, and protein intakes that provide adequate amounts of micronutrients and may reduce the risk of developing certain diet-related chronic diseases	See Table 3.1

Concept **Checkpoint 3.1**

1. What is the difference between an RDA and an AI?
2. Describe how scientists establish the RDA for a nutrient.
3. Explain how an EER differs from an RDA or AI.
4. Discuss how dietitians, pharmaceutical companies, and the FDA use nutrient standards.

3.2 Major Food Groups

Learning Outcome

1 List major food groups, and identify foods that are typically classified in each group.

The DRIs are not practical for planning menus, so nutrition experts develop more consumer–friendly food (dietary) guides. In general, such guides classify foods into major food groups according to their natural origins and key nutrients. Major food groups are usually grains, dairy products, fruits, vegetables, and protein–rich foods. In most instances, dietary guides also provide recommendations concerning amounts of foods from each group that should be eaten daily. The following points identify major food groups and summarize key features of each group.

- **Grains** include products made from wheat, rice, and oats. Pasta, noodles, and flour tortillas are members of this group because wheat flour is their main ingredient. In general, 1 ounce of a grain food is equivalent to 1 slice of bread, 1 cup of ready–to–eat cereal, or ½ cup of cooked rice, pasta, or cereal such as oatmeal. Although corn is a type of grain, it is often used as a vegetable in meals. Cornmeal and popcorn, however, are usually grouped with grain products.

  Carbohydrate (starch) and protein are the primary macronutrients in grains. In the United States, refined grain products can also be good sources of several vitamins and minerals when they have undergone enrichment or fortification. **Enrichment** is the addition of specific amounts of iron and certain B vitamins to cereal grain products such as flour and rice. In general, enrichment replaces some of the nutrients that were lost during processing. **Fortification** is the addition of any nutrient to food, such as adding calcium to orange juice, vitamins A and D to milk, and numerous vitamins and minerals to ready–to–eat breakfast cereals.

  Dietary guides generally recommend choosing foods made with whole grains instead of refined grains. According to the FDA, whole grains are the intact, ground, cracked, or flaked seeds of cereal grains, such as wheat, buckwheat, oats, corn, rice, wild rice, rye, and barley.[5] Compared to refined grain products, foods made from whole grains naturally contain more fiber as well as micronutrients that are not replaced during enrichment.

- **Dairy foods** include milk and products made from milk that retain their calcium content after processing, such as yogurt and hard cheeses. Dairy foods are also excellent sources of protein, phosphorus (a mineral), and riboflavin (a B vitamin). Additionally, most of the milk sold in the United States is fortified with vitamins A and D.

  Foods and beverages made from soy beans (soy "milk" and soy "cheese") can substitute for cow's milk if they are fortified with calcium and other

Grains include products made from wheat, rice, corn, barley, and oats.

enrichment addition of specific amounts of iron and certain B vitamins to cereal grain products

fortification addition of any of nutrient to food

Dairy products, especially yogurt and hard cheeses, are excellent sources of calcium, protein, phosphorus, and riboflavin. Additionally, milk is often fortified with vitamins A and D.

micronutrients. Ice cream, pudding, frozen yogurt, and ice milk are often grouped with dairy foods, even though they often have high sugar and fat contents. Although cream cheese, cream, and butter are made from cow's milk they are not included in this group, because they have little or no calcium and are high in fat.

Most dietary guides recommend choosing dairy products that have most of the fat removed, such as fat—free or low—fat milk. (Fat—free milk may also be referred to as nonfat or skim milk.) Compared to whole milk, which is about 3.25% fat by weight, low—fat milk contains only 1% fat by weight and is often called "1% milk."

In general, 1 cup of fat—free milk has the calcium content of ⅔ cup of plain, low—fat yogurt or frozen yogurt; 2 cups of low—fat cottage cheese; 1½ ounces of natural cheese such as Swiss or cheddar; or 2.3 ounces of processed cheese. To obtain about the same amount of calcium as in 1 cup of fat—free milk, you would have to eat almost 1⅔ cups of regular vanilla ice cream. This amount of ice cream provides 300 kcal and about 26 g of fat, whereas 1⅔ cups of fat—free milk supplies about 135 kcal and less than 1 g of fat.

Dry beans, peas, eggs, nuts, and seeds are protein-rich foods that can substitute for meat.

- ***Protein—rich foods*** include beef, pork, lamb, fish, shellfish, liver, and poultry. Beans, eggs, nuts, and seeds are included with this group because these protein—rich foods can substitute for meats. One ounce of food from this group generally equals 1 ounce of meat, poultry, or fish; ¼ cup cooked dry beans or dry peas; 1 egg; 1 tablespoon of peanut butter; or ½ ounce of nuts or seeds. One—fourth cup of tofu, a food made from soybeans, can substitute for 1 ounce of meat, fish, or poultry.

  Foods in the protein group are rich sources of micronutrients, especially iron, zinc, and B vitamins. In general, the body absorbs minerals, such as iron and zinc, more easily from animal foods than from plants.

  Some dietary guides use fat content to categorize meats and other protein—rich foods. According to these guides, low—fat cottage cheese and the white meat of turkey are very lean meats; ground beef that is not more than 15% fat by weight and tuna are lean meats. Pork sausage, bacon, regular cheeses, and hot dogs are examples of high—fat meats.

- ***Fruits*** include fresh, dried, frozen, sauced, and canned fruit, as well as 100% fruit juice. In general, 1 cup of food from this group equals 1 cup of fruit or fruit juice, or ½ cup of dried fruit, such as raisins or apricots.[6] Most fruits are low in fat and good sources of phytochemicals and micronutrients, especially the mineral potassium and vitamins C and folate. Additionally, whole or cut—up fruit is a good source of fiber. Although 100% juice is a source of phytochemicals and can count toward one's fruit intake, the majority of choices from this group should be whole or cut—up fruits.[7] Whole or cutup fruits are healthier options than juices because they contain more dietary fiber.

- ***Vegetables*** include fresh, cooked, canned, frozen, and dried/dehydrated vegetables, and 100% vegetable juice. Vegetables may be further grouped into dark green, orange, and starchy categories. Some guides include dried beans and peas in the vegetable group as well as in the meat and meat substitutes group. In general, 1 cup of food from this group equals 1 cup of raw or cooked vegetables, 1 cup vegetable juice, or 2 cups of uncooked leafy greens, such as salad greens. Many vegetables are good sources of micronutrients, fiber, and phytochemicals. Furthermore, many vegetables are naturally low in fat and energy.

Other Foods

Food guides may include an oils group and a group for empty—calorie foods or beverages. Oils include canola, corn, and olive oils, as well as other fats that are liquid at room temperature. Certain spreadable foods made from vegetable oils,

MY DIVERSE PLATE

Tomatillos

For centuries, the people of Central America have grown and eaten tomatillos ("husk-tomatoes"). After the papery husk is removed, the fruit can be roasted, chopped, and mixed with ground chili peppers to form sauces, such as salsa verde (green sauce). Three medium tomatillos provide about 33 kcal, 2 g fiber, and 12 mg vitamin C.

such as mayonnaise, soft or "tub" margarine, and salad dressing, are also classi— fied as oils. Nuts, olives, avocados, and some types of fish have high fat contents but these kinds of fat are "healthy" fats that do not contribute to heart disease (see Chapter 6). Some food guides group these foods with oils. Oils are often good sources of fat soluble vitamins.

Solid fats, such as beef fat, butter, stick margarine, and shortening, are fairly hard at room temperature. Solid fat is a source of "unhealthy" *saturated* fats that are associated with an increased risk of cardiovascular disease (CVD). Although cream and coconut oil are liquid or soft at room temperature, these foods are classified as solid fats. Chapter 6 discusses how dietary fats can affect health.

Empty—calorie foods generally contain a lot of added sugar, alcohol, and/ or solid fat. Sugary foods ("sweets") include candy, regular soft drinks, jelly, and other foods that contain high amounts of sugar added during processing or preparation. Sugary foods and alcoholic beverages typically supply energy but few or no micronutrients.

It is important to note that the nutritional content of foods within each group often varies widely. For example, 3.5 ounces of fresh sliced apples and 3.5 ounces of fresh orange slices each supply about 50 kcal. However, the apples contribute about 4 mg of vitamin C, whereas oranges supply about 46 mg of the vitamin to diets (Fig. 3.4). Therefore, dietary guides generally recommend that people choose a variety of foods from each food group when planning daily meals and snacks.

solid fats fats that are fairly hard at room temperature

Concept **Checkpoint 3.2**

5. List at least three foods that are generally classified as grain products.
6. What is the difference between nutrient fortification and nutrient enrichment?
7. List at least four foods that are generally classified as dairy products.
8. Why are dry beans often classified with meat?
9. According to the information in this section of Chapter 3, how many cups of dried apricots are nutritionally equivalent to 2 cups of fresh apricots?
10. Most dietary guides classify eggs and nuts with meat. Why?
11. Identify at least two foods that are classified as solid fat.

About 4 mg vitamin C

About 46 mg vitamin C

Figure 3.4 Comparing apples to oranges. The nutritional content of foods within each group often varies widely.

Did You Know?

The Dietary Guidelines form the basis of the federal government's nutrition policy, which serves as a framework for national, state, and local health promotion as well as food and nutrition programs. Dietary Guidelines are also used for menu planning by individuals and health care professionals.[8] Furthermore, food and beverage manufacturers can apply the guidelines to develop healthier products that appeal to consumers.

To revise the 2010 version of the dietary guidelines, officials with the U.S. Department of Health and Human Services (USDHHS) and the U.S. Department of Agriculture (USDA) appointed a Dietary Guidelines Advisory Committee (DGAC) comprised of nationally recognized medical and nutrition experts. DGAC members reviewed the scientific evidence concerning the role of foods in health, before preparing the *Scientific Report of the 2015 Dietary Guidelines Advisory Committee.*[8] This publication contained recommendations for the development of the *2015–2020 Dietary Guidelines for Americans.* In February 2015, the overseeing government agencies made the DGAC report available for the public to read and provide input.

According to the DGAC report, a healthy diet contains more fruits, vegetables, whole grains, low- or nonfat dairy products, seafood, legumes and nuts than the typical diet of the general American population.[8] Additionally, a healthy diet contains fewer refined grains, red and processed meats, sodium, and sugar-sweetened foods and beverages than the typical American eating pattern. Such eating patterns should be flexible so food choices can be varied and individualized to meet a person's preferences, medical needs, and economic situation. The federal government incorporated some but not all of the DGAC's recommendations into the *2015–2020 Dietary Guidelines for Americans.*[9]

TABLE 3.3 *2015–2020 Dietary Guidelines for Americans: Overarching Guidelines*

- Follow a healthy eating pattern across the lifespan.
- Focus on variety, nutrient density, and amount of food.
- Limit calories from added sugars and saturated fats and reduce sodium intake.
- Shift to healthier food and beverage choices.
- Support healthy eating patterns for all.

TABLE 3.4 A Healthy Eating Pattern

Includes:

- A variety of vegetables;
- Fruits, especially whole fruits;
- Grains, especially whole grains;
- Fat-free or low-fat dairy products;
- A variety of protein foods; and
- Oils.

A healthy eating pattern limits:

- Saturated fats and trans fats, added sugars, and sodium.

3.3 Dietary Guidelines

Learning Outcome

1 List at least four overarching guidelines of the *2015–2020 Dietary Guidelines for Americans* and provide recommendations of each one.

Heart disease, cancer, hypertension (chronically elevated blood pressure), and diabetes mellitus (commonly referred to as *diabetes*) are among the leading causes of disability and death among Americans. According to a considerable amount of scientific evidence, risk of these diseases is strongly linked with certain lifestyles, particularly poor dietary choices and lack of regular physical activity. As required by law, the USDHHS and the USDA publish the *Dietary Guidelines for Americans* (Dietary Guidelines), a set of general nutrition–related lifestyle recommendations that are intended for healthy people over 2 years of age.[8] The Dietary Guidelines are designed to promote adequate nutritional status and good health, and to reduce the risk of major nutrition–related chronic health conditions, such as obesity and cardiovascular disease. These guidelines are updated every 5 years.

Table 3.3 indicates the overarching guidelines of the *2015–2020 Dietary Guidelines*, which focus on encouraging healthy eating patterns. Table 3.4 lists key components of a healthy eating pattern, according to the Dietary Guidelines. The following information includes recommendations about each overarching guideline.[8] You can learn more about the Dietary Guidelines by visiting: http://health.gov/dietaryguidelines/2015/guidelines/ .

Follow a Healthy Eating Pattern Across the Lifespan

- All food and beverage choices matter.
- People should choose a healthy eating pattern that has an appropriate number of calories to achieve and maintain a healthy body weight, is nutritionally adequate, and reduces the risk of diet–related chronic diseases.

Focus on Variety, Nutrient Density, and Amount of Food

To meet nutrient needs within calorie limits, choose a variety of nutrient–dense foods from all food groups and consume recommended amounts.

- Consume a variety of vegetables from all subgroups, including dark green, red, and orange, legumes (beans and peas), starchy, and other vegetables.
- Consume a variety of fruits, especially whole fruits.
- Consume grains, at least half of which are whole grains.
- Consume fat–free or low–fat dairy foods, including milk, yogurt, cheese, and/or fortified soy products.
- Eat a variety of protein foods, including seafood, lean meats and poultry, eggs, legumes, nuts, seeds, and soy products.
- Consume oils or cook with oils.

Limit Calories from Added Sugars and Saturated Fats and Reduce Sodium Intake

- Consume less than 10% of daily calories from added sugars. Added sugars contribute calories to foods and beverages, but they lack essential nutrients. For people consuming 2000 kcal per day, the upper limit of 10% of total calories is 200 kcal, the amount of energy in about 12 teaspoons of sugar.
- Consume less than 10% of daily calories from saturated fats.
- Consume less than 2300 mg of sodium per day. Increased sodium intake is associated with increased risk of hypertension and cardiovascular disease. Salt is the major source of sodium in diets.

Shift to Healthier Food and Beverage Choices

- Choose nutrient–dense foods and beverages from all food groups to replace less healthy products.
- Consider cultural and personal preferences when shifting foods and beverages to healthier choices.

Recommendations for Specific Population Groups

Women who are capable of becoming pregnant, are pregnant, or are breastfeeding:

- Consume 8 to 12 ounces of seafood per week from a variety of seafood types. Certain seafood contain fats that may improve an infant's health. Seafood that are rich in these particular fats include salmon, herring, sardines, and trout.
- Do not eat tilefish, shark, swordfish, and king mackerel because they may contain high amounts of the toxic chemical methylmercury.
- Consume iron–rich foods or take an iron supplement, if recommended by a physician or other qualified health care provider. Iron is a "nutrient of public health concern" for pregnant females.
- Do not consume alcohol.

To reduce the risk of birth defects, women who are capable of becoming pregnant should obtain 400 mcg of folic acid each day by consuming fortified foods and/or taking supplements that contain the vitamin.

Support Healthy Eating Patterns for All

- Everyone has a role in creating and supporting healthy eating patterns in multiple settings throughout the country.
- Health professionals and policymakers should use multiple strategies to promote healthy eating and physical activity behaviors across all segments of society. Such strategies can include developing educational resources that inspire individuals to take appropriate actions with regard to their food and beverage choices.

Applying the Dietary Guidelines

The Dietary Guidelines include several food and nutrition–related messages for consumers, such as "Consume more nutrient–dense vegetables" (Table 3.5). Table 3.6 suggests practical ways people can apply the Dietary Guidelines' recommendations to their usual food choices. However, making recommended dietary and other lifestyle changes does not always reduce risk factors for disease.

TABLE 3.5 Selected Messages from *2015-2020 Dietary Guidelines for Americans*

- Increase the variety of protein foods consumed and incorporate about 8 ounces per week of various seafood into meals. Young children should eat less seafood than older children and adults.
- Consume more nutrient-dense vegetables.
- Choose more nutrient-dense fruits for snacks, desserts, or in side dishes.
- Choose enriched grain products and make at least half your grains whole grains.
- Choose lower fat versions of milk, yogurt, and cheese.
- Compare sodium in foods and choose the foods with the lowest sodium content.
- Drink water instead of sugary drinks.
- Choose foods that provide potassium, dietary fiber, calcium, and vitamin D, which are "nutrients of public health concern," because Americans tend to consume them in limited amounts.
- Achieve or maintain a healthy body weight.
- Consuming three to five 8-oz cups of coffee per day (up to 400 mg/day of caffeine) is acceptable within a healthy eating pattern.
- Consume as little cholesterol as possible while following a healthy diet.
- If one consumes alcohol, the beverage should be consumed in moderation and only by adults of legal drinking age. "Moderation" is up to one drink per day for women and up to two drinks per day for men. People should not begin to drink alcohol or drink more for any reason. Furthermore, certain individuals should not consume alcohol, especially pregnant women.

| 2015–2020 Dietary Guidelines for Americans

For example, a man who has hypertension may find that his blood pressure remains dangerously elevated after several months of exercising, limiting his salt intake, and maintaining a healthy weight for his height. In this case, genetic factors may be influencing the man's health more than his lifestyle, and medica— tion may be necessary to reduce his blood pressure.

TABLE 3.6 Applying the Dietary Guidelines to One's Usual Food Choices

If One Usually Eats:	Consider Replacing with:
White bread and rolls	Whole-wheat bread and rolls
Sugary breakfast cereals	Low-sugar, high-fiber cereal sweetened with berries, bananas, peaches, or other fruit
Cheeseburger, French fries, and a regular (sugar-sweetened) soft drink	Roasted chicken or turkey sandwich, baked beans, fat-free or low-fat milk, or soy milk
Potato salad or cole slaw	Leafy greens or three-bean salad
Doughnuts, chips, or salty snack foods	Small bran muffin or whole-wheat bagel topped with peanut butter or soy nut butter, unsalted nuts, or dried fruit
Regular soft drinks	Water, fat-free or low-fat milk, or 100% fruit juice
Boiled vegetables	Raw or steamed vegetables (often retain more nutrients than boiled)
Breaded and fried meat, fish, or poultry	Broiled or roasted meat, fish, or poultry
Fatty meats such as barbecued ribs, sausage, and hot dogs	Chicken, turkey, or fish; lean meats such as ground round
Whole or 2% milk, cottage cheese with 4% fat, or yogurt made from whole milk	1% or fat-free milk, low-fat cottage cheese (1% fat), or low-fat yogurt
Ice cream	Frozen yogurt or ice milk
Cream cheese on a bagel	Low-fat cottage cheese (mashed) or reduced-fat cream cheese or pea-nut butter (if appropriate)
Creamy salad dressings or dips made with mayonnaise or sour cream	Oil and vinegar dressing, reduced-fat salad dressings, or dips made from low-fat sour cream or plain yogurt
Chocolate chip or cream-filled cookies	Fruit-filled bars, oatmeal cookies, or fresh fruit
Salt added to season foods	Herbs, spices, or lemon juice

Concept **Checkpoint 3.3**

Respond to the following points according to recommendations of the Dietary Guidelines (2015–2020 version).

12. What are two overarching guidelines of the Dietary Guidelines?
13. A healthy person who is 23 years of age should limit his sodium intake to less than _____ per day.
14. List at least three of the key recommendations of the Dietary Guidelines.
15. Replace solid fats with _____.
16. Consume less than _____% of total calories from saturated fat.
17. Consume less than _____ % of total calories from added sugars.
18. What percentage of your intake of grains foods should be whole grains?
19. An adult woman who drinks alcohol and is not pregnant should limit her alcohol intake to no more than _____ drinks per day.
20. Adult men who drink alcohol should limit their alcohol consumption to no more than _____ drinks per day.
21. Which nutrients are "of public health concern" in the American diet?

3.4 Food Guides

Learning Outcomes

1 Use MyPlate to develop nutritionally adequate daily menus.

2 Compare MyPlate with the Exchange System.

For over 100 years, the USDA has issued specific dietary recommendations for Americans. In 1943, the USDA issued the first food guide based on RDAs for the general public to use. By the mid–1950s, the USDA simplified the original food guide to include only four food groups: milk, meat, fruit and vegetable, and bread and cereal. The recommendations of the "Basic Four" provided the foun– dation for an adequate diet while supplying about 1200 to 1400 kcal/day. Extra servings of food could be added to the basic diet plan for people who had higher energy needs.

In 1992, the USDA introduced the Food Guide Pyramid (Fig. 3.5). Unlike earlier dietary guides, the Food Guide Pyramid incorporated knowledge about the health benefits and risks associated with certain foods and ranked food groups according to their emphasis in menu planning. The Food Guide Pyramid displayed the groups in a layered format with grain products at the base to establish the foundation for a healthy diet. Fruit and vegetable groups occupied the next layer of the Food Guide Pyramid, followed by a layer shared by the milk and milk products, and meat and meat substitutes groups. Fatty and sugary foods formed the small peak of the Pyramid, a visual reminder that people should limit their intake of these foods.

Although the Food Guide Pyramid became a familiar feature on many pack– aged foods, the USDA released the *MyPyramid Plan* in 2005 (Fig. 3.6). The MyPyramid Plan was a *food guidance system*, which was based on *Dietary Guidelines for Americans, 2005*. In addition to providing foods and nutrition information, the MyPyramid.gov website emphasized the importance of physical activity and enabled consumers to monitor their activity levels. In 2011, the USDA replaced the MyPyramid Plan with *MyPlate*, another interactive dietary and menu planning guide accessible at a website.

| Figure 3.5 **Food Guide Pyramid.**

| Figure 3.6 **MyPyramid Plan.**

MyPlate

MyPlate (www.choosemyplate.gov) includes a variety of food, nutrition, and physical activity resources for consumers that are based on the recommenda– tions of the Dietary Guidelines. MyPlate differs from the two previous USDA food guides in that it no longer has six food groups depicted by boxes or stripes within a pyramid (Fig. 3.7). MyPlate focuses on five different food groups: fruits, vegetables, protein foods, grains, and dairy.[10] According to the USDA, "oils" is not a food group.[11] The government agency, however, notes the need for some fat in the diet.

To learn more about MyPlate's five food groups, visit www.choosemyplate.gov and click on "MyPlate" in the menu bar to obtain a list of food groups. Click on each food group to find practical information about foods in the group, including how much food should be eaten, scientifically supported health benefits of foods, and helpful food–related tips. The site also has information and tips concerning weight management and calories, as well as physical activity.

Choosemyplate.gov has a wide variety of helpful interactive tools, including "SuperTracker," an excellent tool for developing nutritionally adequate daily food plans, and recording and monitoring dietary intake and physical activity habits.

| Figure 3.7 **MyPlate.**

MyPlate USDA's interactive Internet dietary and menu planning guide

The "Food Tracker" feature of SuperTracker enables people to determine the energy and nutrient contents of their favorite recipes.

Major Sources of Empty Calories

Empty calories include energy from alcoholic beverages and foods that contain high amounts of added sugars and/or solid fats. Many commonly eaten foods include various amounts of empty calories. According to the USDA, the foods and beverages that supply the most empty calories in Americans' diets are:

- Cakes, cookies, pastries, and doughnuts
- Sugar—sweetened soft drinks, sports drinks, and fruit drinks
- Cheese (source of solid fat)
- Pizza (source of solid fat)
- Ice cream[10]

Tips for "Building a Better Plate" The "Ten Tips" page of the MyPlate web—site includes some helpful information and tips to help consumers make healthier food selections:

- Make half of your grains whole grains.
- Add more vegetables to your day.
- Focus on fruits.
- Enjoy your food but eat less.
- Vary your protein routine.

Using MyPlate for Menu Planning

MyPlate has 12 different nutritionally adequate daily food patterns that sup—ply from 1000 to 3200 kcal/day (http://www.choosemyplate.gov/MyPlate—Daily—Checklist). Each pattern can be individualized to meet various personal characteristics, including age, sex, physical activity level, and food likes and dislikes.

MyPlate dietary patterns include foods and beverages that contain little or no empty calories. After a person consumes recommended amounts of nutritious foods from each food group (and oils), a small number of calories remain. The 2000 kcal dietary pattern, for example, has only 260 kilocalories remaining, which is less than the energy in two 12—ounce sugar—sweetened soft drinks. People can use up these remaining calories by choosing foods that contain a lot of solid fat and/or added sugars (empty—calorie foods), or healthy foods such as fresh fruits and vegetables.

To use MyPlate as a personalized menu planning guide, visit http://www.choosemyplate.gov and click on "SuperTracker" and then "Create Your Pro—file." Fill in boxes that request information, including your age, sex, weight, height, and estimated level of physical activity. After you provide this infor—mation, MyPlate estimates your daily energy needs and indicates how much food you should eat from each of the food groups daily to meet your recom—mended energy level. Table 3.7 indicates MyPlate's food intake recommenda—tions for average healthy young adults who consume 1800 to 3200 kilocalories per day.

TABLE 3.7   MyPlate: Recommendations for Average, Healthy 20-Year-Old Adults

MyPlate Guidelines (Daily)	Women	Men
Kilocalories	1800–2400	2600–3200
Fruit	2 cups	2–2.5 cups
Vegetables	2.5–3 cups	3.5–4.0 cups
Grains	6–8 oz	9–10 oz
Protein foods	5.0–6.5 oz	6.5–7 oz
Dairy	3 cups	3 cups
Oils	5–7 tsp	8–11 tsp

Overall, MyPlate can be helpful for planning menus because it promotes food variety, nutritional adequacy, and moderation. You can also use MyPlate to evaluate the nutritional quality of your daily diet by recording your food and beverage choices, classifying your choices into food groups, and estimating your intake of servings from each food group.

A computer and Internet access are necessary to use the program. Many people, particularly older adults, are unfamiliar with personal computers and may find the interactive www.choosemyplate.gov website challenging and frustrating to use. You may encounter some difficulties when using MyPlate to evaluate your diet's adequacy. How do you classify menu items that combine small amounts of foods from more than one group, such as pizza, sandwiches, and casseroles? A slice of pizza, for example, has thin crust made with wheat flour (grains), tomato sauce (vegetable), and cheese (dairy). The first step is to determine the ingredients and classify each into an appropriate food group. Estimate the number of cups or ounces of each ingredient and record the amounts contributed from a particular food group. The slice of pizza may provide ¼ cup of a vegetable, 2 ounces of grains, and ¼ cup of dairy. Another problem you may have when using MyPlate is judging portion sizes without keeping handy a battery of measuring cups and a scale for weighing foods. Figure 3.8 provides convenient ways to estimate typical portions using familiar objects, including a tennis ball and bar of soap.

The USDA has also developed MyPlate menu planning tools for children and pregnant or breastfeeding women. These guides can also be accessed at www.choosemyplate.gov. For information about MyPlate guides for various life stages, see Chapter 13.

MyPlate for Losing Weight

The "My Weight Manager" page at https://www.supertracker.usda.gov/ provides information about planning nutritionally adequate diets for persons who are trying to lose weight. If you would like to lose weight, start by obtaining your personalized daily food plan at https://www.supertracker.usda.gov/ . Click on "Create Your Profile." In the box for "Weight," fill in your present weight; in the box for height, fill in your height. If you are too heavy for your height, the program will let you know and provide a food plan that will help you reach a healthy weight for your height (see Chapter 10). One way to reduce your calorie intake without sacrificing the nutritional adequacy of your diet is

Dairy group   Vegetable group   Grain group

Classifying foods that combine ingredients from different food groups is challenging. This slice of pizza, for example, has crust (grains), tomato sauce and tomatoes (vegetable), and cheese (dairy).

to eat smaller amounts of empty—calorie foods or eliminate them altogether. Additionally, you can increase the amount of time that you are physically active each day.

MyPlate: Physical Activity Although you may be busy while performing daily activities, you may not be moving your body enough to strengthen your muscles and prevent unwanted weight gain. To obtain important health benefits, you should engage in moderate or vigorous physical activity every day.[12] Choosemyplate. gov includes some information about physical activity, including examples of activities that are moderate or vigorous (http://www.choosemyplate.gov/physical—activity). Chapter 11 provides more information about physical activity and the importance of a physically active lifestyle.

Other Food Guides

The USDA's original Food Guide Pyramid inspired the development of other food pyramids for people who follow cultural and ethnic food traditions that differ from the mainstream American ("Western") diet. The "Nutrition Matters" feature at the end of Chapter 3 discusses various cultural, ethnic, and religious influences on American dietary practices. The "Nutrition Matters" feature also includes illustrations of the traditional Latin American Diet (see Fig. 3.16) Mediterranean Diet (see Fig. 3.17), and the Asian Diet Pyramids (see Fig. 3.18). Health Canada, the federal agency responsible for helping Canadians achieve better health, also has a food guide, "Eating Well with Canada's Food Guide". Go to this website: http://hc—sc.gc.ca/fn—an/food—guide—aliment/index—eng. php , to access this interactive guide.

Do Americans Follow Dietary Recommendations?

Analysis of government food consumption data indicates that most Americans do not follow the Dietary Guidelines.[13] In 2003–2004, the typical diet of Americans who were 2 years of age and older did not provide recommended amounts of fruit, vegetables, whole grains, and fat—free or low—fat milk.[13] Furthermore,

Figure 3.8 Estimating portion sizes. You can use familiar items such as these to estimate portion sizes.

Computer mouse = 1/2 to 2/3 cup
(baked potato, ground or chopped food)

Tennis ball = 1/2 to 2/3 cup
(medium or small fruit)

4 dice = 1 oz cheese

the diet generally contained too much added sugar, solid fats, and sodium. It is apparent that the public needs to learn more about the importance of choosing a variety of foods and applying MyPlate to everyday menu planning.

What Is the Exchange System?

Many chronic diseases require special diets to prevent or delay complications. Diabetes, for example, is easier to control when the person's diet has about the same macronutrient composition from day to day. The **Exchange System** is a valuable tool for estimating the energy, protein, carbohydrate, and fat content of foods. The system was originally developed by a committee of the Academy of Nutrition and Dietetics and the American Diabetes Association for planning diets of people with diabetes, a condition characterized by abnormal carbohydrate metabolism. Because the Exchange System makes it relatively easy to plan nutritious calorie—reduced meals and snacks, it is also useful for people who are trying to lose weight.

The Exchange System categorizes foods into three broad groups: carbohydrates, meat and meat substitutes, and fats.[14] The foods within each group have similar macronutrient composition, regardless of whether the food is from a plant or animal. For example, the carbohydrate group includes fruits, vegetables, and grains, as well as milk products. Nuts and seeds are grouped with fats. Meats and meat substitutes are grouped according to their fat content. Cheeses are in the meat and meat substitutes group because of their high protein and fat content. Thus, the Exchange System classifies foods differently than MyPlate does.

Within each of the three major food groups, the Exchange System provides *exchange lists* of specific types of foods. The specified amount of a food listed in an exchange list provides about the same amount of macronutrients and calories as each of the other specified amounts of foods in that list. According to the fruit list, for example, an orange is equivalent to a small apple, a kiwifruit, one—half of a fresh pear, or one—half of a large grapefruit. This equality allows people to plan a wide variety of nutritious menus by exchanging one food for another within each list. For more information about the Exchange System, you can visit

Exchange System method of classifying foods into lists based on macronutrient composition

Did You Know?

Many kinds of fresh fruit make quick and easy snacks that can be carried in backpacks, purses, and briefcases. Fresh fruit such as apples, oranges, tangerines, kiwifruit, and grapes can be kept for a few days at room temperature in a fruit bowl. You can store fresh fruits for longer periods by placing them in the refrigerator. Banana peels, however, turn dark brown when the fruit is refrigerated, so it is best to store bananas at room temperature, but refrigerated bananas are still good to eat.

Baseball or human fist = 1 cup (large apple or orange, or 1 cup serving of ready-to-eat cereal)

Small yo-yo = 1 standard bagel or English muffin

Bar of soap or deck of cards = 3 oz meat

the Academy of Nutrition and Dietetics' website (www.eatright.org) to order easy—to—read publications such as *Eating Healthy with Diabetes* or the *ADA Guide to Eating Right When You Have Diabetes.*

Carbohydrate counting ("counting carbs") is another meal planning technique that people with diabetes can use to control their blood sugar lev— els. The American Diabetes Association offers information about counting carbohydrates (http://www.diabetes.org/food—and—fitness/food/what—can— i—eat/understanding—carbohydrates/carbohydrate—counting.html). You will learn more about diabetes in the section of Chapter 5 that discusses this serious disease in detail.

Concept **Checkpoint 3.4**

22. List four tips for "building a better plate," according to MyPlate.
23. Explain how to use MyPlate to evaluate the nutritional adequacy of an individual's daily food choices.
24. According to the USDA, which foods supply most of the empty calories in Americans' diets?
25. Describe how the Exchange System differs from MyPlate.

3.5 Food and Dietary Supplement Labels

Learning Outcomes

1 Use the Nutrition Facts panel to make more nutritious food choices.

2 Identify nutrition-related claims the FDA allows on food and dietary supplement labels.

Consumers can use information on food labels to determine ingredients and to compare energy and nutrient contents of packaged foods and beverages. In the United States, the FDA regulates and monitors information that can be placed on food labels, including claims about the health benefits of ingredients. Today, nearly all foods and beverages sold in grocery stores must have labels that provide the product's name, manufacturer's name and address, and amount of product in the package (Fig. 3.9a). Producers and sellers of fresh and frozen fruits and vegetables; fresh poultry, fish, and shellfish; and a few other food items must declare the product's *country of origin* either on the packaging or where the product is located in stores. Furthermore, products that have more than one ingredient must display a list of the ingredients in descending order according to weight.

Nutrition Facts Panel

Consumers can find specific nutrition—related information about many packaged foods simply by reading the products' labels. The FDA requires food manufactur— ers to use a special format, the **Nutrition Facts panel,** to display information about the energy and nutrient contents of products (Fig. 3.9b). The Nutrition Facts panel indicates the amount of a serving size, in household units as well as grams, and the number of servings in the entire container.

Serving size is shown in household and metric units

Identity of the food

Content's net weight (or volume)

(a)

Servings per container

To reduce risk of heart disease, choose foods that are low in saturated fat, trans fat, and sodium

Consider limiting your intake of foods with added sugars included among the first few items in the ingredients list

List of ingredients

Manufacturer's name and address

Consume adequate amounts of fiber and these micronutrients

Proposed Label (FDA 2014)

Nutrition Facts

8 servings per container

Serving size   2/3 cup (55g)

Amount per 2/3 cup

Calories   **230**

% DV*	
12%	**Total Fat** 8g
5%	**Saturated Fat** 1g
	Trans Fat 0g
0%	**Cholesterol** 0mg
7%	**Sodium** 160mg
12%	**Total Carbs** 37g
14%	**Dietary Fiber** 4g
	Sugars 1g
	Added Sugars 0g
	Protein 3g
10%	**Vitamin D** 2mcg
20%	**Calcium** 260mg
45%	**Iron** 8mg
5%	**Potassium** 235mg

* Footnote on Daily Values (DV) and calories reference to be inserted here.

(b)

Figure 3.9 What's in a food? (a) Nearly all packaged foods and beverages sold in grocery stores must have labels that provide specific information, including the manufacturer's name and address. (b) The Nutrition Facts panel displays information about energy and nutrient contents of food products.

As of January 2016, the FDA requires food manufacturers to provide information about the food's total fat, saturated fat, trans fat, cholesterol, sodium, total carbohydrate, fiber, sugars, protein, vitamin A, vitamin C, calcium, and iron contents in the Nutrition Facts panel. Additionally, the panel must display the total amount of energy and energy from fat, indicated as numbers of calories, in a serving. The Nutrition Facts panel, however, does not translate the total number of calories from fat into a percentage.

The panel uses grams (g) and milligrams (mg) to indicate amounts of fiber and nutrients in a serving of food. Food manufacturers can also include amounts of polyunsaturated and monounsaturated fats, as well as potassium and other micronutrients, in the Nutrition Facts panel. If the manufacturer has fortified the food with the nutrients or made claims about the product's fat content, listing these particular food components is required.

Foods such as fresh fruits and vegetables, fish and shellfish, meats, and poultry are not required to have Nutrition Facts labels. However, many food suppliers and supermarket chains provide consumers with information about their products' nutritional content on posters or shelf tags displayed near the foods. In the future, fresh foods such as raw meats are likely to include Nutrition Facts panels on their labels.

Early in 2014, the FDA proposed an updated version of the Nutrition Facts panel, which is shown in Figure 13.9b. The proposed panel format has some significant changes to the format that was used in January 2016 (see Fig. 13.9a). The new panel displays the number of calories per serving in very bold print, so it is highly visible. Under "Sugars," a new component, "Added sugars," differentiates between ingredients that are added to foods or beverages to sweeten them, such as high–fructose corn syrup, from sugars that are naturally in a food or beverage, such as those in fruit and cow's milk. Such information is helpful for people who want to monitor their empty–calorie intakes and compare foods for their added sugar contents. Serving sizes are not necessarily consistent for similar foods but are based on portion sizes that people typically consume and not how much they should eat. The proposed Nutrition Facts panel no longer provides information about the number of calories from fat. This is because FDA officials recommend that consumers should be more concerned about eating less unhealthy saturated and trans fats instead of choosing foods that are low in total fat. Furthermore, the FDA no longer requires manufacturers to include information about the vitamin A and C contents of packaged foods, but they must indicate amounts of potassium and vitamin D in their products. This change reflects public health concerns that many Americans have less than adequate intakes of these micronutrients.

Daily Values

Daily Values (DVs) set of nutrient intake standards developed for labeling purposes

Nutrient standards such as the RDA and AI are sex–, age–, and life stage–specific. For example, the RDA for vitamin C is 75 mg/day and 65 mg/day for nonsmoking 18–year–old males and females, respectively. The vitamin's RDA increases to 80 mg/day for 18–year–old pregnant females. Because the RDAs and AIs are so specific, it is not practical to provide nutrient information on food labels that refers to these complex standards. To help consumers evaluate the nutritional content of food products, FDA developed the **Daily Values (DVs)** for labeling purposes. Compared to the RDAs, the DVs are a more simplified and practical set of nutrient standards. The adult DV for a nutrient is based on a standard diet that supplies 2000 kcal/day. Not all nutrients have DVs, but they have been established for total fat, total carbohydrate, fiber, and several vitamins and minerals. As of early 2016, there are no DVs for added sugars or trans fat.

Appendix B lists current (as of January 2016) and proposed DVs. A set of DVs that applies to people over 4 years of age is used for foods and beverages that adults consume. Three other sets of DVs are used on labels of foods intended for infants, children between 1 and 4 years of age, and pregnant or breastfeeding women.

Although the DVs are often the highest RDA or AI for a particular nutrient, in many instances, they are based on recommendations of public health experts. For example, the RDA for carbohydrate is 130 g/day for people over 1 year of age. The DV for carbohydrate, however, is 300 g/day (2015 value). This amount reflects the general dietary recommendations that carbohydrate can contribute 60% of a person's total energy intake, or 1200 kcal (300 g × 4 kcal/g of carbohydrate) of a 2000 kcal/day diet. For people older than 1 year of age, no RDA or AI has been set for daily fat intake. However, DV for fat is 65 g/day. This amount meets the general recommendation that fat intake can be about 30% of a person's total energy intake for a 2000 kcal/day diet.

When evaluating or planning nutritious menus, your goal is to obtain at least 100% of the DVs for fiber, vitamins, and minerals each day. On the other hand, you may need to limit your intake of foods that have high %DVs of total fat, saturated fat, and sodium (Fig. 3.10). High intakes of these nutrients may have negative effects on your health. Thus, your goal is to consume less than 100% of the DV for total fat, saturated fat, and sodium each day. The general rule of thumb: A food that supplies 5%DV or less of a nutrient is a low source of the nutrient; a food that provides 20%DV or more is a high source of the nutrient.[15]

Percents of DVs are designed to help consumers compare nutrient contents of packaged foods to make more healthful choices. However, most people do not eat just packaged foods. Fresh fruits and vegetables, as well as most restaurant meals, do not have labels or menus with information about %DVs per serving. Therefore, many consumers will underestimate their nutrient intakes, if they do not consider the contribution that unlabeled foods make to their diets.

It is important to note the description of a serving size and the number of servings per container when using nutritional labeling information to estimate your intakes of energy, fiber, and nutrients in the food. A common mistake people make when using a Nutrition Facts panel is assuming the information applies to the entire package. For example, the Nutrition Facts panel on a package of food indicates there are four servings in the container. If you eat all the container's contents, you must multiply the information concerning calories, fat, and other food components by four. Why? Because you ate four servings and the nutritional information on the Nutrition Facts panel applies to only *one* serving.

Make Your Calories Count, an interactive program developed by the FDA, helps consumers use Nutrition Facts on food labels to plan nutritionally adequate diets while managing calorie intake. You can access the program by visiting the website http://www.fda.gov/food/ingredientspackaginglabeling/labelingnutrition/ucm275438.htm and downloading "Make Your Calories Count," an interactive training module. The FDA also provides "The Food Label and You," a video that you can watch at http://www.fda.gov/food/ingredientspackaginglabeling/labelingnutrition/ucm275409.htm.

What About Restaurant and Vending Machine Foods?

A section of the *Patient Protection and Affordable Care Act* of 2010 requires restaurants and similar retail food establishments with 20 or more locations to list calorie content information for standard menu items on restaurant menus and menu boards.[16] Information about total calories, fat, saturated fat, cholesterol, sodium, total carbohydrates, sugars, fiber, and total protein contents of menu items must be available in writing when the customer requests it. According

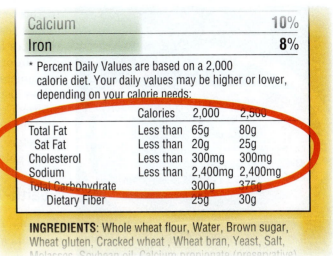

| Calcium | | | 10% |
| Iron | | | 8% |

* Percent Daily Values are based on a 2,000 calorie diet. Your daily values may be higher or lower, depending on your calorie needs:

		Calories	2,000	2,500
Total Fat	Less than		65g	80g
Sat Fat	Less than		20g	25g
Cholesterol	Less than		300mg	300mg
Sodium	Less than		2,400mg	2,400mg
Total Carbohydrate			300g	375g
Dietary Fiber			25g	30g

INGREDIENTS: Whole wheat flour, Water, Brown sugar, Wheat gluten, Cracked wheat , Wheat bran, Yeast, Salt, Molasses, Soybean oil, Calcium propionate (preservative)

Figure 3.10 Nutrients to limit. High intakes of saturated fat and sodium can have negative effects on your health. The appearance of this panel is likely to change when new DVs are published.

Figure 3.11 Label claims. The FDA permits food manufacturers to include certain health claims on food labels.

to this act, companies that maintain 20 or more food vending machines must disclose calorie contents of certain items. The FDA is responsible for developing the rules for providing the nutrition information.

Information about the calorie contents of restaurant foods can help consumers make healthier menu selections. However, the accuracy of the caloric values listed by restaurants can vary.[17] The displayed or published nutrition information may give a close estimate of the food's actual energy and nutrient values, but portions are not exactly the same every time a food is served. Therefore, calorie levels posted at restaurants should be used by consumers as a rough guide for making healthier food choices.

Health- and Nutrition-Related Claims

To make their foods more appealing to consumers, manufacturers often promote products as having certain health benefits or high amounts of nutrients. A health claim describes the relationship between a food, food ingredient, or dietary supplement and the reduced risk of a nutrition-related condition. The FDA permits food manufacturers to include certain health claims on food labels (Fig. 3.11). For example, an allowable health claim may state, "Diets low in saturated fat may reduce the risk of heart disease."

For the FDA to allow a health claim on a product label, the claim should:

- indicate that the product has health benefits only when it is part of a daily diet;

- be complete, easy to understand, honest, and not misleading;

- refer to a product that contains 10% or more of the DV for vitamins A and C, calcium, iron, fiber, or protein, *before* being fortified with nutrients. (This condition does not apply to dietary supplements.);

- be for a product intended for people who are 2 years of age or older;

- use *may* or *might* to describe the relationship between the product and disease. For example, "Diets containing foods that are good sources of potassium and that are low in sodium may reduce the risk of high blood pressure and stroke" is an allowable claim. However, the claim "Reduces the risk of stroke" would not be permitted on a label;

- not quantify any degree of risk reduction. For example, a claim that states, "Reduces risk of cancer by 41%" would not be allowed because it specifies the degree of risk reduction;

- indicate that many factors influence disease.

The FDA requires specific wording for certain health claims that are allowed on labels. Table 3.8 lists some permissible health claims that can be used for labeling purposes. For more information, visit FDA's website at www.fda.gov and search for "qualified health claims."

As of 2015, the FDA will not approve health claims for foods that contain more than 13 g of fat, 4 g of saturated fat, 60 mg of cholesterol, or 480 mg of sodium per serving. For example, calcium is a mineral that strengthens bones and protects them from *osteoporosis*, a condition in which bones become brittle and break easily. Whole milk is a rich source of calcium. Nevertheless, the label on a carton of whole milk cannot include a health claim about calcium and osteoporosis, because the milk contains more than 4 g of saturated fat per serving. In addition, the product must meet specific conditions that relate to the health claim. For example, a claim regarding the benefits of eating a low-fat diet is allowed only if the product contains 3 g or less of fat per serving, which is the FDA's standard definition of a low-fat food.

TABLE 3.8 Examples of Permissible Health Claims for Food Labels (2015)

Dietary Factor/Health Condition	Example of Permissible Health Claim
Certain lipids and heart disease	"While many factors affect heart disease, diets low in saturated fat and cholesterol may reduce the risk of this disease."
Diet and heart disease	"Diets low in saturated fat and cholesterol and rich in fruits, vegetables, and grain products that contain some types of dietary fiber, particularly soluble fiber, may reduce the risk of heart disease, a disease associated with many factors."
Calcium, exercise, and osteoporosis (a disease that weakens bones)	"Regular exercise and a healthy diet with enough calcium help teen and young adult white and Asian women maintain good bone health and may reduce their high risk of osteoporosis."
Sodium (a mineral) and high blood pressure	"Diets low in sodium may reduce the risk of high blood pressure, a disease associated with many factors."
Folate (a B vitamin) and neural tube defects (conditions in which the skull and spine do not form properly before birth)	"Healthful diets with adequate folate may reduce a woman's risk of having a child with a brain or spinal cord defect."
Fruits and vegetables and risk of cancer	"Foods that are low in fat and contain dietary fiber, vitamin A, or vitamin C may reduce the risk of some types of cancer, a disease associated with many factors. Broccoli is high in vitamins A and C, and it is a good source of dietary fiber."

Source: U.S. Food and Drug Administration, Center for Food Safety and Applied Nutrition. *A food labeling guide.* 2013. http://www.fda.gov/food/guidanceregulation/guidancedocumentsregulatoryinformation/labelingnutrition/ucm2006828.htm Accessed: June 9, 2014

Structure/Function Claims

A structure/function claim describes the role a nutrient or dietary supplement plays in maintaining a structure, such as bone, or promoting a normal function, such as digestion. The FDA allows structure/function claims such as "calcium builds strong bones" or "fiber maintains bowel regularity" (Fig. 3.12). Structure/function statements cannot claim that a nutrient, food, or dietary supplement can be used to prevent or treat a serious health condition. For example, the FDA would not permit a claim that a product "promotes low blood pressure," because that claim implies the product has druglike effects and can treat high blood pressure.

Nutrient Content Claims

The FDA permits labels to include claims about levels of nutrients in packaged foods. Nutrient content claims can use terms such as *free*, *high*, or *low* to describe how much of a nutrient is in the product. Additionally, nutrient content claims can use terms such as *more* or *reduced* to compare amounts of nutrients in a product to those in a similar product. This claim is often used for an item that substitutes for a *reference food*, a similar and more familiar food. For example, a "reduced–fat" salad dressing has considerably less fat than its reference food, regular salad dressing.

Table 3.9 lists some legal definitions for common nutrient content claims that were allowed on labels in 2015. Note that a product may contain a small amount of a nutrient such as fat or sugar, yet the Nutrition Facts panel can indicate the amount as "0 g." For example, the Nutrition Facts panel may indicate that a serving of food supplies "0" grams of trans fat, even though the food actually supplies less than 0.5 g of trans fat. As a result, it is possible to consume some trans fats from processed foods even though labels indicate a serving of each food does not contain this type of fat. When the FDA introduces

Figure 3.12 Structure/function claim. Structure/function statements cannot claim that a nutrient, food, or dietary supplement can be used to prevent or treat a serious health condition.

TABLE 3.9   Legal Definitions for Common Nutrient Content Claims (2015)

Sugar	• **Sugar free:** The product provides less than 0.5 g of sugar per serving. • **Reduced sugar:** The food contains at least 25% less sugar per serving than the reference food.
Calories	• **Calorie free:** The food provides fewer than 5 kcal per serving. • **Low calorie:** The food supplies 40 kcal or less per serving. • **Reduced or fewer calories:** The food contains at least 25% fewer kcal per serving than the reference food.
Fat	• **Fat free:** The food provides less than 0.5 g of fat per serving. • **Low fat:** The food contains 3 g or less fat per serving. Two-percent milk is not "low fat," because it has more than 3 g of fat per serving. The term *reduced fat* can be used to describe 2% milk. • **Reduced or less fat:** The food supplies at least 25% less fat per serving than the reference food.
Cholesterol	• **Cholesterol free:** The food contains less than 2 mg of cholesterol and 2 g or less of saturated fat per serving.
Fiber	• **High fiber:** The food contains 5g or more fiber per serving. Foods that include high-fiber claims on the label must also meet the definition for low fat. • **Good source of fiber:** The food supplies 2.5 to 4.9 g of fiber per serving.
Meat and poultry products regulated by USDA	• **Extra lean:** The food provides less than 5 g of fat, 2 g of saturated fat, and 95 mg of cholesterol per serving. • **Lean:** The food contains less than 10 g of fat, 4.5 g of saturated fat, and 95 mg of cholesterol per serving.

the new labeling format, specific amounts of such ingredients, such as trans fat, may need to be shown. To learn more about the FDA's regulations concerning nutrient claims, visit the agency's website (http://www.fda.gov/Food/Ingredients PackagingLabeling/LabelingNutrition/ucm2006873.htm).

Other Descriptive Labeling Terms

According to the FDA, a *light* or *lite* food has at least one–third fewer kilo–calories or half the fat of the reference food. For example, a tablespoon of lite pancake syrup has one–third fewer kcal than a tablespoon of regular pancake syrup, and a tablespoon of light mayonnaise has less than half the fat of regular mayonnaise. The term *light* may also describe such properties as texture and color, as long as the label explains the intent: for example, "light brown sugar." To include the term *natural* on the label, the food must not contain food coloring agents, synthetic flavors, or other unnatural substances (as of February 2016).

Dietary Supplement Labels

According to federal law, every dietary supplement container must be properly labeled (Fig. 3.13). The label must include the term "dietary supplement" or a similar term that describes the product's particular ingredient, such as "herbal supplement" or "vitamin C supplement." Dietary supplement labels are also required to display the list of ingredients, manufacturer's address, and suggested dosage. Furthermore, the label must include facts about the product's contents in a special format—the "Supplement Facts" panel (see Fig. 3.13). The panel pro–vides information about the serving size; amount per serving; and percent Daily Value (%DV) for ingredients, if one has been established. Daily Values (DVs) are standard desirable or maximum intakes for several nutrients, but DVs have not been established for nonnutrient products.

According to the FDA, dietary supplements are not intended to treat, diagnose, cure, or alleviate the effects of diseases. Therefore, the agency does not permit manufacturers to market a dietary supplement product as a treatment or cure for a disease, or to relieve signs or symptoms of a disease. Although such products generally cannot prevent diseases, some can improve health or reduce the risk of certain diseases or conditions. Thus, the FDA allows supplement

Often, the only difference between a creamy salad dressing, such as ranch or blue cheese, and the "light" version of the dressing is the amount of water they contain. Instead of paying more for calorie-reduced bottled salad dress-ings, make your own light salad dressing by adding about ¼ cup water to a jar of regular creamy salad dress-ing, then stir or shake the mixture.

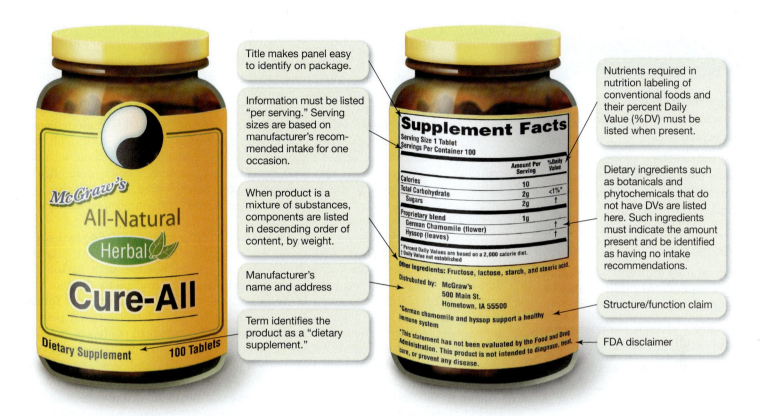

Title makes panel easy to identify on package.

Information must be listed "per serving." Serving sizes are based on manufacturer's recommended intake for one occasion.

When product is a mixture of substances, components are listed in descending order of content, by weight.

Manufacturer's name and address

Term identifies the product as a "dietary supplement."

Nutrients required in nutrition labeling of conventional foods and their percent Daily Value (%DV) must be listed when present.

Dietary ingredients such as botanicals and phytochemicals that do not have DVs are listed here. Such ingredients must indicate the amount present and be identified as having no intake recommendations.

Structure/function claim

FDA disclaimer

Figure 3.13 Supplement Facts label. A nutrient supplement label must list the product's ingredient(s), serving size, amount(s) per serving, suggested use, manufacturer and the company's address, and %DV, if one has been established. If a health claim appears on the supplement's label, the claim must be followed by the FDA disclaimer.

manufacturers to display structure/function claims on labels. Manufacturers of iron supplements, for example, may have a claim on the label that states: "Iron is necessary for healthy red blood cell formation." If the FDA has not reviewed a claim, the label must include the FDA's disclaimer indicating that the claim has not been evaluated by the agency (Fig. 3.14).

The FDA does not require dietary supplement manufacturers or sellers to provide evidence that labeling claims are accurate or truthful before they appear on product containers. However, manufacturers that include structure/function claims on labels must notify the FDA about the claims within 30 days after intro—ducing the products into the marketplace. If FDA officials question the safety of a dietary supplement or the truthfulness of claims that appear on supplement labels, manufacturers are responsible for providing the agency with evidence that their products are safe and the claims on labels are honest and not misleading.

The FDA requires dietary supplement manufacturers to evaluate the purity, quality, strength, and composition of their products before marketing them. The regulations are designed to result in the production of supplements that contain the ingredients listed on the label, are wholesome, contain standard amounts of ingredients per dose, and are properly packaged and accurately labeled.

Organic Food

By the late twentieth century, emphasis on increasing agricultural production resulted in an inexpensive and abundant food supply in the United States. How—ever, the rise of agribusiness also resulted in social, economic, and environmental costs. Rural agricultural communities experienced a dramatic decline in the

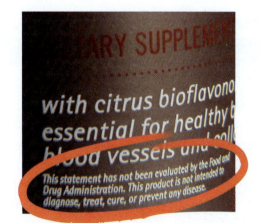

Figure 3.14 Label disclaimer. The FDA permits dietary supplement manufacturers to include certain health-related claims on their product labels. However, the label of products bearing such claims also must display this disclaimer.

Food & Nutrition tip

According to the Environmental Protection Agency, you can reduce your exposure to pesticides in food by:

• washing and scrubbing all fresh fruits and vegetables under running water. However, not all pesticide residues can be removed by washing;

• peeling and trimming fruits and vegetables before eating them;

• trimming fat from meat and skin of poultry and fish, because some pesticide residues accumulate in fat;

• eating a variety of foods; this reduces the likelihood of exposure to a single pesticide;

• eating organically grown foods.

organic foods foods produced without the use of antibiotics, hormones, synthetic fertilizers and pesticides, genetic improvements, or spoilage-killing radiation

number of small farms, as the farms' owners could not compete with the production capabilities and financial resources of large, commercially run farms.

Instead of producing a variety of crops, big farms often focus on growing corn, soybeans, or wheat. These crops require conventional farming methods that include heavy use of fertilizers and products to control pests (*pesticides*). In some parts of the country, large farms also need considerable amounts of water for irrigating crops. As a result, underground water supplies are being depleted in these regions.

The rise in agribusiness helped fuel interest in sustainable agriculture. Sustainable agriculture focuses on producing adequate amounts of food without reducing natural resources and harming the environment.[18] Such agricultural methods promote crop variety, soil and water conservation, and recycling of plant nutrients. Additionally, sustainable agriculture can support small farms, particularly organic farms.

Technically, organic substances have the element carbon bonded to hydrogen (another element) in their chemical structures. Therefore, all foods are organic because they contain substances comprised of carbon bonded with hydrogen. The term *organic*, however, also refers to certain agricultural methods that can promote sustainability. Organic farming and the production of **organic foods** do not rely on the use of antibiotics, hormones, synthetic fertilizers and pesticides, genetic improvements, or ionizing radiation.[19] Table 3.10 compares organic and nonorganic agricultural systems. Although organic farming techniques can benefit the environment, crop yields are typically lower than yields of similar crops grown conventionally.[20]

Over the past 40 years, the popularity of organic foods has increased in the United States as many Americans have become concerned about the environment and the safety and nutritional value of the food supply. Sales of organic foods have increased steadily since the 1990s, even though these products are usually more expensive than the same foods produced by conventional farming methods.[21] According to the Food Marketing Institute, Americans spent an estimated 31.5 billion on organic foods and beverages in 2011.[22]

People who purchase organically grown foods often think the products are better for their health and more nutritious than conventionally produced foods. Few well-designed studies have compared nutrient and phytochemical contents of organically grown foods to their conventionally grown counterparts. Nevertheless, some general trends have been determined. In general, organic food crops are not more nutritious than conventionally grown food crops.[23] Organic

TABLE 3.10   Comparing Organic and Nonorganic Farming Systems

Organic	Nonorganic
Synthetic fertilizers are not allowed.	Limited restrictions on fertilizers
Sewage sludge products are not allowed.	Sludge products may be used on some fields.
Restrictions on use of raw manure on fields used for food crops	Few restrictions on raw manure use for edible crop fields
Synthetic pesticides are not allowed; natural pest management practices are encouraged.	Any government-approved pesticide may be used according to label instructions. Natural pest management practices may also be used.
Genetically modified organisms (GMOs) are not allowed.	Government-approved GMOs are permitted.
Feeding livestock mammal and poultry by-products and manure is not allowed.	Certain mammal and poultry by-products are allowed in livestock feed.
Use of growth hormones and antibiotics in livestock production is not allowed.	Government-approved hormone and antibiotic treatments are permitted.
Food irradiation (a food safety method) is not allowed.	Food irradiation may be used.
Detailed record keeping and site inspections by regulators are required.	Some records are required, but no on-site checks by regulators are necessary.

TABLE 3.11   Organic Labeling Categories

"100% Organic" (may use USDA seal)	100% organic ingredients, including processing aids Must identify organic ingredients
"Organic" (may use USDA seal)	Contains at least 95% organic ingredients Remaining 5% of ingredients are on USDA's allowable list of allowed ingredients Must identify organic ingredients
"Made with organic ingredients" (may not use USDA organic seal)	Contains 70 to 95% certified organic ingredients Must identify organic ingredients

Source: U.S. Department of Agriculture: *Labeling organic products.* (ND). http://www.ams.usda.gov/AMSv1.0/ Accessed: August 4, 2013

crops, however, may contain fewer pesticides than conventionally grown crops.[24] Nevertheless, more research is needed to determine whether there are health advantages to eating organic foods.

Labeling Organic Foods

To protect consumers, the USDA developed and implemented rules for the organic food industry. A food product cannot be labeled "organic" unless its production meets strict national standards. For labeling purposes, organic food manufacturers can use the circular "USDA Organic" symbol on the package (Fig. 3.15). This symbol indicates the products meet USDA's standards for organic food. According to the USDA, there are three organic labeling categories (Table 3.11). Note that certain foods can have the organic symbol on the package, yet they may contain small amounts of nonorganic ingredients. For more information about the government's organic food standards, visit the USDA's National Organic Program's website (http://www.ams.usda.gov/AMSv1.0/nop).

Figure 3.15 Organic food logo. Foods that have been certified "organic" may use the USDA's symbol.

Concept **Checkpoint 3.5**

26. Identify at least one limitation of using %DVs to determine your nutrient intakes.
27. Explain how you can use nutritional information provided on food and dietary supplement labels to become a more careful consumer.
28. What is the difference between a health claim and a structure/function claim? What is a nutrient content claim? Give an example of each type of claim.
29. Discuss the role of the FDA in protecting consumers from false nutrition and health claims on food and dietary supplement labels.

3.6 Using Dietary Analysis Software

Learning Outcomes

1 Explain why different dietary analysis software programs may provide different values for energy and nutrient contents for the same food item.

2 Use the U.S. Department of Agriculture's websites to estimate the nutritional value of various foods.

How much selenium, magnesium, and niacin are in an ounce of Swiss cheese? Have you ever wanted information about nutrients in a food that are not listed on the Nutrition Facts panel? In the past, people relied on food composition

Valencia oranges and other produce may vary in nutrient content depending on numerous factors, including growing conditions.

tables, lists of commonly eaten foods that provide amounts of energy, fiber, macronutrients, and several micronutrients. Today, people can determine the energy and nutrient contents of their food choices by using a dietary analysis software program. Furthermore, people with Internet access can obtain the information from certain websites.

Dietary analysis software and websites can be quick and easy tools for determining nutrient and energy contents of a specific food. However, the values provided by these resources are not necessarily exact amounts. The same type of plant food may vary in nutrient content depending on hereditary factors, age, growing conditions, and production methods. Therefore, scientists generally analyze several samples of a particular food to determine their nutrient contents, and then the researchers average the results. For example, if the amount of energy in three Valencia oranges that each weigh about 4 ounces (120 g) were 55, 60, and 62 kcal, respectively, the value listed in the food composition table for a Valencia orange weighing 4 ounces would be 59 kcal, the average of the three. In many instances, values for certain nutrients are missing. This occurs when accurate data concerning the complete nutrient analysis of the food are unavailable.

The following section discusses some government–sponsored websites that provide practical tools for evaluating food intakes and physical activity habits. The Personal Dietary Analysis feature at the end of this chapter provides an opportunity for you to practice using dietary analysis software.

Government-Sponsored Dietary Analysis Websites

In addition to www.choosemyplate.gov, the USDA sponsors other websites to help you assess the energy and nutrient contents of your food intake. The "What's in the Food You Eat *Search Tool*" (www.ars.usda.gov/Services/docs. htm?docid=17032) is one such site. Another USDA–sponsored site that provides extensive information regarding the energy and nutrient content of food is the National Nutrient Database for Standard Reference. You can access this nutrient database by visiting www.nal.usda.gov/fnic/foodcomp/search. To keep current, USDA–sponsored websites are updated regularly to provide information about new products and serving sizes.

Concept **Checkpoint 3.6**

30. Identify at least two reliable sources of information about the energy and nutrient contents of foods and beverages.

3.7 Nutrition Matters: The Melting Pot

Learning Outcomes

1. Discuss how various ethnic and religious groups influence Americans' dietary patterns.
2. Identify religion-based dietary restrictions.

Wherever you live or travel in the United States, you're likely to find restaurants that serve a wide variety of ethnic fare, such as Italian, Thai, Vietnamese, or Middle Eastern dishes. Although your primary food selection and cooking habits probably reflect your cultural/ethnic heritage, you likely enjoy foods from other cultures and ethnic groups.

This section examines the influences that the dietary practices of certain cultures and ethnic groups have had on the American diet and the possible effects of these practices on health. Traditional ethnic diets are often based on dishes containing small amounts of animal foods and larger amounts of locally grown fruits, vegetables, and unrefined grains. However, these foods are typically the first to be abandoned as immigrants *assimilate,* that is, blend into the general population over time. After an immigrant population has assimilated fully, the prevalence of chronic diseases such as cardiovascular disease, type 2 diabetes, and high blood pressure often increases among them, partly as a result of adopting less healthy eating practices.

Northwestern European Influences

Immigrants from northwestern European regions or countries such as the United Kingdom, Scandinavia, and Germany established the familiar "meat-and-potatoes" diet that features a large portion of beef or pork served with a smaller portion of potatoes. In the past, the potatoes were either boiled or mashed; today, they are usually fried. This mainstream American diet, often referred to as a "Western" diet, provides large amounts of animal protein and fat, and lacks fruits, whole grains, and a variety of green vegetables. Such diets are associated with high rates of serious chronic diseases, particularly CVD and type 2 diabetes, which are discussed in later chapters of this textbook.

Hispanic Influences

The Hispanic (people with Spanish ancestry) population is now the largest minority group in the United States. Many Hispanic–Americans migrated

to the United States from Mexico. The traditional Mexican diet included corn, beans, chili peppers, avocados, papayas, and pineapples. Many supermarkets in the United States sell other plant foods that are often incorporated into Mexican meals, such as fresh chayote, cherimoya, jicama, plantains, and cactus leaves and fruit. Such fruits and vegetables add fiber and a variety of nutrients, phytochemicals, vivid colors, and interesting flavors to Mexican dishes (Figure 3.16).

Authentic Mexican meals are based primarily on rice, tortillas, and beans, depending on the region. However, many non–Hispanic Americans do not like to eat meals limited to these inexpensive yet nutritious plant foods.

Figure 3.16 Latin American Diet Pyramid.
Source: www.oldwayspt.org

To appeal to people with more Western food preferences, "Mexican" fast-food restaurants in the United States often serve dishes that contain large portions of high-fat beef topped with sour cream and cheese. Diets that contain high amounts of these and other solid fats are associated with excess body fat, CVD, and type 2 diabetes.

Italian and Other Mediterranean Influences

The traditional Italian diet of pasta and other grain products, olive oil, fish, nuts, fruits, and vegetables is healthier than the Western diet. Pasta, a product made from wheat flour and water, is the core of the traditional Italian diet. To many Americans *pasta* is spaghetti topped with tomato sauce, meatballs, and grated Parmesan cheese. However, Italians eat a variety of different forms of pasta, such as penne, linguini, acini de pepe, and rotini, along with sauces that are often meatless. Pizza, a dish from southern Italy, is one of the most frequently consumed foods in the United States. Unlike traditional Italian pizza that has a thin crust and is lightly covered with tomatoes, basil (a leafy herb), and mozzarella cheese, many Americans choose thick-crust pizza topped with tomato sauce, plenty of shredded mozzarella cheese, and dotted with fatty pork sausage or pepperoni.

Dietary pyramids or plans developed by governmental agencies or private organizations have plant foods as the core of a healthy diet. The Mediterranean Diet Pyramid shown in Figure 3.17 is based on traditional dietary practices of Greece, southern Italy, and the island of Crete. Grains, fruits, and vegetables, particularly beans and potatoes, form the foundation of this diet. Red meat is rarely eaten. Main dishes often include seafood and poultry, and wine may be included with meals. Although the Mediterranean Diet Pyramid allows as much as 35% of total calories as fat in the diet, much of the fat is from olive oil. Olive oil is a rich source of a type of fat that reduces rather than increases the risk of CVD. Chapter 6 provides more information about oils and fats and their roles in health.

African Heritage Diets

Over the past several decades, the diets of African Americans changed significantly so they now incorporate regional food preferences. In some parts of the United States, for example, the traditional African-American diet includes sweet potato pie, fried chicken, pork, black-eyed peas, and "greens," the nutritious leafy parts of plants such as kale, collards, mustard, turnip, and dandelion. To add flavor, greens may be cooked with small pieces of smoked pork.

Although sweet potatoes, dried peas, and leafy vegetables provide fiber and a variety of vitamins and minerals, fried foods and salt-cured pork products contribute undesirable levels of fat and sodium to the diet. High-fat diets are associated with obesity, and high-sodium diets raise the risk of hypertension. You will learn more about the role of diet in the development of hypertension in Chapters 6 and 9. For more information about African heritage diets and foods, visit http://oldwayspt.org/programs/african-heritage-health .

Asian Influences

Traditional Asian foods, such as Chinese, Japanese, Vietnamese, Thai, and Korean cuisines, are similar and generally feature large amounts of vegetables, rice, or noodles combined with small amounts of meat, fish, or shellfish. The variety of vegetables used in Asian dishes adds color,

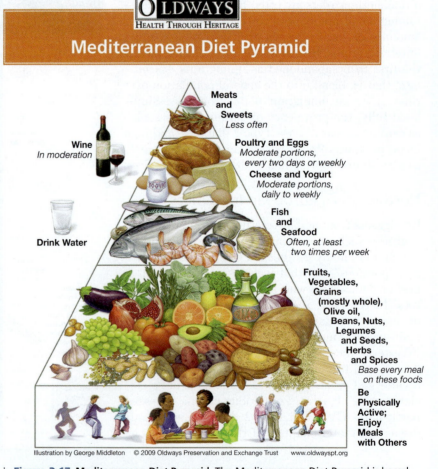

OLDWAYS
HEALTH THROUGH HERITAGE

Mediterranean Diet Pyramid

Meats and Sweets
Less often

Wine
In moderation

Poultry and Eggs
Moderate portions, every two days or weekly

Cheese and Yogurt
Moderate portions, daily to weekly

Fish and Seafood
Often, at least two times per week

Drink Water

Fruits, Vegetables, Grains (mostly whole), Olive oil, Beans, Nuts, Legumes and Seeds, Herbs and Spices
Base every meal on these foods

Be Physically Active; Enjoy Meals with Others

Illustration by George Middleton   © 2009 Oldways Preservation and Exchange Trust   www.oldwayspt.org

Figure 3.17 Mediterranean Diet Pyramid. The Mediterranean Diet Pyramid is based on traditional dietary practices of Greece, southern Italy, and the island of Crete. Source: www.oldwayspt.org.

flavor, texture, phytochemicals, and nutrients to meals. Additionally, Asian dishes often include flavorful sauces and seasonings made from plants, such as soy sauce, rice wine, gingerroot, garlic, scallions, peppers, and sesame seeds. The Asian Diet Pyramid, shown in Figure 3.18, illustrates the traditional Asian dietary pattern, which generally provides inadequate amounts of calcium from milk and milk products. However, using calcium–rich or calcium–fortified foods can add the mineral to diets.

Chinese foods are popular among Americans. Many Americans, however, do not favor dishes that feature seafood and contain large portions of vegetables and grains, because they believe meat should form the basis of a meal. Thus, North American Chinese restaurants that specialize in Cantonese, Szechwan, or Mandarin cuisines typically offer menu items that contain much larger portions of animal foods such as beef and chicken than authentic dishes. Furthermore, American–Chinese foods are often prepared with far greater amounts of fat than are used in true Chinese cooking.

Traditional Chinese food preparation methods, particularly steaming and stir–frying, tend to preserve the vitamins and minerals in fresh vegetables. Stir–frying involves cooking foods in a lightly oiled, very hot pan for a short period of time. Unlike Western methods of deep–fat frying or boiling vegetables, stir–frying vegetables keeps them crisp and colorful.

Rice is the staple food in the traditional Japanese diet. Additionally, fish, poultry, pork, and foods made from soybeans provide protein in this diet. The Japanese people eat sushi, small pieces of raw fish or shellfish that are usually served rolled in or pressed into rice and served with vegetables and seaweed. American–Japanese restaurants often feature sushi, and many non–Japanese Americans like to order the exotic dish.

Some of the longest–lived people in the world reside on Okinawa, a tiny island south of the main Japanese islands. The traditional diet of fresh vegetables, minimal amounts of salt and animal protein (mainly from pork and fish), and moderate amounts of fat may protect the island's population from premature heart disease and stroke. Younger Okinawans have adopted more western dietary practices, such as eating "fast food," and as a result, their life expectancy is not as long as their grandparents.[25]

Not all Japanese are as healthy as the older generations of Okinawans. The people living on the Japanese island of Honshu consume high amounts of salt, which is the principal dietary source of the mineral sodium. High sodium intakes increase the risk of hypertension, and this disease is very common among the Honshu population.

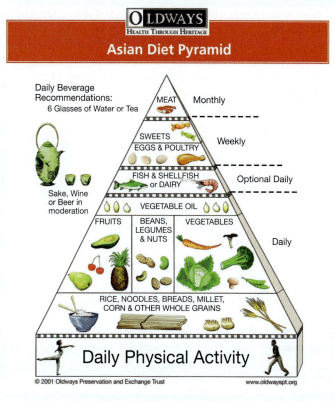

Figure 3.18 Asian Diet Pyramid. The Asian Diet Pyramid dietary pattern generally provides inadequate amounts of calcium from milk and milk products.
Source: www.oldwayspt.org

Native American Influences

In the past, some Native Americans were hunter–gatherers, depending on wild vegetation, fish, and game for food. Other Native Americans learned to grow vegetable crops, including tomatoes, corn, and squash. In general, the traditional Native American diet was low in sodium and fat and high in fiber. During the last half of the twentieth century, many Native Americans abandoned their traditional diets and adopted the typical Western diet. The negative health effects of this lifestyle change have been significant. Before the 1930s, for example, members of the Pima tribe in the southwestern United States primarily ate native foods that included low–fat game animals and high–fiber desert vegetation. By the end of the century, most American

Pima had abandoned their native diets and had adopted a more Western diet. Today, obesity and type 2 diabetes are extremely prevalent among the Pima, whereas in the past, these conditions rarely affected tribal members.

The traditional native Alaskan diet was composed of fatty fish and sea mammals, game animals, and a few plants. Alaskan natives who still follow tra-ditional dietary practices have CVD rates that are lower than those in the general North American population, but those who switched to a more Western diet have developed CVD at rates similar to those of the general population.

Religious Influences

Many religions require members to follow strict food handling and dietary practices that often include the prohibition of certain

foods and beverages (see Table 3.12). According to Jewish dietary laws, for example, meat and poultry products must be kept separate from milk products. Milk products are not used to prepare foods that contain meat or poultry, nor are they served with them. A cheeseburger, for example, is not *kosher*. "Kosher" refers to a specific procedure concerning killing, butchering, and preparation activities that makes food acceptable for the religion's followers to eat. Fruits, grains, and veg-etables are "neutral" foods that can be eaten with meals that contain either meat or dairy products. However, vegetables cooked with meat become a "meat" food and cannot be served with milk; peaches served with cot-tage cheese become a "milk" food and can-not be eaten with meat or poultry. Today many American Jews do not follow their reli-gion's complex dietary laws as closely as their ancestors did.

TABLE 3.12 Religious Influences on Dietary Practices

Religion	Dietary practices*
Buddhist	Meat is avoided; vegetarianism is encouraged.
Eastern Orthodox	Meat and fish restrictions; fasting and specific food abstinence during certain holidays
Hindu	Beef is forbidden, but dairy products are "pure" for consumption. Pork may be restricted. Alcohol is avoided. Fasting is often encouraged.
Islam	Pork; birds of prey; reptiles; insects, except locusts; most gelatins; and alcohol are prohibited (*ha-raam*). Ritual killing of animals that are permitted as food (*ha-lal*) Stimulant beverages (i.e., coffee and tea) are avoided. Fasting from all food and drink (daytime) during month of Ramadan and certain other religious holidays
Jewish	Only kosher foods are acceptable. "Tref" (*trayf*) refers to prohibited foods. Pork and shellfish are prohibited. Eating meat with dairy is prohibited. Consuming blood is forbidden. Raw meat is soaked in cold water to remove blood, salted for 1 hour, and then rinsed. Eggs, fruits, and vegetables can be eaten with either meat or dairy foods. Eggs, however, are inspected to make sure they do not contain blood specks. Only fish with fins and scales can be eaten. Only land animals that have split hooves and chew their cud can be eaten, and only the front half of the cud-chewing animal is used. Ritual killing of certain animals is required. Fasting and specific food restrictions for certain holidays
Mormon	Do not drink alcohol, coffee, and tea Fasting is practiced regularly.
Roman Catholic	Fasting before communion; fasting and specific food abstinence during certain holidays
Seventh Day Adventist	Animal product consumption generally limited to milk, milk products, and eggs (lacto-ovo vegetarianism) Alcohol and beverages containing stimulants are prohibited.

* Some religions have extensive rules governing food-related practices, but many people do not follow their religion's dietary guidelines fully or at all.

Bagels with smoked salmon (*lox*), pickled herring, cream cheese, dill pickles, corned beef, and pastrami are popular among the Ashkenazi, the predominant group of Jews in America. Although many non—Jews enjoy eating these traditional Ashkenazic foods, such items may be too high in sodium and animal fat to be healthy.

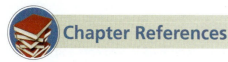

Concept **Checkpoint 3.7**

31. Discuss how immigrants to the United States from Asia and Mexico have influenced the general population's food preferences.

32. Discuss at least two religion-related food restrictions.

Chapter References

See Appendix H.

Summary

3.1 From Requirements to Standards

- A requirement is the smallest amount of a nutrient that maintains a defined level of health. Numerous factors influence nutrient requirements. Scientists use information about nutrient requirements and storage capabilities to establish specific dietary recommendations. The Dietary Reference Intakes (DRIs) are various energy and nutrient intake standards for Americans. An Estimated Average Requirement (EAR) is the amount of the nutrient that meets the needs of 50% of healthy people in a particular life stage/sex group. The Estimated Energy Requirement (EER) is used to evaluate a person's energy intake. The Recommended Dietary Allowances (RDAs) meet the needs of nearly all healthy individuals (97 to 98%) in a particular life stage/sex group. When nutrition scientists are unable to determine an RDA for a nutrient, they establish an Adequate Intake (AI) value. The Tolerable Upper Intake Level (UL) is the highest average amount of a nutrient that is unlikely to harm most people when the amount is consumed daily.

- DRIs can be used for planning nutritious diets for groups of people and evaluating the nutritional adequacy of a population's diet. RDAs and AIs are often used to evaluate an individual's dietary practices. For nutrition labeling purposes, FDA uses RDAs to develop Daily Values (DVs).

3.2 Major Food Groups

- Food guides generally classify foods into groups according to their natural origins and key nutrients. Such guides usually feature major food groups. Some food guides also include groups for oils and empty-calorie foods or beverages.

3.3 Dietary Guidelines

- The Dietary Guidelines is a set of general nutrition-related lifestyle recommendations designed to promote adequate nutritional status and good health, and to reduce the risk of major chronic nutrition-related health conditions.

3.4 Food Guides

- Choosemyplate.gov is an online, interactive food intake and physical activity guide that is based on Dietary Guidelines. Most Americans do not follow the government's dietary recommendations.

- The Exchange System, a tool for estimating the calorie and macronutrient contents of foods, categorizes foods into three broad groups. The foods within each group have similar macronutrient composition. A specified amount of food in an exchange list provides about the same amount of macronutrients and calories as each of the other specified amounts of foods in that list. Carbohydrate counting is a method that people can use for planning menus.

3.5 Food and Dietary Supplement Labels

- Consumers can use information on food labels to determine ingredients and compare nutrient contents of packaged foods and beverages. The FDA regulates and monitors information that can be placed on food labels, including claims about the product's health benefits. Nearly all foods and beverages sold in supermarkets must be labeled with the product's name, manufacturer's name and address, amount of product in the package, and ingredients listed in descending order by weight. Furthermore, food labels must use a special format for listing specific information on the Nutrition Facts panel.

- The Daily Values (DVs) are a practical set of nutrient standards for labeling purposes. The nutrient content in a serving of food is listed on the label as a percentage of the DV (%DV). Not all nutrients have DVs. A dietary goal is to obtain at least 100% of the DVs for fiber, vitamins, and minerals (except sodium) each day.

- The FDA permits food manufacturers to include certain health claims on food labels. However, the agency requires that health claims meet certain guidelines and, in some instances, use specific wording. A structure/function claim describes the role a nutrient plays in the body. Structure/function statements cannot claim that a nutrient or food can be used to prevent or treat a serious health condition.

- Organic foods are produced without the use of antibiotics, hormones, synthetic fertilizers and pesticides, genetic improvements, or food irradiation. In general, organic food crops are not more nutritious than similar conventionally grown foods. More research is needed to determine whether there are health advantages to eating organic foods. A food product cannot be labeled "organic" unless its production meets strict national standards.

3.6 Using Dietary Analysis Software

- Dietary analysis software and websites can be quick and easy tools for determining nutrient and energy contents of a specific food.

3.7 Nutrition Matters: The Melting Pot

- Traditional ethnic diets are often based on dishes containing small amounts of animal foods and larger amounts of locally grown fruits, vegetables, and unrefined grains. However, these foods are typically abandoned as people migrate to other countries and assimilate into the general population. After an immigrant population has assimilated fully, the prevalence of chronic diseases such as cardiovascular disease, type 2 diabetes, and high blood pressure often increases among them, partly as a result of adopting unhealthy eating practices. Many religions require members to follow strict food handling and dietary practices that often include the prohibition of certain foods and beverages.

Recipe for Healthy Living

Mango Lassi

Lassi (*luh-see*) is a simple yogurt-based beverage that originated in India. Lassi is usually made and served before a meal, but the drink can also be a refreshing, nutritious snack. This recipe makes about four ½-cup servings. Each serving supplies approximately 97 kcal, 4 g protein, 9 g digestible carbohydrate, 0.5 g fat, 1 g fiber, 122 mg calcium, and 30 mg vitamin C.

INGREDIENTS:

1 ripe mango
1 cup plain, fat-free yogurt
1 Tbsp sugar
6 ice cubes

PREPARATION STEPS:

1. Wash and peel mango. Remove fruit pulp from mango and discard large seed and peel.

2. Dice mango pulp and place in blender.

3. Add yogurt, sugar, and ice cubes to the blender.

4. Blend ingredients until smooth.

5. Serve immediately or refrigerate for up to 24 hours.

*2000 daily total kcal
**Digestible forms

 Further analyze this and other recipes through activities on Connect at www.mcgrawhillconnect.com.

Personal Dietary Analysis

I. Record Keeping

  A. 24-Hour Dietary Recall

   1. Recall every food and beverage that you have eaten over the past 24 hours. Recall how much you consumed and how it was prepared.

    a. How easy or difficult was it to recall your food intake?

  B. Three-Day Diet Record

   1. Without changing your usual diet, keep a detailed log of your food and beverage intake for 3 days; one of the days should be Friday or Saturday. Use a separate log for each day.

II. Analysis

Using nutritional analysis software, analyze your daily food intakes and answer questions in Part III of this activity. Keep the record on file for future applications.

  A. Computer-Generated Dietary Analysis

   1. Load the software into the computer, or log on to software website.

   2. Choose the DRIs or related nutrient standard from the last pages of this book, based on your life stage, sex, height, and weight.

   3. Enter the information from the 3-day food intake record. Be sure to enter each food and drink and the specific amounts.

   4. The software program will give you the following results:

    a. The appropriate RDA (or related standard) for each nutrient

    b. The total amount of each nutrient and the kilocalories consumed for each day

    c. The percentage intake compared with the standard amount for each nutrient that you consumed each day

   5. Keep this assessment for activities in other chapters.

III. Evaluation of Nutrient Intakes

Remember it is not necessary to consume the maximum of your nutrient recommendations every day. A general standard is meeting at least 70% of the standards averaged over several days. It is best not to exceed the Upper Level (if set) over the long term to avoid potential toxic effects of some nutrients.

  A. For which nutrients did your average intake fall below the recommended amounts, that is, to less than 70% of the RDA/AI?

  B. For which nutrients did your average intake exceed the Upper Level (if a UL has been set)?

IV. MyPlate

This activity determines how your diet stacks up when compared to the amounts of foods from each food group that are recommended by MyPlate.

A. Refer to your 3-day diet record. Classify each food item in the appropriate food group of MyPlate. For each food group, indicate whether you ate the recommended amount daily for your sex, age, height, weight, and physical activity level. Note that some of your food choices—pizza, for example—may contribute to more than one food group. Enter a minus sign (–) if your total falls below the MyPlate recommendation or a plus sign (+) if it equals or exceeds the daily recommendation for each food group.

 Complete this Personal Dietary Analysis activity online at www.mcgrawhillconnect.com.

 ## Critical Thinking

1. Your friend takes several dietary supplements daily, and as a result, his vitamin B–6 intake is 50 times higher than the RDA for the vitamin. You would like to convince him to stop taking the supplements. To support your advice, which nutrient standards would you show him? Explain why.

2. Why should consumers use MyPlate to plan menus instead of the DRIs?

3. How do your added sugars, sodium, and saturated fat intakes compare to the recommendations of the latest Dietary Guidelines?

4. Examine Table 3.6. Which foods in the left–hand column do you eat regularly? Why are those foods listed in that column?

5. The ingredient list on a package of crackers includes vegetable oil. What can you do to learn which type of vegetable oil is in the product?

6. Visit the USDA's website (www.ars.usda.gov/Services/docs.htm?docid=17032) to access "What's in the Foods You Eat *Search Tool*," a database for searching the nutritional content of foods. To practice using this search tool, find the number of kilocalories and the amounts of fiber, vitamin C, iron, and caffeine in 1 cup of raw jicama, 1 cup of 2% milk with added vitamin A, and ¼ cup of dry roasted, salt–added sunflower seed kernels (no hulls).

7. According to a newspaper article, an 8–oz serving of fat–free milk contains 15 mcg of folate (a B vitamin). Another source of nutrition information indicates that an 8–oz serving of fat–free milk contains 12 mcg of folate. Explain why both sources of information can be correct.

Practice Test

Select the best answer.

1. The amount of a nutrient that should meet the needs of half of the healthy people in a particular group is the
   a. Estimated Average Requirement (EAR).
   b. Recommended Dietary Allowance (RDA).
   c. Adequate Intake (AI).
   d. Tolerable Upper Intake Level (UL).

2. Which of the following statements is false?
   a. RDAs are standards for daily intakes of certain nutrients.
   b. RDAs meet the nutrient needs of nearly all healthy people.
   c. RDAs contain a margin of safety.
   d. RDAs are requirements for nutrients.

3. The Estimated Energy Requirement (EER)
   a. has a margin of safety.
   b. does not account for a person's height, weight, or physical activity level.
   c. is based on the average daily energy needs of a healthy person.
   d. reflects a person's actual daily energy needs.

4. A diet is likely to be safe and nutritionally adequate if
   a. average daily intakes for nutrients meet RDA or AI values.
   b. intakes of various nutrients are consistently less than EAR amounts.
   c. nutrient intakes are consistently above ULs.
   d. vitamin supplements are included.

5. Nutritional standards, such as the RDAs, are not
   a. used to develop formula food products.
   b. the basis for establishing DVs.
   c. used to evaluate the nutritional adequacy of diets.
   d. the basis for developing AIs.

6. According to the MyPlate plan, which of the following foods is grouped with dairy products?
   a. cheese   c. butter
   b. eggs   d. cream

7. Protein−rich food sources that also contain high amounts of saturated fat include
   a. peanut butter.   c. nuts.
   b. dry beans.   d. beef.

8. Fruit is generally a good source of all of the following substances, except
   a. fiber.   c. phytochemicals.
   b. vitamin C.   d. protein.

9. The Dietary Guidelines is
   a. revised every year.
   b. a set of general nutrition−related recommendations.
   c. published by the Centers for Disease Control and Prevention.
   d. used to develop DVs.

10. Which of the following foods would be classified as "empty calories" by MyPlate?
    a. chocolate syrup   c. white bread
    b. fat−free milk   d. corn oil

11. Which of the following statements is true?
    a. According to MyPlate, vegetable oils are grouped into the "Fats and Oils" food group.
    b. The MyPlate menu planning guide cannot be indi−vidualized to meet a person's food preferences.
    c. A person can use MyPlate to evaluate his or her diet's nutritional adequacy.
    d. MyPlate was the first food guide developed for Americans.

12. The Exchange System
    a. classifies foods in the same groups as MyPlate.
    b. has exchange lists based on macronutrient contents.
    c. is useful only for people who have diabetes.
    d. incorporates high−protein foods with high−carbohydrate foods.

13. Which of the following information was not provided by the Nutrition Facts panel in 2015?
    a. percentage of calories from fat
    b. amount of carbohydrate per serving
    c. serving size
    d. amount of trans fat per serving

14. Daily Values are

    a. for people who consume 1200 to 1500 kilocalorie diets.
    b. based on the lowest RDA or AI for each nutrient.
    c. dietary standards developed for food—labeling purposes.
    d. used to evaluate the nutritional adequacy of a popu-
       lation's diet.

15. People who follow Islamic dietary rules will not
consume

    a. pork.   c. beef.
    b. rice.   d. milk.

Answers to Quiz Yourself

1. According to the latest U.S. Department of Agriculture food guide, fruits and vegetables are combined into one food group. **False.** (p. 71)

2. According to the recommendations of the *2015–2020 Dietary Guidelines for Americans,* it is acceptable for certain adults to consume alcoholic beverages in moderation. **True.** (p. 69)

3. Last week, Colin didn't consume the recommended amount of vitamin C for a couple of days. Nevertheless, he is unlikely to develop scurvy, the vitamin C deficiency disease. **True.** (p. 64)

4. The Food and Drug Administration develops Dietary Guidelines for Americans. **False.** (p. 68)

5. The Nutrition Facts panel on a food label provides information concerning amounts of energy, fiber, and sodium that are in a serving of the food. **True.** (p. 77)

CHAPTER 4

Body Basics

Quiz Yourself

To test your knowledge of the material covered in Chapter 4, take the following quiz; the answers are on page 127.

1. The atom is the smallest living unit in the body. _____ T _____ F

2. The stomach produces gastric juice that contains hydrochloric acid. _____ T _____ F

3. Digestion begins in the stomach. _____ T _____ F

4. The human intestinal tract cannot digest certain combinations of foods, such as mixtures of simple carbohydrates and proteins. _____ T _____ F

5. Undigested food rots in your stomach, causing toxic materials to build up in your tissues. _____ T _____ F

4.1 Nutrition: Chemistry Foundations

Learning Outcomes

1 Define key basic chemistry terms, including *element, ion, chemical bond,* and *enzyme.*

2 Explain the difference between an acid and a base.

3 Explain the role of enzymes in many chemical reactions.

In Chapter 1, we defined chemistry as the study of the composition and characteristics of matter, and the changes that it can undergo. We also defined human physiology as the study of how the human body functions. Principles of chemistry and human physiology form the foundation for the scientific study of nutrition. The foods you eat and the air you breathe provide nutrients and oxygen, the raw materials (matter) that your cells need to survive and function. By reading Chapter 4, you will learn some basic chemistry concepts to help you understand how the matter in food becomes the raw materials for building, fueling, and sustaining healthy bodies. Additionally, you will learn about body structures and functions so you can understand the roles of nutrients in the body and why these particular chemicals are so important.

Parts of this chapter may seem to be filled with unfamiliar terms and their definitions, but learning the meaning of these terms can help you communicate more effectively with physicians and help you become a wiser consumer of health–related information.

Basic Chemistry Concepts

Do you or does someone you know avoid eating foods that are not labeled organic because they contain chemicals such as additives or pesticides? It is true that chemicals are in your food, but they are not necessarily harmful. Chemicals make up food as well as every other aspect of your environment; air, water, rocks, and other forms of matter contain chemicals. In fact, you are a complex collection of chemicals, much of which is organized into cells. The following sections provide basic information about some chemistry concepts that apply to the study of nutrition.

From Atoms to Compounds

Matter is comprised of atoms that contain certain particles, including protons and electrons (Fig. 4.1). **Protons** are positively charged particles in the *nucleus,* the central region of an atom. **Electrons** are small negatively charged particles that form a cloud surrounding the nucleus. The number of electrons surrounding the nucleus equals the number of protons within the nucleus. Thus, the negative and positive charges cancel out each other, making an atom neutral, which means it has no electrical charge.

More than 100 different types of atoms exist, and each type is an **element,** a substance that cannot be separated into simpler substances by ordinary chemical or physical means. Elements are the "building blocks" of matter. Table 4.1 lists several elements, most of which are essential for human nutrition. An element is essential if the body cannot function normally without it and the element must be supplied by the diet. Note that chemists use letters as symbols to represent elements. For example, the symbols for carbon, nitrogen, and sodium are C, N, and Na, respectively.

protons positively charged particles in the nucleus of an atom

electrons small, negatively charged particles that surround the nucleus of an atom

element each type of atom; substance that cannot be separated into simpler substances by ordinary chemical or physical means

Figure 4.1 An atom. Matter is comprised of atoms that contain particles, including protons and electrons. The nucleus of this hydrogen atom contains one positively charged proton.

TABLE 4.1 Nutrition-related Elements in the Body

Element	Symbol
Hydrogen	H
Oxygen	O
Carbon	C
Nitrogen	N
Calcium	Ca
Phosphorus	P
Potassium	K
Sulfur	S
Sodium	Na
Chloride	Cl⁻
Magnesium	Mg
Iron	Fe
Iodide	I⁻
Copper	Cu
Zinc	Zn
Manganese	Mn
Cobalt	Co
Chromium	Cr
Selenium	Se
Molybdenum	Mo
Fluoride*	F⁻

*Although fluoride is not essential, the mineral helps strengthen teeth and bones.

minerals elements that are found in the Earth's crust

chemical bond attraction that holds atoms together

molecule matter that forms when two or more atoms interact and are held together by a chemical bond

compounds molecules that contain two or more different elements in specific proportions

solution evenly distributed mixture of two or more compounds

solvent primary component of a solution

solute lesser component of a solution that dissolves in solvent

solubility describes a substance's ability to dissolve and form a solution

ion atom or group of atoms that has a positive or negative charge

Minerals are elements, such as calcium, iron, and potassium, that are found in the Earth's crust. Many minerals are essential nutrients. However, not every mineral is in living things or is necessary for life. Your external environment has natural and human—made forms of matter that may contain elements such as mercury (Hg), aluminum (Al), and cadmium (Cd). The human body does not need these minerals to function properly, and they can be quite toxic. Chapter 9 discusses the importance of various minerals to health.

Molecules When atoms interact, they may share electrons and rearrange them—selves, forming a chemical bond. A **chemical bond** is an attraction that holds atoms together and forms a **molecule.** When illustrating the structure of mol—ecules, chemists often use straight lines to show the bonds (Fig. 4.2a).

Molecules can contain the same element or different elements. For example, an oxygen molecule forms when two oxygen atoms bind together, whereas a water molecule forms when two hydrogen atoms bond to an oxygen atom. To identify a particular molecule without using lines to draw its chemical structure, chemists use a chemical formula. The chemical formula for an oxygen molecule is O_2; the subscript "2" indicates the presence of 2 oxygen atoms. The chemical formula for a water molecule is H_2O. The chemical formula for the simple sugar *glucose* is $C_6H_{12}O_6$. Judging from its formula, how many carbon, hydrogen, and oxygen atoms are in a glucose molecule?

Some atoms form single bonds, but a few atoms can form multiple bonds. Each carbon atom (C) has four bonding sites, and as a result, carbon atoms can bond to each other by single, double (Fig. 4.2b), and even triple bonds (Fig. 4.2c). Carbon's ability to bond to other carbon atoms as well as form multiple bonds with a neighboring carbon atom contributes to the formation of a vast array of organic (carbon—containing) compounds. **Compounds** are molecules that contain two or more different elements in specific proportions.

Solutions A **solution** is an evenly distributed mixture of two or more compounds. In living things, water is often the **solvent,** the primary component of solutions. Your body, for example, is about 60% water. A substance that dissolves in the solvent is a **solute.** Many beverages and foods are solutions that have water as the solvent (Fig. 4.3a). A sports drink, for example, is a solution that is mostly water, the solvent. The drink has relatively small amounts of sugar, minerals, colorings, and flavorings (solutes) dissolved in the water.

The **solubility** of a substance describes its ability to dissolve, that is, form a solution, in a solvent. Many naturally occurring substances, including simple car—bohydrates such as sugar and all mineral elements, dissolve in water. Other sub—stances, such as fat, are insoluble and will not dissolve in water (Fig. 4.3b). Your blood has high water content, a characteristic that makes it easier for the body to transport and eliminate water—soluble substances than water—insoluble materials.

Ions When an atom (or group of atoms) gains or loses one or more electrons, it has an electrical charge and is called an **ion** (Fig. 4.4). If an atom gains one electron, it becomes an ion with a negative charge, because electrons are negatively charged.

(a)   (b)   (c)

Figure 4.2 Chemical bonds. Some atoms form single bonds (*a*), but a few atoms can form multiple bonds. Carbon atoms can bond to each other by single, double (*b*), and even triple bonds (*c*).

Figure 4.3 **Solubility.** The solubility of a compound describes how easily it forms a solution. Many substances, including table sugar, dissolve in water. (a) Sports drinks are beverages in which sugar remains dissolved in water. Other substances, such as fat, are insoluble in water and will not dissolve in it. (b) Vinaigrette is an example of a food in which oil and water (balsamic vinegar) do not form a solution. In this particular product, note how the oil separates from the vinegar and forms a layer on top of the darker balsamic vinegar layer.

(a)   (b)

If an atom loses an electron, it becomes an ion with a positive charge, because it has an extra proton and protons are positively charged. A negative charge is indicated with a minus sign ($^-$), and a positive charge is indicated with a plus sign ($^+$) after the chemical symbol or formula. For example, a molecule of ammonia is neutral, that is, has no electrical charge, because it has the same number of protons and electrons. If the molecule loses an electron, it becomes the positively charged ion, ammonium. The formula for the positively charged *hydrogen ion* is simply **H^+**.

When most mineral elements, including sodium and potassium, dissolve in water, they form solutions containing ions that can conduct electricity. Thus, sodium and potassium are called **electrolytes.** Electrolytes have many important functions in the body, including helping to maintain proper fluid balance.

What Are Acids and Bases?   **Acids** are substances that lose H^+ when dissolved in water; **bases** are substances that remove and accept H^+ when dissolved in water. Many of the chemicals you encounter daily are either acidic or basic (alkaline). As you can tell by their names, phosphoric acid in soft drinks and ascorbic acid (better known as vitamin C) are acids. Baking soda and sodium hydroxide, an ingredient of many hair removal products, are bases.

Chemists measure the concentration of hydrogen ions **(pH)** in a watery solu—tion by using the pH scale. The scale ranges from 0 to 14. With each whole number

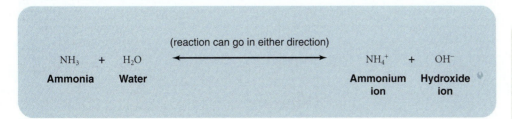

(reaction can go in either direction)

NH_3 + H_2O ⟷ NH_4^+ + OH^-

Ammonia   **Water**   **Ammonium**   **Hydroxide**
                                            ion   **ion**

Figure 4.4 **What is an ion?** An ion is an atom or group of atoms that loses or gains one or more electrons and, as a result, has an electrical charge. In this reaction, ammonia and water react to form the positively charged ammonium ion and the negatively charged hydroxide ion.

H^+ chemical symbol for hydrogen ion

electrolytes ions of minerals that conduct electricity when they are dissolved in water

acids substances that donate hydrogen ions

bases substances that accept hydrogen ions

pH measure of the acidity or alkalinity of a solution

0	0.9 - 3.0	2.3	2.4 - 3.5	4.0	5.0	6.3 - 6.6	7.0	7.4	8.0	9.5	10.0	11.0	13.4	14
Hydro-chloric acid	Gastric juice	Lemon juice	Wine, vinegar, cola, beer	Tomatoes	Black coffee	Milk, urine, saliva	Pure water	Blood	Egg white, seawater	Household bleach, baking soda	Great Salt Lake (Utah)	Household ammonia	Oven cleaner	Sodium hydroxide

← Increasingly acidic   Neutral   Increasingly basic →

Figure 4.5 pH scale. Chemists measure the concentration of hydrogen ions in a watery solution by using the pH scale. This scale indicates the pH values of some substances, including foods. Substances with low pH values are more acidic than substances with high pH values (bases).

increase within the scale, the H^+ concentration decreases 10 times. Examine the pH scale shown in Figure 4.5. Note that black coffee has a pH of about 5.0 and tomatoes have a pH of about 4.0. Thus, tomatoes are 10 times more acidic than black coffee. Although it may seem confusing, a solution with a pH of 2.0 has a *higher* H^+ concentration and is *more* acidic than a solution with a pH of 12.0.

Pure water has equal concentrations of H^+ and OH^-, so it is neither acidic nor basic. Thus, pure water has a pH of 7 and is neutral. By combining an acid with a base, the pH of a solution can become 7.

Your body must maintain its *acid−base balance* to function properly. Under normal conditions, the pH of your blood ranges from 7.35 to 7.45, which is slightly alkaline. To control its pH within normal limits, blood contains buffers—ions or molecules that accept excess OH^- or H^+ when necessary. Acids form naturally as by−products of cellular activity, but if the pH of blood begins to fall, the excess H^+ must be eliminated to prevent *acidosis*, a condition that can be deadly. The lungs remove excess H^+ from blood by means of chemical reactions that result in the release of carbon dioxide (CO_2) and H_2O in exhaled air. Kidneys also partici−pate in the buffering system by removing excess H^+ from the blood when forming urine. As a result, urine is an acidic fluid.

Common household products such as baking soda, household ammonia, and certain oven cleaners are bases.

Did You Know?

Blueberries, raspberries, red cabbage, and strawberries contain the pigment *anthocyanin*. This pigment is used as a natural dye for coloring yarns and can also be used as a crude pH meter. Anthocyanin is red when it is in solutions that have a pH of less than 4; this pigment loses its red color at higher pH values and appears blue-green or green. Aside from being an interesting pigment, anthocyanin has antioxidant activity and may provide health benefits as a result (see Table 1.3).

What Is a Chemical Reaction?

chemical reactions processes that change the atomic arrangements of molecules

Most molecules can undergo **chemical reactions,** processes that change the arrangement of atoms in the molecules. The elements that comprise the mol−ecules that react are never destroyed, but they combine with other elements to

Figure 4.6 **Chemical reaction.** A chemical reaction occurs when vinegar (an acid) combines with baking soda (a base). This reaction forms sodium acetate (a salt), water, and carbon dioxide.

form new molecules or compounds. When elements or compounds combine to form new substances, a synthetic reaction has occurred. The new substances often have physical and chemical characteristics (properties) that are quite dif−ferent from those of the reactants. Decomposition reactions involve the breaking down of molecules. **Digestion,** the process by which large molecules in food are broken down into smaller ones, requires decomposition reactions.

You can observe a simple chemical reaction by combining the reactants vin−egar (an acid) and baking soda (a base). As soon as the vinegar makes contact with the soda, the powdery baking soda disappears and a fizzy liquid forms (Fig. 4.6). This particular reaction produces carbon dioxide gas that forms bubbles in the fizzy liquid and sodium acetate. Thus, carbon dioxide and sodium acetate are two of the products that result when vinegar and baking soda react. Sodium acetate is a **salt,** a substance that forms when an acid reacts with a base. Table salt (sodium chloride) is actually one type of salt. Sodium chloride forms when an acid, such as hydrochloric acid (HCl), reacts with a base, such as sodium hydroxide (NaOH) (Fig. 4.7).

In recipes for baked goods that require baking soda, you will find an acid ingredient such as lemon juice, buttermilk, or cream of tartar (tartaric acid) included to react with the soda. The carbon dioxide gas that forms "raises" the mixture, giving it a light, airy structure after baking.

Metabolism

Metabolism refers to the sum of all chemical reactions that occur in living cells. *Catabolic reactions* involve breaking down molecules. Catabolism, for example, occurs during digestion. *Anabolic reactions* involve synthesizing new compounds. Repairing damaged muscle tissue after injury is an example of anabolism.

Enzymes

Living things contain thousands of chemicals, and life depends upon chemical reactions. However, many of these reactions occur slowly or do not occur spon−taneously. An **enzyme** is a molecule (usually a protein) that *catalyzes* (speeds up) a particular chemical reaction. Enzymes are recyclable; they do not become part of the products of a reaction, and as a result, one enzyme molecule can catalyze many reactions. Figure 4.8 illustrates an enzyme's action.

In general, the names of most enzymes end with −*ase.* Sucrase, for example, is the enzyme that catalyzes the reaction that breaks down the carbohydrate sucrose

$$HCl + NaOH \longrightarrow NaCl + H_2O$$

| Hydrochloric acid | Sodium hydroxide | Sodium chloride (table salt) | Water |

Figure 4.7 **What is a salt?** A salt forms when an acid reacts with a base. For example, sodium chloride (NaCl) and H_2O form when hydrochloric acid (HCl) reacts with sodium hydroxide (NaOH).

digestion process by which large food molecules are mechanically and chemically broken down

salt substance that forms when an acid combines with a base

enzyme molecule (usually a protein) that speeds up a particular chemical reaction

Figure 4.8 **Enzyme action.** In this reaction, the enzyme sucrase is necessary to break down sucrose into glucose and fructose.

Sucrose (table sugar) H_2O Glucose   +   Fructose

Sucrase (enzyme)

Food & Nutrition tip

Gelatin is an animal protein that dissolves in boiled water. As it cools, gelatin holds the water and thickens, forming a gel, a solution that takes the shape of its container. Pineapple, papaya, kiwifruit, and guava naturally contain enzymes that break down gelatin. Therefore, when using gelatin in recipes, don't add fresh or frozen forms of these fruits, because the enzymes will break down gelatin and the mixture will not gel. Heating destroys these enzymes; thus, you can make a molded gelatin salad or dessert that contains canned pineapple. (Foods undergo heating during the canning process.)

(table sugar) to its component simple sugars, glucose and fructose (see Fig. 4.8). Additionally, each enzyme usually has a specific action. For example, sucrase breaks down sucrose, but the enzyme does not affect lactose, the type of sugar in milk.

Enzymes are sensitive to environmental conditions, including pH, temperature, and the presence of certain vitamins and minerals. If the pH or temperature is too high or too low, the enzyme will not function. Raw food contains enzymes, but cook—ing food usually destroys them.

Concept **Checkpoint 4.1**

1. Define the following terms: *electron, proton, element, chemical bond, molecule, compound, solution, solvent,* and *solute.*
2. What is an ion?
3. Explain the difference between an acid and a base.
4. What is pH?
5. What is a chemical reaction?
6. What is an enzyme?
7. What factors can alter an enzyme's activity?

4.2 Basic Physiology Concepts

Learning Outcomes

1. Define *cell, tissue, organ,* and *organ systems.*
2. List the organ systems, identify major organs or tissues in each system, and describe primary functions of each system.

The human body is often compared to a complex machine, such as a car. Like a car, the body has numerous interrelated working parts and requires a source of fuel to operate. Additionally, the body has to be able to cool itself, eliminate waste products, and rely on lubrication to keep operating smoothly. Unlike most machines, however, the human body can make many of its spare parts, enabling the body to repair and maintain itself for long periods. When the body functions properly, this wondrous machine may be taken for granted and expected to perform optimally. Nevertheless, the quality of the fuel that powers the human body can affect performance, much like the quality of gasoline that runs a car.

Anatomy is the scientific study of cells and other body structures; **physiology** is the scientific study of how cells and body structures function. This

anatomy scientific study of cells and other body structures

physiology scientific study of the functioning of cells and other body structures section provides some basic information about human anatomy and physiology, including the organization of the body into systems. By learning about human anatomy and physiology, you may appreciate the complexity of your body and be amazed at the variety of metabolic activities that occur within you to keep you alive, physically active, mentally alert, and healthy.

The Cell

A cell is the smallest living functional unit in an organism. Your body has about 100 trillion cells that can be classified into numerous cell types. Each type of cell has a specific function. For example, muscle cells are necessary for movement, red blood cells transport oxygen, and certain white blood cells protect the body from disease—causing bacteria and viruses.

Most human cells contain several different types of **organelles,** structures that have specific functions (Fig. 4.9). The nucleus, for example, contains **DNA,** the molecule that provides coded instructions for synthesizing proteins. DNA enables the nucleus to control various cellular activities, including cell division and enzyme production. Mitochondria are organelles that play a major role in the generation of energy. Ribosomes are structures involved in the assembly of proteins. The nucleus, mitochondria, and other organelles are surrounded by a watery fluid called cytoplasm. Many chemical reactions take place in the cytoplasm, including some reactions necessary to make proteins. Each human cell has a plasma membrane that defines the boundaries of the cell and holds the cytoplasm in place. The plasma membrane also controls the passage of materials into and out of the cell.

organelles structures in cells that have specific functions

DNA molecule that contains coded instructions for synthesizing proteins

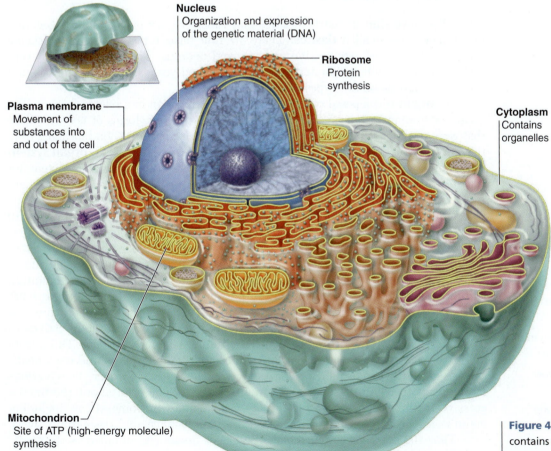

Nucleus
Organization and expression of the genetic material (DNA)

Ribosome
Protein synthesis

Plasma membrame
Movement of substances into and out of the cell

Cytoplasm
Contains organelles

Mitochondrion
Site of ATP (high-energy molecule) synthesis

Figure 4.9 Typical human cell. A typical human cell contains certain structures and various organelles, including mitochondria, ribosomes, and a nucleus.

Figure 4.10 Organization of the human body. Cells in the body are organized into tissues, organs, and organ systems. A living organism is a complete individual comprised of organ systems that function together.

Cell

Tissue
Collection of similar cells

Organ
Collection of various types of tissues with related functions

System
Collection of organs with related functions

Entire body

From Cells to Systems

Cells that have similar characteristics and functions are usually joined together into larger masses called **tissues.** There are four basic types of tissues: epithelial ($ep'-ih-the'-le-al$), connective, muscle, and nervous. The cells that line every body surface, including skin and the inside of blood vessels, are epithelial tissues. Fat, bone, and blood are types of connective tissue.

An **organ** is composed of various tissues that function in a related fashion. The brain, for example, is an organ because it contains different forms of nervous tissue that work together to interpret information from the environment, find meaning from this information, and signal responses, such as muscle movements. An **organ system** is a group of organs that work together for a similar purpose. The urinary system, for example, includes the kidneys and the bladder. Two major functions of the urinary system are filtering blood and excreting wastes in urine. A living organism is a complete individual life form comprised of organ systems that function together. Figure 4.10 illustrates how cells in the body are organized into tissues, organs, and systems.

All systems in your body must work together in a coordinated manner to maintain good health. When one system fails to function correctly, the functioning of the other systems is soon affected. The body's ability to maintain **homeostasis,** an internal chemical and physical environment that supports life and good health, is critical. Internal conditions such as body temperature and blood pressure normally fluctuate throughout the day, but the body strives to maintain such factors within fairly specific limits. Changes in the cell's internal and external environment can disrupt homeostasis, and sickness and even death can result if the abnormality persists. A healthy body, however, uses various mechanisms to regain its normal internal status. As you read about the nutrients, you will recognize how many play crucial roles in homeostasis, including maintaining proper body temperature, acid−base balance, and tissue fluid levels.

Table 4.2 lists each system's major organs or tissues and summarizes their primary functions. The following sections provide a brief description of each organ system.

tissues masses of cells that have similar characteristics and functions

organ collection of tissues that function in a related fashion

organ system group of organs that work together for a similar purpose

homeostasis maintenance of an internal chemical and physical environment that is critical for good health and survival

TABLE 4.2 The Organ Systems of the Human Body

System	Major Organs or Tissues	Primary Functions
Digestive	Mouth, salivary glands, esophagus, stomach, intestines, pancreas, liver, gallbladder	Digestion and absorption of nutrients
Cardiovascular	Heart, blood vessels, blood	Circulation of blood throughout the body
Respiratory	Nose, pharynx, larynx, trachea, bronchi, lungs	Exchange of oxygen and carbon dioxide
Lymphatic and Immune systems	Lymphatic fluid, white blood cells, lymph vessels and nodes, spleen, thymus	Defense and immunity against infectious agents, fluid balance, white blood cell production, absorption of fat-soluble nutrients from intestinal tract
Urinary	Kidneys, bladder	Elimination of salts, water, and wastes; maintenance of fluid balance
Muscular	Muscles	Movement and stability of the body
Skeletal	Bones, tendons, ligaments	Support, movement, protection, and production of blood cells
Nervous	Brain, spinal cord, nerves, sensory receptors	Thought processes, regulation and coordination of many body activities, detection of changes in external and internal environments
Endocrine	Glands or organs that secrete hormones (chemical messengers)	Regulation and coordination of many body activities, including growth, nutrient balance, and reproduction
Integumentary	Skin, hair, nails	Protection and immunity, regulation of body temperature, vitamin D synthesis
Reproductive	Gonads and genitals	Procreation (having children)

Adapted from: Widmaier EP and others: *Vander's human physiology,* 10th ed. Boston: McGraw-Hill, 2006.

Cardiovascular System

The major components of the cardiovascular ("circulatory") system are the heart, blood, and blood vessels (Fig. 4.11). The main function of the cardiovascular system is circulating blood throughout the body. The human heart is a four–chambered muscular pump that keeps blood moving through blood vessels. Blood contains red and white blood cells, nutrients, other substances, and *plasma,* the watery portion of the blood. Blood vessels form a network of tubes that help circulate blood throughout the body. **Arteries** carry blood away from the heart. Arteries branch into smaller and smaller vessels until they form **capillaries,** a network of tiny blood vessels with walls that are only one cell thick. The thin capillary walls enable nutrients and oxygen to move out of the blood and into cells, and carbon dioxide and other waste products to pass from cells and into the blood. After this exchange occurs, the deoxygenated (oxygen–poor) blood enters **veins** for the return trip to the heart.

After entering the right side of the heart, deoxygenated blood is pumped to the lungs, via the pulmonary arteries. In the lungs, red blood cells release carbon dioxide, a cellular waste product, and pick up oxygen from inhaled air. Cells need oxygen to obtain energy. Hemoglobin, an iron–containing protein in red blood cells, carries most of the oxygen in blood. The oxygenated (oxygen–rich) blood then returns to the heart via the pulmonary veins, so it can be pumped to the rest of the body's cells.

| Figure 4.11 Cardiovascular system.

Respiratory System

Lungs, the primary structures of the respiratory system, enable the body to exchange gases, particularly oxygen and carbon dioxide (Fig. 4.12). As mentioned in the previous paragraph blood circulates through the lungs, picks up oxygen from inhaled air, and releases carbon dioxide, a waste product that forms when cells obtain energy. By exhaling, you eliminate carbon dioxide from your body.

arteries vessels that carry blood away from the heart

capillaries smallest blood vessels

veins vessels that return blood to the heart

Figure 4.12 Respiratory system.

Lymphatic System

The lymphatic system helps maintain fluid balance, absorb many fat–soluble nutrients, and defend the body against diseases (*immune* function). This system includes a network of lymphatic vessels and lymph nodes (Fig. 4.13). As blood circulates in the body, some plasma leaks out of capillaries and into spaces between cells. The amount of fluid that surrounds cells must be limited; otherwise, tissue swelling would occur. Under normal conditions, the extra fluid, called **lymph,** collects in tiny lymphatic capillaries and is transported by lymphatic system vessels that eventually drain into major veins near the heart, where it enters the general circulation. The lymphatic system does not have a special organ like the heart that circulates lymph. Muscles in the walls of the lymphatic vessels and skeletal muscle contractions that occur during normal body movements squeeze lymph through the lymphatic system.

Urinary System

The urinary system includes the kidneys and bladder (Fig. 4.14). The major role of the kidneys is filtering unneeded substances from blood and maintaining proper fluid balance. As blood circulates, it passes through the kidneys, two bean–shaped organs that remove waste products as well as excess water and water–soluble nutrients from the bloodstream. This filtration process forms urine that moves from each kidney by a tube for storage in the bladder. Urine is mostly water, but it also contains dissolved substances such as urea, a byproduct of protein metabolism, and excess minerals and water–soluble vitamins.

lymph fluid in the lymphatic system

Muscular System

Muscles are the main organs of the muscular system (Fig. 4.15). Muscles enable movement to occur, and they also provide stability for the body. Furthermore, muscles generate heat that helps maintain normal body temperature.

Figure 4.13
Lymphatic system.

Figure 4.14
Urinary system.

Figure 4.15 Muscular system.

Skeletal System

Bones, tendons, and ligaments are the principal organs of the skeletal system (Fig. 4.16). These structures provide support, movement, and protection for the body. Additionally, bones store excesses of several minerals and produce blood cells.

Nervous System

The brain, spinal cord, and nerves throughout the rest of the body make up the nervous system (Fig. 4.17). The brain produces a variety of intellectual functions and emotional responses, including thoughts, memories, and emotions. The brain also controls and regulates many body functions, including hunger, muscle con—tractions, and physical responses to danger. Nervous system cells (*neurons*) transmit information and responses by electrical and chemical signals.

Endocrine System

The endocrine system is comprised of organs and tissues, including the thyroid gland and pancreas, that produce a variety of chemical messengers called hormones (Fig. 4.18). When released into the bloodstream, a hormone conveys information to cells that are specially equipped to respond (target cells). Hormones regulate a vari—ety of physiological activities, including metabolism, digestion, maintenance of fluid balance, and the maturation of reproductive organs that occurs during puberty.

Figure 4.16
Skeletal system.

Figure 4.17
Nervous system.

Figure 4.18
Endocrine system.

Integumentary System

Hair, nails, and skin, the largest organ of your body, are structures of the integ—umentary system (Fig. 4.19). Skin protects against minor injuries and invad—ing disease—causing agents, such as bacteria. Skin also helps maintain body temperature, primarily by perspiration.

Healthy skin needs many nutrients for its maintenance, including vitamin A, several types of B vitamins, and the mineral zinc. Each day, the dead cells that form the outermost layer of skin are shed, and new skin cells form that will eventually replace them. Because new skin cells are constantly being pro—duced, skin tissue has a high need for nutrients. Therefore, the early signs of many nutritional deficiency disorders often appear as skin abnormalities such as roughened, dry skin.

Reproductive System

The main function of the reproductive system is to produce children (Fig. 4.20). Adequate nutrition is essential for fertility, healthy pregnancies, and healthy newborns. Compared to women whose diets are nutritionally adequate before and during pregnancy, poorly nourished pregnant women have higher risks of miscarriage and stillbirths (infants who are born dead), as well as of giving birth to babies with birth defects and low birth weights. During their first year of life, severely underweight infants are more likely to die than infants whose weights are normal.

Figure 4.19
Integumentary
system.

Figure 4.20 Reproductive
system.

Digestive System

Your cells do not need food to carry out their metabolic activities; they need nutrients that are in food. The primary roles of the digestive system are the breakdown of large food molecules into smaller components (nutrients) and the **absorption** of nutrients into the bloodstream or lymphatic system (Fig. 4.21). Section 4.3 focuses on the process of digestion and absorption.

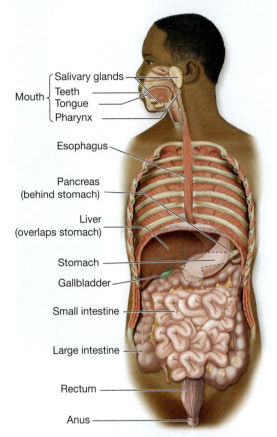

| Figure 4.21 **Digestive system.**

Concept **Checkpoint 4.2**

   8. Define *cell, organelle,* DNA, and *tissue.*
   9. Define *homeostasis.*
   10. List at least six of the organ systems that comprise the human body and indicate at least one major function of each organ system listed.

4.3 Digestion, Absorption, Transport, and Elimination

Learning Outcomes

1 Identify major organs of the digestive system, and describe primary functions of each organ.

2 Identify the accessory organs of the digestive system and the roles these organs play in digestion.

3 Discuss the overall processes of nutrient digestion, absorption, and transport; and waste elimination.

The mouth, esophagus, stomach, and small and large intestines are the major structures of the digestive system, which is often referred to as the **gastrointestinal (GI) tract.** In a living person, the GI tract is a hollow, muscular tube that extends approximately 16 feet from the mouth to the anus (see Fig. 4.21).[1] The length is longer in a *cadaver* (dead body), because there is no muscle tone.

It is important to recognize that many foods need to undergo some processing before they are eaten. Although some nutrients can be lost during food preparation, practices such as removing inedible parts or cooking raw foods often make them more digestible and safe to eat. Additionally, cooking food can enhance the absorption of its nutrients. **Bioavailability** refers to the extent to which the digestive tract absorbs a nutrient and how well the body uses it.

The teeth, tongue, salivary glands, liver, gallbladder, and pancreas are *accessory organs* of the digestive system that assist the GI tract in food digestion, nutrient absorption and distribution, and waste elimination. This section of Chapter 4 describes the digestive system, including accessory organs and their basic functions. More detailed information about digestion and absorption can be found in chapters that discuss specific classes of nutrients, such as Chapters 5, 6, and 7.

Mouth

Digestion actually starts in the mouth. The mouth controls the intake of food; teeth begin the mechanical digestion of food by biting, tearing, and grinding food into smaller chunks that are easier to swallow. The tongue helps direct food to the back of the mouth where it can be swallowed.

absorption process by which substances are taken up from the GI tract and enter the bloodstream or the lymph

gastrointestinal (GI) tract muscular tube that extends from the mouth to the anus

bioavailability extent to which the digestive tract absorbs a nutrient and how well the body uses it

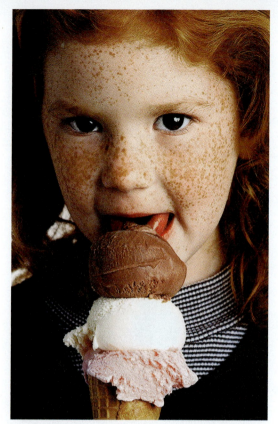

The tongue has regions that are more sensitive to a particular taste.

esophagus tubular structure of the GI tract that connects the pharynx with the stomach

epiglottis flap of tissue that folds down over the windpipe to keep food from entering the respiratory system during swallowing

Chemical digestion refers to the chemical breakdown of foods by substances secreted into the GI tract. As you chew, watery saliva from salivary glands mixes with food and lubricates it. Saliva contains the enzymes *salivary amylase* and *lingual lipase*. Salivary amylase enables a minor amount of starch digestion to occur in the mouth. Lingual lipase does not begin to digest fat until the food reaches the stomach. In addition to playing an important role in digestion, the mouth senses the taste and texture of foods.

When food comes in contact with saliva or other watery fluids, certain molecules in the food dissolve. When these chemicals are in solution, they stimulate sensory structures called *taste buds* that are located primarily on the tongue. Taste buds have specialized cells that help you distinguish sweet, sour, salty, bitter, and umami (*ew−mom′−e*) tastes. Taste buds relay information about the chemicals dissolved in saliva to a part of the brain that identifies the particular taste based on past experiences. The entire tongue can detect all five tastes, but certain areas are more sensitive to specific tastes than other tastes.[1] The tip of the tongue is most likely to detect sweet−tasting foods and beverages; the sides of the tongue are more sensitive to salty and sour items; and the rear portion of the tongue is more likely to detect bitter things than other regions of the organ.

What benefits do you gain from being able to detect various tastes? The sense of taste is important for stimulating appetite and detecting nutrients or toxic substances in substances that enter the mouth. Foods that taste sweet usually contain carbohydrates, major energy sources for your cells. Chemicals that elicit a bitter taste are often poisonous, so you are more likely to eat sweet−tasting foods and reject bitter−tasting ones. The sour taste can indicate the presence of ascorbic acid, more commonly known as vitamin C. You may like foods that taste tart or sour, especially when they are teamed up with sweet ingredients. Sodium ions stimulate your taste buds to detect a salty taste; a food that tastes salty may contain other mineral nutrients as well. The umami or savory taste is often associated with meat and is detected when certain amino acids stimulate taste buds.[1] Foods that produce the umami taste may be protein−rich; protein is another important component of a healthy diet. Recently, scientists have identified a protein in the tongues of rodents that appears to help the animals detect fatty foods. However, researchers have not determined whether human taste buds are capable of sensing the presence of fat in food.[2]

The sense of smell also contributes to your ability to sense the taste of food. As you chew food, it releases chemicals that become airborne and stimulate your nasal passages. Your brain combines such information with taste sensations from your mouth to identify foods' flavors. Thus, favorite foods may seem tasteless and unappealing when you have an upper respiratory tract infection and the inside of your nose is congested.

Esophagus

The **esophagus** (*eh−sof′−ah−gus*) is a muscular tube that extends about 10 inches from the back of the mouth, the pharynx, to the top of the stomach. The primary function of the esophagus is to transfer a mass of swallowed food into the stomach. The entrance to the esophagus is near the voicebox (larynx) and the opening of the windpipe (trachea). The **epiglottis** (*ep−eh−glot′−tis*) is a flap of tough tissue that prevents the food from entering the larynx and trachea (Fig. 4.22). When you swallow, breathing automatically stops and the food normally lands on the epiglottis, making it cover the opening of the larynx. These responses keep swallowed food from entering your trachea and choking you. Now you know why it is not a good idea to talk while you are eating!

Nasal cavity

Food mass

Tongue

Back of the mouth

Epiglottis

Esophagus

Larynx (Voice box)

Trachea (Windpipe)

Epiglottis

Epiglottis

Figure 4.22 What happens when you swallow? The esophagus transfers food into the stomach. The epiglottis prevents the food from entering the larynx and trachea.

Swallowing signals the GI tract that food is being eaten and stimulates **peristalsis** ($per'-uh-stall'-sis$), waves of muscular activity that help propel material through the digestive tract. In the esophagus, each muscular contraction is followed by a brief period of muscle relaxation. Peristalsis moves small amounts of food and beverage from the esophagus into the stomach (Fig. 4.23). Peristalsis is an involuntary response, which means the movements happen without the need to think about them.

Stomach

The stomach is a muscular sac that can expand and hold about 4 to 6 cups of food after a typical meal.[1] The **gastroesophageal sphincter** ($gas'-tro-eh-sof-ah-jee'-al\ sfink'-ter$) is the section of esophagus that is next to the stomach (Fig. 4.24). After food enters the stomach, this sphincter constricts, closing the opening between the esophagus and the stomach.

As food enters the stomach, certain cells within the organ secrete *gastric juice*, a watery solution that contains hydrochloric acid (HCl) and some enzymes. HCl helps convert chemically inactive digestive enzymes to their active forms and makes proteins easier to digest. The acid also kills many dangerous disease-causing microorganisms that may be in food. Note, as shown in Figure 4.5, that gastric juice is very acidic.

Stimulated by the presence of food, the stomach's muscular walls respond with waves of muscular contractions ("mixing waves") and peristalsis.[3] The churning movements mix food with gastric juice, and as a result of this mechanical and chemical activity, some of the protein and fat in food breaks down. At this point, the stomach contents are a semisolid liquid called **chyme** (*kime*). Although the stomach absorbs very few nutrients from chyme, a few drugs, including some alcohol, can pass through the organ's walls and enter the bloodstream.

Stomach walls consist of muscle proteins. So how does the stomach avoid digesting itself? Special cells that line the inside of the stomach produce a thick layer of **mucus.** Mucus is a slippery alkaline substance that protects the stomach from its acid and digestive enzymes. If the layer of mucus breaks down, HCl and gastric enzymes can reach the stomach wall, destroying the tissue. Such destruction can cause one or more sores (ulcers) to form. If the gastroesophageal sphincter does not function properly and relaxes while food is still in the stomach,

Contraction

Food mass

Esophagus

Stomach

| **Figure 4.23** Peristalsis.

peristalsis type of muscular contraction of the gastrointestinal tract

gastroesophageal sphincter section of esophagus next to the stomach that controls the opening to the stomach

chyme mixture of gastric juice and partially digested food

mucus fluid that lubricates and protects certain cells

Figure 4.24 **The stomach and duodenum.**

reflux, the backflow of irritating stomach contents into the esophagus, can occur and cause **heartburn.** For more information about factors that increase the risk of gastrointestinal tract ulcers and heartburn, read the "Nutrition Matters" feature at the end of this chapter.

The *pyloric* (*pie–lor'–ic*) sphincter, a ring of muscular tissue at the base of the stomach, controls the rate at which chyme is released into the small intestine (see Fig. 4.24). Following a meal, the stomach empties in about 3 to 4 hours, depending on the contents and size of the meal.[3] Watery meals such as soups spend less time in the stomach; fatty meals spend more time there. Obviously, larger meals take longer to empty from the stomach than smaller meals.

Did You Know?

When you eat foods or drink beverages, you swallow some air. Burping expels most of this air before it enters the stomach. If some air manages to enter your stomach and small intestine, it mixes with chyme and bubbles through it, often producing rather loud, gurgling sounds that can be embarrassing.

Small Intestine

The small intestine is a coiled hollow tube that extends from the stomach to the large intestine. The organ measures about 16 feet long, because of the effects of muscle tone in living persons.[1] The small intestine is "small" because the tube's diameter is only about 1 inch, about half the width of the large intestine.

The small intestine has three sections (Fig. 4.25). The first, the **duodenum** (*do–wah–dee'–num*), is only about 10 inches long. Within the duodenum, the acidic stomach contents mix with alkaline fluids secreted by the pancreas and gallbladder. This process neutralizes the acidity of chyme and enables enzymes that function in more alkaline conditions to work. The middle segment of the small intestine is the **jejunum** (*jeh–ju'–num*). Most digestion and nutrient absorption occurs in the upper part of the small intestine, primarily in the jejunum.[2] The last portion of the small intestine is the **ileum** (*il'–lee–um*).

A **lumen** is a hollow space in an organ or structure that is surrounded by walls, such as the lumen of the small and large intestines. Each day, the small intestine secretes approximately 1½ quarts (1500 ml) of watery fluids into the lumen. This fluid lubricates the intestinal walls, facilitating the passage of chyme. The cells lining the small intestine also produce mucus that protects the tissue from being damaged by chyme as it moves through the tract.

Many of the major chemical reactions that occur during digestion are *hydrolytic* (*hydro* = water; *lytic* = breakdown), because water molecules are necessary for the reactions to occur. Water in intestinal fluid contributes H^+ and OH^- ions. These ions react with certain nutrients and become part of the products. Sucrose, for example, undergoes hydrolysis in the small intestine (see Fig. 4.8).

The small intestine relies on peristalsis and *segmentation* to help digestion.[3] Segmentation involves regular contractions of ringlike intestinal muscles followed by muscular relaxations to mix chyme within a short portion of the small intestine (Fig. 4.26). The alternating pressure forces chyme to move back and forth within the segment.

As chyme passes through the lumen of the small intestine, enzymes break down the large compounds in chyme and the intestinal cells into smaller fragments

Figure 4.25 **Small intestine.** The small intestine is tightly coiled within the abdominal cavity. Although the appendix may have immune function, you can live without it.

Figure 4.26 **Segmentation.** Segmentation helps mix chyme in the small intestine.

and individual nutrients that can be absorbed. The cells also contain enzymes that are added to chyme and contribute to the digestive process. By the time chyme reaches the middle part of the ileum, most of its nutrient contents have been digested and absorbed. It takes about 3 to 5 hours for chyme to move from the duodenum to the end of the ileum.[3]

The Liver, Gallbladder, and Pancreas

The liver, gallbladder, and pancreas play major roles in digestion, even though chyme does not move through them (Fig. 4.27). The liver processes and stores many nutrients. This organ also makes cholesterol and uses this lipid to make **bile,** a substance that prepares fat and fat−soluble vitamins for digestion and absorption. Bile flows from the liver into the gallbladder, where it is stored until needed. When food and, particularly, fat are in the duodenum, the small intestine sends a hormonal signal to the gallbladder, and as a result, the gallbladder contracts, releasing bile into the duodenum. Chapter 6 provides more information con−cerning bile's role in digestion.

In the United States, many adults develop gallstones within their gallbladders. Gallstones usually consist of cholesterol; they can be small and grainy, like particles of sand, or as large as a coin (Fig. 4.28). When a gallbladder that contains stones con−tracts or a gallstone lodges in one of the ducts that carry bile from the gallbladder to the small intestine, it causes considerable pain in the right upper part of the abdomen. If the stone moves out of the duct, the discomfort ends, but in some cases, the duct remains blocked and bile backs up into the liver or pancreas. When this occurs, surgery to remove the diseased gallbladder is necessary to prevent damage to the liver or pancreas. After sur−gery, bile drips from the liver directly into the small intestine. Having excess body fat increases the risk of gallstones, so keeping your weight at a healthy level can reduce your chances of devel−oping the condition.

The pancreas produces and secretes most of the enzymes that break down carbohydrates, protein, and fat in the GI tract. Additionally, the pancreas secretes *bicarbonate ions* (HCO_3^-) that neutralize HCl in chyme when it enters the duodenum. This is a critical step in the digestion process because the enzymes that function in the small intestine do not work in acidic conditions.

When chyme is in the duodenum, its fat and protein content triggers the release of a hormone *cholecystokinin* (*co′−lee−sis′−toe−ky′−nin*) from small intestinal cells. Cholecystokinin enters the bloodstream and circulates to the pan−creas, where it stimulates the organ to secrete digestive enzymes into the duo−denum. Table 4.3 summarizes major functions of intestinal structures, including the accessory organs.

Absorbing and Transporting Nutrients

The lining of the small intestine is highly folded and covered by tiny, fingerlike projections called **villi** (singular, villus). Each villus has an outer layer of epithe−lial cells called *absorptive cells* (Fig. 4.29). Each absorptive cell has tiny, hairlike

Figure 4.27 Accessory organs of the digestive system. The liver, gallbladder, and pancreas play important roles in digestion. *Ducts* are small tubes that convey fluids, such as bile or pancreatic juice, from one structure to another.

Labels: Liver; Ducts from liver; Common bile duct; Pancreatic ducts; Gallbladder; Duodenum; Pancreas; Jejunum

Figure 4.28 Gallstones. Gallstones can form in the gallbladder. The stones usually consist of cholesterol.

heartburn backflow of irritating stomach contents into the esophagus

duodenum first segment of the small intestine

jejunum middle segment of the small intestine

ileum last segment of the small intestine

lumen open space within a structure such as the small intestine

bile substance that is produced by the liver to prepare fat and fat-soluble vitamins for digestion and absorption

villi (singular, villus) tiny, fingerlike projections of the small intestinal lining that participate in digesting and absorbing food

TABLE 4.3 Digestive System and Accessory Organs

Organ	Major Digestive Functions
Mouth	• Intake of food • Sensory responses to food • Minor chemical digestion of starch
Esophagus	• Transfers food from back of mouth to stomach
Stomach	• Mechanical digestion of food • Produces and secretes HCl • Begins chemical digestion of protein and fat • Secretes chemical messengers that regulate digestion
Small Intestine	• Digestion and absorption
Large Intestine	• Absorption • Elimination of waste
Accessory Organs	
Tongue	• Sensory responses to food, such as taste and texture • Facilitates swallowing
Teeth	• Break food into small pieces
Salivary glands	• Produce saliva
Liver	• Produces and secretes bile • Stores many nutrients
Gallbladder	• Stores and concentrates bile from the liver • Releases bile into duodenum
Pancreas	• Produces and secretes pancreatic juice

Figure 4.29 Small intestinal absorption. The lining of the small intestine is covered with villi, and the surface of each villus is covered with absorptive cells. Absorptive cells move nutrients from chyme into intestinal capillaries or lymph vessels.

microvilli at the end that faces the lumen of the small intestine (see Fig. 4.29). The intestinal folds, villi, and microvilli increase the surface area of the lumen, which helps increase nutrient absorption.

Absorptive cells complete digestion and remove nutrients from chyme and transfer them into capillaries or lymph vessels (see Fig. 4.29). This process occurs in a variety of ways. Some nutrients require the help of transport proteins or pumping mechanisms within the absorptive cell's plasma membrane to enter the cell. Other kinds of nutrients can simply *diffuse* into these cells. Such diffusion happens when the concentration of a particular nutrient is higher in the lumen of the small intestine than in the absorptive cells. In a few instances, a segment of an absorptive cell's plasma membrane surrounds and "swallows" relatively large substances, such as entire protein molecules. This process, for example, enables an infant's intestinal tract to absorb whole proteins in human milk that provide immune benefits.

While digestion is occurring, absorptive cells are shed into the lumen and added to the contents of chyme. The old cells are digested along with chyme. Newly formed absorptive cells constantly replace those that have been shed. The new cells can absorb nutrients from the older cells and recycle some of their contents. However, the small intestine's high cell turnover rate leads to relatively high nutrient needs for these tissues. If the nutrients needed for cell division are lacking, fewer absorptive cells can be replaced, and nutrient *malabsorption* (*mal* = poor) can occur as a result.

After being absorbed, water–soluble nutrients enter the villus's capillary and, eventually, the hepatic portal vein. This vein delivers nutrients directly to the liver, where many undergo processing before they enter the general circulation (Fig. 4.30). Most of the absorbed lipids are coated with a layer that contains protein, forming a **chylomicron** (*ky'–lo–my'–cron*). Chylomicrons move into a **lacteal,** a type of lymphatic system structure in each villus (see Fig. 4.29). Chylomicrons are transported by lymph and eventually enter the bloodstream via a vein near the heart.

About 7.6 to 8.5 quarts (8 to 9 liters) of water from ingested foods and beverages and the secretions of intestinal cells enter into the GI tract daily. Most of the water is absorbed along with other nutrients in the small intestine.[3] Any remaining water and the undigested material that reaches the end of the small intestine must pass through another sphincter before entering the large intestine. This sphincter prevents the contents of the large intestine from reentering the small intestine.

Cystic Fibrosis In the United States, cystic fibrosis (CF) is an inherited incurable disease that is usually diagnosed in early childhood. In CF, certain cells produce thick, sticky mucus that blocks passageways, particularly in the respiratory and digestive systems. People with CF often suffer from serious breathing problems and respiratory infections. The pancreatic ducts of an affected person may also become blocked by thick mucus, which interferes with the organ's ability to deliver digestive enzymes to the small intestine. As a result, the digestion of nutrients, especially fat, is impaired. To overcome the malabsorption problem, patients with cystic fibrosis can take capsules that contain pancreatic enzymes with their meals. The capsules protect the enzymes from being destroyed by stomach acid.

Intestinal villus

Capillary network within villus

1 Nutrients that dissolve in water, such as amino acids, glucose, and minerals, enter the capillary network of the villus.

Hepatic portal vein

Water-soluble nutrient

Water-soluble nutrient

2 Eventually, these water-soluble nutrients are transported from the GI tract to the liver by the hepatic portal vein.

3 The liver has many functions, including monitoring the blood's nutrient contents, detoxifying many harmful substances, making glucose, and storing various nutrients.

| **Figure 4.30 Nutrient transport from the small intestine to the liver.**

Large Intestine

The large intestine is about 5 feet long (in a cadaver)[1], and its major sections are the *colon* and the *rectum* (Fig. 4.31). Under normal circumstances, very little carbohydrate, protein, and fat escape digestion and absorption in the small intestine and enter the large intestine. However, the large intestine has no villi; therefore, little additional absorption other than water and some minerals takes place in this structure. As chyme passes through the large intestine, most of its water content is absorbed. As a result, the residue becomes semisolid and is called stools or *feces*. In addition to containing relatively large amounts of water, feces consist primarily of bacteria that normally live in the large intestine. Feces also contain undigested fiber from plant foods; a small amount of water and fat; and some protein, mucus, and cells shed from the walls of the intestinal tract. Under normal conditions, the large intestine converts chyme to feces within 18 to 24 hours.[3]

Elimination

Feces remain in the **rectum,** a lower section of the large intestine, until muscular contractions move the material into the anal canal and then out of the body through the anus (see Fig. 4.31). The *external anal sphincter* that allows feces to be expelled is

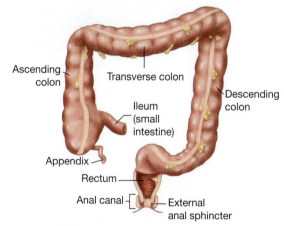

Ascending colon

Transverse colon

Descending colon

Ileum (small intestine)

Appendix

Rectum

Anal canal

External anal sphincter

| **Figure 4.31 Large intestine.**

chylomicron particle formed by small intestinal cells that transports lipids in the bloodstream

lacteal lymph vessel in villus that absorbs most lipids

rectum lower section of the large intestine

omnivore organism that can digest and absorb nutrients from plants, animals, fungi, and bacteria

under voluntary control, so a healthy person can determine when to relax the sphincter and have a bowel movement. Young children must reach the stage of physical and emotional maturity in which they are able to relax or tighten their external anal sphincter voluntarily. The timing of this stage varies but generally occurs in healthy children by 4 years of age.

Inflammatory Bowel Disease Inflammatory bowel disease (IBD) is the general name for a group of diseases that cause inflammation and swelling of the intestines. The inflammation disrupts digestion and nutrient absorption, and damages the intestines. Ulcerative colitis and Crohn's disease are the two most common forms of IBD. The "Real People, Real Stories" feature highlights Matthew Lang, a young man who has ulcerative colitis.

Microbes in Your Digestive Tract

The small intestine of a healthy person usually has few microorganisms residing in its lumen, particularly in the duodenum and jejunum.[4] On the other hand, the large intestine is home to vast numbers of various *species* (types) of bacteria. Under normal conditions, the different bacterial populations (the bacterial *flora*) maintain a balance with each other that is beneficial to their human hosts. Interestingly, the usual composition of the various bacterial species varies from person to person, because of dietary differences. Starvation, antibiotic use, and excessive emotional stress are among the factors that can upset the normal balance of intestinal bacteria and result in intestinal infections.

Intestinal bacteria can metabolize undigested food, make the vitamins K and biotin, which their human hosts can absorb, and produce substances that colon cells can use for energy. As a result of their metabolic activity, intestinal bacteria also produce gases that are expelled through the anus.

Large numbers of intestinal bacteria eventually become a major component of feces. Some species of these bacteria can be harmful if they enter other parts of the body or contaminate food. People should wash their hands after having bowel movements to reduce the likelihood of spreading dangerous microbes from their intestinal tract to others. Chapter 12 discusses microorganisms that cause common food-borne infections and ways to limit your exposure to them.

The Adaptable Digestive Tract

Sometimes popular diet "experts" claim that eating certain combinations of foods, such as meats and fruits together, is unhealthy because the food "rots" in the intestinal tract or one type of food interferes with the digestion of another type. Some people claim the human digestive tract is not designed for the consumption of animal foods and the undigested food blocks the intestinal tract. According to some of these sources, the blockages can be the size of a young child, weighing 40 pounds! Such information is simply not true.

A human being is an **omnivore,** an organism that can digest and absorb nutrients from plants, animals, fungi, and even bacteria. Additionally, the healthy human GI tract responds to dietary changes, such as alterations in the nutritional composition or amounts of food consumed, by increasing the production of various digestive enzymes. Consider this: How would people be able to survive in extreme environments, including deserts and permanently frozen regions, if they were unable to digest foods from a wide variety of sources? And finally, a healthy digestive tract does not become blocked by rotted or undigested food, nor does it store large amounts of feces.

REAL PEOPLE │ REAL STORIES

Matthew Lang

Matthew Lang is a college student who used to take the health of his intestinal tract for granted. When he was 20 and living on campus, he noticed a large amount of blood in his stools after having a bowel movement. Over the next few days, Matthew continued to pass blood in his bowel movements, and he had severe "stomach" cramps. He felt unusually tired, and his friends told him that he "looked pale." After visiting the student health center on campus, Matthew was told that he had *anemia,* a condition characterized by an insufficient number of red blood cells, the cells that transport oxygen in blood to other cells in the body. When the body's cells do not have enough oxygen, they cannot function properly. Matthew's lack of energy and pale skin color are among the signs and symptoms of anemia. His form of anemia was unusual in young men and a sign of chronic blood loss.

Within a few days after visiting the student health center, Matthew had a *colonoscopy,* a procedure in which a *colonoscope,* a long, narrow, flexible tube with a video camera on the end, is inserted into the anal opening and carefully guided through the rectum and colon. The camera enables a physician to see the condition of walls of the rectum and colon. Additionally, the physician can insert small surgical instruments into the colonoscope to perform *biopsies,* the removal of small pieces of abnormal-appearing or damaged intestinal tract tissues. These tissues are sent to a laboratory and studied microscopically for evidence of inflammation or disease.

According to the results of Matthew's biopsy, his colon was inflamed and slightly ulcerated. The young man was told that he had a type of inflammatory bowel disease (IBD) called *ulcerative colitis.* At present, there is no cure for ulcerative colitis, but the condition can be controlled with anti-inflammatory drugs, such as mesalamine (Asacol®). Matthew takes four mesalamine pills a day, and as a result of the treatment, he is able to function normally and feel good.

Medical experts do not know what causes ulcerative colitis, but emotional stress and genetic factors are thought to play major roles in its development. Matthew recalls being very "stressed out" during his sophomore year in college, and the ulcerative colitis was severe enough to send him to the student health center around midterm exams. He notices that his symptoms seem to improve when he is able to relax. Additionally, he has been able to link eating certain foods with "flares," bouts of painful cramping associated with ulcerative colitis. For example, he has determined that consuming red meat, carbonated beverages, and large amounts of cheese and milk seem to trigger his intestinal discomfort.

Matthew recognizes that he will need to monitor his intestinal health, maintain a healthy diet, and probably take medication for the rest of his life. "It's annoying to take all these pills every day, but I'm getting used to it," he said. "I know it's necessary, along with following a good diet for the rest of my life. Having ulcerative colitis has made me realize the benefits of a good diet. Even people who don't have IBD should improve their eating habits. They might feel better, too."

Concept **Checkpoint 4.3**

11. Describe what happens to a cheese sandwich after it is eaten and as it moves through the digestive tract.
12. Provide an example of mechanical digestion and chemical digestion.
13. Identify four different tastes.
14. Eliot choked on a piece of hot dog. Explain why choking can occur while eating.
15. What functional aspect of a healthy digestive system prevents food from becoming "stuck" in the tract?
16. What keeps stomach contents from reentering the esophagus?
17. List the sections of the small intestine. Where does most digestion and absorption occur?
18. How would removal of the pancreas affect digestion?
19. Describe at least two different ways that nutrients can enter villi.

4.4 Nutrition Matters: Gut Reaction

Learning Outcome

1 Identify some common gastrointestinal health problems, and discuss preventive measures and treatments for these conditions.

Even though you may be healthy, you have probably experienced occasional bouts of constipation, vomiting, diarrhea, or heartburn. After being miserable and uncomfortable for a while, you recovered and returned to your usual routine. This section provides general information about common intestinal problems, including peptic ulcers.

Constipation

Many Americans, especially older adults, think they are constipated if they do not have a bowel movement at least once a day. According to the American Gastroenterological Association, it is not necessary to have a daily bowel movement. Although the normal frequency of bowel movements varies individually, a healthy person should have a bowel movement at least every three days.[6] When bowel movements occur less frequently and/or are difficult to eliminate, the condition is called constipation.

Many factors influence the frequency of bowel movements. Lack of dietary fiber; low water intake; anxiety, depression, band other psychological disturbances; and changes in your typical routine, such as taking a long trip or having major surgery, can alter your usual pattern of bowel movements. Furthermore, constipation can result when people regularly ignore their normal bowel urges and avoid making a trip to the bathroom when it's not convenient.

Although occasional constipation is a common health problem, chronic constipation can cause discomfort and may contribute to the development of hemorrhoids and diverticula. Chapter 5 provides more information on these common conditions.

If you feel uncomfortable because your bowel habits have changed or you have hard, dry bowel movements that are difficult to eliminate, discuss the matter with your physician. In many instances, adding more fiber-rich foods to your diet is the first step to becoming more "regular." Chapter 5 provides information about dietary fiber, including rich food sources.

Diarrhea

Diarrhea is a condition characterized by frequent, loose bowel movements. Diarrhea occurs when more water than normal is secreted into the GI tract or the tract absorbs less water than normal. Most cases of diarrhea result from bacterial or viral infections of the intestinal tract. The infectious bacteria or viruses produce irritating or toxic substances that increase the movements (motility) of the GI tract. As a result, the GI tract propels chyme more rapidly through it, absorbing less water than normal in the process. Increased GI motility also enables the large intestine to eliminate the watery feces and the toxic material it contains rapidly.

Loperamide, a medication that is available without a prescription, can be helpful for relieving an occasional bout of mild diarrhea. Cases of severe diarrhea, however, require more immediate medical attention, because frequent watery bowel movements (stools) can deplete the body's fluid volume, causing dehydration and excessive losses of the minerals sodium and potassium. Therefore, treatment of severe diarrhea generally includes drinking replacement fluids that contain sodium, potassium, and simple sugars such as glucose. It's also prudent to avoid eating solid foods until the condition resolves. Prompt treatment of severe diarrhea—within 24 to 48 hours—is especially crucial for infants and older adults, because they can become dehydrated quickly by the loss of body water. In adults, diarrhea that is accompanied by bloody stools or lasts more than 7 days may be a sign of a serious intestinal disease, and a physician should be consulted.

Vomiting

Not long after eating something toxic or drinking too much alcohol, you begin to feel queasy or "sick to your stomach." You soon become well aware that your body has an effective way of removing the harmful food or beverage—vomiting. Although vomiting is an unpleasant experience, it prevents toxic substances from entering your small intestine, where they can do more harm or be absorbed. Vomiting can also be a response to intense pain, food allergies, rotating movements of the head (motion sickness), hormonal changes in pregnancy (morning sickness), and migraine headaches.[7]

Vomiting occurs when the vomiting center in the brain interprets information from various nervous system receptors concerning the physical and chemical conditions of the stomach, small intestine, and bloodstream. When a toxic chemical is detected, the center initiates vomiting by contracting the abdominal muscles, expelling the contents of the stomach and duodenum forcefully out of the body via the mouth.

Vomiting generally does not last more than 24 hours. Repeated vomiting, however, can result in dehydration, especially if it's accompanied by diarrhea. Treatment includes avoiding solid food until the condition resolves. Additionally, sipping small amounts of water or clear liquids, including noncarbonated soft drinks such as sports drinks, can help prevent dehydration. If the affected person is able to retain small amounts of fluid, then he or she can try to drink increasing amounts of fluid until the vomiting subsides completely.

Adults should contact a physician if their vomiting lasts for more than a day and they have signs of dehydration, such as increased thirst, decreased urination, and dry lips and mouth.[7] Contact a physician immediately if the vomit is bloody (looks like coffee grounds) or vomiting is accompanied by other signs and symptoms, such as confusion, fever, or severe abdominal pain (see Table 4.4). Children who suffer from vomiting and/or diarrhea are likely to develop dehydration more rapidly than adults who are suffering from these conditions. Signs of dehydration in young children include sunken eyes, dry lips and mouth, and decreased

TABLE 4.4
Vomiting Danger Signs

Contact a physician when vomiting:
1. lasts longer than a few hours (children under 6 years of age);
2. lasts longer than a day (people over 6 years of age);
3. is accompanied by:
   - blood in vomit (looks like coffee grounds)
   - signs of dehydration
   - diarrhea
   - fever
   - weakness
   - headache or stiff neck
   - severe abdominal pain
   - confusion or decreased alertness

urination. Contact a physician if a child who is less than 6 years of age has vomiting and diarrhea that persists for more than a few hours and shows signs of dehydration.

Heartburn

Many American adults complain of having occasional heartburn ("acid indigestion"), a gnawing pain or burning sensation generally felt in the upper chest, under the breastbone. This discomfort is not the result of a heart problem but is caused by the passage of acidic contents from the stomach into the esophagus ("acid reflux"). Because the esophageal lining does not produce as much protective mucus as the stomach, the acid quickly destroys the tissue, causing pain and, sometimes, bleeding. Many factors can contribute to heartburn or worsen the condition, including being pregnant; smoking cigarettes; having excess body fat; drinking alcohol; and consuming certain foods.

Gastroesophageal Reflux Disease (GERD)

Although many people think heartburn is a trivial health problem, frequent chronic heartburn can be a symptom of **gastroesophageal reflux disease (GERD).** Symptoms of GERD include frequent heartburn and may include nausea, gagging, coughing, or hoarseness. If not treated properly, acid reflux damages the lining of the lower esophagus and contributes to the development of esophageal ulcers (sores) (Fig. 4.32). Such ulcers can damage blood vessels in the wall of the esophagus, causing bleeding. Signs of bleeding from the esophagus and stomach include black, tarry bowel movements and iron—deficiency anemia. In severe cases, the loss of blood from a bleeding ulcer can be deadly.

gastroesophageal reflux disease (GERD) condition that can result when acid reflux damages the wall of the lower esophagus and causes ulcers

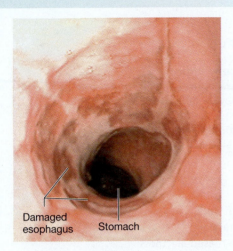

Damaged
esophagus   Stomach

Figure 4.32 Acid reflux damage. An endoscopic view of the esophagus near the opening to the stomach. The reddened areas are signs of damage caused by acid reflux.

People who suffer from GERD have a higher risk of esophageal cancer than people who do not have a history of this condition. If you or someone you know has GERD, typical dietary advice for treating the condition includes consuming smaller, more frequent meals that are low in fat; not overeating at mealtimes; and limiting intake of foods that relax the gastroesophageal sphincter, such as greasy foods, chili powder, onions, garlic, peppermint, caffeine, alcohol, and chocolate.[8] Additionally, you should wait about 2 hours after meals before lying down, because remaining upright reduces the likelihood that stomach contents will push against the gastroesophageal sphincter and move into your esophagus. Table 4.5 lists these and other recommendations for reducing the risk of heartburn and managing GERD. Taking over-the-counter antacids can neutralize excess stomach acid and relieve the discomfort of heartburn within minutes, but these products do not prevent heartburn. People who have GERD can take other medications that inhibit stomach acid production, preventing heartburn.

Peptic Ulcer

A peptic ulcer is a sore that occurs in the lining of the stomach or the upper small intestine. The typical symptoms of a peptic ulcer are deep, dull upper abdominal pain and a feeling of fullness that occur about 2 hours after eating. The pain results when most of the chyme has left the stomach

and the HCl acid that remains comes in contact with and digests the lining of the organ, forming one or more sores. It is not unusual for the sores to damage the wall of a blood vessel, causing bleeding; thus, untreated gastrointestinal ulcers may result in iron–deficiency anemia. Furthermore, an ulcer may erode through the stomach or intestinal wall and allow GI contents to leak into the body cavities, resulting in a potentially life–threatening infection. Therefore, it is important to recognize ulcer symptoms and obtain treatment early.

Physicians detect peptic ulcers by performing a clinical examination called upper endoscopy.[9] The first step of this procedure involves administering a medication that relaxes the patient. Then the physician inserts a special flexible scope into the mouth, down the esophagus, and into the stomach and upper small intestine. The scope is equipped with a video camera that transmits images of the lining of the esophagus, stomach, and upper small intestine to a screen that the physician views for the presence of ulcers, eroded areas, or cancerous tumors. The scope also enables the physician to use tools to treat areas of bleeding or remove pieces of tissue (biopsy) for microscopic examination.

At one time, medical experts thought excessive emotional stress caused peptic ulcers. By the 1990s, however, researchers determined that *Helicobacter pylori* (*H. pylori*), a type of bacteria that can live in parts of the stomach, was responsible for the development of most stomach ulcers. *H. pylori* infection makes the lining of the stomach more susceptible to being damaged by stomach acid. In addition to infection with *H. pylori*, other factors are associated with the development of peptic ulcers, particularly smoking cigarettes, heavy consumption of alcohol, and use of NSAIDs (nonsteroidal anti–inflammatory drugs) such as aspirin, ibuprofen, and naproxen. Table 4.6 lists these and other factors that increase a person's risk of peptic ulcers. Note that stress is still considered a risk factor for ulcer formation. People who have difficulty coping with excess emotional stress are more likely to develop peptic ulcers when compared to people who manage

TABLE 4.5
Recommendations to Reduce the Risk of Heartburn

1. If you have too much body fat, lose the excess weight.
2. Do not lie down within 2 hours after eating a meal.
3. Do not overeat at mealtimes.
4. Avoid smoking cigarettes.
5. Elevate the head of your bed 6 inches higher than the foot of the bed.
6. Do not wear tight belts or clothes with tight waistbands.
7. Learn to recognize foods that cause heartburn.

TABLE 4.6
Factors That Increase the Risk of Peptic Ulcers

Infection with *H. pylori*
NSAIDs
Alcohol consumption
Genetics
Smoking
Emotional stress
Excess acid production

their stress better. Having good stress management skills may explain why some people who are infected with *H. pylori* do not develop these ulcers.

Today, a combination of medical approaches is used for ulcer therapy. People infected with *H. pylori* are given antibiotics, as well as medications that reduce stomach acid production. This treatment is highly effective for combating *H. pylori* infections and healing peptic ulcers.

Current dietary approaches to treatment simply recommend avoiding foods that increase ulcer symptoms; often such foods vary individually. For example, a man who has a history of peptic ulcer may find peppery foods irritating to his stomach, while his friend who is being treated for an ulcer may be able to tolerate the same foods. Today, the combination of medical treatment and lifestyle changes has minimized the need for peptic ulcer patients to make drastic dietary changes.

Irritable Bowel Syndrome (IBS)

As many as 20% of adult Americans suffer from irritable bowel syndrome (IBS), a condition characterized by intestinal cramps and abnormal bowel function, particularly diarrhea, constipation, or alternating episodes of both.[10] Loose stools are often accompanied with mucus, and after bowel movements, the affected person feels as though elimination of stools was incomplete.

The cause of IBS is unknown, but certain foods and beverages, as well as emotional stress, may trigger severe bouts of the disorder. The colons of people with IBS may be more sensitive to nervous stimulation that the colons of people who do not have this condition.[10] Researchers are investigating the role of the nervous system in stimulating these abnormal intestinal tract movements.

Therapy is individualized and may include elimination diets that focus on determining which foods are most likely to contribute to IBS symptoms. Foods often eliminated include dairy products, carbonated beverages, raw fruits, beans, and certain vegetables, especially cabbage and broccoli. Treatment often includes learning stress management strategies, obtaining psychological counseling, and taking antidepressants and other medications. Although irritable bowel syndrome can be uncomfortable and upsetting, the condition does not appear to inflame the tissue of the large intestine or increase the risk of colorectal cancer.[10] For more information about this condition, visit the website www.ibsgroup.org or www.gastro.org.

Concept **Checkpoint 4.4**

20. Explain why diarrhea and vomiting are more dangerous for an 8-month-old baby than for a 20-year-old adult.
21. Describe at least three steps people can take to reduce their risk of heartburn.
22. Discuss at least three steps people can take to reduce their risk of peptic ulcers.
23. Describe common signs and symptoms of irritable bowel syndrome.

Chapter References

See Appendix H.

Summary

4.1 Nutrition: Chemistry Foundations

- Matter is composed of chemicals. Over 100 different types of atoms exist, and each type is an element. Atoms of elements may react with each other to form chemical bonds that hold the atoms together in a new arrangement called a molecule. Molecules that contain two or more different elements are called compounds. A solution is an evenly distributed mixture of two compounds. In living things, water is the solvent, the primary compound of a solution.

- Ions, acids, and bases play important physiological roles in the body. An ion is an atom or group of atoms that has a positive or negative electrical charge. Electrolytes are ions that can conduct electricity. An acid is a molecule that donates hydrogen ions (H^+); a base is a molecule that accepts H^+. Chemists use the pH scale to describe the H^+ concentration of a watery solution.

- Most molecules undergo chemical reactions that change their arrangement of atoms, forming new molecules or compounds. When elements or compounds combine to form new substances, a synthetic reaction has occurred. The new substances often have physical and chemical properties that are quite different from those of the reactants. Decomposition reactions, such as those occurring during digestion, involve the breaking down of molecules. Enzymes are molecules (usually proteins) that speed up rates of chemical reactions. Enzymes do not become part of the products of a reaction and, as a result, can catalyze many reactions.

4.2 Basic Physiology Concepts

- Anatomy is the scientific study of cells and other body structures; physiology is the scientific study of how cells and body structures function. A cell is the smallest functioning unit in a living organism. Cells that have similar characteristics and functions are usually joined together into larger masses called tissues. An organ is composed of various tissues that function in a related fashion. An organ system is a group of organs that work together for a similar purpose.

- The cardiovascular system involves the pumping action of the heart to circulate blood in blood vessels throughout the body. Arteries carry blood away from the heart; veins convey blood back to the heart. The thin walls of capillaries allow nutrients and oxygen to move out of the blood and into cells, and carbon dioxide and other waste products to pass from cells and into the blood.

- The respiratory system enables the body to obtain oxygen and eliminate carbon dioxide. The lymphatic system helps maintain fluid balance, absorb certain nutrients, and defend the body against infectious disease. The urinary system filters and excretes unneeded substances from blood and maintains proper fluid balance.

- The muscular and skeletal systems enable the body to move within its environment and provide support and protection for the body. The nervous system produces intellectual and emotional responses, and controls and regulates many body functions. The endocrine system produces hormones that convey information to target cells; hormones regulate a variety of physiological activities. Hair, nails, and skin are structures of the integumentary system. Skin protects against minor injuries and infectious disease-causing agents, and helps maintain body temperature. The main function of the reproductive organs is to produce children.

- To be healthy, all organ systems must work together in a coordinated manner to maintain homeostasis. When homeostasis is disrupted, the body uses various mechanisms to regain its normal internal status, but sickness and even death can result if the abnormality persists.

- Your cells do not need food to carry out their metabolic activities; they need nutrients that are in food. The primary roles of the digestive system are the breakdown of large food molecules into smaller components (nutrients) and the absorption of nutrients into the bloodstream.

4.3 Digestion, Absorption, Transport, and Elimination

- Digestion is a mechanical and chemical process that breaks down large food components into nutrients that can be absorbed. The mechanical aspects of digestion include the chewing action of teeth as well as involuntary muscular activity, including peristalsis. Chemical digestion includes the actions of enzymes and substances such as hydrochloric acid and bile.

- Digestion begins in the mouth with the mechanical action of teeth and some minor chemical action of salivary amylase. The esophagus conveys food from the mouth to the stomach, where it mixes with gastric juice and is referred to as chyme. The chyme moves from the stomach to the duodenum of the small intestine. In the small intestine, enzymes complete the process of digestion. In the small intestine, cells of villi absorb the end products of digestion and transfer them to blood or lymph. Any remaining undigested material, some water, and intestinal bacteria are eliminated from the body as feces.

4.4 Nutrition Matters: Gut Reaction

- Common gastrointestinal disorders include constipation, heartburn, peptic ulcer, and irritable bowel syndrome. Chronic constipation can cause discomfort and may contribute to the development of hemorrhoids and diverticula. Frequent chronic heartburn can be a symptom of GERD. People with GERD are at risk of esophageal cancer. Peptic ulcers can cause life-threatening bleeding. In addition to infection with *H. pylori,* smoking cigarettes, heavy consumption of alcohol, and use of nonsteroidal anti-inflammatory drugs increase the risk of peptic ulcer. Although irritable bowel syndrome is common, the condition does not result in inflammation of the large intestine.

Recipe for Healthy Living

Egg Salad

Egg salad is an easy-to-make meal or snack. This recipe makes about three ⅓-cup servings. Each serving supplies approximately 144 kcal, 8.5 g protein, 11 g fat, 252 mg cholesterol, 0.84 mg iron, and 190 mg sodium.

INGREDIENTS:

2 Tbsp peeled, finely chopped yellow onion
4 hard-cooked large eggs*
2 Tbsp reduced-fat mayonnaise
1 tsp pickle relish
dash of black pepper

* To hard-cook eggs:

1. Place the eggs in a small saucepan and cover the eggs completely with about 2 inches of water.
2. Heat water and eggs to a boil, then cover the saucepan with its lid, and remove it from the heat.
3. Allow the eggs to remain in the hot water for approximately 20 to 25 minutes (large eggs).
4. Remove eggs from the saucepan and cool by immersing in cold water.

PREPARATION STEPS:

1. Place chopped onion in small mixing bowl.
2. Peel hard-cooked eggs and discard peels. Chop eggs on a cutting board.
3. Add chopped eggs to onions.
4. Add reduced-fat mayonnaise and pickle relish to the egg and onion mixture. Blend together. Mixture should be moist.
5. Serve as a spread on whole-wheat crackers or on rye bread.
6. Egg salad is perishable, so cover any leftover salad and store in the refrigerator for no longer than a day.

Fat
Protein
Carbohydrate

ChooseMyPlate.gov

*2000 daily total kcal

Critical Thinking

1. When your grandmother forgot to buy her heartburn medication, she added a teaspoon of baking soda to a cup of water and drank the solution to relieve her "acid indigestion." Explain why this remedy works, even though physicians do not recommend it (baking soda contains unhealthy amounts of sodium).

2. Why would a person's stomach feel uncomfortably full several hours after eating a bacon–topped double cheeseburger, a large serving of French fries, and a milkshake?

3. Explain why the label for a multivitamin supplement recommends taking the pill with meals, particularly meals that contain some fat.

4. Miguel had a serious condition that required removal of the upper third of his small intestine. Based on this information, is Miguel at risk for developing multiple nutrient deficiencies? Explain why or why not.

5. Your mother complains of having persistent heartburn, but she does not think her discomfort is serious enough to be investigated by her physician. Do you agree or disagree with her attitude about heartburn? Explain your position.

Practice Test

Select the best answer.

1. Which of the following substances is insoluble in water?

   a. fat   c. calcium
   b. sugar   d. sodium

2. Which of the following substances has the lowest pH?

   a. plain coffee
   b. household ammonia
   c. plain water
   d. gastric juice

3. A _____ is a group of similar cells that perform similar functions.

   a. ribosome   c. cytoplasm
   b. tissue   d. system

4. Which of the following organs is an accessory organ of the digestive system?

   a. heart   c. liver
   b. kidney   d. bladder

5. Which of the following statements is false?

   a. Arteries carry blood away from the heart.
   b. Hemoglobin carries most of the oxygen in the blood.
   c. Cells need oxygen to obtain energy.
   d. All arteries carry deoxygenated blood.

6. Mechanical digestion begins in the

   a. mouth.   c. small intestine.
   b. stomach.   d. liver.

7. Two or more atoms that are held together by a chemical bond form a

   a. pH.   c. proton.
   b. molecule.   d. nucleus.

8. A salt forms when an _____ combines with a _____.

   a. electrolyte; proton
   b. acid; base
   c. element; pH
   d. enzyme; mineral

9. Chemical messengers in the body are

   a. enzymes.
   b. cells.
   c. capillaries.
   d. hormones.

10. Tiny, fingerlike projections of the small intestine that absorb nutrients are called

   a. lumen.
   b. villi.
   c. duodenum.
   d. organelles.

11. A lacteal is a

    a. lymph vessel within each villus.

    b. form of carbohydrate in milk.

    c. muscular structure that regulates digestion in the large intestine.

    d. specialized cell.

12. A _____ transports lipids in the bloodstream.

    a. sodium acetate

    b. cholecystokinin

    c. gastrin

    d. chylomicron

13. The stomach secretes

    a. salivary amylase.

    b. hydrochloric acid.

    c. bile.

    d. cholecystokinin.

14. Peristalsis

    a. is a common intestinal infection.

    b. interferes with lipid absorption in the small intestine.

    c. stimulates red blood cell formation in bone marrow.

    d. helps move food/chyme through the digestive tract.

15. Starch digestion begins in the

    a. gastric pouch.

    b. esophagus.

    c. mouth.

    d. gallbladder.

16. Which of the following practices increases the risk of peptic ulcer?

    a. chewing gum

    b. smoking cigarettes

    c. drinking orange juice

    d. eating a low−fiber diet

LEARNSMART®
ADVANTAGE

Get the most out of your study of nutrition with McGraw-Hill's innovative suite of adaptive learning products including McGraw-Hill LearnSmart®, SmartBook®, LearnSmart Achieve®, and LearnSmart Prep®. Visit www.learnsmartadvantage.com.

Answers to Quiz Yourself

1. The atom is the smallest living unit in the body. **False.** (p. 105)

2. The stomach produces gastric juice that contains hydrochloric acid. **True.** (p. 113)

3. Digestion begins in the stomach. **False.** (p. 111)

4. The human intestinal tract cannot digest certain combinations of foods, such as mixtures of simple carbohydrates and proteins. **False.** (p. 118)

5. Undigested food rots in your stomach, causing toxic materials to build up in your tissues. **False.** (p. 118)

CHAPTER 5

Carbohydrates

Quiz Yourself

Do "carbs" cause diabetes or unwanted weight gain? Would sweetening your cereal with honey be a healthier choice than using table sugar? Does eating sugary foods make children hyperactive? Check your knowledge of carbohydrates by taking the following quiz. The answers are found on page 163.

1. Compared to table sugar, honey is a natural and far more nutritious sweetener. _____ T _____ F

2. Ounce per ounce, sugar provides more energy than starch. _____ T _____ F

3. Eating a high-fiber diet may reduce your blood cholesterol level.
_____ T _____ F

4. The average American consumes 80% of his or her energy intake as refined sugars. _____ T _____ F

5. The results of clinical studies indicate that eating too much sugar makes children hyperactive. _____ T _____ F

5.1 Introducing Carbohydrates

Learning Outcomes

1. Identify the two major kinds of carbohydrates in human diets.
2. Explain how plants make carbohydrates.
3. Identify the major role of carbohydrates in the body.

When you are bored, excited, or in a good or bad mood, do you reach for some—thing sweet to eat? Can you imagine celebrating birthdays, weddings, or holidays without cakes, candies, or cookies? If you are like many Americans, you enjoy eating sweets and may even describe yourself as having a "sweet tooth."

Why do humans, even newborn infants, prefer foods that taste sweet? The pleasant and sometimes irresistible taste of sugar is a clue that the food contains **carbohydrates.** Carbohydrates are a class of nutrients that includes starch and table sugar. Without a steady supply of energy, cells cannot function and they die.

Carbohydrates are generally grouped into simple or complex forms. **Simple carbohydrates** ("sugars" or "simple sugars") include *glucose*. Glucose is a very important simple carbohydrate, because it is a primary energy source for human cells. Starches and most kinds of fiber are *complex carbohydrates*, because they contain many simple carbohydrate molecules. Plants make sugars, starches, and fiber by using the sun's energy to combine the carbon, oxygen, and hydrogen atoms from carbon dioxide (*carbo−*) and water (*−hydrate*) (Fig. 5.1). Some of the energy from the sun is stored in the bonds that hold the carbon and hydro-gen atoms together. Human cells can break down some of those bonds, releasing

carbohydrates class of nutrients that includes glucose, a major source of energy for the body

simple carbohydrates group of carbohydrates that includes sugars

Sunlight

Solar energy + Carbon dioxide + Water ⟶ Glucose + Oxygen

Carbohydrates
• Fiber
• Sugars
• Starch

Carbon dioxide

CO_2 **Oxygen**

O_2

Water H_2O

Figure 5.1 Carbohydrates. Plants use the sun's energy to combine carbon, oxygen, and hydrogen atoms from carbon dioxide and water to make glucose. As a result of this process, oxygen gas is released. Plants can use glucose to make fiber, starch, and other sugars.

high-fructose corn syrup (HFCS) caloric sweetener that is often added to food

monosaccharide simple sugar that is the basic chemical unit of carbohydrates

disaccharide simple sugar comprised of two monosaccharides

glucose monosaccharide that is a primary fuel for muscles and other cells; "dextrose" or "blood sugar"

energy that powers various forms of cellular work, including contracting muscles, making vital compounds, and building bone tissue.

On average, each American consumed about 75 pounds of *added* caloric sweeteners, in 2013.[1] Such sweeteners include **high–fructose corn syrup (HFCS),** as well as honey and table sugar. Added caloric sweeteners are "empty calo- ries" that offer little nutritional value other than simple carbohydrates to diets. Although people need some glucose for energy, consuming too much of the simple sugar, as well as the other macronutrients, can lead to extra body fat.

This chapter provides information about the major roles of carbohydrates in the body and rich food sources of carbohydrates, including simple sugars and complex carbohydrates.

Concept **Checkpoint 5.1**

1. What substances do plants need to make carbohydrates?
2. Explain why a plant will die if it is not exposed to light.
3. Why does a human cell need glucose?

5.2 Simple Carbohydrates: Sugars

Learning Outcomes

1 List the three most important dietary monosaccharides for humans.

2 Identify the basic monosaccharide components of sucrose, maltose, and lactose.

3 Explain the difference between a nutritive sweetener and a nonnutritive sweetener.

4 List three nutritive and three nonnutritive sweeteners.

Glucose

Fructose

Galactose

Figure 5.2 Monosaccharides. These chemical symbols for glucose, fructose, and galactose indicate the number and arrangement of carbon, hydrogen, and oxygen atoms. For simplicity, we will omit the atoms and just show the color symbol for each monosaccharide.

You probably are familiar with sugar as the sweet, white, granulated crystals often sprinkled on cereal or into iced tea, but table sugar is only one type of sugar. There are different types of sugars, including forms in milk, blood, and DNA, the genetic material in cells. The simplest type of sugar, the **monosaccharide** (*mono* = one; *saccharide* = sugar), is the basic chemical unit of carbohydrates. A **disaccharide** (*di* = two) is a sugar comprised of two monosaccharides. By combining monosaccharides, plants and animals can form complex carbohydrates.

Monosaccharides

The three most important dietary monosaccharides are glucose, fructose, and galactose. Figure 5.2 shows the chemical structures of glucose, fructose, and galactose, as well as the geometric symbols used to represent them in this text- book. The chemical names of carbohydrates, particularly sugars, often end in *ose*. Gluc*ose*, fruct*ose*, and sucr*ose* are sugars commonly found in foods.

Fruits and vegetables, especially berries, grapes, corn, and carrots, are good food sources of **glucose.** Glucose is the most important monosaccharide in the human body because it is a primary fuel for muscle and other cells. In fact, red blood and nervous system cells, including brain cells, must use glucose for energy under normal conditions. Thus, a healthy body maintains its *blood* *glucose* levels carefully. Glucose is also called dextrose and may be referred to as blood sugar.

Fructose (fruit sugar or levulose) is naturally found in fruit, honey, and a few vegetables, particularly cabbage, green beans, and asparagus. Since fructose tastes much sweeter than glucose and is easily made from corn, food manufacturers use large amounts of high–fructose corn syrup (HFCS) as a food additive to satisfy Americans' demand for "regular" soft drinks, candies, and baked goods. The body has little need for fructose; therefore, most fructose is converted into glucose or fat.

Unlike glucose and fructose, **galactose** is not commonly found in foods. Galactose is a component of lactose, the form of carbohydrate in milk. After a woman gives birth, special glands in her breasts convert glucose into galactose, which is necessary for production of lactose in breast milk.

Disaccharides

Disaccharides include maltose, sucrose, and lactose. **Maltose** (malt sugar) has two glucose molecules bonded together (Fig. 5.3a). Few foods naturally contain maltose. **Sucrose** (table sugar) consists of a molecule of glucose and one of fructose (Fig. 5.3b). **Lactose** (milk sugar) forms when a galactose molecule bonds to a glucose molecule (Fig. 5.3c). Although most animal foods are not sources of carbohydrate, milk and some products made from milk, such as yogurt and ice cream, contain lactose.

Sucrose

Although sucrose occurs naturally in honey, maple syrup, carrots, and pineapples, much of the sucrose in the American diet is refined from sugar cane and sugar beets. The refining process strips away the small amounts of vitamins and minerals in sugar cane and sugar beets. "Raw sugar," turbinado sugar, and some forms of brown sugar are not as fully processed from sugar cane as white sugar. These sweeteners contain a small amount of molasses, which contributes to their flavor, color, and nutritional value. Since refined sucrose has the reputation of being a "junk food," some manufacturers use creative names, such as "granulated cane juice," to disguise the presence of table sugar in their product's ingredient list.

Some people claim that refined white sugar is poisonous and honey is nutritionally superior to table sugar. However, these claims are not true. Table sugar does not contain toxic substances; in fact, it is almost 100% carbohydrate. Table 5.1 compares the nutritional value of honey with certain forms of sucrose. Note that none of the sweeteners is a good source of protein, vitamins, or minerals. The simple sugars in honey are not superior to those that comprise sucrose, and your body does not distinguish whether glucose or fructose came from sugar or honey.

A tablespoon of white table sugar is almost 100% sucrose; a tablespoon of honey has glucose, fructose, water, and a small amount of sucrose. A tablespoon of honey contains more protein and micronutrients than a tablespoon of white sugar, but the amounts are insignificant. For example, you would have to eat a cup of honey to obtain 1 g of protein, 2 mg of vitamin C, and 1.4 mg of iron. That amount of honey supplies over 1000 kcal! Although honey contains phytochemicals, substances in plant foods that may provide health benefits, the amounts are too small to make this sticky sweetener a valuable source of these compounds. Table sugar and honey are sources of empty calories.

fructose monosaccharide in fruits, honey, and certain vegetables; "levulose" or "fruit sugar"

galactose monosaccharide that is a component of lactose

maltose disaccharide comprised of two glucose molecules; "malt sugar"

sucrose disaccharide comprised of a glucose and a fructose molecule; "table sugar"

lactose disaccharide comprised of a glucose and a galactose molecule; "milk sugar"

(a) Glucose **Maltose** Glucose

(b) Glucose **Sucrose** Fructose

(c) Galactose **Lactose** Glucose

| **Figure 5.3** Disaccharides.

Did You Know?

Bees make honey by consuming the sucrose-rich nectar from flowers and digesting most of it into glucose and fructose. The bees regurgitate this material within the beehive, and eventually, it is collected by beekeepers for human processing and packaging.

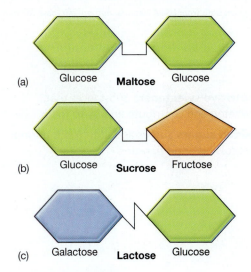

TABLE 5.1 Nutritional Comparison of Selected Sweeteners

Sugar/Syrup 1 Tablespoon	Water %	Kcal	Protein g	Carb g	Vit. C mg	Calcium mg	Niacin mg	Potassium mg	Iron mg	Zinc mg
Honey	17	64	0.06	17.3	0.1	1	0.025	11	0.09	0.05
White granulated sugar	0	49	0	12.6	0	0	0	0	0.01	0
Maple syrup	32	52	0.01	13.4	0	20	0.016	42	0.02	0.29
High fructose corn syrup	24	53	0	14.4	0	0	0	0	0.01	0
Brown sugar	1	52	0.02	13.5	0	11	0.015	18	0.10	0
Molasses	22	58	0	15.0	0	41	0.186	293	0.94	0.06

Source: Data from *USDA National nutrient database for standard reference, release 25.*

nutritive sweeteners substances that sweeten and contribute energy to foods

added sugars sugars added to foods during processing or preparation

Nutritive and Nonnutritive Sweeteners

Sugars are **nutritive sweeteners** because they contribute energy to foods. Each gram of a mono– or disaccharide supplies 4 kcal. **Added sugars** ("added sweeten–ers"), such as sucrose and HFCS, which is chemically similar to sucrose, are often added to foods during processing or preparation. In baked cereal products, added sugars contribute to the browning and tenderness of the food. Sugar also serves as a preservative by inhibiting the growth of molds and bacteria that would otherwise cause food spoilage. If one of the nutritive sweeteners listed in Table 5.2 is the first or second ingredient listed on a product's label, the food probably contains a high amount of added sugar. Table 5.3 indicates the amounts of added sugars that are in typical servings of commonly consumed foods and beverages. The following section provides information about other kinds of sweeteners.

TABLE 5.2 Sugars and Other Nutritive Sweeteners

Brown sugar	Glucose	Polydextrose
Confectioner's or powdered sugar	Granulated cane juice	Raw sugar
Corn sweeteners, corn syrup, high-fructose corn syrup (HFCS), cultured corn syrup	Honey	Sorbitol*
	Invert sugar	Mannitol*
Date sugar	Lactose	Xylitol*
Dextrose	Maltose, high-maltose corn syrup	Table sugar (sucrose)
Evaporated cane juice	Maltodextrin	Turbinado sugar
Fructose (levulose)	Maple syrup	
Fruit juice concentrate or concentrated fruit juice sweetener	Molasses	

* Alcohol forms of sugars

TABLE 5.3 How Much Added Sugar Is in That Food?

Food	Serving Size	Kcal	Approximate Teaspoons Added Sugars
Doughnut, cake, plain	3 ¼" diameter	226	2
Chocolate chip cookies, commercial brand	2 medium (50 g)	239	4
Sugar-frosted cornflakes	¾ cup	114	3
Chocolate-flavored 2% milk	1 cup	158	3
Ice cream, vanilla, light, soft-serve	½ cup	111	2
Chocolate candy bar with almonds	1.76 oz	235	5
Apple pie, double crust	⅙ of an 8" diameter pie	277	4
Snack sponge cake with cream filling	1 cake (43g)	157	4
Yogurt, vanilla low-fat	8 oz	193	4
Cola, canned	12 fl oz	136	8
Fruit punch drink	12 fl oz	175	10
Chocolate milkshake, fast food	16 fl oz	580	10

Source of data: Krebs-Smith SM: Choose beverages and foods to moderate your intake of sugars: Measurement requires quantification. *Journal of Nutrition* 131:527S, 2006.

Alternative Sweeteners

Some people try to control their caloric intake by reducing their consumption of foods and beverages sweetened with nutritive sweeteners such as sugar. **Alternative sweeteners** (also referred to as sugar replacers, sugar substitutes, or "artificial" sweeteners) are substances added to food that sweeten the item while providing few or no kilocalories. Alternative nutritive sweeteners include sugar alcohols: *sorbitol, xylitol,* and *mannitol.* Unlike sugars, sugar alcohols do not promote dental decay. Thus, these compounds are used to replace sucrose in products such as sugar–free chewing gums, breath mints, and "diabetic" candies. Sugar alcohols are not fully absorbed by the intestinal tract, and as a result, they supply an average of 2 kcal/g. However, sugar alcohols may cause diarrhea when consumed.

Nonnutritive sweeteners are a group of synthetic compounds that elicit an intensely sweet taste when compared to the same amount of sugar (Table 5.4). Thus, a very small amount of a nonnutritive sweetener is needed to sweeten a food, and nonnutritive sweeteners supply no energy per serving. Nonnutritive sweeteners may help people control their energy intake and manage their body weight.[4] Consumers, however, need to recognize that most "sugar–free" or "diabetic" foods are not calorie free. Furthermore, results of some studies suggest that artificially sweetened foods and beverages can promote excess calorie consumption. Why? More research is needed, but the taste of products that contain artificial sweeteners may interfere with a person's ability to regulate his or her intake of sugary foods and beverages.[5]

Food & Nutrition tips

Honey can contain spores, the inactive life stage, of the deadly bacterium *Clostridium botulinum* that resist being destroyed by food preservation methods.[2] These spores can become active bacteria within an infant's intestinal tract and produce a poison that is extremely toxic to nerves. According to experts at the Centers for Disease Control and Prevention (CDC), honey should not be fed to children younger than 12 months of age or used to sweeten infant foods because it may cause botulism poisoning.[3] Older children and adults can eat honey without being concerned about botulism, because the mature stomach produces enough acid to destroy the bacterial spores.

Honey and table sugar have similar nutritional value.

alternative sweeteners substances that sweeten foods while providing few or no kilocalories

nonnutritive sweeteners group of synthetic compounds that are intensely sweet tasting compared to sugar

TABLE 5.4   Comparing Nonnutritive Sweeteners

Sweetener	Comparison to Sugar/ Serving*	Brand Name	Kilocalories/ serving
Aspartame	160–220 times sweeter	NutraSweet®, Equal®	Nearly 0
Saccharin	300 times sweeter	Sweet'N Low®, Sugar Twin®, Necta Sweet®	0
Acesulfame-K	200 times sweeter	Sunett®, Sweet One®	0
Neotame	7000–13,000 times sweeter	Neotame	0
Sucralose	600 times sweeter	Splenda®	0
"Stevia," including stevia leaf extracts such as rebaudioside A	250 times sweeter	Truvia®, SweetLeaf®, Rebiana	0
Erythritol	60 to 80% as sweet	Nectresse™	<5

*Source: Position of the Academy of Nutrition and Dietetics: Use of nutritive and nonnutritive sweeteners. *Journal of the Academy of Nutrition and Dietetics,* 112(5): 739, 2012.

Figure 5.4 Warning label for people with PKU. People with PKU need to be concerned about their phenylalanine intake. Artificially sweetened foods that contain aspartame carry this warning on the label because aspartame contains phenylalanine.

The Food and Drug Administration (FDA) has approved the use of the nonnutritive sweeteners saccharin, aspartame, acesulfame−K, sucralose, neotame, and stevia extracts as additives to sweeten foods, as well as other products that may be swallowed, such as mouthwash and toothpaste. Nonnutritive sweeteners do not contribute to dental decay.

In the United States, the safety of nonnutritive sweeteners has been under public and scientific scrutiny for decades. In 1970, the FDA banned the non−nutritive sweetener *cyclamate* after research indicated that the substance caused bladder cancer in mice. In the 1980s, panels of experts at the FDA and the National Academy of Sciences reviewed the scientific evidence and determined that cyclamate did not increase the risk of cancer in humans. Nevertheless, the ban on this food additive continues in the United States. Although *saccharin* has been in use for over 100 years, its safety has also been questioned. Despite the concern, most of the scientific evidence indicates that saccharin is safe when consumed in typical amounts.

Aspartame, better known by its trade names "NutraSweet®" or "Equal,®" con−sists of phenylalanine and aspartic acid, two amino acids, the molecules that com−prise proteins. Some people must avoid aspartame and certain protein−rich foods because they have phenylketonuria (PKU) (*fen′−nul−keet′−en−yur′−e−ah*), a rare inherited disorder that results in abnormal phenylalanine metabolism. If an infant with PKU is not treated with a special diet, phenylalanine and its metabolic by−products accumulate in the child's bloodstream and cause severe brain damage. To alert people with PKU about the presence of aspartame in foods, the FDA requires manufacturers of products containing the nonnutritive sweetener to include a warning on the label (Fig. 5.4). The "Real People, Real Stories" feature in Chapter 7 is about a college student who has PKU.

Since its approval for use as a food additive in 1981, aspartame has been blamed for causing a variety of health problems, including cancer, certain immune system diseases, and chronic headaches. Despite claims to the contrary, no sci−entifically reliable studies have linked aspartame to any health disorder.[4] In 2006, results of a European study involving rats concluded aspartame increased the risk of cancer in the animals.[6] The European Food Safety Authority challenged the findings of this study when the agency determined the conclusions were not

TABLE 5.5 Acceptable Daily Intakes for Nonnutritive Sweeteners

Food/Beverage	Nonnutritive Sweetener	Amount
Diet cola	Aspartame	18 to 19 12-oz cans
Packets	Saccharin	9 to 12 packets
Lemon-lime soft drink	Acesulfame-K	30 to 32 12-oz cans
Diet cola	Sucralose	6 12-oz cans

Source: Mattes RD, Popkin BM: Non-nutritive sweetener consumption in humans: Effects on appetite and food intake and their putative mechanisms. *American Journal of Clinical Nutrition* 89(1):1, 2009.

supported by the data. After a review of the data, the FDA reported that the safety of aspartame has been studied extensively, and at the present time, no links to cancer have been found.[7]

Sucralose, sold under the brand name "Splenda,®" is made from a molecule of sucrose that has been chemically modified to escape digestion and absorption. As a result, sucralose sweetens foods and beverages without increasing their caloric value. Since the sweetener is not digested or absorbed by the intestinal tract, it is excreted in feces unchanged. During normal cooking and storage conditions, sucralose resists destruction by heat, a feature that makes it better for sweetening baked products than aspartame.

Some of the newest nonnutritive sweeteners are made from the leaves of the South American shrub *Stevia rebaudiana* Bertoni. For hundreds of years, people have used extracts of stevia leaves as sweeteners. *Rebiana* is the common name for the chemical in stevia leaves that is responsible for their intense sweetness. The FDA considers rebiana safe for use as an allpurpose sweetener.

Do nonnutritive sweeteners pose a danger to health? A group of international health and safety organizations, including the FDA, have established *Acceptable Daily Intakes* (*ADI*) for certain nonnutritive sweeteners (Table 5.5). According to the Academy of Nutrition and Dietetics, nonnutritive sweeteners are safe when consumed "within acceptable daily intakes, even during pregnancy."[4] Nevertheless, researchers continue to investigate the safety and usefulness of artificial sweeteners.

Concept **Checkpoint 5.2**

4. Identify the three most important dietary monosaccharides.
5. What are the chemical names for blood sugar, table sugar, milk sugar, and malt sugar? Which monosaccharides comprise each molecule of maltose, lactose, and sucrose?
6. What is the difference between a nutritive sweetener and a nonnutritive sweetener?
7. Parents of a child with PKU can give their child either a beverage sweetened with sucralose or one containing aspartame. Which drink should they choose? Explain your answer.

Figure 5.5 Starch and glycogen. (a) *Amylose* and (b) *amylopectin* are forms of starch made by plants. (c) The chains of glycogen are more highly branched than those of starch.

complex carbohydrates (polysaccharides) compounds comprised of 10 or more monosaccharides bonded together

starch storage polysaccharide in plants

glycogen storage polysaccharide in animals

dietary fiber (fiber) nondigestible plant material; most types are polysaccharides

soluble fiber forms of dietary fiber that dissolve or swell in water

insoluble fiber forms of dietary fiber that generally do not dissolve in water

5.3 Complex Carbohydrates

Learning Outcomes

1. Explain the difference between a simple sugar and a polysaccharide.
2. Explain the difference between starch and glycogen.
3. Identify rich food sources of starch, soluble fiber, and insoluble fiber.

Complex carbohydrates (polysaccharides) are comprised of 10 or more monosaccharides bonded together. Plants and animals use complex carbohydrates to store energy or make certain structural components such as stems and leaves. The most common dietary polysaccharides consist of hundreds of glucose molecules and include digestible and nondigestible forms.

Starch and Glycogen

Starch and **glycogen** are polysaccharides that contain hundreds of glucose molecules bound together into large chainlike structures (Fig. 5.5). Plants store glucose as starch, particularly in their seeds, roots, and fleshy underground stems called tubers. Rich food sources of starch include bread and cereal products made from wheat, rice, barley, and oats; vegetables such as corn, squash, beans, and peas; and tubers such as potatoes, yams, taro, cassava, and jicama. Sports drinks and sports or energy bars often include *modified starches* such as maltodextrin and dextrin. Regardless of its source, each gram of starch supplies 4 kcal.

The human body stores limited amounts of glucose as glycogen (see Fig. 5.5c). Muscles and the liver are the major sites for glycogen formation and storage. Although muscles contain glycogen, most animal foods (for example, meat or the flesh of fish and poultry) are not sources of this complex carbohydrate, because muscle glycogen breaks down soon after an animal dies.

Fiber

In addition to storing energy as starch, plants use complex carbohydrates to make supportive structures and protective seed coats that contribute to the fiber content of your diet. Most forms of **dietary fiber (fiber)** are complex carbohydrates comprised of monosaccharides connected by bonds that humans cannot digest. Cellulose, hemicellulose, pectin, gums, and mucilages are carbohydrate forms of fiber; lignin is the only type of fiber that is not carbohydrate. Since fiber is not digested, it moves through the human intestinal tract and contributes to the fecal residue that is eventually eliminated in bowel movements.

There are two types of dietary fiber, **soluble fiber** and **insoluble fiber.** Soluble types of fiber, such as pectins and gums, dissolve or swell in water. Insoluble forms of fiber, such as cellulose and lignin, generally do not dissolve in water. Oat bran and oatmeal, beans, apples, carrots, oranges and other citrus fruits, and psyllium (*sill'−e−um*) seeds are rich sources of soluble fiber; whole-grain products, including brown rice, contain high amounts of insoluble fiber. Table 5.6 provides information about the solubility of various types of fiber, effects of fiber in the body, and major food sources of soluble and insoluble fiber. Although the foods listed in Table 5.6 are rich sources of either soluble or insoluble fiber, plant foods usually contain both forms.

According to food labeling guidelines issued by the FDA, whole grains are the intact, ground, cracked, or flaked seeds of cereal grains (Fig. 5.6). Such grains may include wheat, buckwheat, oats, corn, rice, wild rice, rye, barley, bulgur, millet, and sorghum. If a "whole−grain" product is made from ground, cracked, or flaked cereal grains, the forms must contain the starchy endosperm, oily germ,

TABLE 5.6 Classifying Fiber

Type	Component(s)	Physiological Effects	Food Sources
Insoluble	Cellulose, hemicelluloses	Increases fecal bulk and speeds fecal passage through GI tract	All plants Wheat, rye, brown rice, vegetables
	Lignin	Increases fecal bulk, may ease bowel movements	Whole grains, wheat bran
Soluble	Pectins, gums, mucilages, some hemicelluloses	Delays stomach emptying; slows glucose absorption; can lower blood cholesterol	Apples, bananas, citrus fruits, carrots, oats, barley, psyllium seeds, beans, and thickeners added to foods

| **Figure 5.6** Whole grain product.

and fiber—rich bran seed components in the same relative proportions as they exist in the intact grain.[8] (Figure 1.11 is an illustration of a whole—grain kernel that shows the endosperm, germ, and bran components.)

Although fiber is not digested by humans, soluble and insoluble fiber provide important health benefits. Soluble fiber can help reduce blood cholesterol levels, and insoluble fiber may ease bowel movements. The "Carbohydrates and Health" section of this chapter provides information about the benefits of adding more fiber to your diet and practical ways to increase your fiber intake.

Table 5.7 lists common foods that are sources of dietary fiber. Note that only plant foods provide fiber; animal flesh contains muscle fibers, which are digestible proteins.

| Most plant foods contain both soluble and insoluble fiber.

TABLE 5.7 Dietary Fiber Content of Common Foods

Food	Fiber (g)	Food	Fiber (g)
Split peas, cooked (1 cup)	16.3	Beans, green snap, cooked (1 cup)	4.0
Black beans, cooked (1 cup)	15.0	Banana, sliced (1 cup)	3.9
Oat bran, raw (1 cup)	14.5	Almonds (24 almonds)	3.5
Kidney beans, canned (1 cup)	13.6	Apple, with skin (approx. 4 ½ oz)	3.3
Chickpeas, cooked (1 cup)	12.5	Strawberries, raw, sliced (1 cup)	3.3
Baked beans, canned (1 cup)	10.4	Carrots, raw (1 cup)	3.1
Kellogg's All-Bran cereal (½ cup)	8.8	Orange, raw (1 orange)	3.1
Green peas, cooked (1 cup)	8.8	Barley, cooked (½ cup)	3.0
Raspberries, raw (1 cup)	8.0	Prunes, dried uncooked (5 prunes)	3.0
Blackberries (1 cup)	7.6	Whole-grain bread (1 slice)	1.9
Kellogg's Raisin Bran (1 cup)	6.8	Romaine lettuce (1 cup)	1.2
Broccoli, cooked (1 cup)	5.1	Iceberg lettuce (1 cup)	0.7
Baked potato, with skin (approx. 6 ½ oz)	4.4	White bread (1 slice)	0.7

Source: Data from U.S. Department of Agriculture, Agricultural Research Service, USD Nutrient Data Laboratory: *USDA Nutrient database for standard reference, release 25,* 2012.

Concept **Checkpoint 5.3**

8. What is starch? What is glycogen?
9. What is dietary fiber? Identify at least two rich food sources of soluble fiber and two rich food sources of insoluble fiber.

5.4 What Happens to Carbohydrates in the Body?

Learning Outcomes

1 Describe the major steps involved in digesting and absorbing starches and sugars.
2 Explain how the body regulates blood glucose.
3 Explain what happens when cells do not have glucose to use for energy.

If you eat cooked oatmeal made with milk and sweetened with a little brown sugar for breakfast, what happens to the carbohydrates in these foods? The carbohydrates in oats are primarily starch and fiber; mixing milk and brown sugar with the cereal adds lactose and sucrose. Figure 5.7 summarizes what happens to carbohydrates in the digestive tract.

The small intestine is the main site for carbohydrate digestion and absorption, but a minor amount of starch digestion begins in the mouth, as **salivary amylase** converts some of the oat starch molecules into maltose. Starch digestion stops soon after the food enters the acid environment of the stomach.

In the small intestine, an amylase secreted by the pancreas **(pancreatic amylase)** breaks down the remaining polysaccharides in oat starch into malt—ose molecules. The enzyme **maltase** digests maltose into glucose molecules. The final products of starch digestion, glucose molecules, are absorbed into the intestinal bloodstream and transported to the liver via the hepatic portal vein. Under normal conditions, the process is very efficient and nearly all the starch is digested. The complex carbohydrates that remain are primarily forms of fiber.

The molecules of sucrose in brown sugar and lactose in milk are too large to enter the bloodstream directly from the intestinal tract. The small intesti—nal enzyme **sucrase** splits each sucrose molecule, forming one glucose and one fructose molecule in the process (see Fig. 5.7). Additionally, the enzyme **lactase** breaks down the lactose from milk into glucose and galactose molecules. Intesti—nal cells absorb the monosaccharides, and the hepatic portal vein transports them

salivary amylase enzyme secreted by salivary glands that begins starch digestion

pancreatic amylase enzyme secreted by pancreas that breaks down starch into maltose molecules

maltase enzyme that splits maltose molecule

sucrase enzyme that splits sucrose molecule

lactase enzyme that splits lactose molecule

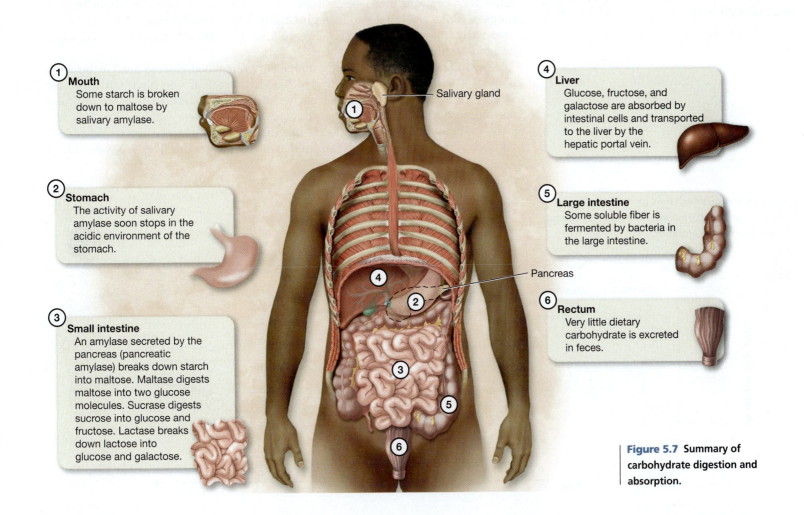

1 Mouth
Some starch is broken down to maltose by salivary amylase.

2 Stomach
The activity of salivary amylase soon stops in the acidic environment of the stomach.

3 Small intestine
An amylase secreted by the pancreas (pancreatic amylase) breaks down starch into maltose. Maltase digests maltose into two glucose molecules. Sucrase digests sucrose into glucose and fructose. Lactase breaks down lactose into glucose and galactose.

Salivary gland

Pancreas

4 Liver
Glucose, fructose, and galactose are absorbed by intestinal cells and transported to the liver by the hepatic portal vein.

5 Large intestine
Some soluble fiber is fermented by bacteria in the large intestine.

6 Rectum
Very little dietary carbohydrate is excreted in feces.

Figure 5.7 Summary of carbohydrate digestion and absorption.

insulin hormone that helps regulate blood glucose levels

glucagon hormone that helps regulate blood glucose levels

to the liver. The liver can use the simple sugars to make glycogen or fat, but if the body needs energy, the organ releases glucose into the bloodstream.

The fiber in oats is not digested by your small intestine, and it eventually enters the large intestine. The "friendly" intestinal bacteria that reside in the large intestine can break down (ferment) the soluble fiber and metabolize the fermentation products for energy. Soluble fiber is sometimes referred to as *viscous fiber*, because it usually forms a gooey, semisolid mass in the intestinal tract that is rapidly fermented by bacterial action. On the other hand, insoluble or fermentation-resistant fiber does not break down completely and, as a result, contributes to softer and easier-to-eliminate bowel movements.[9]

At one time, scientists thought fiber was a nonnutrient because it had no nutritional value. Recent scientific evidence indicates that the body, particularly the cells that line the large intestine, can use by-products produced by the bacterial metabolism of fiber for energy. According to estimates, a gram of fiber adds less than 3 kcal to human diets.[9] The average American who is 2 years of age and older consumes only about 16 g of fiber daily; therefore, fiber contributes relatively little to a typical person's energy intake.[10]

Maintaining Blood Glucose Levels

Glucose is such an important cellular fuel, its blood level is carefully maintained by hormones. Hormones are chemicals that convey messages concerning specific responses to target cells. The pancreas, a digestive system organ shown in Figure 4.27, contains beta cells, clusters of special cells that produce **insulin,** and groups of alpha cells that produce **glucagon.** These two hormones play key roles in regulating blood glucose levels. Figure 5.8 illustrates the effects of insulin and glucagon on blood glucose levels.

If you are healthy, your body maintains your blood glucose level at between 70 and 100 milligrams per deciliter of blood (mg/dl). If you have not eaten for a while, your blood glucose level begins to fall, you start to feel hungry, and your stomach growls. You may grab an apple or a cheese sandwich to eat, and as the carbohydrates in these foods are digested, the glucose from these foods is absorbed into your bloodstream and transported to the liver. As your blood

Figure 5.8 Regulating blood glucose. Insulin and glucagon are key hormones in maintaining normal blood glucose concentration.

glucose level begins to rise, your pancreas responds by secreting insulin into the bloodstream (see Fig. 5.8). Insulin helps regulate blood glucose levels because the hormone enables glucose to enter most cells.

Insulin also influences fat and protein metabolism. The hormone enhances energy storage by promoting fat, glycogen, and protein production. Another effect of insulin's action: you feel satisfied with your snack or meal and are no longer hungry.

If you ignore the hunger signals and do not eat, the alpha cells in your pancreas secrete glucagon. Glucagon opposes insulin's effects by promoting the breakdown of glycogen. This process, called **glycogenolysis** (*lysis* = break down), releases glucose into the bloodstream, which helps maintain your blood glucose level in the normal range (see Fig. 5.8). Glucagon also stimulates liver and kidney cells to produce glucose from certain *amino acids*, the basic molecules that make up proteins. Furthermore, glucagon stimulates **lipolysis** (*lipo* = fat), the breakdown of triglyceride (fat) into *glycerol* and *fatty acids*. As a result, glycerol and fatty acids rapidly enter into the bloodstream. The liver uses glycerol to produce glucose, and most cells, including muscle cells, can metabolize fatty acids for energy. Although the body can convert certain amino acids into glucose, it cannot use fatty acids to make glucose.

What happens to glucose? Its fate depends on the state of your body. If your muscles and other cells that use glucose need energy, glucose enters the cells and is metabolized for energy. When you are well fed and resting, your body stores the extra glucose as glycogen. When glycogen storage reaches maximum capacity, your liver can convert some excess glucose into fat and releases it into the bloodstream. Adipose (*ad'–eh–pose*) (fat) cells remove and store the fat.

Glucose for Energy

Cells metabolize glucose to release the energy stored in the molecule's chemical bonds. As a result of this process, cells form carbon dioxide and water (Fig. 5.9). Glucose is a primary fuel for the body's cells. Furthermore, red blood cells as well as brain and other nervous system cells burn mostly glucose for energy.

Cells need a small amount of glucose to metabolize fat for energy properly. When a person has poorly controlled diabetes, is fasting or starving, or follows a very low–carbohydrate/high–protein diet (the Atkins diet, for example), his or her cells must use greater–than–normal amounts of fat for energy. Under these conditions, there is not enough glucose available for cells to metabolize the fat efficiently, and excessive amounts of *ketone bodies* ("ketones") form as a result. **Ketone bodies** are chemicals that result from the incomplete breakdown of fat. Muscle and brain cells can use ketone bodies for energy, but a condition commonly called *ketosis* occurs when these compounds accumulate in the blood. In severe cases, the excess ketone bodies cause the blood to become acidic, and **ketoacidosis** results. If not treated, ketoacidosis can cause loss of consciousness and even death. The "Type 1 Diabetes" section of this chapter provides more information about ketoacidosis.

The Recommended Dietary Allowance (RDA) for carbohydrate is 130 g/day.[9] This amount of carbohydrate is enough to prevent ketosis. (The RDAs and other DRIs were discussed in Chapter 3.) To estimate your daily carbohydrate intake, complete the Personal Dietary Analysis at the end of this chapter.

Under normal conditions, human cells obtain a small proportion of their energy needs by converting certain amino acids from proteins into glucose. Starvation, however, dramatically alters the body's energy metabolism. Starvation diets lack sources of energy such as glucose and amino acids. The body, however, needs glucose to fuel vital activities such as breathing, transmitting nervous impulses, and pumping blood. To meet the body's energy needs, the starving person's skeletal muscles

glycogenolysis glycogen breakdown

lipolysis fat breakdown

ketone bodies chemicals that result from incomplete fat breakdown

ketoacidosis condition that occurs when the body forms excessive ketone bodies

Glucose + Oxygen → Carbon dioxide + Water + Energy

$$C_6H_{12}O_6 + 6O_2 \longrightarrow 6CO_2 + 6H_2O + Energy$$

Figure 5.9 Releasing energy from glucose. Cells use oxygen to release the energy stored in glucose. As a result of this process, cells produce carbon dioxide and water.

sacrifice components of their proteins for glucose production. Using muscle proteins for energy extends the starving person's survival time, but results in muscle wasting, weakness, and eventually, death. Chapter 7 provides information about proteins.

Concept **Checkpoint 5.4**

10. Sherita ate some whole-wheat crackers with grape jelly for a snack. As this snack passed through her digestive tract, discuss what happened to the starch, sucrose, and fiber in the food.

11. What effects do insulin and glucagon have on blood glucose levels?

12. What is a ketone body? Under what conditions does the body form excessive ketone bodies?

5.5 Carbohydrate Consumption Patterns

Learning Outcomes

1 Identify the primary source of added sugars in American diets.

2 List three practical ways to reduce a person's added sugar consumption.

In developing nations, millions of people rely on diets that supply 70% or more of energy from relatively unprocessed carbohydrates, especially complex carbo—hydrates from whole grains, beans, potatoes, corn, and other starchy vegetables. In industrialized nations, people tend to eat more highly refined starches and added sugars. Nutritionally adequate diets should provide 45 to 65% of total energy from carbohydrates.[9] The typical diet of Americans, 2 years of age and older supplies about 52% of calories from carbohydrates, much of which is sugars added to foods during processing (Fig. 5.10).

According to MyPlate, discussed in Chapter 3, added sugars are grouped with solid fats as empty calories. Adults only have about 120 to 330 empty calories allowed in their personal dietary plans. For example, if your individual dietary plan indicates that you need 2000 kcal daily, then at least 1740 kcal will need to be "spent" consuming foods rich in essential nutrients.[11] The 260 kcal that remain may be depleted by eating foods with added sugars.

In 2012, the average American consumed about 22 teaspoons of added sugars per day, which is 18% of the energy in a diet that supplies 2000 kcal/day.[1] Accord—ing to the Dietary Guidelines, people who follow a 2000 kcal/day diet should limit their intake of added sugars to no more than 12 teaspoons per day (about 200 kcal).

A 12—ounce can of a cola—flavored, sugar—sweetened soft drink contains about 33 g of HFCS, a refined sugar.[12] Each gram of sugar supplies 4 kcal, so this soft drink contributes about 132 kcal to the diet. By drinking only one can of the cola, a person who needs 2000 kcal daily will meet two—thirds of his or her daily limit for the intake of added sugars.

A 12—ounce serving of 100% orange juice supplies about the same amount of sugar as 12 ounces of a sugar—sweetened cola. Because they both contain simple sugars, should you drink regular soft drinks instead of fruit juices? Unlike colas and other soft drinks, 100% fruit juices, such as orange, grapefruit, and cranberry juice, contribute water—soluble vitamins and antioxidant phytochemicals to your diet. According to MyPlate, adults should consume 1 ½ to 2 cups of fruit or fruit equivalents each day.

Average Percentage of Calories per Person (One Day)

33% Fat
15% Protein
52% Carbohydrate
23% Sugars
29% Complex Carbohydrates

Figure 5.10 Average macronutrient intakes. This graph shows the average American's intake of macronutrients as percentages of total kilocalories from macronutrients (2081) on one day in 2009–2010. (Percentage of total energy from alcohol is not included.)
Source: Data from U.S. Department of Agriculture. Agricultural Research Service: *NHANES, 2009–2010, What we eat in America.* Table 1: Nutrient intakes from food: Mean amounts consumed per individual, by gender and age, in the United States, 2009–2010. http://www.ars.usda.gov/SP2UserFiles/Place/12355000/pdf/0910/Table_1_NIN_GEN_09.pdf. Accessed July 30, 2014

The main source of added sugars in Americans' diets is sugar—sweetened beverages, which include carbonated "regular" soft drinks, fruit "ades," flavored vitamin—water drinks, and energy drinks.[13] Although energy drink consumption has increased, carbonated soft drink consumption has declined since 1999–2000. In 2013, however, the average American drank about 42 gallons of carbonated soft drinks, or a little over 15 fluid ounces of these beverages daily, most of which are sweetened with refined sugars.[14] How many fluid ounces of energy drinks and/or sugar—sweetened soft drinks do you consume each day?

Reducing Your Intake of Refined Carbohydrates

Regular soft drinks, energy drinks, cookies, chips, and many other types of processed snack foods contain large amounts of refined carbohydrates, including added sugars. Such foods may satisfy your hunger and thirst, but they may be crowding out more nutritious items from your diet. If you frequently purchase foods and beverages from vending machines, convenience stores, or fast—food restaurants, you are probably eating unhealthy amounts of refined carbohydrates. Some fast—food restaurants and college cafeterias sell yogurt, fresh fruit, and fat—free or low—fat milk as well as unsweetened fruit juices. With a little advance planning, you can prepare your own portable, tasty, and nutritious snacks. For example, place whole fresh fruit or small plastic containers filled with chunks of fresh fruit and pieces of vegetables into your purse or backpack to eat during the day. At home, keep a bowl of fresh grapes, apples, bananas, or other easy—to—eat fruit available for handy snacks, and eat fresh fruit for dessert. Most fruits contain a variety of antioxidants, and they have less fat and more fiber, vitamins, and minerals than pastries or chips.

Food & Nutrition tips

- Replace soft drinks with a naturally calorie-free thirst-quencher: plain water.
- Make plain water more interesting to drink by adding to it a slice of lemon or lime, or a few fresh or frozen berries.
- Add 1 part club soda to 1 part orange or other 100% fruit juice to make a refreshing carbonated drink.
- Read the label for information about juice content when selecting a fruit juice product. Fruit "drinks," "punches," "blends," "cocktails," or "ades" often contain added sugars and only 10% fruit juice.
- Beverage descriptors such as "100% juice" or "pure juice" can be misleading. Read the ingredient list on the label to determine the types of juices used to prepare the product.

Concept **Checkpoint 5.5**

13. What are the main sources of added sugars in American diets?

14. Instead of drinking orange juice, should you choose a beverage called "Orange-Ade"? Explain why or why not.

5.6 Understanding Nutrient Labeling: Carbohydrates and Fiber

Learning Outcome

1 Compare carbohydrate contents of packaged foods by using the Nutrition Facts panel.

Consumers can learn how much total carbohydrate, sugars, and dietary fiber are in packaged foods and beverages by reading the Nutrition Facts panel of a food label. As indicated in Figure 5.11, total grams of carbohydrate in a slice (one serving) of whole—wheat bread is listed, and under it, grams of fiber and sugar. Food labels for high—fiber products, such as whole—grain cereals, may indicate amounts of soluble and insoluble fiber in a serving of the product. In 2014, the FDA proposed a new Nutrition Facts panel that would provide information about the amount of added sugars in foods (see Fig. 3.9b).

According to the label shown in Figure 5.11, 17 g of carbohydrate are in one serving (a slice) of the bread; of this amount, sugars contribute 3 g and

Figure 5.11 Using the Nutrition Facts panel (February 2016). This Nutrition Facts panel is from a package of whole-wheat bread.

fiber supplies 2 g. How can you estimate the grams of starch in the serving of bread? In this example, add the number of grams of sugar with that of fiber and subtract this amount from grams of total carbohydrates, and you will find that starch comprises 12 g of the carbohydrate in the slice of whole—wheat bread. If you are interested in the types of sugars used to make a product, read the ingredient list at the bottom of the panel. In this product, there are three sources of sugar. Can you identify them? Check the nutritive sweeteners listed in Table 5.2 to see if your answers are correct.

Concept **Checkpoint 5.6**

15. According to the Nutrition Facts panel, a serving of ready-to-eat cereal contains 44 g of total carbohydrate, 5 g of dietary fiber, and 10 g of sugars. Estimate the grams of starch in the serving of the cereal.

5.7 Carbohydrates and Health

Learning Outcomes

1 Explain why carbohydrates are not necessarily fattening.

2 Discuss differences between type 1 and type 2 diabetes, including treatments.

3 List at least three signs or symptoms of diabetes.

4 List at least four risk factors for developing type 2 diabetes and ways to reduce the likelihood of developing the disease.

5 List at least four serious health problems associated with poorly controlled diabetes, including poorly controlled diabetes during pregnancy.

6 Compare hyperglycemia with hypoglycemia, and discuss ways to reduce the risk of reactive hypoglycemia.

7 Identify the primary signs of metabolic syndrome, the impact the condition has on health, and how one can reduce the risk of developing the syndrome.

8 Explain the difference between lactose intolerance and milk allergy.

9 Discuss the health benefits of including fiber-rich foods in one's diet.

Carbohydrates seem to get a lot of "bad press." Promoters of low—carbohydrate/high—protein diets often blame sugars and starches for causing unwanted weight gain and diabetes. Many Americans think consuming sugary foods causes depression and hyperactive behavior. On the other hand, "carbs" are welcomed by athletes as an inexpensive and efficient source of energy. What have scientists learned about the roles of carbohydrates in health?

Are Carbohydrates Fattening?

Americans are fatter now than they were 20 years ago. To lose the excess weight, many people follow low—carbohydrate diets, such as the Atkins diet or the Paleo diet. Are carbohydrates responsible for the epidemic of excess body fat in the United States? Are low—carbohydrate diets useful for weight loss?

"Calories do count," because people gain body fat when their intake of food energy from macronutrients and the nonnutrient alcohol exceeds their output of energy for various physiological needs. Regardless of whether people eat a low–carbohydrate, high–fat, or high–protein diet, they will maintain their weight as long as their energy intake matches their energy output.

Foods that contain large amounts of refined carbohydrates, however, do not satisfy hunger as well as those that contain more protein or fat. As a result, a person may become hungrier sooner after eating a meal or snack that contains a lot of added sugars and refined starches than if he or she ate a high–protein, high–fat meal or snack. Thus, people following a high–protein, high–fat diet can lose weight in the short term, because the diet keeps their appetite under control by reducing hunger. On the other hand, diets in which carbohydrates supply more than 70% of a person's energy needs also result in weight loss, particularly when the diets include foods that are rich in fiber and contain plenty of unrefined starches.[15] People following such high–carbohydrate diets generally eat less, because fiber–rich foods tend to be more filling than similar amounts of food that contain a lot of refined carbohydrates.[16]

Metabolism plays a major role in the development of obesity, a chronic health condition characterized by unhealthy amounts of body fat. When a person consumes excess carbohydrate, his or her body converts some of the glucose into fat, but much of the excess is "burned" as a biological fuel. As a result, dietary fat is spared from being used as a fuel and stored in fat cells.[17] Thus, eating too much carbohydrate indirectly contributes to excess body fat.

Combining Carbohydrate with Fat

Foods that contain a lot of added sugars and fats tend to be energy dense. Thus, people can reduce their energy intake by eating fewer energy–dense foods.[18] Fats supply 9 kcal/g compared to only 4 kcal/g of carbohydrates, so adding even small amounts of fat to food can dramatically increase its energy content. People, however, tend to blame carbohydrates for their unwanted weight gain because starches and sugars are often combined with hidden fats such as butter, oil, or shortening (a solid fat) in processed foods. Fats make foods taste rich, creamy, and difficult to resist. Moreover, the sweet taste of sugar masks the bland taste of fat. Although you would not consider eating spoonfuls of plain sugar, flour, shortening, or butter, your mouth waters at the sight of candy bars, fruit pies, doughnuts, and other baked or fried foods. If you are like many people, you probably find it is difficult to resist eating these foods.

Sugar-Sweetened Soft Drinks and Body Weight

During the past 35 years, the percentage of obese Americans rose dramatically. During this same period, Americans substantially increased their consumption of HFCS. Some nutrition scientists think Americans' love of foods and beverages sweetened with HFCS is largely responsible for the population's rising rate of obesity.[19] The rising prevalence of obesity among children is a major public health concern; regular soft drinks are the primary source of added sugar in the diets of American children[20] and high school students.[21] School boards in many communities are so concerned about the epidemic of childhood obesity, they have banned empty–calorie foods, including sugar–sweetened soft drinks, from school cafeterias and vending machines. Is there a connection between consumption of regular soft drinks and excess body fat?

The role that regular soft drink consumption plays in the development of obesity is controversial.[19] Findings from some scientific studies suggest that people who drink regular soft drinks do not reduce their energy intake from solid food accordingly.[22] The reasons are unclear, but the fructose in these beverages may not reduce the urge to eat as does solid food. As a result, consumers of regular soft drinks ("liquid candy") are likely to overeat and have excessive energy intakes. If, for example, you begin to drink three 12–ounce cans of a cola–flavored, sugar–sweetened soft

Many people find it difficult to resist foods that contain a lot of sugar and fat, such as cheesecake.

drink per day, you will obtain about 410 extra kilocalories daily. Unless you increase your daily physical activity level to metabolize the 410 kcal or cut back your food intake by 410 kcal each day, you are likely to gain some weight. By contributing to unwanted weight gain, consumption of regular soft drinks may increase the risk of type 2 diabetes, the most common form of the disease.[25]

Although consumption of regular soft drinks has increased over the past several years, other dietary changes have occurred as well. Americans consume an excess of calories from all foods, and the higher intake contributes to the increased prevalence of obesity in the United States.[26,27] In 2009–2010, adult males consumed an average of 2512 kcal/day, and adult females consumed an average of 1778 kcal/day.[10] These amounts were 361 and 274 kcal higher, respectively, than the average daily calorie intakes of adult males and females about 20 years earlier.[28] Therefore, overall dietary habits may be partly to blame for rising rates of overweight and obesity among the U.S. population.

What Is Diabetes?

Diabetes mellitus (diabetes) is a group of serious chronic diseases characterized by abnormal glucose, fat, and protein metabolism.[29] There are two major types of diabetes mellitus: type 1 and type 2 diabetes. About 5% of people with diabetes have type 1; in the past, this form of diabetes was called "juvenile diabetes" because it was diagnosed more often in children and young adults. Although type 1 diabetes is more likely to occur in children and young adults, the disease can strike at any age.[30] The majority of people with diabetes have type 2, which used to be called "adult–onset diabetes." As in the case of type 1 diabetes, type 2 can affect any person, regardless of age.

The primary sign of diabetes is **hyperglycemia** (*hyper* = excess; *glycemia* = blood glucose), abnormally elevated blood glucose levels. A person's blood glucose levels are usually measured after he or she has not eaten (has fasted) for about 12 hours. Normal fasting blood glucose levels are 70 to 99 mg/dl (Table 5.8). People with **pre–diabetes** ("impaired glucose tolerance") have fasting blood glucose levels that are between 100 and 125 mg/dl. Although a person with pre–diabetes does not have diabetes, he or she has a high risk of cardiovascular disease and eventually developing type 2 diabetes. Individuals who have fasting blood glucose levels of 126 mg/dl or more have diabetes.

> **diabetes mellitus (diabetes)** group of serious chronic diseases characterized by abnormal glucose, fat, and protein metabolism
>
> **hyperglycemia** abnormally high blood glucose level
>
> **pre-diabetes** condition characterized by fasting blood glucose levels that are 100 to 125 mg/dl

TABLE 5.8   Classifying Diabetes Mellitus

Blood Glucose Level (Fasting)	Classification
70 to 99 mg/dl	Normal
100 to 125 mg/dl	Pre-diabetes
126 mg/dl or more	Diabetes

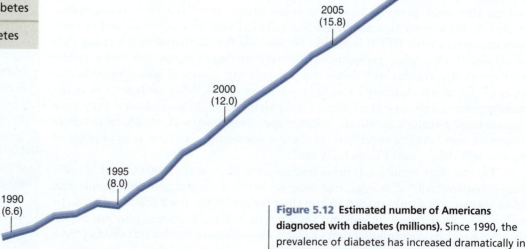

Figure 5.12 **Estimated number of Americans diagnosed with diabetes (millions).** Since 1990, the prevalence of diabetes has increased dramatically in the United States.

Some people with diabetes experience hyperglycemia because their beta cells do not produce any insulin or do not produce enough to meet their needs. In other cases, the affected person produces some insulin, but his or her body does not respond properly to the hormone (*insulin resistance*), and hyperglycemia results. Major signs and symptoms of hyperglycemia include excessive thirst, frequent urination, blurred vision, and poor wound healing (Table 5.9). Over time, untreated or poorly controlled hyperglycemia damages nerves, organs, and blood vessels. In fact, poorly controlled diabetes is a major cause of heart disease, kidney failure, blindness, and lower limb amputations. In 2011, diabetes was the seventh leading cause of death in the United States.[31]

In the United States, the prevalence of diabetes is increasing at an alarming rate (Fig. 5.12). In 2014, an estimated 29.1 million Americans had diabetes; 21.1 million of these persons were diagnosed with diabetes, and the remainder did not know they had the disease.[30] In 2012, an estimated 86 million adult Americans had pre–diabetes. The prevalence of diabetes increases with advancing age; about 26% of Americans who are 65 years of age or older have diabetes.[30] Public health officials are very concerned about the increasing number of children and adolescents who have diabetes, particularly type 2 diabetes.

Type 1 Diabetes

Type 1 diabetes is an *autoimmune* disease that occurs when certain immune system cells malfunction and do not recognize the body's own beta cells. As a result, the immune system cells attack and destroy the beta cells, and the affected person must obtain insulin, usually by injecting the hormone into his or her body, regularly (Fig. 5.13). It is not clear why the immune cells of some individuals malfunction, but genetic susceptibility and environmental factors, particularly exposure to certain viral intestinal infections, are associated with the development of type 1 diabetes.[32] Infants who drink cow's milk–based formulas may have a greater risk of developing type 1 diabetes than breastfed babies.[33] Nevertheless, the association between type 1 diabetes and consuming cow's milk or infant formulas made from cow's milk is controversial. The role of dietary factors in the development of type 1 diabetes continues to undergo scientific study.

People with undiagnosed or poorly managed type 1 diabetes usually develop ketoacidosis. Signs and symptoms of ketoacidosis include excessive thirst, frequent urination, and a blood glucose level of more than 250 mg/dl. Individuals with the condition may also have nausea, vomiting, fatigue, and confusion. The breath of a person with ketoacidosis typically has a "fruity" or acetone odor; acetone is a chemical that is often in fingernail polish remover. Ketoacidosis is a potentially life–threatening condition that requires immediate medical care. If untreated, ketoacidosis can lead to coma (loss of consciousness) and death. Proper management of diabetes, including regular testing of blood glucose levels, is crucial for preventing ketoacidosis.

At present, there is no cure for type 1 diabetes, but the disease can be managed. Stephanie Patton has type 1 diabetes. You can learn about her and how she manages her health by reading the "Real People, Real Stories" feature on page 150.

TABLE 5.9 **Signs and Symptoms of Diabetes Mellitus**

Elevated blood glucose levels
Excessive thirst
Frequent urination
Blurry vision
Vaginal yeast infections (adult women)
Foot pain, abdominal pain
Numbness, especially in the feet
Impotence (male)
Sores that do not heal
Increased appetite with weight loss*
Breath that smells like fruit*
Fatigues easily*
Confusion*

* Typical symptoms of poorly controlled type 1 rather than type 2 diabetes.

(a)

(b)

Figure 5.13 Managing diabetes. Nine-year-old Carson Smith was diagnosed with type 1 diabetes when he was 5 years of age. (*a*) Carson checks his blood glucose at least four times a day. (*b*) After obtaining information about Carson's blood glucose level, his parents determine the amount and type of insulin he needs, and Carson uses a special device to inject the insulin into his body.

Type 2 Diabetes

The most common form of diabetes is type 2 diabetes. Beta cells of people with type 2 diabetes usually produce insulin, but the hormone's target cells are *insulin–resistant* cells, which means they do not respond properly to the hormone and do not allow glucose to enter them. As a result, the level of glucose in the bloodstream becomes abnormally elevated and the typical signs and symptoms of diabetes occur (see Table 5.9).

Over the past 30 years, the number of adults and children with type 2 diabetes has reached epidemic proportions in the United States. Certain people have greater risk of type 2 diabetes than others. Individuals who are physically inactive (sedentary), have excess body fat, and are genetically related to a close family member with type 2 diabetes are more likely to develop the disease than persons who do not have these characteristics. Additionally, Americans who have Hispanic, Native American, Asian, African, or Pacific Islander ancestry are more likely to develop type 2 diabetes than Americans who are not members of these racial/ethnic groups.[30] The American Diabetes Association has an online questionnaire that you can take to assess your risk of type 2 diabetes http://www.diabetes.org/are–you–at–risk/diabetes–risk–test/.

Diabetes During Pregnancy   During pregnancy, a woman with poorly controlled diabetes and her developing offspring (*embryo* or *fetus*) can develop serious health problems. The first 8 weeks of pregnancy are a critical period in a human embryo's development, because its organs are forming. If a woman with diabetes lacks good control of her blood glucose level, her embryo can develop birth defects as a result. By managing her blood glucose properly, however, the pregnant diabetic woman can reduce her chances of giving birth to a baby with birth defects. Additionally, she will be less likely to experience serious health problems, such as high blood pressure, during pregnancy.[34]

As many as 10% of pregnant American women develop a form of diabetes (**gestational diabetes**), usually after the fifth month of pregnancy.[34] Pregnant women who have a family history of type 2 diabetes, are overweight, or have high blood pressure are more likely to experience gestational diabetes than pregnant women who do not have these characteristics. The fetus of a woman with gestational diabetes receives too much glucose from its hyperglycemic mother. As a result of obtaining the excess glucose, the fetus gains weight rapidly and can be abnormally heavy at birth, weighing 9 pounds or more. Giving birth to such a large infant is risky for the mother as well as the infant, because it may prolong the birth process and cause the baby to be injured during delivery.

After giving birth, most women who had gestational diabetes recover and have normal blood glucose levels.[34] Although the new mothers are healthy, they have an increased risk of developing type 2 diabetes later.[34]

A healthy pregnancy typically lasts about 40 weeks. Women with poorly controlled diabetes or gestational diabetes are more likely to have miscarriages (death of an embryo/fetus before the 20th week of pregnancy), stillbirths (delivery of a dead baby), and premature (born before the 37th week of pregnancy) deliveries than women with diabetes who manage their blood glucose properly. Furthermore, women with poorly controlled diabetes or gestational diabetes are more likely to give birth to babies who have difficulty controlling their own blood glucose levels than mothers who do not have diabetes or develop the condition during pregnancy. Thus, pregnant women who have diabetes are encouraged to monitor blood glucose levels carefully to minimize risks to both themselves and their fetuses.

Women who have adequate *prenatal* (before birth) medical care during pregnancy usually undergo screening to detect gestational diabetes. Treatment for women who are diagnosed with gestational diabetes generally includes a special diet to help manage blood glucose levels and regular physical activity. Some

As many as 10% of pregnant American women develop gestational diabetes.

gestational diabetes form of diabetes that pregnant women can develop mothers–to–be will also need to monitor their blood glucose levels and give insulin injections to themselves regularly.

Controlling Diabetes

To avoid or delay serious health complications, people who have diabetes need to achieve and maintain normal or near–normal blood glucose levels. Many people with diabetes rely on daily blood testing to monitor their blood glucose levels (see Fig. 5.13). Physicians can measure *glycated hemoglobin*, also called glycosylated hemoglobin or *hemoglobin A1c* ("HbA1c"), to determine their patients' average blood glucose levels over longer periods. Results of this blood test can provide information about a patient's long–term management of the condition.

Hemoglobin is the compound in red blood cells that carries oxygen. HbA1c is a component of hemoglobin that attracts some glucose that is in blood. About 4.5 to 5.7% of a healthy person's hemoglobin is HbA1c. A person with poorly controlled diabetes often has blood glucose levels that are much higher than normal (Table 5.10). As a result, this individual's hemoglobin will have a higher percentage of HbA1c. Most people with diabetes should strive to maintain their HbA1c level below 7%.[35]

Proper blood glucose management involves monitoring blood glucose levels regularly and carefully following a special diet that usually includes counting grams of carbohydrates. Including physical activity in one's daily routine is also recommended. People with pre–diabetes and type 2 diabetes who are over–weight can often reduce their insulin resistance by losing small amounts of excess body fat.[36] Additionally, exercise increases glucose uptake by muscles, reducing blood glucose levels and improving the body's insulin response. In some instances, however, people with type 2 diabetes need oral medication to stimulate their bodies' insulin production, or they must receive insulin injections.

Promoters of certain weight reduction diets claim that people can lose weight or control diabetes by following *low glycemic index* diets. However, some medical experts question the value of the glycemic index for predicting the body's blood glucose level after eating. To learn more about the glycemic index and gly–cemic load, read the "Nutrition Matters" feature on page 156.

Can Diabetes Be Prevented?

There is no way to prevent type 1 diabetes. By losing some excess body fat and increasing physi–cal activity levels, people with pre–diabetes can prevent or delay the onset of type 2 diabetes and lower their risk of heart disease and stroke.[37] Medical experts refer to these actions as *thera–peutic lifestyle changes (TLC)*.

Certain eating habits may help prevent type 2 diabetes. The typical American diet ("Western diet") contains high amounts of red meat, pro–cessed meats, French fries, high–fat dairy foods, and refined sugars and starches. Some medical experts are concerned that diets that contain excess sugar, particularly fructose, may increase the risk for type 2 diabetes and other serious chronic diseases.[38] Diets that contain more poul–try, fish, and fiber–rich whole grains, fruits, and vegetables are healthier than the Western diet. Such diets may be referred to as "prudent diets." People who follow prudent diets have a lower risk of developing type 2 diabetes than people who consume Western diets.[39,40,41]

TABLE 5.10   Classifying Diabetes According to A1c Values

Diagnosis*	A1c Level
Normal	4.5 to 5.7%
Pre-diabetes	5.7 to 6.4%
Diabetes	6.5% or above

*Any test for diagnosing diabetes requires a second test to confirm the diagnosis, unless the patient has signs and symptoms of diabetes.

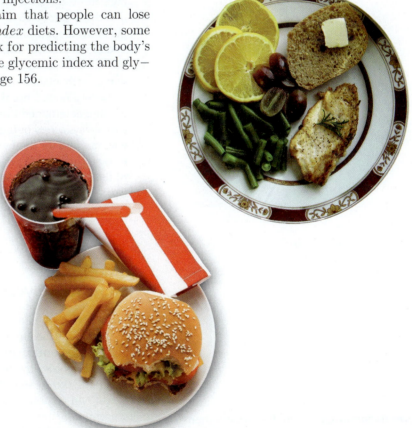

A hamburger with fries is an example of a typical meal for a "Western" diet. Baked chicken served with a variety of fruits and vegetables is an example of a healthier meal.

REAL PEOPLE | REAL STORIES

Stephanie Patton

Although she is only 18 years old, college freshman Stephanie Patton has a long list of accomplishments. "When I was little, I took singing, dancing, and acting lessons," she says. "I loved being on the stage, so I had my parents take me to auditions for local talent shows and theatrical performances. Since I was 7 years old, I've been in over 50 musicals and plays. I appeared in my first beauty pageant at age 10, and I recently competed for the Miss Missouri title. I placed in the top 11, won the preliminary talent award and two college scholarships for community service." Stephanie is majoring in Health Sciences at the University of Missouri-Columbia. While in college, she plans to continue competing for the title of Miss Missouri.

Stephanie manages to balance her college life with her extracurricular activities, but she also has to manage her health and diet. This impressive young lady has type 1 diabetes. Stephanie says, "Just before my fifth birthday, I lost weight and began drinking gallons of juice, water, and milk. At night, I wet the bed. My parents became alarmed, because I have some cousins with type 1 diabetes, and they were worried that I had the disease, too." On her fifth birthday, Stephanie's parents took her to the doctor for a checkup, and her physician told her parents to have her admitted immediately to the local children's hospital. While Stephanie was in the hospital, her parents learned about diabetes and how to take care of their daughter's condition. "At first, my parents gave the insulin shots to me," says Stephanie, "but in a few months, I learned to inject myself and 'count carbs.' An apple was 15 carbs, and my body needed 1 unit of insulin to handle every 15 carbs. I also learned that I had to eat on a set schedule because of the way insulin worked in my body.

"In first grade, the kids avoided me. They didn't understand that you don't 'catch' diabetes like the flu. I was miserable, so my parents placed me in a new school. Since then, I learned that I'm different, and that's OK. I also became determined to educate my friends and the public about diabetes. I was always a very outgoing kid, so after I was diagnosed, my parents started volunteering for the Juvenile Diabetes Research Foundation, and I became one of the organization's child ambassadors. I'd give speeches about the importance of finding a cure for diabetes, and I raised thousands of dollars for this cause. Diabetes doesn't get in my way; I don't let diabetes define who I am."

What Is Hypoglycemia?

If you are healthy and have not eaten for a while, your blood glucose levels decline, and you become hungry. Eating a meal or snack raises your blood glucose. **Hypoglycemia** (*hypo* = low) is a condition that occurs when the blood glucose level is too low to provide enough energy for cells.

Hypoglycemia may be diagnosed when the blood glucose level is less than 70 mg/dl.[42] In response to rapidly declining blood glucose levels, the adrenal glands secrete epinephrine (see Fig. 4.18 [endocrine system] on page 109). You may be more familiar with epinephrine's common name, *adrenaline*. Like glucagon, epinephrine increases the supply of glucose and fatty acids in the bloodstream, but

hypoglycemia condition that occurs when the blood glucose level is abnormally low the hormone can also make a person with hypoglycemia feel irritable, restless, shaky, and sweaty. If the blood glucose level drops too low, the affected person can become confused, and he or she may lose consciousness and die.

Several years ago, popular books and magazine articles warned Americans about the dangers of hypoglycemia and its signs and symptoms. Many peo—ple became convinced that they suffered from the condition. Hypoglycemia is a serious disorder that can affect people with type 1 diabetes who receive too much insulin and those who have certain tumors of the pancreas. The condition, however, rarely affects otherwise healthy persons. Some people develop *reactive hypoglycemia* after they eat highly refined carbohydrates because the pancreas responds by releasing too much insulin. However, these individuals generally have normal fasting blood glucose levels. People with reactive hypoglycemia may feel better if they avoid eating large amounts of sugary foods and eat smaller, more frequent meals that contain a mixture of macronutrients.

Metabolic Syndrome

Do you or does someone you know have a "spare tire," "beer belly," "muffin tops," or an "apple shape"? People who are too fat often have excess abdominal fat, which can be dangerous, especially when it is accompanied by insulin resis—tance, hypertension, and elevated blood lipid (triglyceride and cholesterol) levels.

An estimated 34.3 to 38.5% of adult Americans have **metabolic syndrome,** a condition characterized by three or more of the signs listed in Table 5.11.[43] A **syndrome** is a group of signs and symptoms that occur together and indicate a specific health problem. Compared to people who do not have metabolic syndrome, individuals with this condition have about five times the risk of type 2 diabetes and almost twice the risk of heart and blood vessel (cardiovascular) disease.[44]

Having excess abdominal fat can be harmful to health

TABLE 5.11 Signs of Metabolic Syndrome

Sign	Defining Value
Large waist circumference	≥ 40 inches (men) ≥ 35 inches (women)
Chronically elevated blood pressure (hypertension)	≥ 130 mm Hg systolic (upper value) or ≥ 85 mm Hg diastolic (lower value) or Drug treatment for hypertension
Chronically elevated fasting blood fats (triglycerides)	≥ 150 mg/dl or Drug treatment for elevated triglycerides
Low fasting high-density lipoprotein cholesterol (HDL cholesterol)	< 40 mg/dl (men) < 50 mg/dl (women) or Drug treatment for reduced HDL
High fasting blood glucose	≥ 100 mg/dl or Drug treatment for elevated glucose

Source: Data from Grundy SM and others: Diagnosis and management of the metabolic syndrome: An American Heart Association/National Heart, Lung, and Blood Institute scientific statement: Executive summary. *Circulation* 112:e285, 2005.

metabolic syndrome condition that increases risk of type 2 diabetes and CVD

syndrome group of signs and symptoms that occur together and indicate a specific health problem

Eating more fiber-rich foods, such as whole-grain cereals, may reduce the risk of metabolic syndrome.

lactose intolerance inability to digest lactose properly

Lactose-intolerant people may be able to eat yogurt without experiencing digestive tract discomfort.

Although genetic factors play a major role in the development of metabolic syndrome, excess abdominal fat and insulin resistance are the primary risk factors for the condition.[45] Poor diet, cigarette smoking, and lack of regular physical activity also contribute to the development of the syndrome. People may lower their likelihood of developing metabolic syndrome by increasing their intake of fruits, vegetables, and other fiber—rich foods, such as whole—grain cereals.[44]

Individuals who already have metabolic syndrome may reduce their risk of cardiovascular disease (CVD) by lowering their elevated blood pressure, glucose, insulin, and triglyceride levels. Lifestyle changes that can help manage these levels include losing excess weight, exercising regularly, reducing intakes of salt, saturated fat, and simple sugars.[44] If such changes do not alleviate the condition, medication may be necessary to manage blood pressure and blood lipid levels. Chapter 6 provides more information about cardiovascular disease.

Lactose Intolerance

Millions of Americans suffer from **lactose intolerance** (also referred to as lactose maldigestion or malabsorption), the inability to digest lactose completely. Lactose—intolerant people do not produce enough lactase, the enzyme that breaks lactose into glucose and galactose. Lactose intolerance is not the same as milk allergy, which is an immune system response to cow's milk proteins. Milk allergy is most likely to occur during infancy; lactose intolerance is more likely to occur in adulthood.[46]

When a lactose—intolerant person consumes lactose, the disaccharide is not completely digested and absorbed by the time it enters the large intestine. Bac—teria that reside in the large intestine break down lactose and produce irritat—ing gases and acids as metabolic by—products. As a result, a lactose—intolerant person usually experiences intestinal cramps, bloating, gas, and diarrhea within a couple of hours after consuming milk or other lactose—containing products.

Normally, infants produce lactase, but by the time children are 2 years old, their small intestine begins to produce less of the enzyme. Many older children and adults, particularly those with African, Asian, and Eastern European ances—try, are lactose intolerant and experience some degree of abdominal discomfort after drinking milk.

Milk and milk products are excellent sources of protein, many vitamins, and the minerals calcium and phosphorus. What can people with lactose intolerance do to achieve a nutritionally adequate diet without drinking milk? Lactose—intolerant people are often able to eat hard cheeses and yogurt without experi—encing any digestive tract discomfort. Milk loses most of its lactose content when it is processed to make aged cheeses, such as cheddar and Swiss. The bacteria used to make yogurt convert much of the lactose in milk to lactic acid, and the microbes assist with the digestion of the remaining lactose even after the yogurt is eaten.[47]

Some people with lactose intolerance discover through trial and error that they can consume small amounts of milk without experiencing intestinal dis—comfort. People who cannot tolerate even limited amounts of fresh fluid milk

Did You Know?

People who have severe lactose intolerance should read food labels carefully, because lactose-containing substances may be listed as ingredients. Products contain lactose if they include whey, curds, milk by-products, dry milk solids, and nonfat dry milk powder.

can probably drink milk that has been pre—treated with lactase to reduce its lactose content. Most large supermarkets sell fresh lactase—treated milk in the dairy food section (Fig. 5.14). Also, lactase—containing solutions and pills are available without pre—scription. A lactose—intolerant person simply adds a small amount of the solution to fresh milk before drinking the beverage or takes one of the pills with lactose—containing food. People who cannot tolerate lactose can substitute soy milk for cows' milk, because soy milk does not contain lactose.

Does Sugar Cause Hyperactivity?

If you have ever been in charge of a 7—year—old child's birth—day party or observed third graders preparing for their Halloween celebration, you can understand why people often blame sugary foods for caus—ing unruly and "hyperactive" behavior. Attention deficit hyperactivity disor—der (ADHD) is characterized by impulsivity, hyperactivity, and difficulty paying attention.[48] According to estimates provided by the Centers for Disease Control and Prevention, about 11% of American children have ADHD.[49] Many children do not outgrow the condition by the time they reach adulthood.

Although the cause of ADHD is uncertain, it probably involves genetic and environmental factors. Eating sweets can produce pleasurable sensations, but the results of scientific studies do not indicate that sugar increases chil—dren's physical activity levels, causes ADHD, or otherwise negatively affects their behavior.[48] Birthday and school parties are exciting and happy occasions that typically involve a radical change from a child's usual routine. In these situations, a youngster's excitement and more active behavior is more likely to be the result of the occasion rather than a particular food.

Fiber and Health

Technically, fiber is not an essential nutrient, because the human body can live without it. You can live *better*, however, by adding fiber—rich foods to your diet. Eating high—fiber foods may reduce your risk of obesity, diabetes, certain intestinal tract disorders, and cardiovascular disease, which includes heart disease and stroke. The importance of adequate fiber intake to health is so well recognized that information about a food's fiber content can be found on the food labels of most packaged foods. The following information discusses some roles of fiber in health.

Fiber and the Digestive Tract

"Bloated, constipated, or irregular? Feeling sluggish? You need a laxative!" According to TV advertisements often targeted at older adults, millions of Americans suffer from "irregularity" that can be corrected by taking various over—the—counter remedies. Are serious health problems linked to bowel hab—its? Can making certain dietary changes improve bowel functioning? What causes intestinal gas?

The frequency and ease of bowel movements influence the health of the large intestine. Constipation (infrequent bowel movements) often results in strain—ing to expel feces during bowel movements. Such straining can increase pressure inside the large intestine and force small portions of tissue to form tiny sacs called colonic **diverticula** (Fig. 5.15). In most people, diverticula do not produce symp—toms, but they can become painfully inflamed when bacteria and food particles

Figure 5.14 Lactase-treated milk. Fresh lactase-treated milk is often available near soy milk in the dairy section of supermarkets.

Figure 5.15 Diverticula. In this color-enhanced x-ray, the blue areas are diverticula.

diverticula abnormal, tiny sacs that form in wall of colon

Cross-section of healthy rectum

Cross-section of rectum with hemorrhoids

Rectum

Internal hemorrhoid

External hemorrhoid

Anus

Figure 5.16 **Hemorrhoids.** Hemorrhoids are clusters of swollen rectal veins that can bleed, cause pain, and become itchy.

are trapped within them. When this condition (*diverticulitis*) occurs, the affected person may need surgery to remove the damaged section of large intestine. Hemorrhoids are clusters of small rectal veins that become swollen, making them likely to bleed and cause discomfort and itching (Fig. 5.16). This condition commonly affects adults and may be more likely to occur when a person sits for long periods or strains during bowel movements. Although hemorrhoids are generally not a sign of a serious health problem, you should consult a physician if you experience any bleeding during bowel movements, because it may also be a sign of colorectal cancer, a major cancer site for Americans.

A person's diet, particularly its fiber content, affects his or her bowel habits. Some kinds of fiber in food attract water and swell in the digestive tract, forming a large, soft mass that applies pressure to the inner muscular walls of the large intestine, stimulating the muscles to push the residue quickly through the tract. People who often eat foods that contain adequate amounts of fiber have softer stools and more regular bowel movements, and they are less likely to strain while having bowel movements than people whose diets lack fiber. Thus, people generally do not need to rely on over-the-counter laxatives to treat constipation. Eating more fiber-rich foods is the natural way to become "regular."

Fiber and Colorectal Cancer   In the United States and throughout the world, colon or *colorectal* cancer (cancer of the two lower portions of the large intestine) is one of the most common cancers.[50] In the early 1970s, a group of scientists noted that rural African populations who typically ate high-fiber diets rarely developed colorectal cancer. When these populations moved to urban areas and adopted relatively low-fiber Western diets, their risk of colorectal cancer increased. As a result of these observations, the scientists suggested that high-fiber diets were protective against colorectal cancer. Today, however, it is not known whether diets that provide high amounts of fiber or include fruits and vegetables can reduce the risk of colorectal cancer.[51] Nevertheless, nutrition experts recommend eating high-fiber foods because they provide other important health benefits, such as reducing the risk of cardiovascular disease.[52]

Fiber and Heart Health

Diets rich in fiber, particularly soluble types of fiber, can reduce the risk of cardiovascular disease by reducing blood cholesterol levels. High blood levels of certain forms of blood cholesterol are associated with increased risks of cardiovascular disease. The liver uses cholesterol to make bile, a substance that helps digest fats. The gallbladder stores bile and releases the substance into the small intestine during meals. Instead of eliminating bile along with fecal matter in bowel movements, the intestinal tract breaks it down and absorbs its components, which eventually enter the liver. The liver recycles bile components to make new bile. When you eat oat cereal, the soluble fiber in oats interferes with this recycling process, because it binds to the bile components in the intestinal tract and prevents them from being absorbed. (See Figure 6.12.) Thus, the bile components are eliminated in bowel movements. As a result, blood cholesterol levels drop as the liver removes cholesterol from the blood to make new bile. The FDA permits manufacturers of certain high–fiber cereals to use the American Heart Association's heart–healthy symbol (Fig. 5.17). The "Recipe for Healthy Living" feature of this chapter has a hot oatmeal recipe.

Fiber and Weight Control

If you are trying to lose excess body fat, you may find it helpful to add more fiber–rich foods to your diet. High–fiber foods tend to be "filling" by increas– ing the volume of food eaten, which results in satiety. Additionally, a serving of a high–fiber food generally has lower energy content than the same volume of a low–fiber food. As a result, energy intake usually decreases when people switch their consumption from low–fiber to high–fiber diets.

Increasing Your Fiber Intake

The recommended Adequate Intakes (AIs) for fiber are 38 and 25 g/day for young men and women, respectively, but the typical American diet supplies only about 16g of dietary fiber/day.[10] According to the Dietary Guidelines, fiber is a "nutrient of public health concern." You can estimate your daily fiber intake by completing the Personal Dietary Analysis at the end of this chapter. The "Food & Nutrition Tips" feature on this page provides tips for increasing the fiber content of diets. Eating excessive amounts of fiber may interfere with the intestinal absorption of certain minerals. In rare instances, consuming too much dietary fiber results in intestinal blockage, especially if fluid intake is low.

Intestinal bacteria produce gases when they metabolize fiber; therefore, dietitians recommend that people adjust by gradually increasing their fiber intake. Practices that result in swallowing air, such as eating quickly; drinking carbonated beverages, especially with a straw; and chewing gum, also contribute to intestinal gas.

Figure 5.17 American Heart Association's healthy food symbol.

Food & Nutrition tips

- Read the ingredient label to find out if a bread or cereal product is whole grain; whole grain or bran should be the first ingredient.

- Don't rely on the product's name or appearance. Check the ingredients. Terms such as *100% wheat, multigrain,* or *stone-ground wheat* are misleading, because the product may contain little or no whole grain.

- Brown rice has more fiber and flavor than white rice.

- Substitute whole-wheat pasta for regular pasta, or use half whole-wheat and half regular pasta in pasta dishes.

- Snack on pieces of fresh, frozen, or dried fruit.

- Include more nuts, beans, and seeds in your diet.

- Spread peanut or soy butter on whole-grain crackers for a fiber-filled snack.

- Add frozen, dried, or fresh fruit such as berries, raisins, or bananas instead of sugar or honey to sweeten cereal or plain yogurt.

- Add a small amount of uncooked oatmeal and wheat germ to raw ground meats when making hamburgers or meatloaf.

- Adding bran, wheat germ, and uncooked oatmeal to pancake or waffle batter also enhances the batter's fiber content.

- Good dietary sources of fiber contain at least 2.5 g of fiber per serving.

MY DIVERSE PLATE

ChooseMyPlate.gov

Red Lentils

For thousands of years, people living in Mediterranean countries, the Middle East, India, and other countries of southeastern Asia have eaten lentils, a type of *legume*. Peas and beans are also legumes. Lentils, particularly green varieties, are an excellent source of fiber. Lentils also provide protein, iron, potassium, and folate. Red lentils soften quickly with cooking and can be used in stews, sauces, or dips.

Concept **Checkpoint 5.7**

16. What are the signs and symptoms of type 1 and type 2 diabetes?
17. Lata wants to prevent the development of type 2 diabetes. What health-related lifestyle practices can she follow to reduce her risk of this serious metabolic disease?
18. Identify at least three signs of metabolic syndrome.
19. What is lactose intolerance?
20. List at least three ways to increase dietary fiber intake.
21. Discuss the health benefits of including dietary fiber in meals and snacks.

5.8 Nutrition Matters: Glycemic Index and Glycemic Load

Learning Outcome

1 Explain the difference between the glycemic index and glycemic load.

In the early 1980s, researchers noted that the body digested carbohydrate–rich foods at different rates, and its insulin response to each food varied. Foods that contained large amounts of refined carbohydrates were digested rapidly, and the rapid flow of glucose into the bloodstream raised blood glucose and insulin levels sharply. Other carbohydrate–rich foods that had high fiber contents were digested slowly and did not cause such a dramatic increase in blood glucose and insulin levels. This observation led to the develop–ment of the dietary concepts *glycemic index* and *glycemic load*. Currently, the notion that a food's glycemic index could

influence health has spurred the publication of popular diet books recommending avoiding foods with high glycemic indi–ces, such as potatoes and bread. What is the glycemic index? Should you avoid foods that have high glycemic indices?

The glycemic index (GI) is a way of classifying foods by comparing the rise in blood glucose that occurs after eating a portion of a food that supplies 50 g of digestible carbohy–drate to the rise that occurs after eating a standard source of carbohydrate, such as 50 g of glucose.[53] A related value, the glycemic load (GL), is the grams of carbohydrate in a serving of food multiplied by the food's GI; this figure is then divided by 100. Compared to the GI, the GL may be a more realistic way of rating foods because the value indi–cates the relative rise in blood glucose levels after eating a *typical* serving of a carbohydrate–containing food.

Table 5.12 lists average GIs and GLs of several commonly eaten foods. Note that sucrose and other sugary foods, as well as highly refined starchy foods such as cornflakes, baked pota–toes, and white rice, have high GIs (70 or more). Raw apples, carrots, spaghetti, fat–free milk, and peanuts have low to moderate GIs (less than 70). It is important to note that the

TABLE 5.12 Glycemic Index and Load: Average Values of Selected Foods

Food	Glycemic Index* Value	Glycemic Load** Serving Size	Value
Potato, Russet, baked	158	150 g	33
Jelly beans	114	30 g	22
White rice, medium grain, boiled	107	150 g	29
Bagel, white plain	99	70 g	24
French fries	90	150 g	21
Cola drink	90	1 cup	16
Banana	89	120 g	16
Cornflakes cereal	80	30 g	21
Popcorn, microwave plain	79	20 g	6
Spaghetti, cooked	68	180 g	23
Orange juice	66	1 cup	12
Ice cream, vanilla, low-fat	66	50 g	7
Snickers candy bar	61	60 g	15
Apple, raw	56	120 g	6
Carrots, raw	50	80 g	2
Fat-free milk	46	1 cup	4
Peaches, canned in natural juice	43	120 g	3
Peanuts	10	50 g	0

* Compared to white bread (GI = 100); ** Per serving

Source: Data from Atkinson FS and others: International tables of glycemic index and glycemic load values: 2008. *Diabetes Care* 31(12):2281, 2008.

GL of a food is usually lower than its GI. For example, the GI for 30 g of cornflakes is 80, but the GL value for cornflakes is only 21. Foods with low GLs have values below 15; high GL foods have values of more than 20.

Critics of the GI and GL think the standards have limited usefulness as a menu-planning tool because the values can vary too much. Therefore, the values shown in Table 5.12 may vary significantly, depending on where the food was grown, its degree of ripeness, or the extent of its processing. Additionally, after eating a particular carbohydrate-rich food, the resulting rise in blood glucose level varies among individuals. Furthermore, the values reflect a single food's effect on blood glucose levels. The effect may be reduced when the food is eaten as part of a meal that contains a mixture of macronutrients and fiber.

Despite the criticism directed at the indices, epidemiological studies suggest an association between high GI/GL diets and serious chronic diseases.[54] As people in developing countries abandon traditional diets and eat more high GI/GL foods, they become more likely to develop obesity and type 2 diabetes, as well as cardiovascular disease and certain cancers.[55] Low GI diets may improve blood lipid levels and reduce the risk of cardiovascular disease[56] and improve HbA1c levels.[57] People with diabetes can follow a low GI or low GL diet while monitoring their total carbohydrate intake to control their blood glucose levels.[58] More long-term research is needed before nutrition experts recommend low GI or low GL diets for the general population.

Concept **Checkpoint 5.8**

22. Which of these foods has the lowest glycemic index: plain, white bagel; raw apple; orange juice; or microwave popcorn?

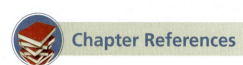

Chapter References

See Appendix H.

Summary

5.1 Introducing Carbohydrates

- Carbohydrates are an important source of energy for the body. Plants use energy from the sun to make carbohydrates from water and carbon dioxide. Some of the energy is stored in the bonds that hold the carbon and hydrogen atoms together. Cells break down those bonds, releasing the energy that powers various forms of cellular work.

5.2 Simple Carbohydrates: Sugars

- The three most important dietary monosaccharides are glucose, fructose, and galactose. Glucose is a primary fuel for muscles and other cells; nervous system and red blood cells rely on glucose for energy under normal conditions. Lactose and sucrose are major dietary disaccharides.

5.3 Complex Carbohydrates

- Starch, glycogen, and most forms of dietary fiber are polysaccharides. Although fiber is not digested by humans, soluble and insoluble fiber provide important health benefits.

5.4 What Happens to Carbohydrates in the Body?

- Glucose is the primary end product of carbohydrate digestion. Hormones, particularly insulin and glucagon, maintain normal blood glucose levels. Insulin enables glucose to enter cells, where the sugar is metabolized for energy. Glucagon stimulates the liver to break down glycogen into glucose molecules and release them into the bloodstream.

5.5 Carbohydrate Consumption Patterns

- People in industrialized nations tend to eat less complex, unprocessed carbohydrates and more highly refined sugars than people living in less-developed countries. Healthy Americans should consume diets that furnish 45 to 65% of energy from carbohydrates, primarily complex carbohydrates. Refined sugar is often blamed for causing obesity, diabetes, and hyperactivity, but tooth decay is the only health problem that is clearly associated with eating carbohydrates. Many adults are lactose intolerant because they do not produce enough lactase, the intestinal enzyme needed to digest the disaccharide.

5.6 Understanding Nutrient Labeling: Carbohydrates and Fiber

- The Nutrition Facts panel provides information about total carbohydrate, sugars, and fiber contents of packaged foods and beverages.

5.7 Carbohydrates and Health

- Foods that contain a lot of added sugars and fats tend to be energy dense. Some nutrition scientists think high intakes of added sugars, especially in regular soft drinks, is largely responsible for Americans' rising rate of obesity.

- Diabetes mellitus is characterized by elevated blood glucose levels. Diabetes can result in cardiovascular disease, kidney failure, blindness, and lower limb amputations. There are two major types of diabetes mellitus, type 1 and type 2 diabetes. Type 2 diabetes is the more common form of the disease. People who are sedentary, have excess body fat, eat Western diets, and have a close relative with type 2 diabetes are at risk of developing this form of the disease.

- Eating fiber-rich foods may reduce your risk of obesity, type 2 diabetes, cardiovascular disease, and certain intestinal tract disorders. High-fiber diets, especially those with ample amounts of insoluble fiber, are associated with lower risk of constipation and hemorrhoids compared to diets that contain little fiber. Additionally, foods that contain soluble fiber may improve cardiovascular health by reducing cholesterol absorption. Plant foods generally contain both forms of fiber.

5.8 Nutrition Matters: Glycemic Index and Glycemic Load

- The glycemic index (GI) and glycemic load (GL) are ways of classifying certain foods by their effect on blood glucose levels. Results of some epidemiological studies suggest an association between high GI/GL diets and serious chronic diseases. However, more long-term research is needed before nutrition experts recommend low GI or low GL diets for the general population.

Recipe for Healthy Living

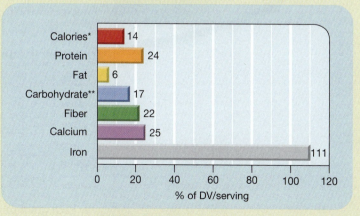

Berry-Good Hot Oatmeal Cereal

This single-serving hot cereal recipe is a very good source of carbohydrate and provides 7 g of fiber. For variety, substitute raisins, frozen or fresh strawberries, or raspberries for the blueberries. A serving of this oatmeal supplies about 280 kcal, 12 g protein, 3 g fat, 51 g digestible carbohydrate, 5.6 g fiber, 250 mg calcium, and 20 mg iron.

- Fat
- Protein
- Carbohydrate

INGREDIENTS:

½ cup frozen or fresh unsweetened blueberries
½ cup quick-cooking, enriched oats
¾ cup fat-free milk
1 tsp sugar
pinch of ground cinnamon (optional)

PREPARATION STEPS:

1. Place ingredients in a microwaveable bowl and stir.

2. Microwave on "high" for about 2 ½ minutes.

3. Stir and top with blueberries before eating.

Cleanup tip: After eating, soak cereal bowl in cold water before washing it.

	% of DV/serving
Calories*	14
Protein	24
Fat	6
Carbohydrate**	17
Fiber	22
Calcium	25
Iron	111

*2000 daily total kcal
**Digestible

 Further analyze this and other recipes through activities on Connect at www.mcgrawhillconnect.com.

Personal Dietary Analysis

1. Refer to the 3-day food log from the "Personal Dietary Analysis" feature in Chapter 3. List the total number of kilocalories you consumed for each day of record keeping. Add the figures to obtain a total, divide the total by 3, then round the figure to the nearest whole number to obtain your average daily energy intake for the 3-day period.

Sample Calculation: _____

Day 1	<u>2500</u> kcal
Day 2	<u>3200</u> kcal
Day 3	<u>2750</u> kcal
Total kcal	<u>8450</u> ÷ 3 days = <u>**2817**</u> **kcal/day**

       (average kilocalorie intake, rounded to the nearest whole number)

Your Calculation: _____

Day 1	_____ kcal
Day 2	_____ kcal
Day 3	_____ kcal
Total kcal	_____ ÷ **3 days** = _____ **kcal/day**

       (average kilocalorie intake, rounded to the nearest whole number)

2. Add the number of grams of carbohydrate eaten each day of the period. Divide the total by 3 and round to the nearest whole number to calculate the average number of grams of carbohydrate consumed daily.

Sample Calculation: _____

Day 1	<u>300</u> g
Day 2	<u>495</u> g
Day 3	<u>475</u> g
Total =	<u>1270</u> g
Total g	<u>1270</u> ÷ 3 days = <u>**423**</u> **g/day**

       (average, rounded to the nearest whole number)

Your Calculation: _____

Day 1	_____ g
Day 2	_____ g
Day 3	_____ g
Total =	_____ g
Total g	_____ ÷ **3 days** = _____ **g of carbohydrate/day**

       (average, rounded to the nearest whole number)

3. Each gram of carbohydrate provides about 4 kcal; therefore, you must multiply the average number of grams of carbohydrate obtained in step 2 by 4 to obtain the number of kcal from carbohydrates.

Sample Calculation: _____

423 g/day × 4 kcal/g = **1692** kcal from carbohydrates

Your Calculation:

_____ g/day × 4 kcal/g = _____ kcal from carbohydrates

4. To calculate the average daily percentage of kilocalories that carbohydrates contributed to your diet, divide the average kilocalories from carbohydrate obtained in step 3 by the average total daily kilocalorie intake obtained in step 1; round the figure to the nearest one-hundredth. Multiply the value by 100, drop decimal point, and add the percent symbol.

Sample Calculation:

1692 kcal ÷ 2817 kcal = 0.60

0.60 × 100 = 60%

Your Calculation:

_____ kcal ÷ _____ kcal = _____

_____ × 100 = _____ %

5. On average, did you consume *at least* the RDA of 130 g of carbohydrate? Yes _____ No _____

6. Did your average carbohydrate intake meet the recommended 45 to 65% of total energy? Yes _____ No _____

a. If your average carbohydrate intake was less than 130 g or below 45% of total calories, list five nutrient-dense, carbohydrate-rich foods you could eat that would boost your intake of carbohydrates.

Foods: _____

7. Review the log of your 3-day food intake. Calculate your average daily intake of fiber by adding the grams of fiber consumed over the 3-day period and dividing the total by 3.

Your Calculation:

Day 1   _____ g

Day 2   _____ g

Day 3   _____ g

Total =   _____ g

Total grams _____ ÷ 3 days = _____ g of fiber daily

a. What was your average daily fiber intake? _____ g

b. Did your average daily fiber intake meet the recommended Adequate Intakes of 38 and 25 g/day for young men and women, respectively? Yes _____ No _____

c. If your response is yes, list foods that contributed to your fiber intake.

d. If you did not meet the recommended level of fiber intake, list at least five foods that you would eat to increase your fiber intake to the recommended level.

 Complete the Personal Dietary Analysis activity online at www.mcgrawhillconnect.com

Critical Thinking

1. One of your friends thinks honey is more nutritious and safer to eat than table sugar. He wants you to avoid table sugar and use only honey as a sweetener. What would you tell this person about the nutritive value and safety of honey compared to sugar?

2. Maria has diabetes, and she just found out that she is in the sixth week of pregnancy. She wants to know what she can do to increase her chances of having a problem—free pregnancy and healthy baby. What would you tell her about the importance of properly managing her blood glucose level during pregnancy?

3. How did you feel about drinking regular soft drinks before reading this chapter? Has your opinion changed? If so, explain how.

4. If you were 25 pounds overweight, explain why you would or would not follow a weight—loss diet that supplied less than 15% of calories from carbohydrate.

5. Consider the fiber content of your diet. Do you consume enough fiber each day? If your fiber intake is adequate, what foods do you eat regularly that contribute soluble and insoluble fiber to your diet? If your fiber intake is low, list foods you would consume to increase your intake of both types of fiber.

6. Jeff experiences intestinal cramps and gas after drinking a glass of milk. He suspects that he has lactose intolerance. What steps can he take to obtain adequate nutrition without eliminating dairy foods from his diet?

Practice Test

Select the best answer.

1. Which of the following substances is a disaccharide?

   a. fructose
   b. sucrose
   c. galactose
   d. glycogen

2. _____ is a primary fuel for muscles and other cells.

   a. Protein
   b. Cholesterol
   c. Glucose
   d. HFCS

3. Which of the following substances is a polysaccharide?

   a. glycogen
   b. glucose
   c. lactose
   d. insulin

4. Which of the following conditions is a common sign or symptom of untreated type 1 diabetes?

   a. migraine headaches
   b. hyperglycemia
   c. diverticula
   d. stomach ulcers

5. Dietary fiber

   a. supplies more energy, gram per gram, than fat.
   b. is not digested by the human intestinal tract.
   c. promotes tooth decay.
   d. is only in animal sources of food.

6. Insoluble fiber

   a. is in beef and pork.
   b. dissolves or swells in water.
   c. is in whole—grain products, including brown rice.
   d. increases the risk of heart disease.

7. _____ is the hormone that enables glucose to enter cells.

   a. Glucagon
   b. Insulin
   c. HFCS
   d. Maltase

8. _____ are the primary source of added sugars in American diets.

   a. Candies
   b. Regular soft drinks
   c. Refined cereals
   d. Canned fruits

9. Type 2 diabetes is

   a. a disease that primarily affects young children.
   b. characterized by severe hypoglycemia.
   c. often associated with excess body weight.
   d. caused by eating refined sugars.

10. Which of the following signs is associated with meta-bolic syndrome?

    a. low blood pressure
    b. high fasting blood glucose
    c. low hemoglobin
    d. high fasting HDL cholesterol

11. Which of the following conditions is clearly associated with eating certain dietary carbohydrates, especially sticky sugars?

    a. tooth decay
    b. type 1 diabetes
    c. attention deficit hyperactivity disorder
    d. hypertension

12. Which of the following substances is an enzyme that breaks down lactose?

    a. galactose
    b. salivary amylase
    c. lactase
    d. lactic acid

13. Which of the following foods is the best source of solu-ble fiber?

    a. raw fruit
    b. whole-grain oat cereal
    c. sports drinks
    d. cooked meat

14. Which of the following foods has a high glycemic index?

    a. nonfat milk
    b. cornflakes cereal
    c. salted peanuts
    d. raw carrots

Answers to Quiz Yourself

1. Compared to table sugar, honey is a natural and far more nutritious sweetener. **False.** (p. 131)

2. Ounce per ounce, sugar provides more energy than starch. **False.** (pp. 132, 136)

3. Eating a high-fiber diet may reduce your blood cholesterol levels. **True.** (p. 154)

4. The average American consumes 80% of his or her energy intake as refined sugars. **False.** (p. 142)

5. The results of clinical studies indicate that eating too much sugar makes children hyperactive. **False.** (p. 153)

LEARNSMART ADVANTAGE

Get the most out of your study of nutrition with McGraw-Hill's innovative suite of adaptive learning products including McGraw-Hill LearnSmart®, SmartBook®, LearnSmart Achieve®, and LearnSmart Prep®. Visit www.learnsmartadvantage.com.

CHAPTER 6

Fats and Other Lipids

Quiz Yourself

What are trans and omega-3 fats, and which foods contain these fats? How much dietary fat is recommended? Should you avoid eating eggs because they contain cholesterol? Test your knowledge of fat and other lipids by taking the following quiz. The answers are found on page 213.

1. To lose weight, use regular, stick margarine instead of butter because it has 25% fewer calories per teaspoon. _____ T _____ F

2. Egg yolks are a rich source of cholesterol. _____ T _____ F

3. Taking too many fish oil supplements may be harmful to health. _____ T _____ F

4. On average, Americans consume 60% of their calories from fat. _____ T _____ F

5. Increasing your intake of saturated fat will reduce your risk of heart disease. _____ T _____ F

McGraw Hill Education **connect** | NUTRITION   www.mcgrawhillconnect.com

A wealth of proven resources are available on Connect® Nutrition including McGraw-Hill LearnSmart®, SmartBook®, NutritionCalc Plus, and many other dynamic learning tools. Ask your instructor about Connect!

6.1 Introducing Lipids

Learning Outcomes

1 Identify the major kinds of lipids, including triglycerides and cholesterol.

2 List at least six functions of lipids in the body.

3 List at least three important functions of lipids in foods.

What do you think when you hear the word *fat* or *cholesterol?* Does "bad," "heart attack," or "deadly" enter your mind? If your answer is yes, are you con—cerned about the amounts and types of fat in your diet? Do you avoid eating eggs because of their cholesterol content? Does your concern have anything to do with having a family history of heart disease?

Lipids are a class of macronutrients that includes fatty acids, triglycerides (*try—glis'—er—eyeds*), phospholipids (*fos—foe—lip'—ids*), and cholesterol. In general, lipids are insoluble in water, but they are soluble in organic solvents such as alcohol and acetone. Consider what happens when you mix vinegar and olive oil to make a vinaigrette salad dressing. Vinegar is 95% water; oil is 100% lipid. Therefore, the oil does not dissolve in water to make a solution. Additionally, oil is less dense than water, so it rises to the top of the vinegar in small globules when added to vinegar. The globules join others to form an oily layer that floats on the vinegar until you shake the mixture. Shaking the ingredients mixes them temporarily. When left undisturbed, the oil and vinegar soon separate; hence the saying, "Oil and water don't mix."

You probably know fat is a major source of energy and eating too much fat can result in excess weight gain, which is unhealthy. Additionally, you may know that cholesterol is associated with heart attacks. However, you may not be aware of the many important roles that fat, cholesterol, and other lipids play in the body (Table 6.1). Lipids are crucial components of the plasma membrane that surround each human cell. In fact, a person cannot claim to be "fat free," because every cell in the body contains fat, as well as other lipids. The layer of fat under your skin (subcutaneous fat) stores energy, insulates you against cold temperatures, protects you against minor bruising, and contributes to your body's contours. In addition to storing energy, the fat deposits in your abdominal region cushion your vital organs from jarring movements and damaging blows.

In food, lipids enhance intestinal absorption of fat—soluble vitamins and phytochemicals. Dietary lipids also provide nonnutritional benefits by contribut—ing to the rich flavor, smooth texture, and appetizing aroma of foods. Whether fat is naturally in food or added to it, the nutrient often makes foods taste more appetizing. For example, if you are used to consuming whole milk that is about 3.25% fat by volume, you will recognize the difference fat makes to "mouth feel" when you drink fat—free milk that contains less than 0.5% fat.

It is not surprising that many Americans are confused about the roles of fat and cholesterol in health. The results from numerous studies conducted over the past 60 years indicate that consuming high amounts of certain lipids may increase the risk of serious health conditions, including obesity,[1] certain cancers,[2] and cardiovascular disease (CVD), which includes heart disease and *stroke* (the loss of blood flow to a part of the brain; "brain attack").[3,4] On the other hand, some fat is essential to good health. By reading this chapter, you will learn about the roles of lipids in your foods and body, as well as their major food sources. Additionally, you will learn how certain lipids may influence your health.

Oil and water do not mix.

TABLE 6.1 Major Functions of Lipids in the Body

Fats and certain other lipids are important for:

- providing and storing energy (fat);
- maintaining cell membranes;
- producing certain hormones;
- insulating the body against cold temperatures;
- cushioning the body against bumps and blows;
- contributing to body contours;
- absorbing fat-soluble vitamins and phytochemicals.

lipids class of nutrients that generally do not dissolve in water

165

1. Although 88-year-old Rose has more body fat than is recommended, she is healthier than her much thinner 88-year-old cousin, Lily. Explain why having excess body fat can be beneficial for older adults.
2. Ingredients for a cake recipe include ½ cup of water. What would happen to the sensory quality of the baked cake if you replaced the water with the same amount of whole milk?

6.2 Fatty Acids, Triglycerides, Phospholipids, and Sterols

Learning Outcomes

1 Explain the differences in the chemical structures of saturated, monounsaturated, polyunsaturated, and trans fatty acids.

2 Identify major food sources of each kind of lipid, including the essential fatty acids, phospholipids, and cholesterol.

3 Discuss the roles of essential fatty acids, phospholipids, and cholesterol in the body.

4 Discuss signs and symptoms of an essential fatty acid deficiency.

Fatty Acids

Most lipids have fatty acids in their chemical structures. Fatty acids provide energy for muscles and most other types of cells. As Figure 6.1 illustrates, a fatty acid is comprised of a **hydrocarbon chain,** a chain of carbon atoms bonded to each other and to hydrogen atoms. The first carbon in the molecule has three hydrogen atoms attached to it. Chemists call this part of the molecule the **omega** (or methyl) **end.** The last carbon in the fatty acid molecule forms an acid group.

In nature, common fatty acids have even numbers of carbon atoms. *Short−chain* fatty acids have 2 to 4 carbons; *medium−chain* fatty acids have 6 to 12 carbons; and *long−chain* fatty acids have 14 to 24 carbons. The molecules shown in Figure 6.1 contain 18 carbons; thus, they are long−chain fatty acids. Chemists identify a fatty acid by its number of carbon atoms and type of bond between carbon atoms in the hydrocarbon chain. Additionally, these factors influence how various fatty acids can affect a person's health.

Saturation

Fatty acids can be saturated or unsaturated. The carbons in the fatty acid chain shown in Figure 6.1a have single bonds between them. Note that each carbon in the chain has two hydrogen atoms attached to it. This is a **saturated fatty acid** because each carbon within the chain is saturated, that is, completely filled with hydrogen atoms.

An **unsaturated fatty acid** has two neighboring carbons within the chain that are missing two hydrogen atoms, and a double bond holds those particular carbons together (Fig. 6.1b). Unsaturated fatty acids can have one or more double bonds within the chain of carbons. The fatty acid illustrated in Figure 6.1b has only one double bond linking two carbon atoms; therefore, it is referred to as a **mono**unsaturated **fatty acid (MUFA).** The fatty acid shown in Figure 6.1c is also unsaturated, but it

hydrocarbon chain chain of carbon atoms bonded to each other and to hydrogen atoms

omega end first carbon of a fatty acid chain that has three hydrogen atoms attached to it

saturated fatty acid fatty acid that has each carbon atom within the chain filled with hydrogen atoms

unsaturated fatty acid fatty acid that is missing hydrogen atoms and has one or more double bonds within the carbon chain

monounsaturated fatty acid (MUFA) fatty acid that has one double bond within the carbon chain

(a) **Saturated Fatty Acid (stearic acid)**

(b) **Monounsaturated Fatty Acid (oleic acid)**

(c) **Polyunsaturated Fatty Acid (alpha-linolenic acid)**

Number 1 carbon   Number 3 carbon

Figure 6.1 Fatty acids. A fatty acid is comprised of a hydrocarbon chain. The omega end contains the first carbon in the molecule; the last carbon in the molecule forms an acid group.

has three double bonds within its hydrocarbon chain. A fatty acid that has two or more double bonds between carbons is a **polyunsaturated fatty acid (PUFA).**

What is the difference between fats and oils? Although both substances contain fatty acids, fats are solid and oils are liquid at room temperature. Compared to foods that contain high amounts of unsaturated fatty acids, foods that are rich sources of long-chain saturated fatty acids tend to be more solid at room temperature. A pat of butter, for example, contains more long-chain saturated fatty acids than a pat of margarine. Thus, butter keeps its shape better than margarine when it is not refrigerated. The "Lipids and Health: Cardiovascular Disease (CVD)" section of this chapter discusses the health effects of eating diets that are rich in saturated or unsaturated fats.

Essential Fatty acids

The body cannot make two polyunsaturated fatty acids, **alpha-linolenic** (*al'-fah lin'-o-len'-ik*) **acid** and **linoleic** (*lin'-o-lay'-ik*) **acid.** These lipids are **essential fatty acids** because they must be supplied by the diet. Alpha-linolenic acid is an **omega-3 fatty acid.** The "3" refers to the position of the first double bond that appears in the fatty acid's carbon chain, when you start counting carbons at the omega end of the molecule (see Fig. 6.1c). Cells use alpha-linolenic acid to synthesize two other omega-3 fatty acids, eicosapentaenoic (*eye'-koss-uh-pen'-tah-ee-no'-ik*) acid (EPA) and docosahexaenoic (*doe'-koss-uh-hex'-uh-ee'-no'-ik*) acid (DHA). Linoleic acid is an *omega-6 fatty acid*. Cells can convert linoleic acid to arachidonic (*a'-rak'-ih-don'-ik*) acid (AA). The body uses EPA, DHA, and AA to make several compounds that have hormone-like functions, including *prostaglandins*. Prostaglandins produce a variety of important effects on the body, such as stimulating uterine contractions, regulating blood pressure, and promoting the immune system's inflammatory response. Figure 6.2 shows relationships among the essential fatty acids.

Essential fatty acids are necessary in small amounts for good health. Infants require DHA and EPA for nervous system development, and babies do not grow

polyunsaturated fatty acid (PUFA) fatty acid that has two or more double bonds within the carbon chain

alpha-linolenic acid an essential fatty acid

linoleic acid an essential fatty acid

essential fatty acids lipids that must be supplied by the diet

omega-3 fatty acid type of polyunsaturated fatty acid

Figure 6.2 Essential fatty acids. Alpha-linolenic acid and linoleic acid are not synthesized by the body; they must be supplied in the diet. The body uses these essential fatty acids to make DHA, EPA, and AA.

properly when their diets lack essential fatty acids. Other signs of essential fatty acid deficiency include scaly skin, hair loss, and poor wound healing. The Adequate Intake (AI) for alpha−linolenic acid is 1.6 g/day for men and 1.1 g/day for women. The AI for linoleic acid is 17 g/day for men and 12 g/day for women who are 19 through 50 years of age.[5] These amounts can be met by eating 2 to 3 tablespoons of vegetable fat daily, especially products made with canola and soybean oils, and meals that contain fatty fish, such as salmon and tuna, at least twice a week.

In the United States, essential fatty acid deficiency is uncommon because most Americans eat plenty of fat, especially linoleic acid. This omega−6 fatty acid is in vegetable oils often used for frying foods and making margarines and salad dressings. Additionally, whole−grain products contain linoleic acid. Certain fish are rich sources of omega−3 fatty acids, including DHA and EPA (see Table 6.6). Many Americans eat relatively small amounts of omega−3 fatty acids. The "Lipids and Health: Cardiovascular Disease (CVD)" section of this chapter pres− ents more information about essential fatty acids and their health effects.

Trans Fats

Trans fats are unsaturated fatty acids that have at least one *trans* double bond in their chemical structure rather than the more common *cis* configuration. The trans double bond enables the hydrocarbon chain to be relatively straight. The cis double bond, however, forms a kink in the hydrocarbon chain (Fig. 6.3).

trans fats unsaturated fatty acids that have a trans double bond

Figure 6.3 *Cis* and *trans* double-bond arrangements. Unsaturated fatty acids usually have "kinks" where double bonds are in the carbon chain. (*a*) Oleic acid, a cis fatty acid, has the hydrogen atoms of the double-bonded carbons on the same side of the molecule, resulting in a kink. (*b*) Elaidic acid, a trans fatty acid, has the hydrogen atoms of the double-bonded carbons on opposite sides, resulting in a straighter arrangement of the fatty acid chain. For simplicity, most of the hydrogen atoms in these molecules are not shown.

Whole milk and whole milk products, butter, and meat naturally contain small amounts of trans fats. However, processed foods and margarines contribute the largest share of trans fat in the American diet. Most of the trans fat in processed food (artificial trans fat) results from the **hydrogenation** process. *Partial hydrogenation* is a food manufacturing process that adds hydrogen atoms to some unsaturated fatty acids in liquid vegetable oil. The hydrogenation process also converts many of the oil's naturally occurring cis fatty acids into trans fatty acids. Structurally, a trans fatty acid resembles a saturated fatty acid and provides properties of long–chain saturated fatty acids to foods that contain them. Thus, fats that contain a high proportion of trans fatty acids are more solid at room temperature than those with a high proportion of cis fatty acids. As a result of the partial hydrogenation process, vegetable oil can be made into shortening or shaped into sticks of margarine. Shortening is often used to prepare deep–fat fried foods and cakes, pastries, and frostings.

Foods made with partially hydrogenated fat can be stored for longer periods of time than foods that contain cis fatty acids. Why? Trans fatty acids are less likely to undergo *oxidation*, a chemical process that alters the compound's structure. When oxidized, the fat in food becomes rancid and develops an unappetizing odor and taste. Unsaturated fatty acids that have the cis double–bond arrangement, especially polyunsaturated fatty acids, are very susceptible to oxidation. Instead of relying on trans fats to extend the shelf life of products, manufacturers can preserve fat and other ingredients in foods by adding antioxidants to them. Certain food additives, vitamins, and plant pigments function as antioxidants (see Chapter 8).

Although the body can use trans fatty acids for energy, these lipids are not essential, and medical researchers have not discovered any positive health effects from consuming them.[6] In the body, trans fats raise blood cholesterol levels, which may increase the risk of heart disease.[7]

As American consumers have become more aware of the potential health problems associated with trans fat consumption, many food manufacturers have removed ingredients that contain artificial trans fats from their products. Responding to consumer concerns, some fast–food chains voluntarily stopped using rich sources of artificial trans fat during food preparation. In 2013, officials with the Food and Drug Administration (FDA) announced a ban on the addition of trans fats to processed foods. The FDA, however, will allow food manufactures to gradually phase out their use of trans fats.

The use of a synthetic lipid, *interesterified (in'–ter–eh–stear'–ih–fide')* oil, to replace artificial trans fats in processed foods may also have undesirable health effects.[8] More research is needed to determine the long–term safety of consuming foods that contain interesterified oil. Processed foods that include "fully hydrogenated" or "interesterified" oil in their ingredient lists are sources of interesterified fat.

Triglycerides

A **triglyceride** has three fatty acids attached to glycerol (*glis'–er–ol*), a three–carbon compound that is often referred to as the "backbone" of the triglyceride (Fig. 6.4). Triglycerides comprise about 95% of lipids in your body and food. Triglycerides are often referred to as fats and oils. The body stores energy as triglycerides (fat).

Most triglycerides contain mixtures of unsaturated and saturated fatty acids. In a particular food, such as olives or cheese, the unsaturated and saturated fats occur in different proportions, but one type of fatty acid (saturated, monounsaturated, or polyunsaturated) often predominates. Table 6.2

Did You > Know?

Cooks often use shortening to make pie crust because the partially hydrogenated fat results in a flaky, tender crust. When making pie dough, oil can be substituted for shortening, but it produces a crumbly texture that may be undesirable.

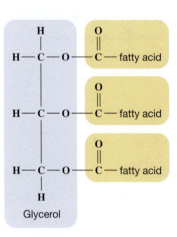

| Figure 6.4 Triglyceride.

hydrogenation food manufacturing process that adds hydrogen atoms to liquid vegetable oil, forming trans fats

triglyceride lipid that has three fatty acids attached to a three-carbon compound called glycerol

TABLE 6.2 Comparing Fats and Oils: Saturated, Monounsaturated, and Polyunsaturated Fatty Acids

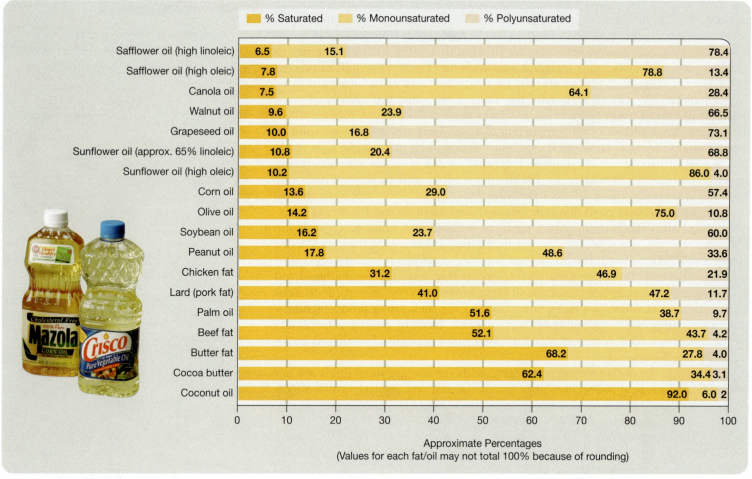

Oil/Fat	% Saturated	% Monounsaturated	% Polyunsaturated
Safflower oil (high linoleic)	6.5	15.1	78.4
Safflower oil (high oleic)	7.8	78.8	13.4
Canola oil	7.5	64.1	28.4
Walnut oil	9.6	23.9	66.5
Grapeseed oil	10.0	16.8	73.1
Sunflower oil (approx. 65% linoleic)	10.8	20.4	68.8
Sunflower oil (high oleic)	10.2	86.0	4.0
Corn oil	13.6	29.0	57.4
Olive oil	14.2	75.0	10.8
Soybean oil	16.2	23.7	60.0
Peanut oil	17.8	48.6	33.6
Chicken fat	31.2	46.9	21.9
Lard (pork fat)	41.0	47.2	11.7
Palm oil	51.6	38.7	9.7
Beef fat	52.1	43.7	4.2
Butter fat	68.2	27.8	4.0
Cocoa butter	62.4	34.4	3.1
Coconut oil	92.0	6.0	2

Approximate Percentages
(Values for each fat/oil may not total 100% because of rounding)

Source: Data from U.S. Department of Agriculture, Agricultural Research Service, USDA Nutrient Data Laboratory: *USDA national nutrient database for standard reference, release 26*, 2013.

Did You Know?

Lard is pork fat. In some parts of the United States, lard is used to make biscuits, pie dough, and refried beans. Lard is high in saturated fat (41%), but it is not as highly saturated as butter (68%).

compares the percentages of saturated, monounsaturated, and polyunsaturated fatty acids in commonly eaten fats. Note that the fat in beef and dairy products contains more saturated than unsaturated fatty acids; olive oil is a rich source of monounsaturated fatty acids; and liquid corn oil contains a greater proportion of unsaturated than saturated fatty acids. Certain animal foods, especially beef and dairy foods such as cheese, cream, and butter, contain higher percentages of saturated fatty acids than most plant fats. Exceptions are tropical oils such as coconut and palm oils. Tropical oils contain more saturated than unsaturated fatty acids. Fats and oils that contain high amounts of saturated or unsaturated fatty acids are commonly called saturated fats or unsaturated fats.

Why is it important to understand the differences between saturated, unsaturated, and trans fats, and identify foods that contain high amounts of these fats? Populations that consume diets rich in saturated fat and trans fat ("unhealthy fat") have a higher risk of cardiovascular disease than popula-tions whose diets contain more unsaturated than saturated fat.[9] The "Lipids and Health: Cardiovascular Disease (CVD)" section of this chapter provides more information about this topic.

Phospholipids

A **phospholipid** is chemically similar to a triglyceride, except that one of the fatty acids is replaced by chemical groups that contain phosphorus and, often, nitrogen. Phospholipids are naturally found in plant and animal foods. **Lecithin** (*less'−uh−thin*) is the major phospholipid in food; egg yolks, liver, wheat germ, peanut butter, and soybeans are rich sources of lecithin.

Unlike triglycerides, phospholipids are partially water soluble because the phosphorus−containing portion of the molecule is **hydrophilic** (*hydro* = water; *philic* = loving); that is, it attracts water (Fig. 6.5). A phospholipid molecule also has a **hydrophobic** (*phobic* = fearing) portion that avoids watery substances and attracts oily ones. By having both hydrophilic and hydropho-bic regions, a phospholipid can serve as an **emulsifier,** a substance that keeps water−soluble and water−insoluble compounds mixed together (Fig. 6.6). Manufacturers may add emulsifiers to foods to keep oily and watery ingre-dients from separating during storage. Processed foods, such as cheese food, salad dressing, and ice cream, often have phospholipids added as emulsifying agents. Egg yolk, for example, naturally contains phospholipids and is used to emulsify oil and vinegar when making mayonnaise or mixing oil and milk in cake batters.

In the body, phospholipids are major structural components of cell mem-branes. Cell membranes are comprised of a double layer that is mostly phos-pholipids (Fig. 6.7). The chemical structure of the phospholipids enables the membrane to be flexible and function properly. Phospholipids are also needed for normal functioning of nerve cells, including those in the brain. Phospholipid deficiencies among adults are uncommon, because the lipids are in a variety of foods and bodies of healthy adults synthesize these compounds.

Lecithin contains **choline** (*co'−leen*), a water−soluble compound that nerves use to produce the neurotransmitter *acetylcholine* (*ah−see'−till−co'−leen*). A neurotransmitter is a chemical that transmits messages between the

phospholipid type of lipid that is chemically similar to a triglyceride

lecithin major phospholipid in food

hydrophilic part of molecule that attracts water

hydrophobic part of molecule that avoids water and attracts lipids

emulsifier substance that helps water-soluble and water-insoluble compounds mix with each other

choline water-soluble compound in lecithin

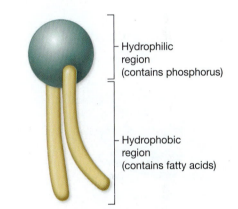

Hydrophilic region (contains phosphorus)

Hydrophobic region (contains fatty acids)

Figure 6.5 Phospholipids have a hydrophilic and a hydrophobic region.

Phospholipid (emulsifier)

Oil

Water

Water around hydrophilic shell

Oil emulsified in water

Hydrophilic portion of phospholipid

Hydrophobic portion of phospholipid

Figure 6.6 Emulsification. Phospholipids act as emulsifiers.

Figure 6.7 **Phospholipids in cell membranes.** Human cell membranes are comprised of a double layer of phospholipids. Cholesterol and proteins are embedded in the membrane.

cholesterol sterol in animal foods and precursor for steroid hormones, bile, and vitamin D

nerve cells. Nutritionists classify choline as a vitamin—like nutrient, because deficiency symptoms can occur under certain conditions.[10] The results of scientific studies, however, do not support claims that lecithin supplements improve the physical performance[11,12] or memory of healthy people.[13] Chapter 8 provides more information about choline.

Sterols

Sterols have carbons arranged in rings, which makes them a more chemically complex type of lipid than a triglyceride or a phospholipid (Fig. 6.8). **Cholesterol** is the most well—known sterol. Many people think that cholesterol is unhealthy and foods that contain the lipid should be avoided, but it is a very important nutrient. Cholesterol is a component of every cell membrane in your body (see Fig. 6.7). Although cholesterol is not metabolized for energy, cells use the lipid to synthesize a variety of substances, including vitamin D, and steroid hormones such as estrogen and testosterone. The liver uses cholesterol to make bile, an emulsifier that facilitates lipid digestion.

Although triglycerides are widespread in foods, cholesterol is found only in animal foods. Egg yolk, liver, meat, poultry, whole milk, cheese, and ice cream are rich sources of cholesterol (Table 6.3). Even if you do not eat animal foods, your body produces cholesterol, primarily in the liver. If your body makes too much cholesterol, the excess can increase your risk of CVD.

Plant Sterols and Stanols

Plants make small amounts sterols (plant sterols and stanols) that have chemical structures that are similar to cholesterol. Although plant sterols and stanols are not well absorbed by the human intestinal tract, these substances compete with cholesterol for absorption by the digestive tract. This competition reduces the amount of cholesterol that is absorbed. As a result, plant sterols and stanols are added to certain foods, beverages, and dietary supplements because they may lower elevated blood cholesterol levels, a risk factor for heart disease. Cholesterol—lowering margarine—like spreads such as Benecol® and TakeControl® and other manufactured food products that contain plant sterols and stanols are functional foods, because they have been developed specifically to provide beneficial health effects (see Chapter 3).

Figure 6.8 **Cholesterol.** Cholesterol is a complex organic molecule. For simplicity, this illustration shows only the molecule's alcohol group (OH) and carbon atoms.

TABLE 6.3 Approximate Cholesterol Content of Some Foods/Serving

Food	Serving Size	Cholesterol (mg)
Liver	3 oz	234
Egg	1 large	186
Egg yolk	1	186
Sardines	3 oz	121
Single-patty cheeseburger	1	111
Beef	3 oz	88
Turkey, ground	3 oz	84
Danish fruit-filled pastry	2 ½ oz	81
Shrimp	6 large, breaded and fried	80
Ham	3 oz	80
Ice cream, soft-serve	½ cup	78
Ground beef, lean (15% fat)	3 oz	77
Salmon	3 oz	75
Turkey, dark meat	3 oz	71
Egg noodles	1 cup	53
Chicken breast	3 oz	49
Hot dog	1	44
Chocolate milkshake	16 oz	43
Whole milk	1 cup	34
Cottage cheese	1 cup	32
Cheddar cheese	1 oz	30

Concept **Checkpoint 6.2**

3. What are the major lipids in food and the body?
4. What is the difference between a saturated and an unsaturated fatty acid? What is the difference between a monounsaturated and a polyunsaturated fatty acid?
5. Identify at least one food that is a rich source of saturated fat, monounsaturated fat, and polyunsaturated fat.
6. Identify the two essential fatty acids.
7. What structural characteristic distinguishes a trans fatty acid from a cis fatty acid? Identify at least two foods that are rich sources of trans fat.
8. What is an omega-3 fatty acid?
9. A recipe mixes ¼ cup of oil with ¾ cup of milk. What common food could you add to keep the oil and milk emulsified?
10. Which foods contain cholesterol? List at least three functions of cholesterol in the body.

6.3 What Happens to Lipids in the Body?

Learning Outcomes

1 Discuss the digestion, absorption, and transport of lipids in the body.

2 Describe effects of enterohepatic circulation on cholesterol metabolism.

3 Explain the primary role of adipose cells.

Figure 6.9 summarizes some key steps in fat digestion and absorption. Triglycerides and phospholipids need to be broken down by special enzymes called **lipases** before they can be absorbed. When you eat a cheeseburger and French fries, an inactive lipase in saliva mixes with the food. As the food enters the stomach, the organ's acid environment activates the lipase, enabling some lipid breakdown to occur. The small intestine, however, is the primary site of lipid digestion.

As the fatty chyme leaves the stomach and enters your small intestine, it stimulates certain intestinal cells to release the hormone **cholecystokinin** (*kol′−e−sis′−toe−kye′−nin*) **(CCK).** CCK signals the pancreas to secrete digestive enzymes, including *pancreatic lipase*, into the duodenum of the small intestine. **Pancreatic lipase** digests triglycerides by removing two fatty acids from each triglyceride molecule. This action converts most triglycerides into *monoglycerides*. A **monoglyceride** has a single fatty acid attached to the glycerol backbone of the molecule. Some triglycerides are completely broken down into glycerol and fatty acid molecules.

The process of digesting phospholipids is similar to that of digesting triglycerides. The enzyme *phospholipase* removes two fatty acids from a phospholipid molecule. The remaining structure contains the lipid's phosphate region (see Fig. 6.5). Cholesterol does not undergo digestion; small intestinal cells can absorb cholesterol directly from food. Glycerol, fatty acids, monoglycerides, cholesterol, and phospholipid fragments are the end products of lipid digestion.

Bile

Another function of the hormone CCK is stimulating the gallbladder to contract. This action forces some bile into the duodenum, where it mixes with chyme. Bile contains **bile salts,** compounds that enhance digestion and absorption by keeping lipids dispersed in small particles, increasing their surface area (see Fig. 6.9). As a result, pancreatic lipase gains greater access to the lipid molecules and digests them more readily. If bile is not secreted into the duodenum, lipids clump together in large fatty globules, making lipid digestion less efficient.

Bile enhances digestion by keeping fats and oils in chyme dispersed in the watery environment of the small intestine (emulsification). Bile salts have hydrophilic "heads" and hydrophobic "tails" (refer to Fig. 6.5). The tails are oriented inward, so they surround the lipid particle, while the heads face outward and toward the watery components of chyme. This action forms a **micelle** (see Fig. 6.9). As a result of micelle formation, lipids in chyme remain separated in small particles, which increases the ability of pancreatic lipase to gain access to and digest them.

What Are Lipoproteins?

Under normal conditions, the small intestine digests and absorbs nearly all of the triglycerides and phospholipids in food, but only about 50% of the dietary cholesterol is absorbed. After being absorbed, short− and medium−chain fatty acids can enter the bloodstream directly. Most long−chain fatty acids, glycerol,

---

lipases enzymes that break down lipids

cholecystokinin (CCK) hormone that stimulates the gallbladder to release bile and pancreas to secrete digestive enzymes

pancreatic lipase digestive enzyme that removes two fatty acids from each triglyceride molecule

monoglyceride single fatty acid attached to a glycerol backbone

bile salts components of bile that enhance lipid digestion and absorption

micelle lipid-rich particle that is surrounded by bile salts; transports lipids to absorptive cells monoglycerides, and phospholipid fragments are reassembled into triglycerides and phospholipids within the absorptive cells of the small intestine. Cholesterol and the reassembled triglycerides are coated with a thin layer of protein, phospholipids, and cholesterol to form chylomicrons (see Fig. 6.9). A *chylomicron* (*ky'−low−my'−kron*) is a type of *lipoprotein*. **Lipoproteins** are water−soluble structures that transport lipids through the bloodstream. Chylomicrons are too large to be absorbed directly into the bloodstream. These lipoproteins must pass through the larger openings of *lacteals* (*lak'−te−als*), lymphatic system vessels in each villus (see Fig. 4.29).

lipoprotein water-soluble structure that transports lipids through the bloodstream

| Figure 6.9 **Lipid digestion and absorption.**

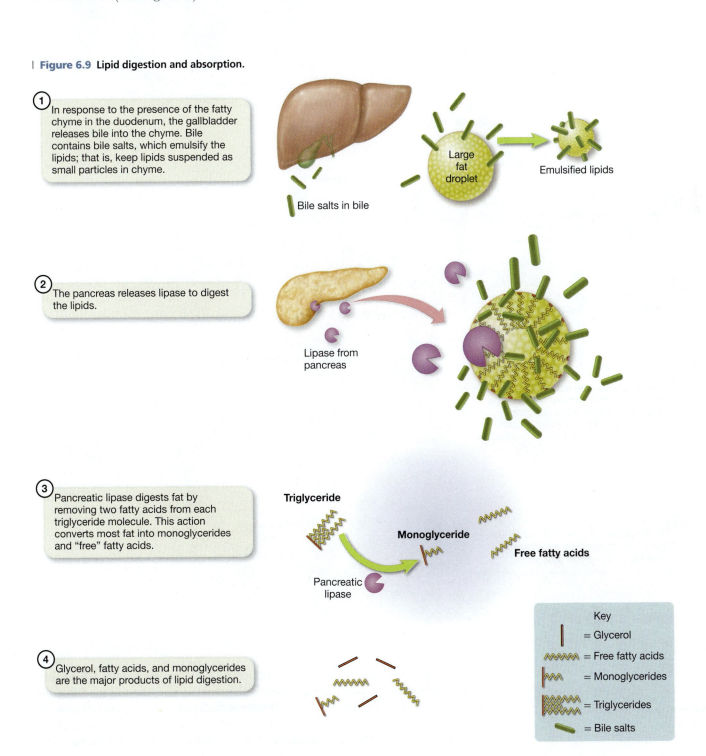

1. In response to the presence of the fatty chyme in the duodenum, the gallbladder releases bile into the chyme. Bile contains bile salts, which emulsify the lipids; that is, keep lipids suspended as small particles in chyme.

Bile salts in bile

Large fat droplet

Emulsified lipids

2. The pancreas releases lipase to digest the lipids.

Lipase from pancreas

3. Pancreatic lipase digests fat by removing two fatty acids from each triglyceride molecule. This action converts most fat into monoglycerides and "free" fatty acids.

Triglyceride

Monoglyceride

Free fatty acids

Pancreatic lipase

4. Glycerol, fatty acids, and monoglycerides are the major products of lipid digestion.

Key

| = Glycerol

= Free fatty acids

= Monoglycerides

= Triglycerides

= Bile salts

Figure 6.9 Lipid digestion and absorption. *(continued)*

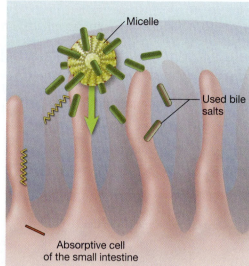

(5) Bile salts surround the fatty acids and monoglycerides to form a water-soluble particle called a micelle. Micelles transport the lipids to the edge of the absorptive cell. These cells remove the monoglycerides and fatty acids from micelles. The used bile salts that remain can continue to form new micelles.

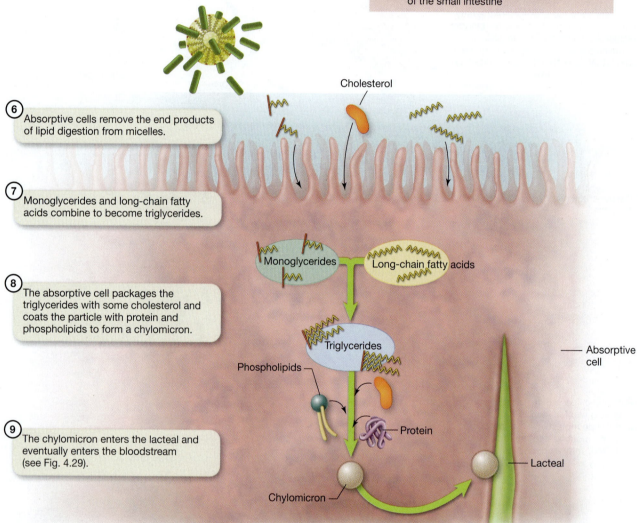

(6) Absorptive cells remove the end products of lipid digestion from micelles.

(7) Monoglycerides and long-chain fatty acids combine to become triglycerides.

(8) The absorptive cell packages the triglycerides with some cholesterol and coats the particle with protein and phospholipids to form a chylomicron.

(9) The chylomicron enters the lacteal and eventually enters the bloodstream (see Fig. 4.29).

lipoprotein lipase enzyme in capillary walls that breaks down triglycerides

The lymphatic system transports chylomicrons to the thoracic duct, where they enter the bloodstream through the left subclavian vein in the chest (Fig. 6.10). As chylomicrons circulate through the body, **lipoprotein lipase,** an enzyme in the walls of capillaries, breaks down their load of triglycerides into fatty acids and glycerol. Nearby cells can pick up the fatty acids and glycerol molecules to use for energy. Ten

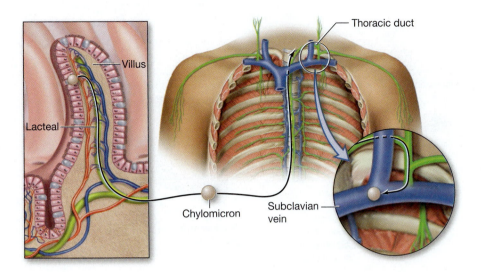

- Thoracic duct
- Villus
- Lacteal
- Chylomicron
- Subclavian vein

Figure 6.10 **Journey into the general circulation.** The lymphatic system transports chylomicrons from the small intestine to the thoracic duct, where they enter the bloodstream through the left subclavian vein in the chest.

to 12 hours after a meal, most chylomicrons have been reduced to small cholesterol—rich remnants. The liver clears these remnants from the bloodstream and uses their contents to synthesize new lipids and other lipoproteins that are released into the general circulation. Figure 6.11 provides a summary of lipid digestion and absorption.

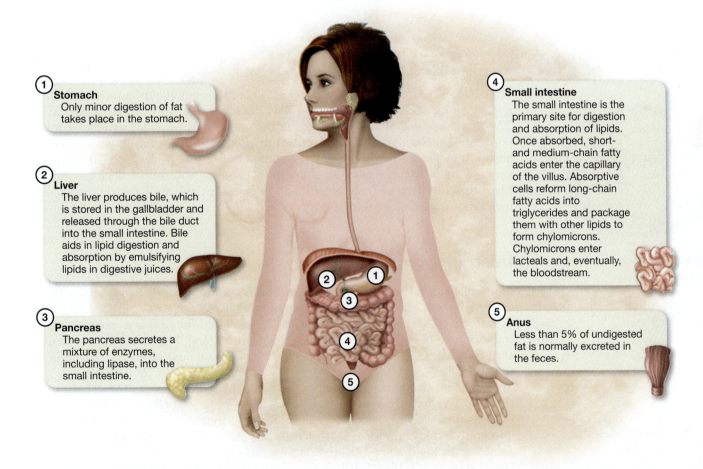

1 **Stomach**
Only minor digestion of fat takes place in the stomach.

2 **Liver**
The liver produces bile, which is stored in the gallbladder and released through the bile duct into the small intestine. Bile aids in lipid digestion and absorption by emulsifying lipids in digestive juices.

3 **Pancreas**
The pancreas secretes a mixture of enzymes, including lipase, into the small intestine.

4 **Small intestine**
The small intestine is the primary site for digestion and absorption of lipids. Once absorbed, short- and medium-chain fatty acids enter the capillary of the villus. Absorptive cells reform long-chain fatty acids into triglycerides and package them with other lipids to form chylomicrons. Chylomicrons enter lacteals and, eventually, the bloodstream.

5 **Anus**
Less than 5% of undigested fat is normally excreted in the feces.

Figure 6.11 **Summary of lipid digestion and absorption.** This illustration summarizes the basic steps of lipid digestion, absorption, transport, and elimination.

| Figure 6.12 **Enterohepatic circulation.** Enterohepatic circulation is the process of recycling bile salts.

Figure 6.13 **Adipose cells.** A primary function of an adipose cell is storing a fat droplet.

enterohepatic circulation process that recycles cholesterol in the body

adipose cells fat cells; specialized cells that store fat

Recycling Bile Salts

Most bile salts are absorbed in the ileum, where the compounds enter the bloodstream and travel to the liver. The liver uses the bile salts to make new bile. The process of recycling bile from the intestinal tract is called **enterohepatic** (*ent'−eh−roe−hih−pah'−tik*) **circulation** (Fig. 6.12). Interfering with enterohepatic circulation can reduce blood cholesterol levels, because the liver must use cholesterol to make new bile salts. Plants contain substances, such as soluble fiber, that interfere with cholesterol and bile absorption (see Table 5.6 for common food sources of soluble fiber).

Using Triglycerides for Energy

Most cells can metabolize fatty acids for energy. Fat is more energy dense than carbohydrate or protein: A gram of fat supplies 9 kcal, whereas a gram of carbohydrate or protein provides only 4 kcal. Thus, a high−fat food is a more concentrated source of energy than a high−carbohydrate food. For example, you would need to eat 2 ½ tablespoons of sugar to obtain the amount of energy in 1 tablespoon of oil.

In many instances, your body does not need the energy from the fat in the food you have just eaten. **Adipose** (*ad'−eh−pose*) **cells,** commonly called fat cells, remove fatty acids and glycerol from circulation and reassemble them into triglycerides for storage. Most cells in your body contain triglycerides, but adipose cells are designed to store large amounts of fat (triglycerides). As illustrated in Figure 6.13, a fat droplet comprises most of an adipose cell's volume. When your body needs energy, adipose cells break down some stored triglycerides into fatty acid and glycerol molecules, and release these substances into your bloodstream. Muscle and other cells then remove the fatty acids from circulation and metabolize them. The liver clears the glycerol molecules from the bloodstream and converts them into glucose molecules that cells can also use for energy.

Eating too much fat contributes to unwanted weight gain, but consuming too much energy from protein and carbohydrates also increases body fat. Why? The body can convert excess glucose and certain amino acids into fatty acids that are used to make triglycerides. Additionally, the nonnutrient alcohol stimulates triglyceride synthesis, and excess body fat can accumulate as a result of alcohol consumption. Alcohol has many other effects on the body, some of which are beneficial to cardiovascular health. To learn more about alcohol and assess your use of the substance, read "Nutrition Matters: Drink to Your Health?" on page 195. For more information about energy metabolism, see Chapter 11 and Appendix C.

A slice of an extra-cheese, thick-crust pizza (1/10 of the pie) provides about 17 g fat, which is 26% of the Daily Value for fat (2000 kcal/day).

Concept **Checkpoint 6.3**

11. Describe what happens to the fat in a piece of fried chicken as it undergoes digestion and absorption in a healthy person's intestinal tract. In your description, include the roles of bile, CCK, pancreatic lipase, villi, and chylomicrons.
12. Explain why high-fiber diets can reduce the concentration of cholesterol in a person's blood.
13. Why can an obese person survive starvation for a longer period than a thin person?

Food & Nutrition tip

To lower the fat content of their products, manufacturers of "lite" spreads may have water as the first ingredient. Therefore, replacing the margarine, butter, oil, or shortening in a recipe with a reduced-fat spread could alter the product's taste, texture, and appearance. It is a good idea to read the reduced-fat spread's label to determine whether the product is suitable to use in recipes.

6.4 Lipid Consumption Patterns

Learning Outcomes

1 Recall the percentage of fat in the typical American diet and the AMDR for fat.

2 Discuss Dietary Guidelines recommendations for fat and cholesterol intakes.

In 1987–1988, Americans who were 2 years of age and older each consumed an average of 54 pounds of fat.[14] In 2009–2010, each member of this population consumed an average of about 62 pounds of fat per year, which is an increase of almost 15%, compared to the earlier period.[15] Fat contributes 33% of the average American's daily energy intake. Although there is no RDA or AI for total fat (for people over 1 year of age), the Acceptable Macronutrient Distribution Range (AMDR) for the macronutrient is 20 to 35% of total calories.[5] According to the Dietary Guidelines, people should consume diets that include rich sources of polyunsaturated and monounsaturated fatty acids, such as fish, nuts, and vegetable oils.[16] Furthermore, adults should consume less than 10% of their total calories from saturated fatty acids, keep their cholesterol intake to as little as possible, while following a healthy eating pattern. Trans fat intake should also be as low as possible.[16]

In 2009–2010, the typical American diet supplied about 11% of a person's total daily energy intake from saturated fat.[15] To estimate your average percentage of total energy from fat as well as your average saturated fat intake per day, complete the "Personal Dietary Analysis" activity at the end of this chapter.

14. Fat contributes what percentage of total energy in the typical American diet?
15. What is the AMDR for fat?
16. According to the Dietary Guidelines, what is the recommendation for saturated fat intake (percentage of total calories)?

6.5 Understanding Nutritional Labeling: Lipids

Learning Outcomes

1 Use the Nutrition Facts panel to determine amounts of total fat and various types of fatty acids in a serving of a packaged food.

2 Compare total fat and saturated fat contents of packaged foods.

As of 2015, you can determine how much total fat, saturated fat, trans fat, and cholesterol are in most packaged food products by reading the Nutrition Facts panel. As you can see in Figure 6.14, grams of total fat in one serving of bread (a slice) are shown, and under it, the number of grams of the different fats that comprise the total amount. The panel indicates that there are 2 g of total fat in each slice, and of that amount, 1 g is polyunsaturated fat. According to the panel, there are 0 g of saturated, trans, and monounsaturated fats in a slice of the bread. You may be asking yourself, why do the amounts of the various types of fat not add up to 2 g? What happened to the other 1 g of fat? In 2015, if a serving food had less than 0.5 g of a specific type of fat, the amount could be reported as 0 g. When the fractions of fat are added together, however, the total amount, in this example, is 2 g. By reading the list of ingredients shown at the bottom of the panel, you will note that soybean oil is the main source of fat in this bread.

As of 2015, the Nutrition Facts panel also provides information about the cholesterol content of a food. In the panel, the amount of cholesterol in a serving is shown below that of total fat. According to information listed on the Nutrition Facts panel shown in Figure 6.14, a slice of whole-grain bread provides 0 mg of cholesterol.

In 2014, the FDA proposed a new Nutrition Facts panel format that did not indicate calories from fat. Compare the Nutrition Facts panel shown in Figure 6.14 with the proposed format shown in Figure 3.9b.

Nutrition Facts
Serving Size 1 slice (38 g)
Servings Per Container 18

Amount Per Serving

Calories 100
Calories from Fat 20

	% Daily Value*
Total Fat 2g	3%
Saturated Fat 0g	0%
Trans Fat 0g	
Polyunsaturated Fat 1g	
Monounsaturated Fat 0g	
Cholesterol 0mg	0%
Sodium 180mg	7%
Total Carbohydrate 17g	6%
Dietary Fiber 2g	8%
Sugars 3g	
Protein 4g	

Figure 6.14 **Nutrition Facts panel (February 2016).** This Nutrition Facts panel from a package of whole-wheat bread displays the amount of total fat, as well as the amounts of saturated, unsaturated, trans fat, and cholesterol, in one serving.

17. According to the Nutrition Facts panel, a serving of potato chips supplies 150 kcal, and there are 9 g of fat in the serving of chips. Calculate the number of kcal from fat in a serving of the chips.

6.6 Lipids and Health: Cardiovascular Disease (CVD)

Learning Outcomes

1. Explain the process of atherosclerosis.
2. List at least three modifiable risk factors and three nonmodifiable risk factors for atherosclerosis.
3. Distinguish HDL cholesterol from LDL cholesterol.
4. Discuss dietary and other lifestyle actions that can reduce the risk of atherosclerosis.

> **cardiovascular disease (CVD)** group of diseases that affect the heart and blood vessels
>
> **coronary artery disease (CAD)** a major form of CVD
>
> **atherosclerosis** long-term disease process in which plaques build up inside arterial walls

Cardiovascular disease (CVD) includes diseases of the heart and blood vessels. According to estimates, more than one in three adult Americans has one or more forms of CVD.[17] Heart disease (**coronary artery disease, or CAD**) and stroke, the most common forms of CVD, are among the top four leading causes of death in the United States. In 2011, heart disease and strokes were responsible for about 28% of deaths in the United States.[18]

From Atherosclerosis to Cardiovascular Disease

Most cases of heart disease and stroke result from **atherosclerosis** ($athero$ = lipid containing; $sclerosis$ [$skleh-ro'-sis$] = hardening), a chronic process that negatively affects the functioning of arteries. Normal arteries have a smooth lining (Fig. 6.15.1). When something in the bloodstream, such as excess choles— terol or glucose, compounds from cigarette smoke, or certain bacteria, irritates the lining of an artery, a cascade of events begins that results in atherosclerosis. The body's immune system responds to the irritation by producing inflammation

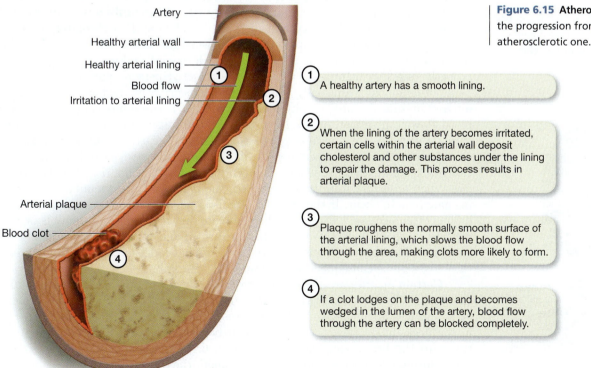

Figure 6.15 **Atherosclerosis.** This illustration depicts the progression from a normal arterial lining to an atherosclerotic one.

Artery
Healthy arterial wall
Healthy arterial lining
Blood flow
Irritation to arterial lining
Arterial plaque
Blood clot

1. A healthy artery has a smooth lining.

2. When the lining of the artery becomes irritated, certain cells within the arterial wall deposit cholesterol and other substances under the lining to repair the damage. This process results in arterial plaque.

3. Plaque roughens the normally smooth surface of the arterial lining, which slows the blood flow through the area, making clots more likely to form.

4. If a clot lodges on the plaque and becomes wedged in the lumen of the artery, blood flow through the artery can be blocked completely.

Figure 6.16 **Healthy and atherosclerotic arteries.** Note the differences between the cross section of a healthy artery (*a*) and that of an artery nearly completely blocked as a result of atherosclerosis (*b*).

(a) Lumen of the artery — Artery wall

(b) Plaque — Arterial wall — Lumen of the artery — Blood clot

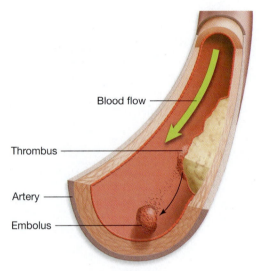

Blood flow

Thrombus

Artery

Embolus

Figure 6.17 **Embolus formation.** A thrombus or part of a plaque that breaks free from where it formed and travels through the bloodstream is an embolus.

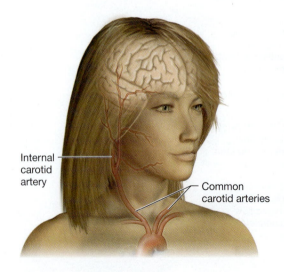

Internal carotid artery

Common carotid arteries

Figure 6.18 **Carotid arteries.**

within the artery. Inflammation can stimulate healing, but the process can also trigger certain cells within the arterial wall to deposit cholesterol under the artery's lining. As a result, **arterial plaque** forms (Fig. 6.15.2). In addition to cholesterol, arterial plaques contain fat, components of dead cells, and calcium. Plaque interferes with circulation in the affected area of the artery, because it narrows and may even block the opening through which blood flows (*lumen*). Furthermore, plaque roughens the normally smooth surface that lines the artery. The rough lining slows blood flow in the area and makes clots more likely to form (Fig. 6.15.3). If a plaque ruptures (tears open), repairing the damage also involves clot formation, and such blood clots can be life threatening (Fig. 6.15.4). Figure 6.16 shows cross sections of a healthy artery and one that is almost completely blocked by plaque.

Blood must be able to clot, especially when blood vessels have been injured; otherwise, a person could bleed to death from a minor bruise. In some instances, however, clots form too readily at the injury site. A **thrombus** is a fixed bunch of clots that remains in place and disrupts blood flow. If a thrombus partially closes off the lumen of an artery that nourishes the heart, the affected section of the heart muscle is unable to receive enough oxygen and nutrients to function properly (see Fig. 6.16b). As a result, the affected person typically experiences bouts of chest pain, especially when his or her heart beats faster, such as during intense emotional states or physical activities. If a thrombus completely blocks blood flow to a section of the heart muscle, the muscle dies and a **myocardial infarction** (*my′–eh–card′–e–al in–farc′–shun*) (heart attack) occurs. Sudden death can result from a severe myocardial infarction. A stroke can happen when a clot blocks an artery in the brain and brain cells that are nourished by the vessel die. When an artery to a limb is blocked, the tissue in the extremity dies, causing gangrene to occur. If the affected area is large, amputation of the gangrenous limb is often necessary to prevent life–threatening infection. A thrombus or part of a plaque that breaks free from where it formed and travels through the bloodstream is an **embolus** (Fig. 6.17). An embolus that lodges in an artery can create the same serious consequences as a stationary thrombus.

Certain arteries are more likely to be damaged by atherosclerosis; in addition to the blood vessels of the heart and brain, the blood supply in the kidneys, eyes, and legs is vulnerable. When atherosclerosis occurs in the *carotid arteries* in the neck, blood flow to the brain can be decreased and clots can form that travel to the brain, causing a stroke (Fig. 6.18). Although atherosclerosis can begin during adolescence and young adulthood, the disease usually does not produce signs or symptoms of CVD until decades later.

Arteriosclerosis

In addition to interfering with blood flow, plaques reduce the flexibility of arteries, causing **arteriosclerosis** (*arterio* = artery), a condition commonly called "hardening of the arteries." Arteriosclerosis contributes to the development of **hypertension,** a chronic condition characterized by abnormally high blood pressure levels that persist even when the person is relaxed. Hypertension is a major risk factor for atherosclerosis and heart disease. The heart of a person with hypertension must work harder to circulate blood through abnormally stiff arteries. Furthermore, elevated blood pressure can cause hardened arteries to tear or burst, causing serious bleeding problems and even sudden death, depending on the artery's size and location.

Lipoproteins and Atherosclerosis

Lipoproteins transport cholesterol and triglycerides in the bloodstream, so these structures play major roles in the development of atherosclerosis. In addition to chylomicrons, the body makes three major types of lipoprotein (Fig. 6.19). Each type carries different proportions of protein, cholesterol, triglycerides, and phospholipids.

The protein content of a lipoprotein contributes to its density. A chylomicron, for example, is the largest and least dense kind of lipoprotein. Compared to the other types of lipoproteins, chylomicrons carry much more fat and very little protein. **High–density lipoprotein (HDL)** is the smallest and densest kind of lipoprotein, because it transports more protein and less lipids than the other lipoproteins. HDL conveys lipids away from tissues and to the liver, where they can be processed and eliminated (Fig. 6.20). Thus, the cholesterol carried by HDL (HDL cholesterol) is often called "good" cholesterol because it does not contribute to plaque formation.

Low–density lipoprotein (LDL) transports more cholesterol than HDL in the bloodstream. LDL is needed to transport lipids to tissues, where the nutrients are used to make cell structures and vital compounds (see Fig. 6.20b). The cholesterol carried by LDL (LDL cholesterol) is often referred to as "bad" cholesterol,

---

arterial plaque lipid-filled deposits that form under the lining of certain arteries

thrombus fixed bunch of clots that remains in place

myocardial infarction heart attack

embolus thrombus or part of a plaque that breaks free and travels through the bloodstream

arteriosclerosis condition that results from atherosclerosis and is characterized by loss of arterial flexibility

hypertension abnormally high blood pressure levels that persist

high-density lipoprotein (HDL) lipoprotein that transports cholesterol away from tissues and to the liver, where it can be eliminated

low-density lipoprotein (LDL) lipoprotein that carries cholesterol into tissues

Figure 6.19 **Major lipoproteins.** The composition of a lipoprotein contributes to its size and density.

(a)

(b)

Figure 6.20 HDL, LDL, and oxidized LDL. Lipoproteins transport lipids in the bloodstream. (*a*) The liver releases protein "shells" into the bloodstream that pick up cholesterol and other lipids from cells. When filled with lipids, the shells are called high-density lipoprotein (HDL). (*b*) LDL transports cholesterol and other lipids to tissues. (*c*) Oxidized LDL cholesterol is harmful because it is taken up by arterial cells that form plaque.

(c)

because LDL conveys the lipid to tissues, including cells in the arterial walls that make atherosclerotic plaques. However, there are different types of LDL, and not all forms of the lipoprotein are unhealthy.

Some LDLs are smaller and denser than others. People with high levels of small dense LDLs are more likely to develop atherosclerosis than are people with low levels of these particular LDLs.[19] Additionally, chemically unstable substances ("free radicals") can damage LDL, especially small, dense LDLs. The damage results in oxidized LDL cholesterol, which is taken up by the plaque-forming arterial cells (see Fig. 6.20c). Cigarette smoking increases the production of oxidized LDL cholesterol.[20]

A third major class of lipoproteins, **very-low-density lipoprotein (VLDL),** may also contribute to atherosclerosis. VLDL carries a larger amount of triglycerides than cholesterol (see Fig. 6.19). Excessive alcohol and refined carbohydrate intakes stimulate VLDL production in the liver. As blood triglyceride levels increase, HDL cholesterol tends to decrease. As a result, high triglyceride levels may contribute to the development of CVD.

Risk Factors for Atherosclerosis

The National Heart, Lung, and Blood Institute has identified risk factors for atherosclerosis.[21] The more risk factors a person has, the greater his or her likelihood of developing CVD. Table 6.4 lists major risk factors and indicates which ones are nonmodifiable or modifiable. A nonmodifiable risk factor cannot be changed.

very-low-density lipoprotein (VLDL) lipoprotein that carries much of the triglycerides in the bloodstream

TABLE 6.4   Atherosclerosis: Major Risk Factors

Nonmodifiable Risk Factors
Family history of CVD Increasing age

Modifiable Risk Factors
Hypertension Pre-diabetes or diabetes Elevated blood cholesterol (especially LDL cholesterol) Excess body fat Physical inactivity Tobacco use or exposure to tobacco smoke

Nonmodifiable Risk Factors

Advancing age is a major risk factor for CVD. The risk of atherosclerosis increases for men after age 45 and for women after age 55. Having a family history of CVD also influences one's risk of the disease. A person's risk increases when he or she has a father or brother who was diagnosed with CVD before 55 years of age. Furthermore, one's risk increases when he or she has a mother or sister who was diagnosed with CVD before 65 years of age. Characteristics such as age and family history of CVD cannot be modified, but controlling other risk factors, such as smoking and hypertension, can reduce the risk of atherosclerosis.[21]

Genetics and CVD   Genetics (family history) is a major risk factor for athero‐sclerosis and CVD. A person's genes, for example, may code for various physical conditions that increase risk of heart disease, such as hypertension and diabetes. Additionally, genes may influence the way in which the circulatory and immune systems respond to diet. Thus, some people may be protected against the devel‐opment of atherosclerosis, whereas other persons with similar diets develop seri‐ous arterial plaques early in life and die prematurely of CVD as a result.

Until recently, much of the research examining the role of diet in the development of atherosclerosis focused on the association between lipids and CVD. Nevertheless, some people with no apparent CVD risk factors still had heart attacks, strokes, and related blood vessel diseases. In many cases, affected individuals were under 40 years of age. This puzzling observation led to the discovery that the amino acid **homocysteine** ($ho'-mo-sis-teen$) may be associated with CVD. Amino acids are the chemical units that comprise proteins. Although homocysteine is an amino acid, the substance is not found in human proteins, and higher‐than‐normal blood levels of homocysteine can be toxic. High blood levels of homocysteine may injure arterial walls and contribute to atherosclerosis.[22] A few people have a rare genetic abnormality that causes the amino acid to accumulate in their bloodstream. These indi‐viduals have a higher risk of premature CVD than persons who do not have the genetic defect. Cells use two vitamins, B–6 and folate, to convert homo‐cysteine into safer compounds. Deficiencies of certain B vitamins can also cause homocysteine levels to become elevated. Some medical experts think an elevated blood homocysteine level may be a "marker" in blood that indicates a person has CVD. Nevertheless, more studies are needed to determine whether elevated blood homocysteine plays a role in the development of CVD among the general population.

Major risk factors for CVD include advanced age, excess body fat, and physical inactivity.

homocysteine amino acid that may play a role in the development of atherosclerosis

Modifiable Risk Factors

Several major risk factors for atherosclerosis involve lifestyle choices that can be modified. Hypertension, diabetes, excess body fat, and elevated blood cholesterol are modifiable risk factors that can be influenced by diet and exercise. Many people, for example, can reduce their chances of developing atherosclerosis by avoiding tobacco use, limiting their intake of saturated fat, exercising regularly, and maintaining a healthy body weight.

Nearly one in three adult Americans has hypertension, chronically elevated blood pressure.[17] Hypertension is often referred to as a "silent disease," because people with the condition frequently feel healthy and do not have obvious symptoms that indicate trouble within their circulatory system. The condition, however, is quite serious because it damages arterial walls and increases the risk of stroke, heart failure, and kidney disease. Chapter 9 presents information about hypertension, including healthy blood pressure values (see Table 9.10). Chapter 9 also discusses ways to reduce the likelihood of developing the condition.

Diabetes is another modifiable risk factor for atherosclerosis. Adults who have diabetes are two to four times more likely to die of heart disease or stroke than adults without diabetes.[23] Chapter 5 discusses diabetes in detail. Excess body fat, especially in the abdominal region, increases the risk of type 2 diabetes and hypertension; Chapter 10 focuses on sensible ways to lose body fat. Physical inactivity also contributes to excess body fat. Chapter 11 provides suggestions for becoming more physically active. Elevated blood lipids, particularly certain lipoproteins, are a risk factor for atherosclerosis. The "Reducing the Risk of Atherosclerosis: Dietary Changes" section of this chapter presents ways people can modify their diets to reduce their chances of developing atherosclerosis.

Tobacco use is another major risk factor for atherosclerosis that is modifiable. Compared to nonsmokers, smokers have two to four times the likelihood of developing heart disease and having a stroke.[24] Smokers expose other people in their environment to secondhand smoke, which is a combination of the smoke from the burning end of a cigarette and the exhaled air of the person who is smoking. Exposure to secondhand smoke is a risk factor for heart disease.[25] If you smoke, simply improving your diet is unlikely to reduce your risk of atherosclerosis; therefore, if you smoke, make every effort to quit using tobacco products. If you do not smoke, avoid breathing secondhand smoke.

Emotional stress, particularly anger, also plays a role in the development of atherosclerosis.[21] Although individuals respond to stress differently, chronic stress generally causes physical changes in the body that can damage arteries and contribute to atherosclerosis. Furthermore, people who are "stressed out" may make unhealthy food choices, drink too much alcohol, and get inadequate exercise.

It is important to understand that a risk factor is not the same as a *cause* of disease. AIDS, for example, is caused by human immunodeficiency virus (HIV); a person cannot develop AIDS without being infected with HIV. Atherosclerosis, however, is an extremely complex disease process. In most cases, no single cause for the condition can be identified. Instead, having one or more risk factors increases a person's chances of developing the condition.

Assessing the Risk of Atherosclerosis

You may not be able to prevent having a heart attack or stroke some day, but there is plenty of scientific evidence that suggests you can forestall CVD and live a longer, more satisfying life by reducing or eliminating modifiable risk factors for atherosclerosis. Diet, for example, influences the likelihood of atherosclerosis and is highly modifiable.

Smoking is a major risk factor for atherosclerosis. Furthermore, smoking exposes nonsmokers to cigarette smoke, which is also a risk factor for heart disease. If you smoke, simply improving your diet is unlikely to reduce your risk of heart disease; therefore, make every effort to quit using tobacco products.

Medical Testing

To determine your risk of atherosclerosis, it is a good idea to have regular medical checkups in which a physician checks your blood pressure and listens to blood flow in your carotid arteries to assess whether the arteries are becoming blocked (see Fig. 6.18). The physician may request a lipoprotein profile to assess your total serum cholesterol level as well as serum HDL cholesterol, LDL cholesterol, and triglyceride levels. Although this textbook generally refers to "blood cholesterol" or "blood lipids," the amount of lipids in serum or plasma rather than whole blood is usually measured. Serum is the liquid portion of blood; plasma is similar to serum except that it contains clotting factors.

Table 6.5 presents classifications for healthy and unhealthy blood lipid levels. The desirable range for total cholesterol is less than 200 mg/dl. In 2009–2012, American adults had an average total blood cholesterol level of 196 mg/dl.[26] Do you know what your blood cholesterol level is? Even if it is below 200 mg/dl, you may still have a high risk of atherosclerosis. Why? Although knowing the concentration of cholesterol carried by all lipoproteins is important, the amounts of certain lipoproteins in your blood, particularly LDL and HDL, are more critical risk factors. As mentioned earlier, LDL carries cholesterol to cells and HDL transports cholesterol away from cells.

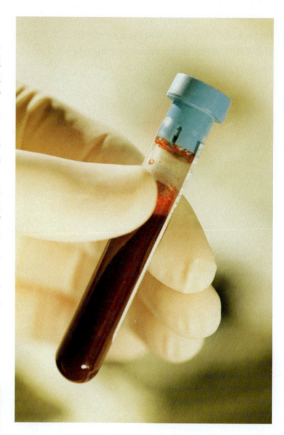

TABLE 6.5 Classification of Blood Lipid Levels

Total Cholesterol (mg/dl)	Classification
< 200	Desirable
200 to 239	Borderline high
≥ 240	High risk

LDL Cholesterol (mg/dl)	Classification
< 100	Optimal
100 to 129	Near optimal
130 to 159	Borderline high risk
160 to 189	High risk
≥ 190	Very high risk

HDL Cholesterol (mg/dl)	Classification
< 40 (for men); < 50 (for women)	High risk
≥ 60	Low risk

Triglycerides (mg/dl)	Classification
< 150	Normal
150 to 199	Borderline high risk
≥ 200	High risk

Source of data: American Heart Association, *Levels of cholesterol.* http://www.heart.org/HEARTORG/ GettingHealthy/FatsAndOils/Fats101/Levels-of-Cholesterol_UCM_305051_Article.jsp.

high-sensitivity C-reactive protein (hs-CRP) protein produced primarily by the liver in response to inflammation

People with a high ratio of total cholesterol to HDL cholesterol usually have too much LDL cholesterol in their blood and an increased risk of heart disease and stroke. A healthy ratio of total cholesterol to HDL cholesterol is less than 4:1.[27] To calculate your risk of having a heart attack during the next 10 years, use the risk assessment tool at http://cvdrisk.nhlbi.nih.gov/calculator.asp.

Someday, scientists may be able to locate genes that are involved in the process of atherosclerosis and develop a blood test that identifies biological markers produced by the abnormal genes. Thus, young people could undergo testing to determine their risk of atherosclerosis well before the signs and symptoms of the condition appeared. Until then, it is wise to have regular health checkups that include blood pressure and lipid measurements (*lipoprotein profile*). Ask your physician for a copy of the laboratory results, and keep them along with others in your personal "medical file" for future reference.

C-reactive Protein Chronic inflammation is involved in the development of CVD. The liver responds to certain kinds of inflammation by producing and releasing **high-sensitivity C-reactive protein (hs-CRP)** into the bloodstream. People with high levels of hs-CRP are more likely to develop CVD.[28] Thus, elevated hs-CRP may be a marker for atherosclerosis, like homocysteine. If you have a family history of premature CVD, consider having your homocysteine and hs-CRP levels measured.

Coronary Calcium Cigarette smoking and elevated total blood cholesterol level in early adulthood are significantly associated with the formation of *coronary calcium*, calcium deposits in arteries of the heart later in life.[20] High amounts of coronary calcium are associated with increased risk of atherosclerosis. Computerized tomography (CT) scans, special computerized images that show the body's internal structures, can detect coronary calcium deposits. A CT scan, however, involves exposure to ionizing radiation, so physicians generally reserve its use for other diagnostic purposes.

Reducing the Risk of Atherosclerosis: Dietary Changes

Specific recommendations for consumption of various types of fat are primarily based on the results of epidemiological studies that examined the effects of dietary lipids on blood lipids and risk of CVD. Populations that consume diets rich in saturated fats generally have higher rates of heart disease than populations that eat less saturated fat. Saturated fat alters the structure of liver cell membranes so they no longer function properly. As a result, the liver removes less cholesterol from the bloodstream.[29] Most saturated fatty acids increase blood cholesterol levels by raising concentrations of both LDL and HDL cholesterol. Trans fats also raise blood cholesterol levels. However, trans fats raise LDL cholesterol while reducing beneficial HDL cholesterol levels.[29]

Monounsaturated fatty acids generally lower LDL cholesterol without reducing HDL cholesterol levels. Foods rich in monounsaturated fat include peanuts and peanut oil, canola oil, olives and olive oil, almonds, and avocados.

Diets containing high amounts of polyunsaturated fatty acids may reduce blood levels of total cholesterol and LDL cholesterol. In some individuals, however, polyunsaturated fat also reduces beneficial HDL cholesterol. Nevertheless, polyunsaturated fatty acids tend to be beneficial because they do not promote atherosclerosis. Foods rich in polyunsaturated fat include corn, soybean, and cottonseed oils, as well as some types of sunflower and safflower seed oils (see Table 6.2).

MY DIVERSE PLATE

Ghee (Indian Clarified Butter)

Ghee is a solid fat that is used for cooking, primarily in India. Traditionally, ghee was made from the milk of a type of buffalo that was native to India and Pakistan, but milk from other animals can be used. To make ghee, butter is heated until its water content evaporates completely and the solids (primarily lactose and some proteins) brown and sink to the bottom. After heating, the fat is strained to remove the solids. Scientists are exploring whether certain lipids in ghee have antioxidant activity in cells.

As mentioned earlier, the Dietary Guidelines recommend limiting saturated fat intake to less than 10% of total energy intake by replacing foods that are rich sources of saturated fat with foods that contain high amounts of unsaturated fat.[16] People should limit their trans fat intake as much as possible. You can reduce your trans fat intake by eating fewer solid fats, especially foods made with partially hydrogenated oils, such as stick margarine.

What About Omega-3 and Omega-6 Fats?

The typical American diet provides far more omega–6 foods than foods that contain omega–3 fatty acids.[30] The primary omega–6 fatty acid, linoleic acid, increases inflammation and blood clotting. Some inflammation is necessary because it attracts immune system cells to disease–causing microorganisms that have entered the body. Inflammation, however, can also damage the inside of arteries. Clotting is also an important function of blood, but excess blood clotting can increase the risk of strokes, heart attacks, and other serious blood vessel disorders. In 2009, experts with the American Heart Association issued an advisory statement indicating that consuming 5 to 10% of energy in the form of omega–6 fatty acids *reduces* the risk of heart disease.[31] The role of omega–6 fats in preventing this major cause of death among Americans is controversial among medical experts. Thus, more research is needed to clarify the pros and cons of following diets that contain high amounts of these par–ticular fatty acids.

Salmon is a rich source of omega-3 fatty acids, including DHA and EPA.

Food & Nutrition tips

- Eat seafood, especially fatty fish, two times a week. Before cooking, marinate fresh fish in olive or canola oil that has been seasoned with a small amount of garlic, pepper, and lemon juice. The light coating of oil on fish can help keep the food from drying out during cooking.

- Bake, grill, or broil fish.

- Add water-packed tuna to salads, or mix tuna with a little olive oil and spread on toast.

- If you don't want the flavor of olive oil in a food, use canola oil, soybean oil, or soft margarines made from these oils for frying or sautéing.

- Sprinkle chopped walnuts on salads, yogurt, or cereal, or simply eat the nuts as a snack.

Eating foods that supply omega–3 fatty acids reduces the risk of heart dis–ease to a greater extent than does eating foods with omega–6 fatty acids.[30] The body incorporates omega–3 fatty acids into cell membranes and uses these lipids to make compounds that can reduce inflammation, serum triglycerides, and blood clotting. Table 6.6 lists foods that are sources of omega–3 fatty acids, includ–ing several species of fish. Certain fatty fish are rich sources of DHA and EPA, long–chain omega–3 fatty acids.

Alpha–linolenic acid is an omega–3 fatty acid that the body can convert to DHA and EPA (see Figure 6.2). Flaxseeds, soybeans, and walnuts are good sources of alpha–linolenic acid. However, the body can only make small amounts of DHA and EPA from alpha–linolenic acid. Therefore, it is important to include other sources of these long–chain fatty acids in your diet.

TABLE 6.6 Food Sources of Omega-3 Fats

Fish/Shellfish
Herring, salmon, sablefish, anchovies, tuna, bluefish, sardines, catfish, striped bass, mackerel, trout, shark, swordfish, halibut, pollock, flounder, shrimp, mussels, crab
Oils
Flaxseed, walnut, canola, soybean
Nuts and Seeds
Walnuts, flaxseeds
Other
Algae

To obtain beneficial long–chain omega–3 fatty acids such as DHA, the Dietary Guidelines recommend that Americans eat at least 8 ounces of various seafood, a week.[16] Because large species of fish can contain high amounts of the toxic compound *methylmercury*, young children, pregnant and breastfeeding women, and women who are likely to become pregnant should not eat shark, king mackerel, tilefish, and swordfish.[16] Shrimp, canned light tuna, salmon, pollock, and catfish are low in methylmercury. According to the Dietary Guidelines, women who are pregnant or breastfeeding can safely consume up to 12 ounces of low–mercury fish and shellfish weekly (see Chapter 3). The "Recipe for Healthy Living" feature of this chapter has an easy recipe made with salmon.

What if you do not like to eat fish? Are fish oil supplements safe? Fish oil supplements can reduce elevated triglyceride levels, but doses higher than 3 g/day may interfere with blood clotting and increase the risk of strokes. Therefore, check with your physician before you embark on a campaign to increase the omega–3 fatty acid content of your diet by taking fish oil supplements. The "Food & Nutrition Tips" on page 191 provides some ideas for increasing your intake of omega–3 fatty acids from dietary sources.

Should People Avoid Eggs?

Eggs are a relatively economical source of protein and many micronutrients. However, egg yolks are the most concentrated source of cholesterol in the typical American diet. The yolk of a large egg contains 5 grams of fat and about 190 mg of cholesterol. To reduce their cholesterol consumption, many Americans eat fewer fresh eggs than in the past. Whole eggs, however, are often hidden in commonly eaten foods such as salad dressings, noodles, frozen custards, sauces, and baked goods.

Does eating egg yolks and other cholesterol–rich animal foods raise the risk of atherosclerosis? Studies designed to determine the effects of dietary cholesterol on blood cholesterol levels have provided mixed results.[32] In gen–eral, the cholesterol in food does not have as much effect on blood cholesterol levels of healthy people as the saturated fat does. Why? In a healthy person, the liver produces less cholesterol when large amounts of cholesterol are eaten. On the other hand, eating large amounts of saturated fat increases the liver's cholesterol production. Because foods that are high in cholesterol are often rich sources of saturated fat, dietary cholesterol was blamed for raising blood cho–lesterol levels. Egg yolks, however, have almost twice as much unsaturated fat as saturated fat.

Egg whites have no fat or cholesterol. For those who must limit their cho–lesterol intake, egg whites can often be used in recipes that call for whole eggs. Products that substitute for whole eggs are available in supermarkets.

Is It Safe to Eat Butter?

Many Americans have replaced butter with partially hardened vegetable oil mar–garines because of concern over butter's cholesterol and saturated fat content. In the late 1990s, however, news reports alerted Americans that eating trans fat in margarine was more harmful than consuming the natural lipids in butter. If you use margarine, should you be concerned about its trans fat content and switch to using butter?

Compared to butter, a serving of margarine provides more unsaturated fat and less saturated fat and cholesterol. However, margarine made from par–tially hardened vegetable oil contains considerable amounts of unhealthy trans

Did You Know?

Chicken eggs normally contain very low amounts of omega-3 fatty acids. By feeding hens ground flaxseed, farmers can increase the amount of omega-3 fatty acids in eggs. In supermarkets, such omega-3 enriched eggs are often sold beside cartons of regular eggs. Expect to pay more for the enriched eggs.

fat.[33] The amount of saturated and trans fat in soft margarines is less than the amount in hard "stick" margarines or butter. You can reduce your intake of trans fats by using soft ("tub") or liquid margarines, or trans fat–free spreads that resemble margarine, instead of stick margarine or butter. However, if you enjoy butter, occasionally having some is unlikely to clog your arteries. The "Food & Nutrition Tips" feature on this page suggests ways to reduce your trans fat intake.

Did You Know?

About 80% of stick margarine is fat—the same percentage of fat as in butter. A pat of stick margarine (approximately a teaspoon) also supplies about the same amount of energy as a pat of butter—35 kcal.

Food & Nutrition tips

- Read the Nutrition Facts panel and the ingredient list on the label when choosing processed foods, especially margarine. Compare margarines to find the product with 0 g of trans fat. Margarines that have "liquid" vegetable oil as the first ingredient generally have less trans fat than stick margarines.

- Avoid products that include "interesterified" (fully hydrogenated) oil, partially hydrogenated fat, or shortening in the ingredient list.

- Eat fewer commercially prepared baked goods, snack foods, and fried fast-food items.

- Purchase brands of microwave popcorn that have little added fat or no trans fats. Buy plain popcorn, and to pop the kernels, use a small amount of hot oil in a covered saucepan or use a hot-air machine.

- Commercial frostings that are made with vegetable shortenings are likely to be high in hydrogenated oils. Remove most of the frosting from a serving of cake before eating it. (Frosting is primarily sugar and fat—empty calories.) You can make your own frosting by mixing soft margarine or smooth peanut butter with a little milk, powdered sugar, and vanilla flavoring.

- Pastry dough may be made with shortening. Replace shortening with oil or soft margarine to make your own pastry dough "from scratch." The pastry, however, will be crumbly instead of flaky.

Will Weight Loss and Exercise Help?

Excess body fat, especially around the midsection of the body, is associated with unhealthy LDL cholesterol and triglyceride levels. Physical inactivity and excess energy consumption contribute to unwanted weight gain. Performing moderate–intensity physical activity nearly every day and balancing energy intake with energy expenditure each day can help people achieve and maintain healthy body weights. Taking such steps can also reduce elevated LDL cholesterol and triglyceride levels.

Food Selection and Preparation

You can change your food selection and preparation practices to reduce the amount of unhealthy fat in your diet. Fatty meats such as rib steaks are often more tender and expensive than leaner cuts such as chuck roasts. Certain cooking

When foods such as chicken or fish are breaded and fried, the breading soaks up fat, greatly increasing the food's energy value.

methods, however, can increase the tenderness of lean cuts of meat. Moist cooking methods, such as pot roasting or tightly covering the baking dish with foil, help tenderize meats without adding fat. In addition to using a moist cooking method, reduce the oven temperature from 350°F to less than 325°F. The meat will take longer to cook, but it is less likely to toughen and dry out. After cooking, avoid eating the visible fat that remains. For example, trim away much of the fat from the meat and do not use pan drippings to make sauces or gravies. Steaming meats and vegetables is a cooking method that does not require adding fat during preparation. Stir—frying pieces of raw vegetables, meat, fish, shellfish, and poultry in small amounts of hot vegetable oil cooks them quickly and preserves micronutrients. Additionally, when you brown ground beef in a pan, drain much of the fat before you add other ingredients to the meat.

Dipping raw foods in batter and deep—fat frying them adds considerable amounts of fat to your diet, because breading serves as a sponge that soaks up oil. If you prepare breaded fried foods, place the items on paper towels after cooking them to soak up as much excess fat as possible. Some people think the breading is the "best part" of a fried food, but removing some or all of the breading before eating the item can reduce your overall fat intake. Although it is easy to peel greasy breading from fried fish, much of the fat that you eat is hidden in foods and beverages. For example, do you drink 2% milk? Fat comprises only 2% of the milk's volume, but the lipid contributes 37% of the beverage's calories. Fat—free milk actually contains less than 0.5% fat by volume, and fat contributes essentially no energy to the beverage.

What about the fat content of the cream cheese, margarine, or butter that you spread on a piece of toast? About 90% of the calories in cream cheese and about 100% of the calories in butter and margarine are from fat. Vegetable oils are almost 100% fat, so fat contributes all the energy in most salad dressings. Fried foods, chips, and salad dressings are high in fat; bacon, sausage, hot dogs, luncheon meats, and hard cheeses are also fatty foods. Nuts, including peanuts and almonds, have high fat contents, but they generally contain high amounts of healthy monounsaturated fats.

Instead of striving to eliminate all fatty foods from your diet, try reducing your intake of them, especially solid fats. For example, if you drink 2% or whole milk, switch to 1% or fat—free milk. Nearly all the lipids in fat—free milk have been removed; that is why it tastes watery to people who are not accustomed to drinking it. Except for energy and lipid content, the nutritional value of fat—free milk is basically the same as that of whole and 2% milks. The "Food & Nutrition Tips" feature on page 193 provides more practical suggestions for reducing your saturated fat intake.

Fat Replacers   In response to consumer demand for more fat—reduced and fat—free foods, manufacturers may use synthetic fat replacers to substitute for some or all of the fat in their products. The ideal synthetic fat is safe, provides little or no energy, mimics natural fat's contribution to the taste and texture of food, and withstands typical cooking temperatures. Oatrim, Simplesse, and Olean are brands of fat replacers, but few manufactured foods contain these synthetic substances.

People who are concerned about their energy intake should recognize that fat—reduced and fat—free foods are not "calorie free." Moreover, food manufacturers often increase the amounts of added sugars in these products to improve taste and compensate for reduced fat content. Nevertheless, fat replacers can help people reduce their total fat intake.[35]

Food & Nutrition tips

• Reduce your intake of fried foods, including French-fried potatoes.

• Purchase lean meats and trim visible fat from meat before cooking. Before eating cooked meat, trim and discard any remaining visible fat.

• Try replacing some fatty foods with reduced-fat or fat-free alternatives. For example, substitute plain, fat-free yogurt in recipes that call for sour cream. Place a spoonful of the yogurt, instead of butter or sour cream, on a baked potato.

• Because most nuts are rich sources of healthy unsaturated fats, replace foods that contain saturated fat with nuts. For example, use peanut or soy nut butters instead of cheese or luncheon meat in sandwiches. Some nut butters contain trans fats and added sugars, so read the Nutrition Facts panel and ingredients list before selecting these products.

• Replace some or all of the solid fat in recipes for baked goods with vegetable oil or unsweetened applesauce. In general, 1 cup of applesauce can replace 1 cup of fat.

• Pretzels, air-popped popcorn, and most fruits and vegetables are low fat and generally more nutrient-dense than chips, cookies, pastries, and candy bars.

• Patronize fast-food restaurants that offer low-saturated fat menu items such as salads without added cheese and meat, baked or broiled chicken and fish, low-fat yogurt, and bean burritos.

• Use less salad dressing on salads. When in restaurants, order salad dressings "on the side" so you can control the amount that is added.

• Replace butter in recipes with trans fat–free margarines (60% oil). Use olive or canola oils in recipes that call for "vegetable oil."

| Plain yogurt is a low-fat substitute for sour cream.

Other Dietary Modifications

In addition to modifying your fat intake, you can reduce your risk of CVD by making other dietary changes. Eating foods that are rich sources of fiber, particularly soluble fiber (see Chapter 5), can reduce LDL cholesterol levels without lowering beneficial HDL cholesterol levels. If your triglyceride level is too high (> 150 mg/dl), consider cutting back on your intake of refined carbo–hydrates by eating less candy and pastries and drinking fewer sugar–sweetened soft drinks.

Drinking small amounts of alcohol (1 to 2 drinks/day) can raise beneficial HDL cholesterol levels. Consuming too much alcohol, however, contributes to hypertension and damages every organ of the body. Furthermore, excess alco–hol consumption has devastating effects on society, as well as on personal safety and relationships. If you consume several alcoholic beverages regularly, consider reducing your intake to no more than one serving per day.

Dietitians and other nutrition experts often promote the traditional Mediterranean diet for healthy eating as well as reducing elevated blood lipid levels and the risk of CVD. The Mediterranean diet (see Fig. 3.17) recommends eating more fish and seafood, and smaller amounts of red meat; using heart—healthy unsaturated fatty acids; engaging in regular physical activity; and drinking a glass of wine daily. This diet also emphasizes phytochemical—rich fruits, vegetables, beans, and nuts. Table 6.7 summarizes ways certain actions, such as dietary manipulations and other therapeutic lifestyle changes, may alter a person's blood lipid levels.

What If Lifestyle Changes Do Not Work?

Some people are unable to lower their risk of CVD significantly by making dietary changes, exercising regularly, and losing excess body fat. If your blood lipids are too high and the levels have remained elevated even after you have made these lifestyle modifications, it is important to discuss additional treatment options with your physician. Millions of Americans take a class of prescription drugs called *statins* to reduce their elevated blood lipid levels. Statins interfere with the liver's metabolism of cholesterol, effectively reducing LDL cholesterol and triglyceride levels as a result. Statins are relatively safe when taken as directed.[36]

TABLE 6.7 Ways to Lower Your Risk of CVD

Action	Potential Benefits
Increase physical activity level.	Raises HDL levels
Lose excess body fat.	Lowers elevated triglycerides, blood pressure, and risk of type 2 diabetes; may increase HDL
Quit smoking.	May raise HDL and lower LDL levels
Make specific dietary changes:	
Reduce intake of saturated fats and avoid trans fats.	Raises HDL and lowers LDL
Replace saturated fats with polyunsaturated and monounsaturated fats.	Lowers LDL
Include some omega-3 and omega-6 fats. (Discuss the need for fish oil supplements with your physician.)	Reduces triglycerides; may raise HDL and reduce blood pressure
Replace margarine or butter with spread made from plant sterols/stanols.	Reduces LDL
Eat more whole-grain, fiber-rich foods, especially those containing soluble fiber.	Reduces total cholesterol and LDL without altering HDL
Consume foods that contain antioxidant nutrients and certain phytochemicals, such as red grapes and red wine (see Table 1.3). Dietary supplements of these compounds are not recommended.	Reduces risk of heart disease, but the mechanism is unclear
Reduce alcohol and sugar intake.	Lowers triglyceride levels

Concept Checkpoint 6.6

18. Define *atherosclerosis, arteriosclerosis, arterial plaque, thrombus,* and *embolus.* Discuss the series of physiological changes that occur in arteries and contribute to the development of CVD.
19. List three kinds of fish that often contain high amounts of methylmercury.
20. List at least two major risk factors for atherosclerosis that are nonmodifiable and at least five that are modifiable.
21. Bernard's HDL cholesterol level is 62 mg/dl. Based on this information, does Bernard have a high risk or low risk of CVD? Explain your answer.
22. What is "hs-CRP"? What can you learn about your risk of heart disease and stroke from having a lipoprotein profile performed on your blood?
23. Suggest at least four ways people can reduce their intakes of saturated and trans fats and increase their intakes of unsaturated fats.
24. What is a statin?

6.7 Nutrition Matters: Drink to Your Health?

Learning Outcomes

1 Identify amounts of beer, wine, and distilled spirits in a standard drink.

2 Classify people who drink alcohol according to their usual pattern of consumption.

3 Identify factors that affect alcohol metabolism.

4 Discuss alcohol's effects on health.

What do beer, wine, vodka, whiskey, sake (*sak'−e*), koumiss (*koo'−mis*), and kefir (*keh−feer'*) have in common? These beverages contain *ethanol*, a two−carbon compound that chemists classify as an alcohol. Alcohols such as ethanol, glycerol, and cholesterol are organic molecules that have one or more *hydroxyl* (*OH*) groups in their chemical structures (Fig. 6.21). This textbook refers to ethanol simply as "alcohol."

Figure 6.21 Ethanol. Ethanol is a simple two-carbon compound.

$$CH_3 — CH_2 — OH$$

Ethanol

Offering wine in religious ceremonies, toasting the bride and groom with champagne at a wedding, or barhopping with friends on their 21st birthdays—for many Americans, alcohol consumption is a part of celebrating religious rites and life's milestones. When consumed in moderation, alcoholic beverages can make social situations more enjoyable. Many people, however, experience serious problems as a result of their drinking habits. This section focuses on alcohol metabolism, as well as the chemical's effects on the body.

Alcohol Production

Throughout the world, people have been producing and drinking alcoholic beverages for thousands of years. The chemical process that results in alcohol is not complicated and occurs naturally. The process requires certain microbes, warm conditions, and a source of simple sugars. Although some types of bacteria produce alcohol, commercial alcoholic beverage production relies on *yeast*, one−celled fungi (*fun'−ji*) that break down (*ferment*) simple sugars in the absence of oxygen to obtain energy and the metabolic waste product, alcohol. Grains, fruit, and potatoes—just about anything

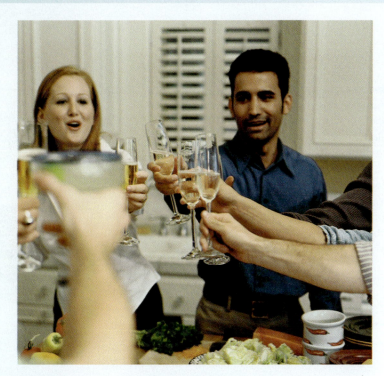

TABLE 6.8
Approximate Alcohol, Carbohydrate, and Energy Contents of Alcoholic Beverages*

Beverage	Amount (fl oz)	Kcal	Alcohol (g)	Carbohydrates (g)
Beer				
Regular	12.0	139	13	11
Lite	12.0	103	11	5
Table Wines	5.0	114	14	5
Distilled Spirits				
Gin, rum, vodka, whiskey	1.5	96	14	0

* Protein and fat contribute little or nothing to the caloric content.

Source: U.S. Department of Agriculture.

Figure 6.22 What's a standard drink? A standard drink is approximately 12 ounces of beer, 1½ ounces of liquor, or 5 ounces of wine.

that contains simple sugars—will ferment under the proper conditions. Yeast will even ferment lactose in milk.

Alcohol is soluble in water, and alcoholic beverages generally contain a considerable amount of water. Beers are typically 3 to 6% alcohol, wines contain about 8 to 14% alcohol, and wine coolers are generally less than 5% alcohol by volume. Alcohol is poisonous (*toxic*), and yeast die when the concentration of alcohol in the fermenting solution reaches 14 to 16%. The distilling process increases the alcohol concentration of an alcoholic beverage. Distilled spirits (hard liquors) such as whiskey, bourbon, and vodka are generally 40 to 50% alcohol. You can determine the percentage of alcohol in hard liquor by dividing the "proof" declaration on the label by two. Tequila, for example, is "80 proof," or 40% alcohol.

Although each gram of alcohol provides 7 kcal, alcohol is not a nutrient; it is a mindaltering drug that is often classified as a food. Beer and wine contain simple carbohydrates and small amounts of certain minerals and B vitamins. Distilled spirits have essentially no nutritional value other than water. Mixing distilled spirits with juices, cocktail mixes, or other flavorings increases the alcoholic beverage's energy content and may add some nutrients, particularly simple sugars, depending on the ingredients in the mixer. Table 6.8 indicates the grams of alcohol and carbohydrates in certain alcoholic drinks, as well as their caloric content. A standard drink (approximately 12 ounces of beer, 5 ounces of wine, or 1½ ounces of liquor) contains 13 to 14 grams of alcohol (Fig. 6.22).

How the Body Processes Alcohol

Alcohol requires no digestion and readily passes through the tissues lining the inside of the mouth, esophagus, stomach, and small intestine. When alcohol is consumed with meals, food delays its absorption from the stomach and slows the rate at which the drug enters the bloodstream. To reduce alcohol's harmful effects, the body detoxifies the simple chemical by converting it into less damaging compounds. Detoxification begins in the stomach, where the enzyme gastric alcohol dehydrogenase metabolizes up to 20% of the alcohol. Most of the remaining alcohol passes through the small intestinal wall and circulates to the liver, the primary site for metabolizing alcohol. Since alcohol is a poison, the liver shifts its metabolic focus from macronutrient metabolism to alcohol detoxification when the compound enters its tissues.

The liver relies on two biochemical pathways to metabolize alcohol. When relatively low doses are consumed, the enzyme alcohol dehydrogenase converts most of the alcohol to acetaldehyde, a substance that is more toxic than alcohol. Another enzyme, aldehyde dehydrogenase, reacts with acetaldehyde to form acetate, which can also be harmful. Acetate, however, can be metabolized to carbon dioxide (CO_2) and water (H_2O), or the molecule can be used to synthesize fatty acids and cholesterol (Fig. 6.23).

If a person consumes excessive amounts of alcohol such as during a drinking binge, the alcohol overwhelms the liver's ability to metabolize the drug using the dehydrogenase pathway. When this occurs, the second method of processing alcohol, the microsomal ethanol oxidizing system (MEOS), takes over. Unlike the alcohol dehydrogenase pathway, MEOS wastes energy in the form of body heat that dissipates into the environment. Thus, alcoholics typically gain little weight from their energy intake when alcohol supplies most of their energy.

Factors That Influence Alcohol Metabolism You may have noticed that a few of your friends who drink can "hold their liquor" better than others. Why are some people able to drink more alcohol at one time than others? Several factors account for the variability. In addition to the amount and timing of alcohol consumption, personal characteristics such as sex, body size and composition, age, and prior drinking history affect the body's detoxification rate. For example, a healthy person who weighs 154 pounds (70 kg) metabolizes about 1 alcoholic drink per hour. Drinking caffeinated beverages, exercising, or taking vitamins does not increase this rate. To sober up, the drinker must stop consuming alcohol and give his or her liver time to metabolize the drug.

Alcohol is not stored in the body. Until the liver can detoxify the toxic chemical, it circulates in the bloodstream and diffuses into the watery fluids within and surrounding cells. The lungs and perspiration eliminate some of the alcohol; that's why you can smell alcohol when you're around someone who's been drinking. The kidneys also filter some of the drug from the bloodstream and eliminate it in urine. To determine whether someone is legally intoxicated as a result of drinking alcohol, law enforcement officials use special devices to analyze the alcohol in blood, urine, or expired air to estimate the person's blood alcohol concentration (BAC). BAC is reported as a percentage that indicates the amount of alcohol in the blood. In the United States, a BAC of 0.08% is the legal limit for intoxication for automobile operators who are 21 years of age or older.

Men and women have different physical responses to alcohol. Women tend to become more impaired than men do after drinking the same amount of alcohol, even when differences in body weight are taken into account. The reasons for these sexual differences are unclear, but they probably involve physiological factors including body size and composition. The average man is larger than the average woman, and larger people can often drink more alcohol without showing ill effects than smaller individuals, because they have bigger livers that detoxify more alcohol at a time. Additionally, a healthy 150-pound man typically has more body water than a healthy 150-pound woman. After the man drinks a beer, the alcohol diffuses out of his bloodstream and into the water compartments of his body. The woman's body has less water, so more alcohol remains in her bloodstream after she drinks a beer. As a result, her BAC rises faster, and she becomes more intoxicated after drinking the same amount of alcohol as her male counterpart (Fig. 6.24). Compared to men who drink heavily, women have a higher risk of serious health problems, especially damage to their liver, brain, and heart, when they abuse the same amounts of alcohol.[37]

Prior alcohol exposure also influences the rate of alcohol metabolism. People who drink regularly develop tolerance. Tolerance occurs as the levels of liver enzymes needed to metabolize alcohol increase, and as a result, the rate of alcohol metabolism increases. Consequently, the regular drinker needs to consume more alcohol at a time to achieve the same mind-altering effects as a person who drinks infrequently. Tolerance can lead to alcohol dependence (alcoholism).

Figure 6.23 Alcohol metabolism: Major metabolic steps. This diagram simplifies the major chemical steps involved in the metabolism of low doses of alcohol.

Figure 6.24 Alcohol consumption and BAC. This table shows the relationship between the number of alcoholic drinks consumed within the same period and BACs for healthy men and women. For example, a 170-pound man will have his BAC reach 0.05% after he has three drinks, whereas a 137-pound woman will have her BAC reach 0.05% after drinking only two drinks. However, alcohol's effects on individuals can vary. In the United States and Canada, a person is legally intoxicated when his or her BAC is 0.08% or higher.

Classifying Drinkers

In 2012, slightly more than 50% of Americans who were 12 years of age or older reported being current alcohol drinkers during the 30 days prior to the survey.[38] Almost one–quarter of the current drinkers engaged in binge drink– ing at least once, and 6.5% of current drinkers drank heavily during this period.

What is "moderate drinking" or "binge drinking"? Although there is no universally accepted definition for "light," "moderate," or "heavy" drinking, medical practi– tioners and alcohol researchers often follow the classification guidelines listed in Table 6.9. Binge drinking is a form of heavy drinking, but the definition of binge drinking often differs according to sex. According to the Centers for Disease Control and Prevention, binge drinking is defined as hav– ing four or more drinks during an occasion (about 2 hours) for females and five or more drinks during an occasion for males.[39] Regardless of their backgrounds, binge drinking is a common practice among Americans.

As a college student, you may have observed binge drinking or engaged in the practice. In 2012, Americans who were 21 to 25 years of age were more likely to binge drink than Americans in other age groups.[38] Youthful binge drink– ing is a serious public health concern because the behavior is often associated with driving while drunk. Furthermore, the practice may increase a person's later risk of alcoholism and can result in death.

TABLE 6.9
Classifying Drinkers

Level	Amount of Alcohol Consumed (Standard Drinks)
Abstainer	None or fewer than 12 drinks/year
Light	1 to 13 drinks/month
Moderate	4 to 14 drinks/week
Heavy	3 or more drinks/day
Binge drinker	5 or more drinks/about 2 hours (males)
Binge drinker	4 or more drinks/about 2 hours (females)

Source: Modified from: Dufour MC: What is moderate drinking? Defining "drinks" and drinking levels. *Alcohol Research & Health* 23(1):5, 1999.

Binge drinking has become an expected "rite of pas– sage" for American youth celebrating their 21st birthday. The practice of trying to consume 21 drinks quickly while celebrating "power hour" ("21 for 21") can have deadly consequences. On March 15, 2004, Jason Reinhardt was celebrating his 21st birthday with friends in a bar. Jason rapidly drank 16 shots of alcohol. Although he managed to return to his friends' house and go to bed, his lifeless body was discovered a few hours later. The young man's blood alcohol concentration was 0.361, well within the deadly range. What makes binge drinking so dangerous?

Binge drinking increases a person's BAC rapidly and to a point at which signs of alcohol poisoning occur. An individual suffering from alcohol poisoning is confused, "passes out" and cannot be aroused (*comatose*), breathes slowly and irregularly, and has pale or bluish skin. Alcohol poisoning can cause the heartbeat to slow down and the lungs to stop functioning, resulting in death. Additionally, if a comatose person vomits, his or her stomach contents can enter the lungs, causing the person to choke to death. Jason died in his sleep from alcohol poisoning. His breathing rate slowed, his heartbeat became irregular, and his organs gradually shut down while he slept. Thus, it is important to recognize that alcohol poisoning is a life-threatening condition. If you suspect someone has consumed a deadly amount of alcohol, don't waste time trying to estimate how many drinks that person has drunk; call 911 immediately.

The three teenagers who died in this automobile had consumed alcohol before the accident.

Assessment: What Are Signs and Symptoms of Alcohol Abuse

These questions incorporate many common signs and symptoms of alcoholism. This test is intended to help you determine if you or someone you know needs to find out more about alcoholism; it is not intended to be used to establish the diagnosis of alcoholism.

YES	NO		YES	NO	
❑	❑	1. Do you ever drink heavily when you are disappointed, under pressure, or have had a quarrel with someone?	❑	❑	14. Have you sometimes failed to keep promises you made to yourself about controlling or cutting down on your drinking?
❑	❑	2. Can you handle more alcohol now than when you first started to drink?	❑	❑	15. Have you ever had a DWI (driving while intoxicated) or DUI (driving under the influence of alcohol) violation, or any other legal problem related to your drinking?
❑	❑	3. Have you ever been unable to remember part of the previous evening, even though your friends said that you did not pass out?	❑	❑	16. Do you try to avoid family or close friends while you are drinking?
❑	❑	4. When drinking with other people, do you try to have a few extra drinks when others won't know about them?	❑	❑	17. Are you having more financial, work, school, and/or family problems as a result of your drinking?
❑	❑	5. Do you sometimes feel uncomfortable if alcohol is not available?	❑	❑	18. Has your physician ever advised you to cut down on your drinking?
❑	❑	6. Do you sometimes feel a little guilty about your drinking?	❑	❑	19. Do you eat very little or irregularly during the periods when you are drinking?
❑	❑	7. Are you in more of a hurry to get your first drink of the day than you used to be?	❑	❑	20. Do you sometimes have the "shakes" in the morning and find that it helps to have a "little" drink, tranquilizer, or medication of some kind?
❑	❑	8. Has a family member or close friend ever expressed concern or complained about your drinking?	❑	❑	21. Have you recently noticed that you can't drink as much as you used to?
❑	❑	9. Have you been having more memory blackouts recently?	❑	❑	22. Do you sometimes stay drunk for several days at a time?
❑	❑	10. Do you often want to continue drinking after your friends say they've had enough?	❑	❑	23. After periods of drinking, do you sometimes see or hear things that aren't there?
❑	❑	11. Do you usually have a reason for the occasions when you drink heavily?	❑	❑	24. Have you ever gone to anyone for help about your drinking?
❑	❑	12. When you're sober, do you sometimes regret things you did or said while drinking?	❑	❑	25. Do you ever feel depressed or anxious before, during, or after periods of heavy drinking?
❑	❑	13. Have you tried switching brands or drinks, or following different plans to control your drinking?	❑	❑	26. Have any of your blood relatives ever had a problem with alcohol?

Any "yes" answer indicates that you may be at greater risk for alcoholism. More than one "yes" answer may indicate the presence of an alcohol-related problem or alcoholism and the need for consultation with an alcoholism professional. To find out more, contact the National Council on Alcoholism and Drug Dependence in your area.

Source: National Council on Alcoholism and Drug Dependence, Inc.

Alcohol Dependence and Abuse

A person who is *dependent* on alcohol (an alcoholic) has an uncontrollable need to drink; is unable to limit his or her alcohol consumption; suffers withdrawal symptoms, such as shakiness and anxiety, when alcohol is unavailable after a period of heavy drinking; and experiences *tolerance* to the drug. Tolerance develops over time as the drinker's body becomes better able to metabolize the alcohol. As a result, the alcohol-dependent person needs to consume more of the drug to obtain the same effects that he or she experienced prior to becoming dependent. About 17% of men and about 8% of women who drink alcohol become dependent on the drug at some point in their lives.[40] A self-assessment you can take to indicate whether you are at risk of alcoholism appears on page 199.

Many people are not dependent on alcohol, but they abuse the drug (drink in excess) and are at risk of alcoholism. The alcohol abuser experiences problems at home, work, and school that are associated with his or her drinking habits. Both abusers and alcoholics engage in behaviors that place themselves and others in danger, such as drinking and driving.

Alcohol and Health

Alcohol is a central nervous system depressant. Mild alcohol intoxication often produces pleasant sensations and relaxed inhibitions. Consuming large amounts, however, depresses normal motor functioning, including breathing, and death can result. Excessive alcohol use is the third leading lifestyle-related cause of death in the United States.[41] The drug is often involved in motor vehicle accidents, falls, and drownings, as well as acts of violence and abuse. An estimated 88,000 Americans die each year as a result of excessive alcohol use.[41] Thousands of other people suffer physical injuries and have damaged interpersonal relationships related to excess alcohol consumption.

The potentially harmful physiological effects of abusing the drug vary from person to person, primarily because of differences in overall health, drinking habits, and genetic background. Alcohol affects every cell in the body, and when consumed in excess, the drug damages every system in the body, particularly the gastrointestinal, nervous, and cardiovascular systems. Figure 6.25 summarizes major damaging physiological effects of alcohol.

Alcohol and the Gastrointestinal Tract If you have consumed distilled spirits without adding mixers, you probably felt a burning sensation as the alcohol entered your throat and stomach. This sensation is an indication of alcohol's irritating effects on the lining of your gastrointestinal tract. Not surprisingly, chronic drinking contributes to intestinal ulcer formation, particularly in the esophagus and stomach. An ulcer is a sore. Intestinal ulcers can cause chronic bleeding and may penetrate through the intestinal wall. When this occurs, intestinal contents leak into the abdominal cavity, causing serious and often deadly infections. Although the reasons are unclear, chronic alcohol

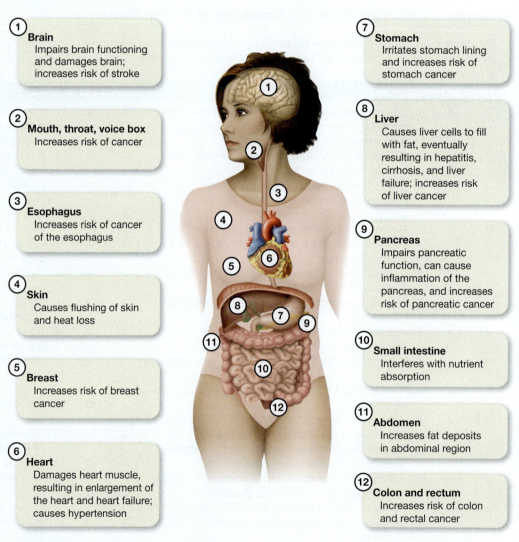

1 **Brain**
Impairs brain functioning and damages brain; increases risk of stroke

2 **Mouth, throat, voice box**
Increases risk of cancer

3 **Esophagus**
Increases risk of cancer of the esophagus

4 **Skin**
Causes flushing of skin and heat loss

5 **Breast**
Increases risk of breast cancer

6 **Heart**
Damages heart muscle, resulting in enlargement of the heart and heart failure; causes hypertension

7 **Stomach**
Irritates stomach lining and increases risk of stomach cancer

8 **Liver**
Causes liver cells to fill with fat, eventually resulting in hepatitis, cirrhosis, and liver failure; increases risk of liver cancer

9 **Pancreas**
Impairs pancreatic function, can cause inflammation of the pancreas, and increases risk of pancreatic cancer

10 **Small intestine**
Interferes with nutrient absorption

11 **Abdomen**
Increases fat deposits in abdominal region

12 **Colon and rectum**
Increases risk of colon and rectal cancer

Figure 6.25 Some of alcohol's effects on the body. Chronic alcohol abuse seriously damages several organs and increases the risk of various cancers.

consumption increases the risk of *alcoholic pancreatitis*, a painful and sometimes fatal condition characterized by inflammation and destruction of the pancreas.

People who consume alcohol have an increased risk of cancers of the digestive system. Such cancers include mouth, throat, esophagus, liver, colorectal, and pancreatic cancers.[42]

Alcohol and the Brain Alcohol's effects on the central nervous system, especially the brain, appear within a few minutes of having a drink. Alcohol acts as a depressant, slowing the transmission of messages between nerve cells (neurons). At low BACs ($< 0.06\%$), the drinker is relaxed and less inhibited socially as regions of the brain that control decision making and reasoning ability are depressed. If the person continues to drink and his or her BAC increases to between 0.08 and 0.15%, the person loses control over voluntary muscles, particularly muscles that move the lips, eyes, and limbs. As a result, the drinker's speech is slurred, his or her eyes have difficulty focusing on objects, and the person's ability to drive or operate any heavy equipment is seriously compromised. When the drinker's BAC reaches 0.20 to 0.30%, his or her brain is unable to process information. Higher BACs usually result in loss of consciousness ("passing out"). Moreover, coma and even death can occur as the brain loses control over lung and heart functioning. Table 6.10 lists BAC levels and typical nervous system effects that can occur at each level.

Alcohol can disrupt the ability of neurons in the brain to transmit messages. Long-term consumption of excessive amounts of alcohol can cause the neurons to shrink, and the brain develops other structural abnormalities. Confusion and memory loss are common signs of the extensive brain damage that occurs in a chronic heavy drinker.

Alcohol and the Liver In addition to harming the brain, alcohol can damage the liver. Some acetaldehyde that forms when alcohol is metabolized enters the complex series of biochemical pathways that eventually produce carbon dioxide, water, and ATP, the primary energy storage molecule for cells. The liver, however, also uses acetaldehyde to make fatty acids

TABLE 6.10
Typical Effects of Alcohol at Various BAC Levels (Adults)

Blood Alcohol Concentration	Typical Physiological and Psychological Effects
0.02–0.03	Increased sociability, slightly elevated mood, and mild relaxation May experience mild "light-headed" sensation
0.04–0.06	Sense of warmth, well-being, and relaxation Reduced inhibitions, resulting in exaggerated emotional and behavioral responses to situations Highly elevated mood Minor impairment of reasoning
0.07–0.09	Slight loss of balance, may have difficulty carrying on a conversation, slower than normal reaction time Highly elevated mood Reduced ability to make reasonable decisions and control one's behavior
0.10–0.15	Major impairment of muscular coordination, slurred speech, delayed reaction time, hearing and visual impairment Depressed mood and increased anxiety Severely impaired ability to understand information and make reasonable decisions
0.16–0.20	Disoriented May need assistance to stand and walk May experience nausea and vomiting; can choke on vomit May blackout, that is, not recall what has occurred when sober again
0.25–0.30	In a stupor (severely impaired intellectual, physical, and sensory functions) High risk of choking to death from inhaling vomit High risk of accidental injuries May pass out
0.35–0.40 and higher	Onset of coma (become unconscious and unable to be awakened for a long period of time) Death due to respiratory arrest

Adapted from: Oklahoma University: *Blood alcohol content calculator.* 2009. www.ou.edu/oupd/bac.htm. Accessed: August 23, 2013

(a)

(b)

Figure 6.26 Liver cirrhosis. The photograph on the left (*a*) shows a normal liver; the one on the right (*b*) shows a liver damaged by alcoholic cirrhosis.

for synthesizing triglycerides (see Fig. 6.23). Even after a single bout of heavy drinking, fat accumulates in liver cells and causes a condition called "fatty liver." Fatty liver is reversible; if the affected person avoids alcohol for an extended period, the liver metabolizes the fat, and the organ eventually heals itself. If the person continues to drink, the buildup of fat destroys his or her liver cells, and tough scar tissue replaces them. This irrevers-ible condition is called *liver cirrhosis* or hardening of the liver (Fig. 6.26). Alcoholics are prone to develop *hepatitis*, inflam-mation of the liver. Hepatitis can cause cirrhosis and increases the risk of liver cancer.

The scarred regions of an alcoholic's liver have no func-tion other than holding the organ together. Under normal conditions, a healthy liver can regenerate sections of itself, but when destruction of liver cells is extensive, the organ begins to fail. In this situation, the affected person will die unless he or she undergoes liver transplantation. Chronic alcohol abuse is a major cause of liver failure among adult Americans.

Alcohol and the Cardiovascular System When con-sumed in low to moderate intakes (1 to 2 drinks/day), alcohol may reduce the risk of heart disease.[43] Excess consumption, however, can damage heart muscle and elevate blood pressure to dangerous levels. As a result, chronic alcoholics often have enlarged but weakened hearts and suffer strokes.

Alcohol and Cancer Compared to people who do not consume alcohol, chronic drinkers are more likely to develop certain cancers. Alcohol causes changes to cells that increase the drinker's risk of oral cavity, esophageal, stomach, liver, pancreatic, and colorectal cancer. Women who consume two or more drinks daily have a higher risk of breast cancer than women who avoid alcohol or drink

less than two drinks per day. Heavy drinkers who smoke tobacco products have a much greater risk of developing cancers of the oral cavity and esophagus than people who drink less and do not smoke.

Alcohol and Drug Interactions People who drink alco-hol while taking other drugs, including prescription medi-cations and over–the–counter remedies, need to recognize that alcohol's harmful effects may be amplified by the medications. Additionally, alcohol may interact with other drugs, causing serious side effects that do not occur when a drug is consumed alone. For example, combining alcohol with products that contain the pain–reliever acetamino-phen can cause severe liver damage and even death.

Effects of Alcohol on Nutritional Status When con-sumed in moderation, alcohol stimulates the appetite. Alco-hol, however, lowers blood glucose levels and raises blood triglycerides. Chronic, excessive alcohol intake can have adverse effects on the drinker's nutritional intake and sta-tus. Many alcoholics consume a considerable portion of their energy as alcohol, which often displaces nutrient–dense foods from their diets and increases their risk of malnu-trition. Even when an alcoholic consumes nutritious meals while drinking, the alcohol interferes with the absorption, metabolism, and storage of various vitamins and increases the excretion of certain nutrients, particularly fat and the mineral magnesium.

Poor diets contribute to deficiencies of vitamin A, vitamin C, and the B vitamins thiamin and folate among alcoholics. It is not unusual for chronic alcoholics to become thiamin deficient and develop *Wernicke–Korsakoff syn-drome*, a brain disorder characterized by mental confusion, memory loss, and uncoordinated muscular movements. The person with this condition typically staggers when trying to walk. Taking thiamin supplements can resolve some signs of the syndrome, but the person must avoid drinking alcohol while being treated.

Although chronic alcohol abuse is associated with an increased risk of bone loss and fractures, light to moder-ate alcohol drinkers tend to have stronger bones and lower risk of fractures than nondrinkers, especially among women who are past child bearing age.[44] More research, however, is needed to determine the effects of alcohol on bone health.

Alcohol and Body Water Billboard and commercial advertisements for alcoholic beverages often show sweaty, physically active young adults gulping down beer or liquor to relieve their thirst. These ads are misleading. Alcohol is not a good thirst quencher, because it is a diuretic that suppresses the production of antidiuretic hormone (ADH) by the pituitary gland. Without ADH's action, the kidneys produce more urine, and the body loses water and cer-tain vitamins and minerals along with it. If a dehydrated drinker consumes even more alcohol to relieve thirst, this

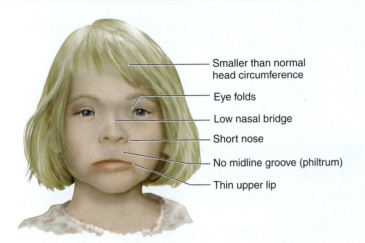

- Smaller than normal head circumference
- Eye folds
- Low nasal bridge
- Short nose
- No midline groove (philtrum)
- Thin upper lip

Figure 6.27 **Fetal alcohol syndrome.** Physical deformities and developmental delays are characteristics of fetal alcohol syndrome (FAS), a type of fetal alcohol spectrum disorder.

TABLE 6.11
Who Should Avoid Alcohol?

Women who suspect they are pregnant, know they are pregnant, or are trying to become pregnant

People who plan to drive or use heavy machinery

People taking certain over-the-counter or prescription medications

People with medical conditions that alcohol can aggravate

Recovering alcoholics

People younger than 21 years of age

Source: Adapted from National Institute on Alcohol Abuse and Alcoholism. *Moderate & binge drinking.* http://www.niaaa.nih.gov/alcohol-health/overview-alcohol-consumption/moderate-binge-drinking. Accessed: October 27, 2013

response only increases his or her water losses. Drinking water and other nonalcoholic drinks is the best way to keep the body well hydrated.

Fetal Alcohol Spectrum Disorders
When a pregnant woman drinks alcohol, her embryo/fetus also "drinks" alcohol, because the drug passes freely from the mother's bloodstream into the embryo/fetus's bloodstream. Alcohol is most devastating when it affects an embryo, because organs develop during the first 2 months after conception. Unfortunately, many women are not aware that they are pregnant during this early stage of their child's prenatal (before birth) development, and they may drink socially or binge drink. Alcohol is toxic to cells, including rapidly dividing embryonic cells. An infant born with a *fetal alcohol spectrum disorder (FASD)* has some degree of developmental abnormalities as a result of its mother's consumption of alcohol during pregnancy. *Fetal alcohol syndrome (FAS)* is a devastating form of FASD. A child with FAS is born with certain facial and heart defects, as well as extensive, irreversible damage to its nervous system that causes intellectual disability (Fig. 6.27). Children with FAS also experience delayed and abnormal physical development.

The amount of alcohol that can be safely consumed by a pregnant woman has not been determined. Therefore, if you or someone you know is trying to conceive or is pregnant, you or that person should "play it safe" and avoid alcohol. The risks are too high to justify even one drink. Table 6.11 identifies people, including pregnant women, who should not drink alcohol.

Health Benefits of Alcohol

Consuming light to moderate amounts of alcohol raises HDL cholesterol levels; reduces blood levels of fibrinogen, an important blood-clotting factor; and decreases platelet stickiness.

Platelets are cell fragments involved in the blood-clotting process. Reducing the likelihood of blood clot formation lowers the risk of heart attack and certain types of strokes.

Some medical researchers think drinking beer and red wine is healthier than consuming white wines or spirits. Although the alcohol in beer is the same as that in wine and distilled spirits, red wine and beer have higher levels of certain antioxidants and B vitamins than other alcoholic beverages, which may explain their health benefits.[43] (Moderate alcohol consumption was defined as no more than 2 drinks/day for men and no more than 1 drink/day for women.) Purple grape juice, which is used to make red wine, contains the same antioxidants as the wine and appears to protect against heart disease as well. The role of moderate alcohol consumption in coronary artery disease prevention is controversial. Drinking small amounts of alcohol seems to reduce the risk of heart disease, but consuming moderate to excessive amounts of alcohol is associated with increased risks of addiction, hypertension, heart failure, cancer, liver cirrhosis, and motor vehicle accidents. More research is needed to determine if alcohol alone or other compounds present in certain alcoholic beverages provide beneficial effects on health when consumed in moderation.

Alcohol and Physical Performance

Although some athletes may think consuming a small amount of alcohol before a competitive event might help relieve anxiety, alcohol reduces eye-hand coordination and slows reaction times even when BACs are relatively low (0.02 to 0.05%). Studies indicate conflicting findings concerning the effects of low to moderate amounts of alcohol on strength and endurance. In some instances, low to moderate intakes of alcohol reduce endurance and have negative effects on strength, but in other cases, this level of alcohol consumption produces no detrimental effects on strength and endurance. Alcohol can contribute to dehydration, which impairs muscular performance and causes heat injuries such as heat exhaustion and heat stroke. Chronic alcohol abuse causes muscular wasting that affects skeletal as well as heart muscle. Obviously, such effects will have negative effects on muscular mass, strength, and endurance.

According to the American College of Sports Medicine, athletes should learn about alcohol's effects on health and avoid consuming excess alcohol during the 48 hours before an event. After exercise, and until his or her body recovers its normal fluid status, the athlete should focus on consuming nonalcoholic beverages.

Where to Get Help for Alcohol Abuse or Dependence

If you think you are abusing alcohol or are dependent on the drug, seek help from your personal physician. For information about alcohol abuse, you can contact the National Drug and Alcohol Treatment Referral Routing Service at 1–800–662–HELP. You can also visit the websites of Alcoholics Anonymous (www.aa.org), the Substance Abuse and Mental Health Services Administration (http://www.samhsa.gov), or Al–Anon/Alateen (www.al–anon.alateen.org).

Concept **Checkpoint 6.7**

25. Summarize the effects of alcohol on the body, including the liver.
26. What is BAC? What is the legal limit for BAC in the United States?
27. Samuel drinks three 12-ounce cans of beer daily. Based on this information, is Samuel a light, moderate, heavy, or binge drinker?

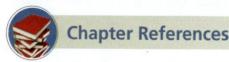

Chapter References

See Appendix H.

Summary

6.1 Introducing Lipids

- Lipids are needed for energy, proper growth and development, nerve functioning, maintenance of healthy skin and hair, and the production of bile and several hormones. Major lipids are triglycerides, phospholipids, and sterols. In addition to being a source of fuel, body fat contributes to body contours, insulates the body against cold temperatures, and protects against damaging blows.

6.2 Fatty Acids, Triglycerides, Phospholipids, and Sterols

- Triglycerides, an important fuel for the body, comprise most of the lipid content of your food and body. Lipids can be sources of the essential fatty acids. Furthermore, the fat in food enhances absorption of fat-soluble vitamins and phytochemicals. Dietary lipids also contribute to the appealing flavor, texture, and aroma of foods.

Although consuming some lipids is essential for health, high amounts may increase your risk of serious health conditions, including obesity, certain cancers, and CVD.

- Most lipids have fatty acids in their chemical structures. Fatty acids can be saturated or unsaturated, and unsaturated fatty acids can be either monounsaturated or polyunsaturated. The body cannot synthesize the omega-6 fatty acid linoleic acid or the omega-3 fatty acid alpha-linolenic acid; these essential fatty acids must be supplied by the diet. The typical American diet provides omega-6 fat than omega-3 fat. Fatty fish, canola and soybean oils, walnuts, and flaxseed are rich sources of the omega-3 fats.

- Trans fatty acid molecules have a different configuration than cis fatty acid molecules. This difference enables fats that contain a high proportion of trans fatty acids to be more solid at room temperature than fats with a high proportion of cis fatty acids. Most of the trans fat in food results from the hydrogenation process. Partial hydrogenation partially hardens the oil so that it can be made into shortening or shaped into sticks of margarine. Diets that contain high amounts of trans fats are associated with an increased risk of heart disease and stroke.

- A triglyceride has three fatty acids attached to glycerol. Triglycerides comprise about 95% of lipids in the body and in food. Triglycerides usually contain mixtures of unsaturated and saturated fatty acids, but one type of fatty acid (saturated, monounsaturated, or polyunsaturated) tends to predominate. In general, animal fats contain higher percentages of saturated fatty acids than plant fats. Important exceptions are the highly saturated coconut and palm oils.

- Phospholipids have both hydrophilic and hydrophobic regions, and as a result, they are partially soluble in water and can serve as emulsifiers. Phospholipids are the major structural component of cell membranes and are needed for proper functioning of nerve cells, including those in the brain. Lecithin is the major phospholipid in food; egg yolks, liver, wheat germ, peanut butter, and soybeans are rich sources of this compound.

- The sterol cholesterol is a component of every cell membrane. Cells use cholesterol to make a variety of substances, including vitamin D, bile, and steroid hormones such as estrogen and testosterone. Cholesterol is found only in animal foods. Plants synthesize sterols and stanols that are not well absorbed by humans. Plant sterols and stanols, however, may be beneficial to health because they interfere with cholesterol absorption.

6.3 What Happens to Lipids in the Body?

- The triglycerides and phospholipids in food undergo digestion primarily in the upper part of the small intestine. Cholesterol is not broken down and is absorbed through the intestinal wall. Before leaving the small intestine, triglycerides, cholesterol, and other lipids are coated with a layer that contains protein to form chylomicrons. Chylomicrons enter the lymphatic system of the small intestine and eventually reach the bloodstream. The liver uses lipids to make various lipoproteins, substances that transport lipids in the bloodstream. Enterohepatic circulation enables the liver to recycle bile salts to make new bile.

- Triglycerides and carbohydrates are major sources of cellular energy. If energy is not needed, adipose cells remove fatty acids and glycerol from circulation and use them to synthesize triglycerides for storage. When energy is needed, adipose cells break down some stored triglycerides and release glycerol and fatty acids into the bloodstream.

6.4 Lipid Consumption Patterns

- Fat contributes 33% of the average American's daily energy intake. According to the Dietary Guidelines, fat should comprise 20 to 35% of total energy intake; the AMDR for fat is 20 to 35% of total calories.

6.5 Understanding Nutritional Labeling: Lipids

- Consumers can use nutrient labels to determine how much total fat, saturated fat, and trans fat are in packaged food.

6.6 Lipids and Health: Cardiovascular Disease (CVD)

- CVD affects the heart and blood vessels. In the United States, heart disease is the leading cause of death. Atherosclerosis is a long-term process that can result in CVD. Numerous risk factors are associated with atherosclerosis; some risk factors are nonmodifiable, but many are related to lifestyle practices that can be altered. Smoking cigarettes, eating certain fats, and being physically inactive are lifestyle practices that increase a person's risk of atherosclerosis and CVD.

- Blood lipid levels can have a major influence on the risk of atherosclerosis. Having high blood levels of HDL cholesterol is healthier than having high LDL cholesterol levels, because elevated LDL cholesterol contributes to atherosclerosis, whereas elevated HDL cholesterol reduces the risk of this condition.

- Exercising and replacing saturated and trans fats with unsaturated fats may reduce LDL levels and increase HDL levels. On the other hand, physical inactivity and eating high amounts of saturated fat may raise LDL and blood triglyceride levels, increasing one's risk of atherosclerosis. Healthy people, however, generally do not experience an increase in their blood cholesterol levels when they eat cholesterol in foods.

- Although oils, fatty spreads, and salad dressings are obvious sources of dietary fat, much of the fat we eat is not visible. Saturated fat contributes much of the calories in fatty meats, luncheon meats, sausage, hot dogs, hard cheeses, and whole milk. If people make dietary modifications, lose excess weight, and exercise regularly, and their blood lipid levels still remain elevated, they should discuss additional treatment options with their physicians. Millions of Americans take prescription statin medications to reduce their elevated blood lipid levels.

6.7 Nutrition Matters: Drink to Your Health?

- Alcohol (ethanol) is a water-soluble, two-carbon compound that is toxic to cells. Beers are typically 3 to 6% alcohol, and wines contain about 8 to 14% alcohol by volume. Each gram of alcohol provides 7 kcal, but alcohol is not a nutrient; it is a mind-altering drug. A standard drink (approximately 12 ounces of beer or wine cooler, 5 ounces of wine, or 1½ ounces of liquor) contains 13 to 14 grams of alcohol.

- Alcohol requires no digestion and readily passes through the tissues lining the inside of the mouth, esophagus, stomach, and small intestine. The body detoxifies alcohol by converting the chemical into less damaging compounds. Until the liver has had enough time to metabolize all the alcohol that has been consumed, the amount of the drug that remains circulates in the bloodstream. In the United States, a blood alcohol concentration of 0.08% is the legal limit for intoxication for automobile operators who are 21 years of age or older. Binge drinking is a major public health problem in the United States.

• Although drinking light to moderate amounts of alcohol raises HDL, excessive amounts of the drug damages every system in the body, particularly the gastrointestinal, nervous, and cardiovascular systems. Alcohol has especially devastating effects on an embryo. Infants born with fetal alcohol syndrome (FAS) have certain facial and heart defects, as well as extensive, irreversible damage to their nervous systems that causes intellectual disability. Therefore, pregnant women should not drink alcohol.

Recipe for Healthy Living

Salmon Salad Sandwiches

Are you tired of eating burgers? Try something different that's easy to prepare and a rich source of omega-3 fatty acids: salmon salad sandwiches. You can use canned salmon or leftover baked salmon to make the salad. This recipe makes enough salad for two sandwiches. Each sandwich provides approximately 312 kcal, 11 g fat, 23 g protein, 4.2 g fiber, and 230 mg calcium.

INGREDIENTS:

    1 cup canned or cooked salmon
    2 Tbsp pickle relish
    2 Tbsp minced (finely chopped) sweet onion
    2 Tbsp lite mayonnaise
    4 slices whole-wheat bread
    1 slice fresh tomato (optional)
    1 piece leaf lettuce (optional)

PREPARATION STEPS:

1. If using canned salmon, drain fluid from salmon. In a bowl, break up salmon with a fork, including the small bones. Add other ingredients to the salmon and mix until well blended.

2. Toast slices of whole-wheat bread.

3. Spread ½ cup of salad on one slice of the toasted bread. Add a fresh tomato slice and/or piece of leaf lettuce, if desired.

 Further analyze this and other recipes through activities on Connect at www.mcgrawhillconnect.com.

*2000 daily total kcal

Personal Dietary Analysis

1. Refer to the 3-day food log from the "Personal Dietary Analysis" feature in Chapter 3. List the total number of kilocalories you consumed for each day of record keeping. Add the figures to obtain a total, divide the total by 3, then round the figure to the nearest whole number to obtain your average daily energy intake for the 3-day period.

Sample Calculation:

Day 1	<u>2000</u> kcal
Day 2	<u>1700</u> kcal
Day 3	<u>2350</u> kcal

Total kcal <u>6050</u> ÷ 3 days = <u>2017</u> **kcal/day**
(average kilocalorie intake, rounded to the nearest whole number)

Your Calculation:

Day 1	_____ kcal
Day 2	_____ kcal
Day 3	_____ kcal

Total kcal _____ **÷ 3 days =** _____ **kcal/day**
(average kilocalorie intake, rounded to the nearest whole number)

2. Add the number of grams of fat eaten each day of the period. Divide the total by 3 and round to the nearest whole number to calculate the average number of grams of fat consumed daily.

Sample Calculation:

Day 1	<u>50</u> g
Day 2	<u>57</u> g
Day 3	<u>42</u> g
Total =	<u>149</u> g

Total grams <u>149</u> ÷ 3 days = 50 g/day (average)

Your Calculation:

Day 1	_____ g
Day 2	_____ g
Day 3	_____ g
Total =	_____ g

Total grams _____ **÷ 3 days =** _____ **g of fat/day**
(average, rounded to the nearest whole number)

3. Each gram of fat provides about 9 kcal; therefore, you must multiply the average number of grams of fat that you ate daily (step 2) by 9 to obtain the average number of kilocalories from fat.

Sample Calculation:

<u>50</u> g/day × 9 kcal/g = <u>450</u> kcal from fat

Your Calculation:

_____ g/day × 9 kcal/g = _____ kcal from fat

4. To calculate the average percentage of calories that fat contributed to your diet, divide the average number of calories from fat obtained in step 3 by the average total daily calorie intake obtained in step 1 and round to the nearest one-hundredth. Multiply the value by 100, drop the decimal point, and add the percent symbol.

Sample Calculation:

<u>450</u> kcal ÷ <u>2017</u> kcal = 0.22

0.22 × 100 = <u>22</u>%

Your Calculation:

_____ kcal ÷ _____ kcal = _____

_____ × 100 = _____ %

5. Did your average daily fat intake meet the U.S. Dietary Guidelines recommended 20 to 35% of total energy?
Yes _____ No _____

6. If your average fat intake was more than 35% of your total energy intake, which foods contributed to your intake of fats?

Foods: _____

7. Review the log of your 3-day food intake. Calculate your average daily intake of saturated fat by adding the grams of saturated fat consumed over the 3-day period and dividing the total by 3.

Your Calculation:

Day 1 _____ g

Day 2 _____ g

Day 3 _____ g

Total = _____ g

Total g _____ ÷ 3 days = _____ g of saturated fat daily

a. What was your average daily saturated fat intake? _____ g

b. Was your average daily intake less than the Dietary Guidelines recommended limit for an adult (less than 10% of total calories)? _____ Yes _____ No

c. If your average saturated fat intake was greater than the recommended limit, list foods that contributed to your intake. _____

Using Nutrient Labels: Fats

1. Remove the labels from two different packaged foods that contain fat. Using information from each of the product's Nutrition Facts panel, answer the following questions.

   a. Name of product #1 _____

   Name of product #2 _____

   b. How many kcal are in one serving of each food?

   Product 1   _____ kcal
   Product 2   _____ kcal

   c. How many grams of fat, saturated fat, and trans fat are in a serving?
   Product 1

   _____ grams of fat

   _____ grams of saturated fat

   _____ grams of trans fat

   Product 2

   _____ grams of fat

   _____ grams of saturated fat

   _____ grams of trans fat

   d. Calculate the percentage of total kcal/serving that are from saturated fat. First, multiply the number of grams of saturated fat by 9 (number of kcal per gram of fat). Then, divide the number of kcal contributed by saturated fat by the total number of kcal per serving. (The Nutrition Label uses the term "Calories" for kcal.) To obtain the percentage, move the decimal point two places to the right, remove the decimal point, and insert % symbol.

   Product 1 _____ grams of saturated fat × 9 kcal = _____ kcal of saturated fat/serving

   _____ % total kcal/serving contributed by saturated fat

   Product 2 _____ grams of saturated fat × 9 kcal = _____ kcal of saturated fat/serving

   _____ % total kcal/serving contributed by saturated fat

   e. Read the list of ingredients for each product. If the food contains saturated fat and trans fat, identify ingredients that contributed saturated fat or trans fat to the product.

   Saturated fat ingredients in Product 1 _____

   _____

   Trans fat ingredients in Product 1 _____

   _____

Saturated fat ingredients in Product 2 _____

_____

Trans fat ingredients in Product 2 _____

_____

connect NUTRITION — Complete the Personal Dietary Analysis activity online at www.mcgrawhillconnect.com

Assessment: Evaluating Your Solid Fat Intake

Do You Consume:	Rarely or Never	1 to 2 Times/ Week	3 to 5 Times/ Week	Daily
1. Bacon, hot dogs, sausage, salami, bologna, or other fatty luncheon meat?	0	1	2	3
2. Whole milk?	0	1	2	3
3. 2% milk?	0	1	2	3
4. Ice cream or milkshakes?	0	1	2	3
5. Sour cream or cream cheese?	0	1	2	3
6. Fatty cuts of pork or beef?	0	1	2	3
7. Hard cheeses, such as cheddar or Swiss?	0	1	2	3
8. Butter?	0	1	2	3
9. Stick margarine?	0	1	2	3
10. Gravy, cheese sauce, or cream-based sauce?	0	1	2	3
11. Buttered popcorn or "rinds"?	0	1	2	3
12. Biscuits, croissants, doughnuts, Danish pastries, pies, cakes, or cookies?	0	1	2	3
13. Products made with lard?	0	1	2	3
14. Cream in your coffee or tea?	0	1	2	3
15. Pizza?	0	1	2	3
16. Creamed soups such as cream of potato soup or New England clam chowder?	0	1	2	3
TOTAL	____	____	____	____

Scoring: Add points in each column and then add those figures together. (The higher the total points, the higher your solid fat intake.)

My "Solid Fat Score" is _____

If your score is 30 or more: Your solid fat intake is probably too high. Note which of these fatty foods you eat more than three times per week. Consider reducing your intake of these items and replacing them with foods that do not contain solid fat.

Critical Thinking

1. Calculate your risk of having a heart attack by completing the American Heart Association's risk calculator at https://www.heart.org/gglRisk/main_en_US.html. Based on your results, should you be concerned about your risk of CVD? If you are concerned, discuss steps you can take to reduce your risk of atherosclerosis and CVD.

2. Do you avoid fried foods and look for "lite" and "fat−reduced" foods when shopping for groceries? If your answer is no, explain why not.

3. Plan a meal that supplies 20 to 35% of energy from fat. The meal should include foods from the major food groups and provide 700 to 900 kcal.

4. Prepare a pamphlet that provides information about risk factors for CVD. In addition to English, you may prepare the pamphlet in Spanish, French, Vietnamese, or another modern language.

5. Develop a lesson for middle−school−aged children that describes atherosclerosis and the role that personal choices (lifestyles) play in the development of the disease.

6. If you drink alcohol, consider filling out the "What Are Signs and Symptoms of Alcohol Abuse" questionnaire on page 199 to assess your alcohol consumption habits. According to this assessment, are you an alcohol abuser or an alcoholic? If your answer is yes to either classification, what can you do to obtain help?

Practice Test

Select the best answer.

1. Fats in foods
   a. add taste and contribute to "mouth feel."
   b. are digested and absorbed in the stomach.
   c. carry water−soluble nutrients.
   d. need to be eliminated to have a healthful diet.

2. Solid fats generally have a high proportion of _____ fatty acids.
   a. unsaturated
   b. saturated
   c. polyunsaturated
   d. monounsaturated

3. A saturated fatty acid has
   a. one double bond within the hydrocarbon chain.
   b. two double bonds within the hydrocarbon chain.
   c. no double bonds within the hydrocarbon chain.
   d. three or more double bonds within the hydrocarbon chain.

4. Which of the following statements is true?
   a. Certain fish are rich sources of omega−3 fatty acids.
   b. Omega−3 fatty acids increase the risk of cardiovascular disease.
   c. Trans fats are rich sources of omega−3 fatty acids.
   d. The human body converts dietary fiber into omega−3 fatty acids.

5. Trans fatty acids are
   a. naturally in many foods.
   b. a by−product of the hydrogenation process.
   c. essential to good health.
   d. found primarily in fatty fish.

6. Phospholipids
   a. do not have fatty acids in their chemical structures.
   b. lack glycerol in their chemical structures.
   c. do not occur naturally.
   d. are partially water−soluble.

7. Cholesterol is
   a. metabolized for energy.
   b. found only in animal foods.
   c. not made by the human body.
   d. harmful to health.

8. The primary site of triglyceride digestion and absorption is the
   a. stomach.
   b. liver.
   c. small intestine.
   d. gallbladder.

9. Lipoproteins

   a. are water-insoluble.
   b. transport lipids in the bloodstream.
   c. contain glucose.
   d. are toxic to cells.

10. Modifiable risk factors for atherosclerosis include

    a. family history.
    b. age.
    c. tobacco use.
    d. racial/ethnic background.

11. Homocysteine is a(n)

    a. form of folate.
    b. lipid that lowers blood pressure.
    c. possible marker for cardiovascular disease.
    d. essential amino acid.

12. Alcohol metabolism is not influenced by a person's

    a. sex.
    b. level of caffeine consumption.
    c. prior history of alcohol use.
    d. body size and composition.

13. After her college graduation party, Jade's BAC was 0.16%. This level is _____ times the legal limit.

    a. 5
    b. 4
    c. 3
    d. 2

Answers to Quiz Yourself

1. To lose weight, use regular, stick margarine instead of butter because it has 25% fewer calories per teaspoon. **False.** (p. 191)

2. Egg yolks are a rich source of cholesterol. **True.** (p. 190)

3. Taking too many fish oil supplements may be harmful to health. **True.** (p. 190)

4. On average, Americans consume 60% of their energy from fat. **False.** (p. 179)

5. Increasing your intake of saturated fat will reduce your risk of heart disease. **False.** (p. 186)

Proteins

Quiz Yourself

How much protein is recommended for optimal health? Can people obtain enough protein by eating only plant foods? What happens if you eat more protein than your body needs? Before reading Chapter 7, take the following quiz to test your knowledge of protein. The answers are on page 255.

1. Animal foods such as meat and eggs are almost 100% protein. _____ T _____ F

2. Foods made from soybeans can be sources of high-quality protein. _____ T _____ F

3. Americans typically consume more protein from animal sources than from plant foods. _____ T _____ F

4. Registered dietitians generally recommend that healthy people take amino acid supplements to increase their protein intake. _____ T _____ F

5. People can nourish their hair by using shampoo that contains protein. _____ T _____ F

connect | NUTRITION   **www.mcgrawhillconnect.com**

A wealth of proven resources are available on Connect® Nutrition including McGraw-Hill LearnSmart®, SmartBook®, NutritionCalc Plus, and many other dynamic learning tools. Ask your instructor about Connect!

7.1 What Are Proteins?

Learning Outcomes

1 List the primary function of proteins in the body.

2 Identify the basic structural unit of proteins and its components.

3 Classify an amino acid as essential or nonessential.

Since ancient times, many people have believed that eating animal foods, par—ticularly meat, was necessary for good health and optimal physical performance. Milo of Croton, an ancient Greek Olympian wrestler with extraordinary strength, reportedly consumed about 20 pounds of meat daily. Although accounts of Milo's superhuman capacity for eating meat are unreliable, modern athletes often make protein—rich foods and protein supplements the foundation of their diets. Fur—thermore, it is not unusual for nonathletes to associate meat with protein and a lack of protein with poor muscular development and weak muscular strength.

Many Americans think a meal is not adequate unless it contains large por—tions of meat. Although it is true that meat is a rich source of protein, other foods, including those from plants, are often overlooked as sources of protein. The beef patty of a cheeseburger provides protein, as well as the melted cheese that tops the burger and the bun that makes the sandwich convenient to eat.

Proteins are complex organic molecules that are chemically similar to lipids and carbohydrates because they contain carbon, hydrogen, and oxygen atoms. Proteins, however, contain nitrogen, the element cells need to make a wide array of important biological compounds. Plants, animals, bacteria, and even viruses contain hundreds of proteins.

Protein is an important class of nutrients, but it is not more valuable to your health than other nutrients. Nutrients work together in your body like members of a well—trained basketball team on the playing court. Making one player the star while neglecting to develop the other athletes' skills can have disastrous effects on the team's success. Similarly, overemphasizing one class of nutrients in your diet, such as protein, while ignoring other nutrients, can lead to nutritional imbalances that result in serious health problems. By reading this chapter, you will learn about the roles of proteins in your body and their major food sources. You will also learn how proteins influence your health.

Proteins in the Body

Proteins are necessary for muscle development and maintenance, but the more than 200,000 different proteins in your body have a wide variety of functions, including those shown in Table 7.1.[1] Skin, blood, nerve, bone—all cells in your body—contain proteins. Structural proteins such as *collagen* are in your car—tilage, ligament, and bone tissue. *Keratin* is another structural protein; it is in your hair, nails, and skin. Contractile proteins in your muscles enable you to move, and transport proteins carry many substances in the bloodstream. Proteins are also necessary for your blood to clot properly.

Certain hormones, such as insulin and glucagon, are proteins. Hormones and neurotransmitters are chemical messengers that regulate body processes and responses, such as growth, metabolism, and hunger. *Neurotransmitters* send signals from one nerve cell to another. Some neurotransmitters are proteins.

proteins large, complex organic molecules made up of amino acids

TABLE 7.1 Proteins in the Body

The body uses proteins to make or function as:
New cells and many components of cells
Structures such as hair and nails
Enzymes
Lubricants
Clotting compounds
Antibodies
Compounds that help maintain fluid and pH balance
Certain hormones and neurotransmitters
Energy source (minor, under usual conditions)

Arterial end
Fluid forced into tissue
spaces by blood pressure
generated by pumping
action of the heart

Protein

Blood cell

Capillary

Venous end
Fluid drawn into bloodstream
by the proteins as blood pressure
declines in the capillaries

(a) **Normal tissue**

(b) **Swollen tissue (edema)**

Figure 7.1 Normal fluid balance and edema. Under normal conditions, blood pressure is high enough at the arterial end of a capillary bed to force fluid into the tissue space that surround capillaries. At the venous end of the capillary bed, blood pressure is lower, and proteins in the bloodstream help draw fluid back into the capillaries. (*a*) As a result of the balance between blood pressure and proteins in the bloodstream, the tissues contain normal amounts of fluid. (*b*) When blood pressure is greater than the counteracting force of the proteins in the bloodstream, fluid remains in the tissues, causing edema.

Nearly all enzymes are proteins. Enzymes speed up the rate of (*catalyze*) chemi‑cal reactions without becoming a part of the products (see Fig. 4.8). Additionally, infection‑fighting **antibodies** are proteins. Although cells can use proteins for energy, normally they metabolize very little for energy, conserving the nutrient for other important functions that carbohydrates and lipids are unable to perform.

In the bloodstream, proteins transport nutrients and oxygen. Proteins in blood, such as *albumin*, also help maintain the proper distribution of fluids in blood and body tissues (Fig. 7.1). The force of blood pressure moves watery fluid out of the bloodstream and into tissues. Blood proteins help counteract the effects of blood pressure by attracting the fluid, returning it to the bloodstream. During starvation, the level of protein in blood decreases, and as a result, some water leaks out of the bloodstream and enters spaces between cells. The resulting accumulation of fluid in tissues is called **edema** (*eh–dee'–mah*).

Proteins also help maintain **acid–base balance,** the proper pH of body fluids. To function properly, blood and tissue fluids need to maintain a pH of 7.35 to 7.45, which is slightly basic.[1] (To review the concept of pH, see Chapter 4.) Metabolic processes can produce acidic or basic by‑products. If a particular body fluid becomes too acidic or too basic, cells can have difficulty functioning and may die. A **buffer** can protect the pH of a solution. Proteins can act as buf‑fers, because they have acidic and basic components. For example, if cells form an excess of hydrogen ions (H^+), the pH of tissues decreases. To help restore the pH level to within the normal range, the basic portions of protein molecules bind to the excess H^+, neutralizing the excess ions and raising the pH.

Amino Acids

Proteins are comprised of smaller chemical units called **amino acids.** The human body contains proteins made from 20 different amino acids (see Appendix D). To understand how the body uses amino acids, it is necessary to learn some basic chemistry that relates to these compounds.

antibodies infection-fighting proteins

edema accumulation of fluid in tissues

acid-base balance maintaining the proper pH of body fluids

buffer substance that can protect the pH of a solution

amino acids nitrogen-containing chemical units that comprise proteins

Each amino acid has a carbon atom that anchors a hydrogen atom and three different groups of atoms: the **amino** or **nitrogen–containing group,** the **R group,** and the **acid group.** The chemical structure of the amino acid alanine shown in Figure 7.2 indicates these three groups. Note that the nitrogen atom is in the amino group. The R group varies with each type of amino acid, so it identifies the molecule as a particular amino acid, such as *serine* or *lysine*. When the nitrogen–containing group is removed, the R group, acid group, and anchor–ing carbon atom form the "carbon skeleton" of an amino acid (see Fig. 7.2). The carbon skeleton is an important component of an amino acid, because the body can convert the carbon skeletons of certain amino acids to glucose and use the simple sugar for energy.

Classifying Amino Acids

Traditionally, nutritionists classify amino acids as either nonessential or essential according to the body's ability to make them. A healthy human body can make 11 of the 20 amino acids. These compounds are the **nonessential amino acids.** The remaining nine amino acids are **essential amino acids** that must be supplied by foods, because the body cannot synthesize them or make enough to meet its needs. Sometimes, nonessential and essential amino acids are referred to as "dispensable" and "indispensable" amino acids, respectively. Table 7.2 lists amino acids according to their classification as essential and nonessential.

Several nonessential amino acids are "conditionally essential," which means they become essential in certain situations. For example, cells can make cysteine from methionine and serine. If a person's methionine and serine intake is inade–quate, his or her body cannot make enough cysteine to meet its needs and dietary sources of the amino acid are necessary.

Figure 7.2 Amino acid: Basic chemical structure. Alanine has the typical chemical features of an amino acid—the nitrogen-containing or amino group, R group, and acid group.

TABLE 7.2 Amino Acids

Essential		Nonessential	
Histidine	Threonine	Alanine	Cysteine*
Isoleucine	Tryptophan	Aspartic acid	Glutamine*
Leucine	Valine	Asparagine	Glycine*
Lysine		Glutamic acid	Proline*
Methionine		Serine	Tyrosine*
Phenylalanine		Arginine*	

* Under certain conditions, this amino acid can become essential.

Concept **Checkpoint 7.1**

   1. What is the chemical unit that makes up a protein?
   2. List at least four different functions of proteins in the body.
   3. Identify the three groups of atoms that make up a typical amino acid.
   4. What is the "carbon skeleton" of an amino acid?
   5. How many different kinds of amino acids are needed to make human proteins? How many of these amino acids are essential?

amino or **nitrogen-containing group** portion of an amino acid that contains nitrogen

R group part of amino acid that identifies the molecule as a particular amino acid

acid group acid portion of a compound

nonessential amino acids group of amino acids that the body can make

essential amino acids amino acids the body cannot make or make enough to meet its needs

7.2 Proteins in Foods

Learning Outcomes

1. Explain the difference between a high-quality protein and a low-quality protein.
2. Identify foods that are rich sources of high-quality proteins.
3. List at least three amino acids that are often "limiting amino acids" in plant foods.

People often associate animal foods with protein, but beans, nuts, seeds, grains, and certain vegetables are good sources of protein, too. In fact, nearly all foods contain protein, but no naturally occurring food is 100% protein. Protein comprises only about 20 to 30% of the weight of a piece of beef; 25% of the weight of drained, water–packed tuna fish; and only 12% of an egg's weight. Nevertheless, animal foods generally provide higher amounts of protein than similar quantities of plant foods. A 3–ounce serving of broiled lean ground beef supplies 23 g of protein; a 3–ounce serving of steamed broccoli or cooked carrots provides only about 1 g of protein. In general, most plant foods provide less than 3 g of protein per ounce. Table 7.3 lists some commonly eaten foods and their approximate protein content per serving.

TABLE 7.3 Approximate Protein Content of Some Commonly Eaten Foods/Portion

Food	Serving Size	Protein g/serving
Chicken, breast, roasted, meat only	4 oz	34
Ham, lean, cooked	4 oz	30
Hamburger, 80% lean, broiled	4 oz	29
Pepperoni pizza, regular crust, 14" pie	2 slices (200 g)	25
Tuna, canned, water-packed, drained	4 oz	22
Miso (soybean product)	½ cup	16
Lasagna with meat sauce	8 oz	15
Cottage cheese, 2% low-fat	4 oz	13
Milk, fat-free	1 cup	8
Peanut butter	2 Tbsp	8
Tofu, regular	½ cup	8
Bagel, plain	1 (3 ½" diam)	7
American processed cheese	1 oz	7
Baked beans, vegetarian	½ cup	6
Egg, hard cooked	1	6
Vanilla ice cream	1 cup	4
White rice	1 cup	4
Peas, green	½ cup	4
Banana	1	1

Certain parts of plants contain more protein than other parts. Seeds, tree nuts, and legumes supply more protein per serving than servings of fruit or the edible leaves, roots, flowers, and stems of vegetables. Tree nuts include walnuts, cashews, and almonds; **legumes** are plants that produce pods that have a single row of seeds, such as soybeans, peas, peanuts, lentils, and beans (Fig. 7.3). A 3–ounce serving of almonds, dry–roasted peanuts, or sunflower seed kernels supplies about 20 g of protein. Many seeds and nuts, however, pack a lot of calories from fat. Snack on just 3 ounces of almonds, dry–roasted peanuts, or sunflower seed kernels, and you will add almost 500 kcal to your diet!

Peas, lentils, and most kinds of beans contain more protein and complex carbohydrate than fat. Eating a 3–ounce serving of vegetarian baked beans, for example, adds about 4 g of protein, 14 g of carbohydrate, and less than 1 g of fat to your diet. Although soybeans contain more fat than carbohydrate, soy fat is high in unsaturated fatty acids. The health ben–efits of unsaturated fatty acids are discussed in Chapter 6.

Figure 7.3 Legumes. Legumes, such as these soybeans, are plants that produce pods that have a single row of seeds.

Protein Quality

Foods differ not only in the amount of protein they contain but also in their pro–tein quality. A **high–quality (complete protein)** contains all essential amino acids in amounts that support protein deposition in muscles and other tissues, as well as a young child's growth.[2] High–quality proteins are well digested and absorbed by the body. Meat, fish, poultry, eggs, and milk and milk products contain high–quality proteins. Egg protein generally rates very high for protein quality because it is easy to digest and has a pattern of essential amino acids that closely resembles that needed by humans.

A **low–quality (incomplete protein)** lacks one or more of the essential amino acids or contains inadequate amounts of these nutrients. Furthermore, the human digestive tract does not digest low–quality protein sources as efficiently as foods containing high–quality protein. The essential amino acids that are in relatively low amounts are referred to as *limiting* amino acids, because they reduce the protein's ability to support growth, repair, and maintenance of tis–sues. In most instances, tryptophan, threonine, lysine, and the sulfur–containing amino acids methionine and cysteine are the limiting amino acids in foods.[3]

Most plant foods are not sources of high–quality proteins. *Quinoa (keen'–wa)* and soy protein are exceptions. Quinoa is botanically related to sugar beets and spinach, but the quality and amount of protein in quinoa seeds are superior to those of many cereal grains.[4] Cooked quinoa is often used as a cereal (see "Recipe for Healthy Living" at the end of this chapter). The quality of soy protein is comparable to that of most animal proteins.[5] Processed soybeans are used to make a variety of nutritious foods, including soy milk, infant formula, and meat substitutes. Furthermore, eating foods made from soybeans may reduce the risk of chronic diseases, such as certain cancers.[5] More research, however, is needed to determine the long–term health benefits of eating diets that contain soy products.

Understanding the concept of protein quality is important. Regardless of how much protein is eaten, a child will fail to grow properly if his or her diet lacks essential amino acids. The "Vegetarianism" section of this chapter explains how you can obtain these and other essential nutrients by eating only plant foods.

legumes plants that produce pods with a single row of seeds

high-quality (complete) protein protein that contains all essential amino acids in amounts that support the deposition of protein in tissues and the growth of a young person

low-quality (incomplete) protein protein that lacks or has inadequate amounts of one or more of the essential amino acids

7.3 What Happens to Proteins in the Body?

Learning Outcomes

1. Explain how cells make proteins.

2. Describe what happens to excess amino acids in the body.

3. Explain what happens to proteins as they undergo digestion and absorption in the human digestive tract.

4. Explain the concept of nitrogen balance and identify conditions in which the body is in a state of positive or negative nitrogen balance.

5. Calculate a person's RDA for protein based on his or her body weight.

peptide bond chemical attraction that connects two amino acids together

polypeptide protein comprised of two or more amino acids

peptides small chains of amino acids

gene portion of DNA

In a television crime series, police in a major city are investigating what could be a homicide. A man has been reported missing by his parents, who suspect foul play and their daughter—in—law's involvement in their son's disappearance. While knocking on the door of the missing man's house, police notice some dried blood on the front porch. The man's wife, who lives in the house, tells police that the blood is from her injured dog. How can police know she is telling the truth? The blood holds important clues. Every organism synthesizes proteins— including those in blood—that are unique. Samples of the blood can be analyzed to determine whether it contains proteins from a dog or another animal, such as a human. We will leave it to your imagination to finish this story, but we will examine a real—life story: how human cells make proteins.

How the Body Uses Amino Acids to Synthesize Proteins

Your body makes proteins by following information coded in your DNA, or deoxy—ribonucleic (*de—ox′—e—rye′—bow—new—klay′—ik*) acid, the hereditary material in a cell's nucleus. To make proteins, cells assemble the 20 amino acids in specific sequences according to the information provided by DNA. To understand this process, imagine proteins as various chains made from 20 different amino acid "beads." Figure 7.4 illustrates some of these beads and how they can be assembled into chains. Note that each bead has two metal wires that are used to link it with another bead. To make a copy of a particular beaded chain, you would follow directions for connecting the beads in a specific order and length by hooking the metal wires of each bead together. Consider the vast variety of beaded chains comprised of different bead sequences and chain lengths that you could make from just 20 different beads.

In living things, the beaded chains are proteins that contain amino acids. An amino acid can connect to another amino acid by a **peptide bond,** a chemi—cal attraction between the acid group of one amino acid and the amino group of another amino acid (Fig. 7.5). A **polypeptide** forms when two or more amino acids

Amino acids

Amino acid

Peptide bond

Figure 7.4 Amino acids form proteins. Each type of bead represents a specific amino acid in human proteins. The "hook" that connects the beads represents a peptide bond.

join to form a chain (see Figure 7.4). **Peptides** are small chains of amino acids that usually contain fewer than 15 amino acids. Dipeptides and tripeptides are compounds that consist of two and three amino acids, respectively. Most naturally occurring proteins are polypeptides comprised of 50 or more amino acids.

Figure 7.6 summarizes the basic steps of protein synthesis. Protein synthesis begins with DNA in the cell's nucleus. DNA is a twisted, two–stranded molecule referred to as a double helix. To begin the process, a section of the DNA double helix unwinds, exposing a gene. A **gene** is a portion of DNA that contains infor-mation concerning the order of amino acids that comprise a specific protein. *Mes-senger ribonucleic acid (mRNA)*, a compound that is chemically similar to DNA, is formed by *transcription* (see Fig. 7.6). The actual production of a protein occurs in the cytoplasm, so mRNA leaves the nucleus and moves to ribosomes—the protein–manufacturing sites in the cytoplasm. Ribosomes translate the gene's coded instructions for adding amino acids to the polypeptide chain. During this translation process, *transfer ribonucleic acid (tRNA)* conveys specific amino acids, one at a time, to the ribosomes. At the ribosomes, the amino acid from tRNA is added to the last amino acid, causing the peptide chain to grow longer. After the mRNA is read completely, the ribosome releases the polypeptide, and then the new protein gener-ally undergoes further processing at other sites within the cytoplasm.

Diets that contain low–quality protein can result in poor growth, slowed recovery from illness, and even death. These situations occur because protein syn-thesis in cells cannot proceed when the supply or "pool" of amino acids does not

Figure 7.5 Peptide bond. A dipeptide forms when two amino acids bond and a molecule of water is released in the process.

Figure 7.6 Protein synthesis. This illustration summarizes the basic steps of protein synthesis.

1. Protein synthesis begins when a section of DNA unwinds, exposing a single portion (a *gene*). The gene contains coded information about the order of amino acids that comprise a specific protein.

2. The gene undergoes *transcription,* that is, the sequence of its amino acids is copied in a special manner, forming *messenger RNA (mRNA)* in the process.

3. mRNA transfers the information concerning the amino acid sequence from the nucleus to *ribosomes,* protein manufacturing sites in the cytoplasm.

4. During the *translation* process, ribosomes "read" mRNA. The coded instructions indicate which amino acid to add to the polypeptide chain and its sequence.

5. Each specific *transfer RNA (tRNA)* molecule conveys a particular amino acid to the ribosome.

6. At the ribosome, the amino acid that has been delivered by tRNA attaches to the peptide chain, lengthening it.

7. When the translation process is complete, the ribosome releases the polypeptide, and the new protein generally undergoes further processing at other sites within the cytoplasm.

DNA

mRNA

Cell Nucleus

TRANSCRIPTION

Gene

Cytoplasm

Ribosome

Amino acids

tRNA

Peptide chain

Amino acid

tRNA

TRANSLATION

Iron-containing unit

Polypeptide chains

Figure 7.7 Shaping of a protein. A hemoglobin molecule has four peptide chains associated with an iron-containing unit.

Figure 7.8 Sickle cell anemia. This microscopic view of red blood cells shows (a) normal disc-shaped cell and (b) sickle cell that contains abnormal hemoglobin.

(a)

(b)

Normal protein

Heat, acid, alcohol, whipping

Denatured protein

| **Figure 7.9 Denaturation.**

denaturation altering a protein's natural shape and function by exposing it to conditions such as heat, acids, and physical agitation

pepsin gastric enzyme that breaks down proteins into smaller polypeptides

have one or more of the essential amino acids needed for constructing the polypeptide chain. When this happens, production of the protein stops. The partially made polypeptide chain is dismantled, and its amino acids are returned to the pool.

When assembly of the new protein has been completed, the polypeptide acid chain coils and folds into a three-dimensional shape that is characteristic of that particular protein. In some instances, more than one polypeptide chain curls around each other to form large protein complexes. For example, hemoglobin, a protein in red blood cells, is comprised of four polypeptide chains coiled together (Fig. 7.7). The shape of a protein is important because it influences the compound's activity in the body.

Occasionally, the wrong amino acid is introduced into the amino acid chain during the protein synthesis process. Cells usually check for such errors and replace the amino acid with the correct one. If the DNA code is faulty, however, the wrong amino acid will be inserted into the chain consistently, forming an abnormal polypeptide. Such errors often cause genetic defects that have devastating, even deadly, effects on the organism. *Sickle cell anemia*, for example, is an inherited disease characterized by abnormal hemoglobin. Cells in red bone marrow synthesize hemoglobin by following DNA instructions concerning proper amino acid sequencing. If the DNA codes for the insertion of the wrong amino acid in two of hemoglobin's four polypeptide chains, the resulting protein is defective and does not function correctly. Figure 7.8a shows a red blood cell that contains normal hemoglobin; the red blood cell shown in Figure 7.8b has the defective hemoglobin associated with sickle cell anemia. Crescent-shaped red blood cells cannot transport oxygen efficiently. As a result, the abnormal cells can clog small blood vessels, causing pain, organ damage, and premature death. Sickle cell anemia is a common genetic disorder that generally affects people with African, Caribbean, or Mediterranean ancestry.

Protein Denaturation

A protein undergoes **denaturation** when it is exposed to various conditions that alter the macronutrient's natural folded and coiled shape (Fig. 7.9). We often cook protein-rich foods to make them more digestible and safe to eat, but heat also causes the proteins in foods to unfold. The protein in raw egg white, for example, is almost clear and has a jellylike consistency. When you cook egg white, it becomes white and firm as its proteins become denatured. Other treatments often used during food preparation also denature proteins, including whipping or exposing them to alcohol or acid. Wine, for example, is often used in marinades, because the alcohol it contains denatures proteins in meat, helping tenderize it. Adding acidic lemon juice to milk denatures ("curdles") the proteins in milk. In your stomach, hydrochloric acid denatures food proteins, making them easier to digest. Denaturation does not "kill" a protein (because proteins are not living), but the process usually permanently alters the protein's shape and functions. Once an egg white has been cooked or milk has curdled, the food cannot return to its original state.

Protein Digestion and Absorption

When you eat oatmeal mixed with milk for breakfast, the large proteins in these foods must be digested before undergoing absorption. Protein digestion begins in the stomach, where hydrochloric acid denatures food proteins and **pepsin,** an enzyme, digests proteins into smaller polypeptides. Soon after the polypeptides enter the small intestine, the pancreas secretes protein-splitting enzymes, including trypsin (*trip'-sin*) and chymotrypsin (*ki'-mo-trip'-sin*). *Trypsin* and *chymotrypsin* break down polypeptides into shorter peptides and amino acids. Enzymes released by the absorptive cells of the small intestine break down most of the shortened peptides into dipeptides, tripeptides, and individual amino acids. Within the absorptive cells, di— and tripeptides are broken down into amino acids. Thus, amino acids are the end products of protein digestion. After being absorbed, the amino acids enter the hepatic portal vein and travel to the liver, where they may enter the general circulation.

By the time cells obtain amino acids from blood, they cannot distinguish the ones that were originally in oat proteins from those that were in milk proteins. The cells, however, now have all the amino acids they need to make human pro— teins. Protein digestion and absorption is very efficient: Very little dietary pro— tein escapes digestion and is eliminated in feces. Figure 7.10 summarizes protein digestion and absorption.

Protein Turnover

Not all protein must be supplied by the diet. **Protein turnover,** the process of breaking down old or unneeded proteins into their component amino acids and recycling them to make new proteins, occurs constantly within cells. Amino acids that are not incorporated into proteins become part of a small amino acid pool, a readily available supply of amino acids that cells can use for future protein syn— thesis. The amino acid pool is an *endogenous*, or internal, source of nitrogen. The body obtains about two—thirds of its amino acid supply from endogenous sources and the remainder from *exogenous* (dietary) sources.

protein turnover cellular process of breaking down proteins and recycling their amino acids

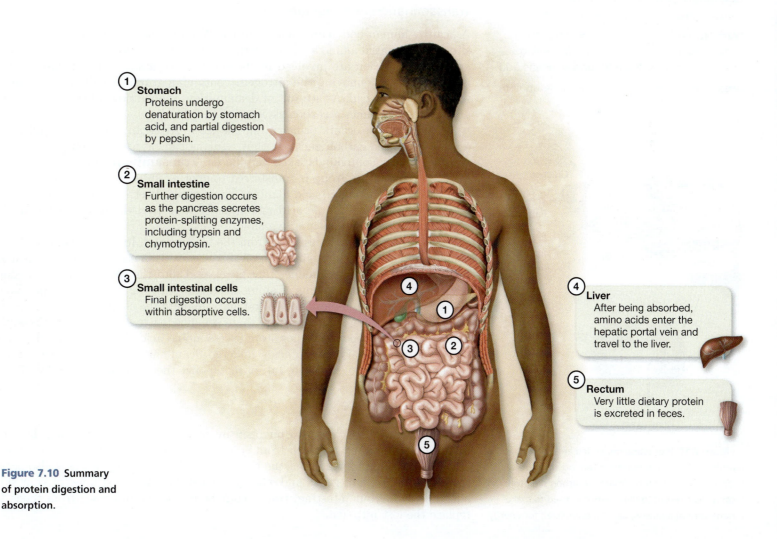

1 Stomach
Proteins undergo denaturation by stomach acid, and partial digestion by pepsin.

2 Small intestine
Further digestion occurs as the pancreas secretes protein-splitting enzymes, including trypsin and chymotrypsin.

3 Small intestinal cells
Final digestion occurs within absorptive cells.

4 Liver
After being absorbed, amino acids enter the hepatic portal vein and travel to the liver.

5 Rectum
Very little dietary protein is excreted in feces.

Figure 7.10 Summary of protein digestion and absorption.

DEAMINATION

Glutamic acid
(amino acid)

TRANSAMINATION

Carbon skeleton

Pyruvic acid

Alanine
(amino acid)

Figure 7.11 Deamination and transamination. Deamination is the process of removing the nitrogen-containing group from an unneeded amino acid. Transamination occurs when the nitrogen-containing group is transferred to another substance to make an amino acid.

deamination removal of the nitrogen-containing group from an amino acid

transamination transfer of the nitrogen-containing group from an unneeded amino acid to a carbon skeleton to form an amino acid

urea waste product of amino acid metabolism

Figure 7.12 Processing unneeded amino acids. In the liver, unnecessary amino acids are deaminated, and the remaining carbon skeletons can be converted to glucose or fat, used to make nonessential amino acids, or metabolized for energy.

Transamination and Deamination

A healthy human body can make 11 of the 20 amino acids. The liver is the main site of nonessential amino acid production. Chemical reactions called deamination and transamination are involved in the synthesis of amino acids. **Deamination** is the process of removing the nitrogen-containing group (usually NH_2) from an unneeded amino acid. As a result of deamination, the amino acid that gives up its amino group becomes a carbon skeleton (Fig. 7.11).

Deamination occurs primarily in the liver. After an amino acid undergoes deamination, the carbon skeleton that remains can be used for energy or converted to other compounds, such as glucose. **Transamination** occurs when the nitrogen-containing group is transferred to another substance to make an amino acid. To make the amino acid alanine, for example, liver cells remove the amino group (NH_2) from glutamic acid and transfer it to pyruvic acid (see Fig. 7.11). Transamination reactions are reversible.

Liver cells remove excess NH_2 from the bloodstream, forming ammonia (NH_3), a highly poisonous waste product (Fig. 7.12). The liver can use the ammonia to make **urea,** a metabolic waste product that is released into the bloodstream. The kidneys filter urea, small amounts of ammonia, and *creatinine* (a nitrogen-containing waste produced by muscles) from blood and eliminate the compounds in urine.

If you consume more protein than you need, what happens to the extra amino acids? The body does not store excess amino acids in muscle or other tissues. The unnecessary amino acids undergo deamination, and cells convert the carbon skeletons into glucose or fat, or metabolize them for energy (see Fig. 7.12).

Nitrogen Balance

Although your body conserves nitrogen by recycling amino acids, each day you lose some protein and nitrogen from your body. Urinary elimination of urea and creatinine accounts for most of the lost nitrogen. Daily nitrogen losses also occur as your nails and hair grow, and when you shed the outermost layer of your skin and cells from your intestinal tract. Your body uses amino acids from foods to replace the lost nitrogen.

Normally, an adult's body maintains its protein content by maintaining **nitrogen balance (equilibrium),** that is, balancing nitrogen intake and protein turnover with losses. During certain stages of life or physical conditions, however, nitrogen intake and retention do not equal nitrogen losses. When the body is in a state of **positive nitrogen balance,** it retains more nitrogen than it loses as proteins are added to various tissues. In this case, a person must eat more protein to satisfy the increased need for the nutrient. Positive balance occurs during periods of rapid growth such as pregnancy, infancy, and puberty, and when people are recovering from illness or injury. Hormones such as insulin, growth hormone, and testosterone stimulate positive nitrogen balance. Performing weight (resistance) training also leads to nitrogen retention.[6] When the body is in a state of **negative nitrogen balance,** the body loses more nitrogen than it retains and protein intake is less than what the body needs. Negative balance occurs during starvation, serious illnesses, and severe injuries. Recovery from the illness or injury results in positive nitrogen balance until nitrogen equilibrium is restored. Figure 7.13 illustrates the concept of nitrogen balance and lists conditions that result in positive and negative nitrogen balance.

nitrogen balance (equilibrium) balancing nitrogen intake with nitrogen losses

positive nitrogen balance state in which the body retains more nitrogen than it loses

negative nitrogen balance state in which the body loses more nitrogen than it retains

How Much Protein Do You Need?

The Estimated Average Requirement (EAR) for protein is 0.66 g of protein/kg of body weight.[3] The EAR for protein increases during pregnancy, breastfeeding, periods of rapid growth, and recovery from serious illnesses, blood losses, and burns. Recall from Chapter 3 that scientists use EARs to establish Recommended Dietary Allowances (RDAs). A healthy adult's RDA for protein is 0.8 g/kg of body weight.[3] By reviewing DRI tables (last pages of this book), you will note that the RDAs for protein vary during certain ages and conditions.

Positive Nitrogen Balance

- Growth
- Pregnancy
- Recovery from illness/injury
- Increased levels of the hormones insulin, testosterone, and growth hormone
- Resistance exercise

Nitrogen Equilibrium

- Healthy adult meets protein and energy needs

Negative Nitrogen Balance

- Inadequate protein intake or digestive tract diseases that interfere with protein absorption
- Increased protein losses resulting from certain kidney diseases or blood loss
- Bed rest, fever, injuries, or burns
- Increased secretion of thyroid hormone or cortisol (a "stress hormone")

Figure 7.13 Nitrogen balance. This diagram illustrates the concept of nitrogen balance and lists conditions that result in positive and negative nitrogen balance. Note that nitrogen balance occurs when nitrogen intake plus turnover equals nitrogen losses.

To determine your RDA for protein, multiply your weight in kilograms by 0.8 grams. If you are underweight or overweight, use a healthy weight for your height when making this calculation (see the body mass index chart in Chapter 10). For example, a healthy man who is 5−feet, 10−inches tall and weighs 75 kilograms (his weight in pounds divided by 2.2) should consume 60 grams of protein daily (75 kg × 0.8 g) to meet his RDA for the nutrient. The "Personal Dietary Analy−sis" at the end of this chapter can help you estimate your daily protein intake.

Concept **Checkpoint 7.3**

9. Explain the basic steps involved in protein synthesis.
10. Define denaturation, deamination, and transamination.
11. Describe conditions that can cause the body to be in negative nitrogen balance. Describe conditions in which the body is in positive nitrogen balance.
12. A healthy young woman weighs 143 pounds. Calculate her RDA for protein.
13. Explain what happens to proteins in beans as they undergo digestion and absorption in the human digestive tract.

7.4 Protein Consumption Patterns

Learning Outcomes

1 Compare the percentage of calories that protein contributes in the typical American diet to the AMDR for protein.

2 Identify foods groups that contribute most of the protein in the typical American diet.

In 2009–2010, protein comprised about 15% of the typical American's total energy intake for a day.[7] For healthy adults, this level of consumption is within the Acceptable Macronutrient Distribution Range (AMDR), which is 10 to 35% of energy from protein.[3] In 2010, Americans generally ate about the same percent−age of total daily calories from protein as they did in the early 1900s.[8] Ameri−cans, however, consumed more protein from meat, fish, and poultry than from grains. In 1909, grain products contributed approximately 37% of Americans' typical protein intake. At that time, meat, fish, and poultry accounted for 31% of the protein in the American diet. In 2010, grain products supplied only 20% of Americans' protein intake, whereas meat, fish, and poultry provided most of the protein (43%) in the diet (Fig. 7.14).[8]

MyPlate: Recommendations for Protein Intake

Animal sources of protein are often rich sources of saturated fat. According to the Dietary Guidelines and the MyPlate food plan, Americans should choose lean or low−fat meat and poultry.[9] The leanest cuts of beef include round, and top round, loin, and top sirloin steaks, as well as chuck and arm roasts.

Ham, bacon, sausage, frankfurters, and deli meats generally contain high amounts of saturated fat and sodium.

Figure 7.14 Protein consumption patterns. In 2010, Americans ate more protein from meat, fish, and poultry than they did in the early 1900s.

Before cooking a piece of beef, you can reduce its fat content by trimming the visible fat away from the meat. When buying ground beef, consider choosing "extra lean" products. The label on a package of extra lean ground beef should state that the meat is at least 90% lean. When cooked, extra lean ground beef can taste "dry." You can improve the taste of the beef by adding a small amount of "heart healthy" olive oil to the raw meat before shaping it into hamburger pat-ties. The leanest cuts of pork include pork loin, tenderloin, and center loin.

You can choose lean turkey, roast beef, or low—fat luncheon meats for sandwiches, instead of processed meat products. Processed meat products, such as ham, bacon, sausage, frankfurters, and bologna and salami, generally contain a lot of saturated fat, and they also have high amounts of added sodium. Excessive sodium intakes are associated with increased risk of hypertension. If you decide to purchase processed meats, check the Nutrition Facts panels on products' labels to compare fat as well as sodium contents.

The MyPlate plan also recommends varying your protein choices. For example, consider eating fish that are rich sources of beneficial omega—3 fatty acids, such as salmon, trout, and herring. You can also replace main menu items that contain meat with dishes made with dry beans, peas, or foods made from soybeans. Additionally, consider snacking on nuts, such as peanuts, almonds, cashews, walnuts, and pecans, instead of pieces of meat or cheese.

Did You Know?

Humans use nearly every part of an animal for food. "Meat" is muscle tissue; "tripe" is from the stomach of cattle; "prairie or Rocky Mountain oysters," "lamb or calf fries," and *huevos del toro* are testicles of male sheep or cattle; and "sweetbreads" are the thymus glands of calves and lambs. In some cultures, people even consume the tongues, brains, and blood of certain animals.

Concept **Checkpoint 7.4**

14. What is the AMDR for adult protein intake?

15. Describe how Americans' food sources of protein have changed since the early 1900s.

16. Consider your usual food choices. Using the recommendations of the MyPlate food guide, discuss ways you can reduce your intake of protein from animal foods.

Figure 7.15 Nutrition Facts panel (as of February 2016). The Nutrition Facts panel provides information about a product's protein content.

Nutrition Facts

Serving Size 1 slice (38 g)
Servings Per Container 18

Amount Per Serving

Calories 100
Calories from Fat 20

	% Daily Value*
	3%
Total Fat 2g	0%
Saturated Fat 0g	
Trans Fat 0g	
Polyunsaturated Fat 1g	
Monounsaturated Fat 0g	0%
Cholesterol 0mg	7%
Sodium 160mg	6%
Total Carbohydrate 17g	8%
Dietary Fiber 2g	
Sugars 3g	
Protein 4g	
	10%
Vitamin A	0%
Vitamin C	10%
Calcium	8%
Iron	

* Percent Daily Values are based on a 2,000 calorie diet. Your daily values may be higher or lower, depending on your calorie needs:

	Calories	2,000	2,500
Total Fat	Less than	65g	80g
Sat Fat	Less than	20g	25g
Cholesterol	Less than	300mg	300mg
Sodium	Less than	2,400mg	2,400mg
Total Carbohydrate		300g	375g
Dietary Fiber		25g	30g

INGREDIENTS: Whole-wheat flour, Water, Brown sugar, Wheat gluten, Cracked wheat, Wheat bran, Yeast,Salt, Molasses, Soybean oil, Calcium propionate (preservative), Mono–and diglycerides, Lecithin

7.5 Understanding Nutritional Labeling

Learning Outcomes

1 Explain how to use the Nutrition Facts panel to determine the grams of protein in a serving of a packaged food.

2 Explain how you can use the ingredient list on a food label to determine the quality of the protein in the product.

You can determine how much protein is in a packaged food product by reading the Nutrition Facts panel on the label. As you can see in Figure 7.15, one serving of whole–wheat bread contains 4 g of protein. The panel does not provide infor–mation about a product's protein quality, but you can judge from the list of ingredients. This particular brand of bread, for example, contains proteins from various cereal grains and some seeds, but its ingredients do not include sources of *high–quality proteins* such as eggs, milk, or processed soybeans. The "Proteins: Economical Considerations" section of this chapter explains how you can use plant proteins to obtain high–quality protein.

Concept **Checkpoint 7.5**

17. Discuss how you can use information on a food product's label to determine whether the food is a source of high-quality protein.

7.6 Proteins: Economical Considerations

Learning Outcomes

1 Describe ways people can reduce the amount of meat in their diet without sacrificing protein quality.

2 Explain how using mixtures of foods with complementary proteins can help reduce animal protein intake.

If you are like most Americans, your daily protein intake is higher than the RDA. Furthermore, animal foods contribute the largest share of the protein in your diet. In fact, animal foods, including eggs and milk products, sup–ply almost two–thirds of the protein in the American diet.[8] Some of these foods, however, are among the most expensive items on our grocery lists, and you may be able to reduce your food costs if you eat less of them. Fur–thermore, you may reap substantial health benefits by reducing your animal protein intake and increasing your consumption of plant foods.

Animal foods are among the best dietary sources of essential amino acids, so is it safe to eat less animal protein? Yes! One way you can lower your intake is to include only one animal source of protein in a meal and reduce its serving size. For example, if your breakfast is a 6–ounce slice of ham with two large fried eggs, you are obtaining over 500 kcal and almost 60 g of high–quality protein. That is enough protein in one meal to meet the

RDA for a person who weighs 132 pounds. Instead of eating such a large serving of ham with the fried eggs, have 3 ounces of ham without the eggs, or skip the ham and eat just the eggs. Two fried eggs supply 12.5 g of high—quality protein and only 180 kcal.

An easy way to reduce your meat consumption is to replace meat with other high—quality protein sources. Eggs, milk, cheese, and yogurt are animal sources of high—quality protein that you can substitute for meat, fish, or poultry items in your diet. For example, simply have a cheese sandwich instead of eat—ing a submarine sandwich made with various luncheon meats and cheeses. If you are interested in eating less fat, a serving of low—fat cottage cheese or low—fat yogurt makes a protein—rich substitute for the "sub" or cheese sandwich.

Another way to reduce the amount of animal food in your diet and your food costs is to make meals that contain less animal protein and more plant protein. Many commonly eaten menu items provide the proper amounts and mixtures of essential amino acids without relying heavily on animal products. Throughout the world, people with limited access to meat and other animal foods rely heavily on recipes that combine small amounts of animal protein with larger portions of certain plant proteins. Proteins in animal foods contain enough essential amino acids to extend or "beef up" the lower—quality plant proteins in dried peas, beans, cereals, and other grain products. Pasta made from white flour, for example, contains cereal (wheat) proteins that have limiting amounts of lysine. By mixing large amounts of cooked pasta with smaller amounts of lysine—rich meat, seafood, chicken, or cheese, the proteins in the animal foods enhance the quality of the wheat proteins. As a result, the body can use the amino acids in pasta for growth, repair, and maintenance of tissues.

Pancakes, waffles, crepes, and cornflakes with milk are examples of break—fast foods that extend egg and milk proteins with large amounts of cereal proteins. Many popular Asian dishes mix small amounts of chicken, beef, or seafood with large portions of rice; Italian dishes often combine pasta with small amounts of cheese or meat sauce. Serving meals that extend the high—quality protein in animal foods is an economical way to feed large numbers of people. For example, you can use 1 pound of ground meat to make a single hamburger for each of your four friends. However, you will have enough chili con carne to feed six or more friends if you combine that pound of ground meat with three cans of kidney beans and a couple of large cans of tomatoes. The ground meat has plenty of cysteine and methionine, the essential amino acids that are low in kidney beans. By mixing plant and animal sources of protein together in chili con carne, the beef protein extends the quality of the protein in the kidney beans. Although the chili recipe calls for adding tomatoes to the meat and beans, tomatoes are botanically classified as fruit, so they add very little protein to the dish. (Imagine eating chili con carne without tomatoes!) If you want to extend the chili even more, add cooked macaroni to the mixture. Macaroni is made from wheat, so it contains cereal proteins that are enhanced by the proteins in the meat and beans. For more practical ways to "stretch" your food dol—lars without sacrificing the nutritional quality of your diet, read the "Nutrition Matters" at the end of this chapter.

Animal foods are among the most expensive items on our grocery lists.

Food & Nutrition tip

Commercially canned beans often have considerable amounts of salt added to them. Consider purchasing canned or frozen beans that have little or no added salt. Dried beans do not have salt added to them, but they take a long time to cook, unless you soak them for several hours before cooking. The soaking process softens the beans, reducing cooking time and making them more digestible and less likely to contribute to intestinal gas.

Combining Complementary Proteins

Although research findings indicate that it is not necessary to consume all essential amino acids during a meal for the body to utilize them for growth, certain plant—based recipes ensure that these compounds are consumed dur—ing a day. **Complementary combinations** are mixtures of certain plant foods that provide all essential amino acids without adding animal proteins. However,

complementary combinations mixing certain plant foods to provide all essential amino acids without adding animal protein

Traditional Asian dishes, such as beef stir-fry, combine small amounts of animal protein with larger amounts of cereal and vegetable proteins.

to make dishes that contain complementary amino acid combinations, you must know which plant foods are good protein sources and which essential amino acids are limiting or low in those plant foods. Most plant foods are poor sources of one or more essential amino acids, particularly tryptophan, threonine, lysine, and methionine. Green peas, for example, are good sources of lysine, but they contain low amounts of tryptophan and methionine. Cereal grains such as wheat, rice, and corn are good sources of tryptophan and methionine, but they tend to be low in lysine. Wheat germ, however, is a rich source of lysine. Legumes are low in methionine. Seeds such as sesame and sunflower seeds are generally low in lysine. Walnuts, cashews, almonds, and other tree nuts also contain low amounts of lysine. Although most fruits and some kinds of vegetables are poor sources of protein, they add appealing colors and textures as well as vitamins, minerals, and phytochemicals to plant−based meals.

Many cultures have traditional foods that combine complementary plant proteins. For example, a peanut butter sandwich combines two foods that supply complementary plant proteins. Peanuts are a fair source of lysine. Bread con−tains some methionine, but the grain product is very low in lysine. Serving the two foods together as a peanut butter sandwich provides adequate amounts of these essential amino acids. Table 7.4 lists some other foods that are examples of complementary protein combinations. When menu planning, you can combine a variety of legumes, grains, tree nuts, and seeds with vegetables to prepare dishes that provide adequate mixtures of the essential amino acids. Figure 7.16 shows three categories of plant proteins (legumes, grains, and tree nuts and seeds) that make complementary combinations when one or more foods from at least two different groups are mixed together.

Not every mixture of plant foods creates a complementary combination. For example, making a fruit salad by combining apples, grapes, and oranges will not provide a complementary mixture of essential amino acids. Fruits are nutritious foods, but they are generally poor sources of protein. Combining Boston, iceberg, and romaine varieties of lettuce with carrots and onions makes a tasty salad, but simply mixing leafy greens with other vegetables does not make a complemen−tary combination, because vegetables have small amounts of protein that tend to contain low amounts of essential amino acids. However, adding sunflower seed kernels, kidney or black beans, cashews, and bread cubes to the salad boosts the amount of protein and provides a complete mix of amino acids. To increase the essential amino acid content of the salad even further, you can add a small

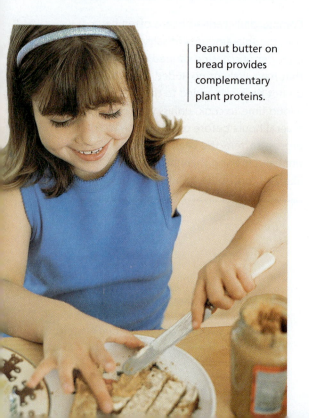

Peanut butter on bread provides complementary plant proteins.

TABLE 7.4 Complementary Protein Dishes

Red beans and rice
Peanut or soy nut butter on bagel, sprinkled with wheat germ
Hummus (mashed chickpeas/garbanzo beans) with sesame seeds
Hummus on whole-grain pita bread
Black beans and cornmeal tortilla
Split pea soup with toasted whole-wheat bread
Meatless kidney bean chili with macaroni
Cornmeal tortilla with black bean salsa
Peanut butter on whole-grain crackers, sprinkled with wheat germ
Green beans with brown rice and cashews

Seeds and Tree Nuts

Primary limiting amino acid:
Lysine

- Sesame seeds, sunflower seed kernels, pumpkin seeds
- Cashews, pistachios, walnuts, pine nuts, almonds

Grains

Primary limiting amino acid:
Lysine

- Wheat and products made from wheat flour
- Rice, oats, millet, barley, bulgur
- Corn and products made from corn

Legumes

Primary limiting amino acids:
Methionine
Tryptophan

- Peas
- Peanuts and peanut butter
- Soybeans, soy products, and other beans

Figure 7.16 Complementary combinations. To ensure an adequate mix of amino acids, combine one or more foods from at least two of the plant food groups shown in this illustration (legumes, grains, and seeds and tree nuts).

Food & Nutrition tips

The following information describes popular soybean foods and tips for how to use them in menu planning.

- Plain tofu has little flavor, so it can be added to a variety of foods, including stir-fried vegetables and scrambled eggs.

- Tempeh is a fermented soybean and grain mixture that can substitute for meat in sandwiches and casseroles.

- Soy nuts are roasted soybeans that are often eaten as a snack. Ground soy nuts form a spread that is used like peanut butter.

- Soy milk is made from crushed soybeans. Soy milk is usually fortified with calcium and vitamins A, D, B-12, and riboflavin. Regular soy milk can substitute for cow's milk as a beverage or in recipes. Soy milk cheeses and yogurt are also available.

- Texturized soy protein (TSP) is made from soybean flour. A TSP product that resembles ground beef can be used to replace half or all of the ground beef in meatloaf, meatball, chili, taco, or meat sauce recipes.

- Soy protein concentrate is a high-protein, high-fiber refined soybean product that is used to boost the protein content of foods.

amount of hard—cooked egg, shredded cheese, or bits of *tofu*, a soybean prod— uct, to it. If you are interested in trying foods made from soybeans, the "Food & Nutrition Tips" feature on this page provides information about some of the more popular foods made from soybeans.

Concept **Checkpoint 7.6**

18. Give examples of common foods that are high-quality substitutes for meat and foods that extend a source of high-quality protein.

19. Does a recipe that combines apples and oranges with peanuts provide a complementary mixture of proteins? Explain why or why not.

20. A recipe mixes cereals made from wheat, rice, and corn. What plant foods could you add to this combination of cereals to make the recipe a source of high-quality protein?

7.7 Vegetarianism

Learning Outcomes

1 Describe different forms of vegetarianism.

2 Discuss pros and cons of vegetarian diets.

vegetarians people who eat plant-based diets

semivegetarian (or flexitarian) vegetarian who eats animal products, except red meat

lactovegetarian vegetarian who consumes milk and milk products for animal protein

ovovegetarian vegetarian who eats eggs for animal protein

lactoovovegetarian vegetarian who consumes milk products and eggs for animal protein

vegan vegetarian who eats only plant foods

Are you or is anyone you know vegetarian? If you are vegetarian, do you eat any animal foods? **Vegetarians** rely heavily on plant foods and may or may not include some animal foods in their diets. About 2.3% of American adults do not eat meat, fish, or poultry; about 1.4% of adults avoid eating any foods from animal sources.[10]

There are many different types of vegetarian diets, including some that contain animal foods. A **semivegetarian** (or **flexitarian**), for example, avoids red meat but consumes other animal foods, including fish, poultry, eggs, and dairy products. Other vegetarians have more restrictive diets, particularly when choosing whether to eat animal foods. A **lactovegetarian** (*lacto* = milk) consumes milk and milk products, including yogurt, cheese, and ice cream, to obtain animal protein. An **ovovegetarian** (*ovo* = egg) eats eggs, and a **lactoovovegetarian** consumes milk products and eggs. A **vegan,** or total vegetarian, eats only plant foods. Table 7.5 lists types of vegetarian diets.

Vegetarians have various reasons for eating few or no animal products. Many vegetarians have religious, ethical, and other philosophical beliefs that do not support the practice of killing and eating animals. For others, vegetarianism is a matter of concern for the environment and economics; plant foods are generally less expensive than animal foods. Some vegetarians believe that humans are not physically able to digest animal foods. This is not true. The omnivore's intestinal tract is able to obtain nutrients from both plants and animals, and humans are omnivores. Nevertheless, eating more plant than animal sources of protein may provide important health benefits.

A vegan, or total vegetarian, might enjoy this dish: couscous with vegetables and chickpeas. Couscous is a grain product.

TABLE 7.5 Types of Vegetarian Diets

Type of Vegetarian Diet	Animal Foods Included
Semivegetarian (flexitarian)	All except red meats
Lactovegetarian	Milk and milk products No animal flesh or eggs
Ovovegetarian	Eggs but no other animal foods
Lactoovovegetarian	Milk and milk products and eggs but no other animal foods
Vegan	No animal foods
Fruitarian	No animal foods (nuts and seeds only)
Macrobiotic	No animal foods (will eat organically-grown whole grains, fruits and vegetables, and soups made with vegetables, seaweed, grains, beans, and miso)

Is Vegetarianism a Healthy Lifestyle?

Vegetarian diets are often lower in saturated fat and energy than "Western" diets that contain animal foods, particularly plenty of red meat. Compared to people who eat meat, vegetarians tend to have a lower risk of metabolic syndrome, which is associated with increased risk of type 2 diabetes and cardiovascular disease (CVD).[11] Furthermore, vegans tend to be leaner than nonvegans.[12] It is difficult, however, to pinpoint diet as responsible for vegetarians' health status. Why? Vegetarians often adopt other healthy lifestyle practices, such as exercising regularly; practicing relaxation activities, such as meditation; and avoiding tobacco products and excess alcohol.

Compared to the typical American diet, vegetarian diets provide more fiber, phytochemicals, folic acid (a B vitamin), vitamins E and C, and the minerals potassium and magnesium.[12] Furthermore, vegetarian diets often supply less saturated fat and cholesterol than diets that include animal foods.

In general, plant foods have low energy density: They add bulk to the diet without adding a lot of calories. Thus, vegetarians may feel "full" soon after eating a meal of plant foods, and they may not consume as much energy and nutrients as they need. Poorly planned plant–based diets may not contain enough energy; high–quality protein; omega–3 fatty acids; vitamins B–12, D, and riboflavin; and minerals zinc, iron, and calcium to meet a person's nutritional needs.[10,12] Humans digest animal proteins to a greater extent than plant proteins.[13] Therefore, vegetarians may need to increase their protein intakes by about 10%. Total vegetarians, including vegan athletes, can obtain adequate amounts of the essential amino acids by eating processed soybean products and foods that combine complementary plant proteins.

Vegetarians who do not consume fish may need to obtain DHA and EPA (omega–3 fatty acids) by eating certain algae or taking pills that contain the algae. Plant foods contain little or no vitamin B–12, and there are few dietary sources of vitamin D other than fortified cow's milk. Furthermore, mineral nutrients such as calcium and iron are more available from animal than from plant foods. Plants often contain phytochemicals that interfere with the body's absorption of minerals, particularly iron, zinc, and calcium.

Vegans can obtain vitamin B–12, vitamin D, iron, zinc, and many other micronutrients by consuming fortified foods such as soy and rice beverages, "Red Star" vegetarian nutritional yeast, and breakfast cereals. Vegetarians can also take a multiple vitamin/mineral supplement to provide dietary "insurance." Table 7.6 summarizes the nutritional advantages and possible nutritional disadvantages of vegetarian diets.

Children have higher protein and energy needs per pound of body weight than an adult. Since plant foods add bulk to the diet, vegan children are likely to eat far less food than adult vegans because they become full sooner during meals. Thus, very young vegans may be unable to eat enough plant foods to meet their protein and energy needs. Therefore, it is very important for parents or other caretakers to plan nutritionally adequate diets for vegetarian children and monitor the youngsters' growth rates.

Vegan women who breastfeed their infants may produce milk that is deficient in vitamin B–12, particularly if the mothers' diets lack the vitamin. These infants of vegan mothers have a high risk of developing severe developmental delays associated with neurological damage, especially when breast milk is their only source of vitamin B–12.[14] Pregnant vegan women should consult with their physicians about the need to take a vitamin B–12 supplement to reduce the likelihood of having a baby who is deficient in this nutrient. Additionally, vegan mothers who breastfeed their infants may need to provide the babies with a source of vitamin B–12 as well.

Many American teenagers and young adults are adopting vegetarian diets. Switching from the typical Western diet to vegetarianism can be a healthy

MY DIVERSE PLATE

Miso

Miso, a seasoning paste made from fermented soybeans, is a staple of traditional Japanese diets. Miso is added to soup (misoshiru) and vegetables. Two tablespoons of miso supply about 70 kcal, 4 g protein, 2 g fat, and 1280 mg sodium. Although miso adds flavor to foods, the paste is very salty; therefore, it should be used in small amounts.

 Did You Know?

There is nothing inherently "bad" about eating small portions of red meat. Red meat is a good source of zinc and iron, minerals that are often less bioavailable from plant foods.

TABLE 7.6 Vegetarian Diets: Nutritional Aspects

Advantages	Possible Disadvantages
High in: Vitamins C, E, and folic acid	**Low in:** Vitamins B-12, D, and riboflavin
Phytochemicals	Zinc, iron, and calcium
Fiber	Omega-3 fatty acids
Magnesium and potassium	Certain essential amino acids
Low in: Fat (saturated)	Energy
Cholesterol	

Commercially prepared vegetarian foods are often available in the frozen food section of supermarkets.

practice for teens; vegetarian youth often eat more fruits and vegetables and less fat than their nonvegetarian peers. On the other hand, female vegetarian teenagers may have a higher risk of unhealthy weight control practices and eating disorders, such as *anorexia nervosa*, than young people who eat meat.[15] Anorexia nervosa ("anorexia") is a serious psychological disorder that can result in starvation and suicide. The Chapter 10 "Nutrition Matters" provides more information about anorexia nervosa and other eating disorders.

Meatless Menu Planning

Many common menu items can be converted into vegetarian foods by removing the meat, fish, or poultry. For example, pizza and lasagna can be prepared without meat and still provide plenty of protein from the cheese as well as the crust or pasta. Stir—fried foods can also be a reliable source of protein without adding meat, fish, or poultry. To stir—fry, heat a small amount of peanut or canola oil in a frying pan and add cooked rice and pieces of raw vegetables. While the mixture is heating, add a beaten egg to it and stir so the egg cooks thoroughly. Before serving the dish, sprinkle cashews or sunflower seed kernels over the hot rice and vegetable mixture. Table 7.7 presents more meatless menu suggestions.

Commercially prepared vegetarian foods that substitute for meat, fish, and poultry items are often available in the frozen food section of supermarkets. These vegetarian products can look and taste like their nonvegetarian counterparts, but they generally do not contain cholesterol and may be lower in saturated fat. Such foods include soy—based sausage patties or links, soy hot dogs, "veggie" burgers, and soy "crumbles" that look like bits of cooked ground beef. Asian restaurants usually offer vegetarian dishes. Some "Western — style" restaurants offer vegetarian menu items, or their cooks can modify menu items by substituting meatless sauces, omitting meat from stir—fries, and adding vegetables or pasta in place of meat.

With careful planning, vegetarians can overcome the nutritional limitations of a plant—based diet and consume adequate diets.[10] If you are interested in learning more specific details about vegetarian cookery and menu planning, contact a registered dietitian (RD) or university extension nutritionist in your area. The MyPlate website also offers suggestions for planning nutritionally adequate meatless meals. For more information, visit http://www.choosemyplate.gov and click on "Tips for Vegetarians."

TABLE 7.7 Meatless Menu Ideas

- Cooked pasta with marinara sauce and grated Parmesan or part-skim mozzarella cheese
- Vegetable lasagna with layers of thinly sliced zucchini, mushrooms, and bell peppers
- Vegetable stir-fry with bits of tofu and cheese
- Grilled vegetable kabobs served over cooked rice and black beans
- Black or red bean burritos
- Bean and corn tacos

7.8 Protein Adequacy

Learning Outcomes

1 Discuss potential health problems that may occur with excessive protein intake.

2 Explain why protein-energy malnutrition is a serious nutritional state, especially for young children.

If some protein is necessary for proper growth and good health, can eating extra amounts of the nutrient make you *extra* healthy or physically fit? Intuitively, the idea of eating more protein to improve your health seems logical, but protein is no different from the other nutrients. If your diet contains adequate amounts of protein, then eating "more is not better."

In many parts of the world, the lack of foods containing high—quality proteins is a serious problem, particularly for young children. Protein deficiency interferes with a child's normal growth and development, and contributes to many childhood deaths. The following sections examine protein malnutrition.

Excessive Protein Intake

Heart disease and cancer are the leading causes of death in developed countries, including the United States. In these nations, the typical Western diet that con—tains high amounts of meat protein and saturated fat is associated with increased risk of certain chronic diseases, particularly heart disease and colorectal cancer,[16] and possibly prostate cancer.[17] Consumption of red meat, pork, and processed meats may increase the risk of pancreatic cancer;[18] processed, smoked, and/or salted meats increase the risk of stomach cancer.[19] More research, however, is needed to clarify the role of high—protein diets in the risk of certain cancers.

High—protein diets are generally not recommended for healthy individuals. Results of some studies indicate that diets that contain high amounts of animal protein may lead to higher—than—normal urinary losses of the mineral calcium.[20] Such losses may be more likely to occur when people, particularly older adult women, consume diets that are low in calcium and contain more animal than vegetable proteins.[20] Some nutrition experts suspect that diets that supply a lot of animal protein are associated with osteoporosis, a condition characterized by thin bones that fracture easily. Chapter 9 discusses dietary and other factors that contribute to osteoporosis.

Excess amino acid or protein intake can lead to dehydration, because the kidneys need more water to dilute and eliminate the toxic waste products of amino acid metabolism in urine. Dehydration is a potentially life—threatening condition in which the body's water level is too low. People with liver or kid—ney diseases may need to avoid protein—rich diets and amino acid supplements because metabolizing the excess amino acids is a burden to their bodies.

Some weight loss diets promote large servings of protein-rich foods.

What About High-Protein Weight-Loss Diets?

Certain popular weight—loss diets, such as the Atkins, Protein Power, and Paleo diets, promote high intakes of protein. While following high—protein diets to lose weight, people often report decreased feelings of hunger and increased sense of fullness (satiety) after meals. Protein may contribute to satiety to a greater extent than fat or carbohydrate.[21] Chapter 10 provides information about the safety and effectiveness of various popular weight—loss diets.

What About Protein or Amino Acid Supplements?

Healthy people may adapt to protein intakes that are higher than the AMDR for the macronutrient and not experience health problems as a result. However, taking protein or amino acid supplements is not recommended for healthy per—sons, especially if the products supply individual amino acids. Why? The human digestive system is designed to digest large protein molecules from the mixture of proteins that naturally occurs in foods. Consuming supplements that supply large amounts of individual amino acids can upset intestinal cells' ability to absorb other amino acids.

For thousands of years, humans have obtained amino acids by eating plants and animals. The use of amino acid and protein supplements as sources of the nutrient is a relatively recent development, and little is known about the long—term safety of using these products. Chapter 11 provides more information about protein needs of physically active people and examines the evidence concerning the value and safety of using certain foods and dietary supplements to enhance physical performance.

Protein Deficiency

Although food insecurity exists in the United States, protein deficiency is uncommon. (See the Chapter 1 "Nutrition Matters" for information about food insecurity.) People suffering from alcoholism, anorexia nervosa, or certain intestinal tract disorders are at risk of protein undernutrition. People with low incomes, especially those who are elderly, are also at risk of protein deficiency. Many elderly Americans have limited incomes and must make difficult choices concerning their expenses. If you were old, chronically ill, and on a low fixed income, what would you think was more important: purchasing nutritious foods or costly prescription medications that control your serious health problems?

Protein Energy Malnutrition

Undernutrition, the lack of food, is often widespread in poor nations in which populations endure frequent famine resulting from crop failures, political unrest, or civil wars. In these countries, **protein—energy malnutrition (PEM)** affects people whose diets lack sufficient protein as well as energy. The failure to con—sume nourishing food also results in vitamin and mineral deficiencies.

When food is limited, it is often more difficult for children to obtain nutri—tionally adequate diets than for adults to do so. Why? Adults may be able to consume enough plant proteins to meet their protein and energy needs, but chil—dren have smaller stomachs and higher energy and protein needs per pound of body weight than adults. They are unable to eat enough plant foods to meet their relatively high protein and other nutrient requirements.

In children, being underweight is often a sign of PEM. According to the World Health Organization (WHO), 17% of children were underweight through—out the world in 2012.[22] Impoverished children in southern Asia and much of Africa are most likely to be underweight, and the effects of undernutrition are especially devastating for the very young. Children whose diets lack sufficient protein and energy do not grow and are very weak, irritable, and vulnerable to

protein-energy malnutrition (PEM) condition that results from diets that provide inadequate amounts of protein and energy dehydration and infections, such as measles, that can kill them. If these children survive, their growth may be permanently stunted and their intelligence may be lower than normal because undernutrition during early childhood can cause per—manent brain damage.

Forms of PEM   At one time, nutrition experts thought there were only two types of PEM, **kwashiorkor** and **marasmus.** The distinctions between these conditions, however, are often blurred, because protein deficiency is unlikely when a person's energy intake is adequate. Nevertheless, dietitians generally consider *kwashior—kor*, *marasmic kwashiorkor*, and *marasmus* as forms of PEM.

Kwashiorkor (*qwash′—e—or′—kor*) primarily occurs in developing countries where mothers commonly breast—feed their infants until they give birth to another child. The older youngster, who is usually a toddler, is fairly healthy until abruptly weaned from its mother's milk to make way for the younger sibling. Although the toddler may obtain adequate energy by consuming a traditional diet of cereal grains, the diet lacks enough complete protein to meet the youngster's high needs, and he or she soon develops signs of protein deficiency. Children affected by kwashiorkor have stunted growth (see Fig. 1.15); unnaturally blond, sparse, and brittle hair; and patches of skin that have lost their normal coloration. Children with kwashiorkor have some subcu—taneous (under the skin) fat and swollen cheeks, arms, legs, and bellies that make them look well fed, but their appearance is misleading. An important function of certain proteins in blood is to maintain proper fluid balance within cells and blood vessels, as well as between cells. During starvation, levels of these proteins decline, resulting in edema, which can make the protein—deficient child look plump and over—fed instead of thin and undernourished. In many cases, the child suffering from kwashiorkor does not obtain enough energy and eventually develops maras—mic kwashiorkor, a condition characterized by edema and wasting (Fig. 7.17). *Wasting* is the loss of organ and muscle proteins as the body tears down these tis—sues to obtain amino acids for energy metabolism.

Severe PEM causes extreme weight loss and a condition called marasmus (*mah—raz′—mus*), which is commonly referred to as starvation (Fig. 7.18). Obvious

Figure 7.17 Mild to moderate protein-energy malnutrition. This Nigerian child is suffering from marasmic kwashiorkor. Note the edema in the child's abdomen and feet. The inset photo shows "pitting" edema—swollen tissues that become deformed when pressed with a finger. These photos were taken during the Nigerian civil war that occurred in the late 1960s.

kwashiorkor form of undernutrition that results from consuming adequate energy and insufficient high-quality protein

marasmus starvation

Figure 7.18 Severe protein-energy malnutrition. This photo of a Nigerian person suffering from marasmus was taken during the civil war that occurred in the late 1960s.

signs of marasmus are weakness and wasting. The marasmic person is so thin that his or her ribs, hips, and spine are visible through the skin. People suffering from marasmus avoid physical activity to conserve energy, and they are often irritable. If marasmus is not treated with a nutritious diet, death results.

Concept Checkpoint 7.8

24. In the United States, which groups of people are most likely to suffer from protein-energy malnutrition?
25. Why is protein-energy malnutrition a devastating condition for young children?
26. Police bring a 2-year-old child into a hospital; the child is so underweight, his bones are visible through the skin. The police report indicates the child was severely neglected by his parents. According to this information, is this child suffering from kwashiorkor, severe protein-energy malnutrition, or sickle cell anemia? Choose one of these conditions and explain why you selected it.

7.9 Food Allergies, Celiac Disease, and PKU

Learning Outcomes

1. Explain the cause of a food allergy, identity foods that are most likely to cause food allergies in vulnerable people, and list three common signs or symptoms of a food allergy.

2. Explain what causes celiac disease, identify foods that a person with celiac disease must avoid, and list three common signs or symptoms of the disease.

3. Explain the cause of phenylketonuria and discuss how the condition is treated.

4. Distinguish between nutrigenetics and nutrigenomics.

There is no question that cells need amino acids to function properly. In some instances, however, certain amino acids or proteins cause havoc in the body, resulting in serious health problems and even death. The following sections take a closer look at three protein—related conditions that affect the lives of millions of Americans. By following special diets, people with these conditions can live normal and productive lives. This section also includes information about *nutritional genomics*, the science that explores ways genes interact with dietary choices and the environment.

What Is a Food Allergy?

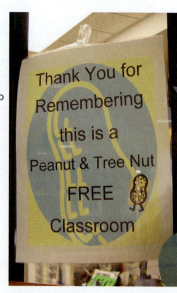

This sign on the door of an elementary school classroom lets people know to avoid bringing anything containing peanuts and tree nuts into the room.

Thank You for Remembering this is a Peanut & Tree Nut FREE Classroom

Have you ever experienced an allergic reaction after eating certain foods or drinks? A food allergy is an inflammatory response that results when the body's immune system reacts inappropriately to one or more harmless substances (*allergens*) in the food. In most instances, the allergen is a protein. Some people with food allergies experience swelling of their lips and tongue as they eat the food and the allergens come in contact with their mouth. Other people do not have a physical reaction to the food until a few hours after eating it. In these cases, a protein in the food that is eaten does not undergo digestion, and the small intestine absorbs the whole molecule. Immune system cells in the small intestine recognize the food protein as a foreign substance and try to protect the body by mounting a defen— sive response. As a result of the immune response, the person who is allergic to that food experiences typical signs and symptoms.

Common signs and symptoms of food allergies include *hives*, red raised bumps that usually appear on the skin; swollen or itchy lips; skin flushing; a scaly skin rash (eczema); difficulty swallowing; wheezing and difficulty breath— ing; and abdominal pain, vomiting, and diarrhea. Allergic reactions generally occur within a few minutes to a couple of hours after eating the offending food. In severe cases, sensitive people who are exposed to food allergens can develop *anaphylactic shock*, a serious drop in blood pressure that affects the whole body. Anaphylaxis (*an—a—pha—lax'—is*) can be fatal, unless emergency treatment is provided. Genetics play a major role in the risk of food allergies; people who have family histories of allergies to foods or other environmental triggers are more likely to develop these conditions.

Although any food protein has the potential to cause an allergic reaction in a susceptible person, the most allergenic proteins are in cow's milk, eggs, peanuts and other nuts, wheat, soybeans, fish, and shellfish. Allergic responses to non— protein food dyes or other food additives such as *sulfites* can also occur. Sulfites are a group of sulfur—containing compounds that result from the metabolism of certain amino acids. Sulfites can be found naturally in foods, but the compounds are often added to wines, potatoes, and shrimp as a preservative.[23] People who suffer from asthma often develop breathing difficulties after consuming food treated with sulfites. Other sulfite—sensitive people report skin flushing (redness and warmth), hives, difficulty swallowing, vomiting, diarrhea, and dizziness after consuming foods that contain the compounds.

In the United States, approximately 5% of young children suffer from food allergies.[24] Since 1997, the prevalence of food allergies among children under 18 years of age has been increasing in the United States. Children with food allergies are more likely than other children to experience other allergies and asthma. Most youngsters outgrow their food allergies by the time they are 5 years old. Allergies to nuts, seafood, and wheat, however, usually are not outgrown. About 1 in 25 adults in the United States has one or more food allergies.[24]

Accurate diagnosis of a food allergy should be undertaken by an immunol— ogist, a physician who specializes in the diagnosis and treatment of allergies. Skin testing is a reliable way to identify allergens. Although hair analysis, cytotoxic or electrodermal testing, and kinesiology are promoted by alternative medical prac— titioners to diagnose allergies, these are unproven diagnostic methods.[25]

Treatment of food allergies involves strict avoidance of the offending foods. Parents or caregivers of young children with food allergies should read food labels carefully to check for allergens listed among ingredients. Additionally, they should educate teachers and other adults who associate with the allergic child about the importance of not exposing the youngster to specific foods. In 2004, the U.S. Congress passed the Food Allergen Labeling and Consumer Protection Act, which required food manufacturers to identify potentially allergenic ingredients, such as soy, milk, and peanuts, on product labels (Fig. 7.19).[26]

Figure 7.19 Allergen labeling.

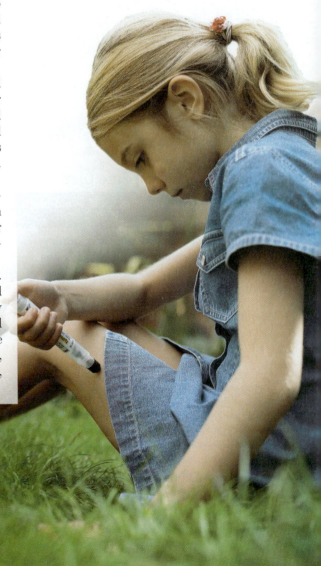

Emergency treatment for anaphylaxis often involves injecting a medication that prevents or blunts the allergic response. This child is using an *autoinjector pen,* a special syringe, to inject herself with a dose of the medication.

Figure 7.20 Gluten-free foods. Gluten-free foods are often available in supermarkets.

TABLE 7.8   Gluten-Free Diet

People with celiac disease should avoid foods that contain:
wheat, including wheat, enriched, durum, graham, and semolina flours; farina, wheat bran, wheat germ, cracked wheat, wheat protein
barley
rye
triticale
Unless contaminated with any of the above foods, products that contain the following ingredients are generally safe to eat for people with celiac disease:
arrowroot, buckwheat, cassava, corn, flax, oats (small amounts), millet, nuts, quinoa, rice, sorghum, soy, tapioca

What Is Celiac Disease?

Celiac (see'—lee—ak) disease is a common inherited condition that results in poor absorption of nutrients (malabsorption) from the small intestine. People with the disease cannot tolerate foods that contain gluten, a group of related proteins in wheat, barley, and rye. Gluten provides the chewy texture and stiff structure of breads and other baked products made from wheat, barley, and rye. After a person with celiac disease eats foods or is exposed to substances that contain gluten, a component of the protein stimulates the body to mount an immune response in the small intestine that inflames or destroys villi. (Villi are the tiny, fingerlike projections of small intestine that absorb nutrients [see Fig. 4.29].) Even though the affected person's food intake may be nutritionally adequate, malnutrition results because his or her intestinal tract lacks healthy villi.

The signs and symptoms of celiac disease vary from person to person but usually include abdominal bloating, chronic diarrhea, and weight loss. Children with this condition also experience poor growth due to nutrient malabsorption and protein malnutrition. Some people have no obvious signs or symptoms of the disease, despite the damage occurring to their small intestines. Serious health problems such as anemia (a blood disorder), osteoporosis (weak bones), infertility, liver disease, and intestinal cancer can result from untreated celiac disease.

In the United States, about 1 in 133 people has celiac disease.[27] Although the tendency to develop the disease is probably inherited, environmental factors often play a role by triggering the condition. A serious viral infection or severe emotional stress, for example, may activate the disorder in a genetically susceptible person.

No single medical test is effective in determining whether a person has celiac disease. However, blood testing and intestinal biopsies are often used to diagnose the condition. The biopsy involves removing tiny pieces of tissue from the small intestine. The tissue samples undergo microscopic examination to evaluate the condition of the villi. The presence of damaged villi can help confirm the diagnosis of celiac disease.

There is no cure for celiac disease, but persons with the condition can achieve and maintain good health by following a special gluten—free diet very carefully. Many supermarkets carry a variety of gluten—free foods (Figure 7.20). Table 7.8 lists foods that must be avoided by people with celiac disease as well as those that are safe for them to consume. Although people with the condition can eat corn, rice, and soy products, these foods may be contaminated with gluten if they are processed in factories that also manufacture wheat products. Because gluten may be used to make medications, dietary supplements, and lipsticks, people with celiac disease should read ingredient lists to determine whether such "hidden" sources of gluten are present. The U.S. Food and Drug Administration (FDA) has rules for the use of the claim "gluten—free" on product labels (see http://www.fda.gov/forconsumers/consumerupdates/ucm363069.htm).

Katie Adams was diagnosed with celiac disease when she was in college. The "Real People, Real Stories" feature on page 241 introduces Katie and describes how she manages her diet to avoid signs, symptoms, and complications of celiac disease.

REAL PEOPLE | REAL STORIES

Katie Adams

When Katie Adams was an American college student, she had the opportunity to attend England's renowned Cambridge University during her junior year. Within a few months after Katie began her studies in England, she began to experience frequent bouts of abdominal pain not long after eating. Making matters even worse, she suffered from nearly constant diarrhea. Although her weight was at a healthy level when she first went to England, she began to lose pounds despite eating adequate amounts of food.

Eventually, Katie reached the point at which she could no longer ignore her health problems. While at Cambridge, she was examined by a physician who thought her signs and symptoms were the result of celiac disease. Although Katie was unfamiliar with the disease, she decided to forgo being tested for the condition until she returned to the United States.

After coming home from England, Katie underwent specialized testing by a physician who diagnoses and treats conditions affecting the intestinal tract. This testing detected the presence of antibodies to proteins in gluten. She also underwent an endoscopic examination of her upper gastrointestinal tract. This exam enabled the gastroenterologist to see the condition of her small intestine and remove a small part of the damaged tissue to view under a microscope. As a result of these definitive tests, Katie was diagnosed with celiac disease. The only treatment for celiac disease is complete avoidance of gluten-containing foods.

Eating out is especially difficult for people with celiac disease, because of restaurants' widespread inclusion of breads, rolls, pasta, and desserts made from wheat flour in menus. Katie learned how to locate the few restaurants in her community that cater to people with celiac disease by having kitchens that are dedicated to gluten-free food preparation.

Today, Katie maintains her good health by continuing to avoid gluten. Although her diet is very restrictive, she knows from experience that if she "cheats" by eating even a small amount of food that contains gluten, she'll get sick again. After such occasions, she returns to following a gluten-free diet, and within several days, her intestinal tract heals itself.

According to Katie, people who are unfamiliar with celiac disease should take the condition seriously and accommodate the special dietary needs of people who have the disease. For example, if you invite someone with celiac disease to share a meal or snack with you, wash your hands after you prepare foods that contain gluten and don't offer those foods to the person. Additionally, prepare some gluten-free foods for your guest who has celiac disease to eat safely. She says, "It's discouraging when people think I'm simply a 'picky eater' and just making life hard for them. The more people who understand celiac disease, the easier my life becomes!"

What Is PKU?

Phenylketonuria (*fen'–il–keet'–n–your'–e–ah*) or PKU is a rare genetic metabolic disorder that affects about 1 in 10,000 to 1 in 15,000 infants in the United States.[28] PKU usually occurs when cells are unable to produce an enzyme that converts the essential amino acid phenylalanine (*fen–il–al'–ah–neen*) to other compounds. As a result, phenylalanine or its toxic by–products build up in tissues and damage cells, including nerve cells in the brain. If PKU is not diag–nosed and treated within a few weeks of birth, the affected infant can develop intellectual disability within the first year of life.

To diagnose PKU, physicians generally rely on a simple blood test that is conducted on infants within 48 hours after their birth. In the United States, more than 98% of newborns undergo testing for PKU and several other treatable inher–ited diseases.[29] Infants who have PKU are generally given special formulas that lack phenylalanine. Phenylalanine is essential for growth and development; therefore, young children can consume a small amount of the amino acid. As the children grow and mature, fruits, vegetables, and special low–protein foods can be added to their formula diet. However, children and adults with the disorder need to avoid foods that are rich sources of phenylalanine, such as nuts, milk products, eggs, meats, and other animal foods. Additionally, people with PKU should not consume diet soft drinks and other foods and beverages containing the alternative sweetener aspartame, because the sweetener is a source of phenylalanine (see Chapter 5 for information about aspartame).

Throughout their lives, individuals with PKU may need to follow the restrictive diet, especially if they cannot take medication that helps their body metabolize phenylalanine. Furthermore, people with the disorder need to undergo frequent blood tests to make sure they are maintaining a healthy concentration of phenylalanine in their bodies. Monitoring blood phenylalanine is especially important during pregnancy. An expectant woman who has PKU must carefully control her phenylalanine level to avoid exposing her embryo/fetus to excessive amounts of the amino acid. If she fails to control the concentration of phenylala–nine in her blood, she can give birth to a baby with severe birth defects, includ–ing a smaller–than–normal brain. The "Real People, Real Stories" on page 243 features Dallas Clasen, a college student who has PKU.

What Is Nutritional Genomics?

nutritional genomics science that investigates the complex interactions among gene functioning, dietary choices, and the environment

nutrigenetics study of how a person's genetic makeup affects the way his or her body responds to food

nutrigenomics study of how nutrients and other food components can affect one's genetic expression

Human DNA has approximately 23,000 genes that code for protein synthesis ("the human genome").[30] **Nutritional genomics** is a relatively new science that investigates the complex interactions among gene functioning, dietary choices, and the environment. Nutritional genomics includes **nutrigenetics,** the study of how a person's genetic makeup affects the way his or her body responds to food. For example, people who are genetically vulnerable to develop celiac disease are healthy until they consume foods that contain gluten. Nutritional genomics also involves **nutrigenomics,** the study of how nutrients and other food compo–nents can affect a person's *genetic expression*. Gene expression results in pro–tein synthesis. As mentioned earlier, newborns with a particular genetic defect develop PKU when they consume amounts of phenylalanine that are harmless to babies who do not have the defect. By providing a diet that is low in phenylala–nine to newborns with PKU, the infants develop normally.

REAL PEOPLE | REAL STORIES

Dallas Clasen

Dallas Clasen is majoring in engineering at the University of Wisconsin-Platteville. In addition to keeping up with his coursework, he runs cross country at school and participates in triathlons. Like most college students, Dallas is very busy, but unlike most students, he has to pay very close attention to his diet. Dallas was born with a rare inherited metabolic disorder, an inborn-error of metabolism called phenylketonuria (PKU).

A few days after birth, Dallas underwent standard newborn blood testing. The results of the test indicated that the level of phenylalanine in his blood was about 40 times higher than the normal amount, a sign of PKU. To avoid developing severe brain damage and other physiological effects of PKU, Dallas was cared for by a physician who specializes in treating children with the disorder. The primary treatment for PKU is a low-phenylalanine diet.

Most foods that are rich sources of protein, especially high-quality animal proteins, contain more phenylalanine than people with PKU can tolerate. Thus, from the time Dallas was a week old, he has consumed a formula that does not contain the amino acid. In addition to the formula, Dallas can eat limited amounts of grain products and most fruits and vegetables. He also consumes special low-phenylalanine foods that resemble "regular" foods but are not available in supermarkets. As part of Dallas's college meal plan, he has access to the special foods through the university's food service.

Foods that are eaten away from home can present problems for people with PKU. When at a restaurant, Dallas usually orders French fries or "sub" sandwiches that are made with vegetables but do not contain any cheese or meat. Instead of drinking milk, Dallas drinks his special formula or sports drinks that do not contain the nonnutritive sweetener aspartame (see Chapter 5). He is so accustomed to his special diet, he thinks meat looks "gross." In addition to following the special diet, Dallas takes Kuvan®, a prescription medication that stimulates the enzyme that converts phenylalanine to tyrosine. He takes 14 capsules after breakfast with apple juice. The medication does not help everyone with PKU, but it allows Dallas to consume more foods that contain phenylalanine. "I can eat double the amount of the amino acid," Dallas says. To determine whether his special diet and medication are working, each week Dallas pricks his finger and allows a few drops of blood to soak into a special paper. Then he sends the paper to a laboratory that checks the level of phenylalanine in his blood.

In the past, children with PKU were often allowed to eat regular foods after they were about 6 years of age. However, the importance of continuing the low-phenylalanine diet became evident when many of the children experienced learning and behavioral problems as they matured. Dallas is aware of the consequences that can occur if he does not limit his phenylalanine intake, and he accepts the need to follow the special diet for the rest of his life. "Being on a strict diet has not only made me disciplined, it has taught me to do whatever is needed to always take good care of myself," says Dallas. "I have learned that we are all different, anyway. So, accept who you are!"

Nutrigenetics

Genes

Influence →

Nutrient Needs

Example:
• Variation in human nutrient requirements

low   high

average

Metabolism

Examples:
• Diabetes and obesity development

Nutrigenomics

Nutrients or food components

Influence →

Genetic Expression

Examples:
• Excess vitamin A during pregnancy causes birth defects in embryo

• Alcohol consumption during pregnancy causes birth defects in embryo

• Food allergies and intolerances in vulnerable persons

| **Figure 7.21** Nutritional genomics.

Nutritional genomics may explain why special diets or dietary supplements can have different effects on the health of different individuals (Fig. 7.21). A young man, for example, may develop kidney stones while taking a daily dietary supplement that contains 1000 mg vitamin C. However, another man who is the same age and takes the same amount of vitamin C each day does not form kidney stones. Thus, the effectiveness of a specific diet, dietary supplement, medication, or lifestyle intervention may largely depend on one's genes. In the future, physicians may be able to consider such individual differences to provide more personalized treatments.

Genetic Testing Kits

Several biotechnology companies sell at−home genetic test kits for individuals to collect a small amount of saliva and mail the saliva sample to the company for genetic analysis. As a result of the saliva analysis, the company develops an "optimal health" plan based on the person's genetic makeup. Consumers, however, are encouraged to use caution when considering purchasing at−home genetic testing kits, because the industry of nutrigenetic testing is not well regulated.[31] People who are interested in having genetic testing should consult their physician.

Concept **Checkpoint 7.9**

27. List three common signs or symptoms of food allergy and celiac disease.
28. Discuss what parents of infants with PKU can do to help their children grow and develop normally.
29. Explain how nutritional genomics may be used to improve a person's health.

7.10 Nutrition Matters: Stretching Your Food Dollars

Learning Outcomes

1 Discuss practical ways to save money when purchasing food.

2 Compare similar foods to determine the most economical product.

Are you concerned about the high cost of food? If you are, how can you lower your food costs without sacrificing proper nutrition? You can trim food costs, and preserve and even improve the nutritional quality of your diet, by analyzing your food buying practices and making a few changes. This section focuses on ways you can eat well for less. Please note that the pricing of products reflects food costs during the winter of 2014 in a major Midwestern city, but you should find them useful for comparing current prices where you live.

Where and What You Buy

Where you buy foods and beverages and what you decide to purchase are major factors in determining your overall food expenditures. If you frequently purchase meals and snacks from vending machines, convenience stores, fast-food outlets, and other restaurants, you may be spending too much on such "convenience" foods. In general, the less time you spend preparing food, the more money you will spend by having someone at a commercial outlet prepare the food for you. Even if a fast-food restaurant hamburger seems like a bargain because it is "only $1.00," you are likely paying a premium for the French fries and soft drink that you purchase to accompany the sandwich. From a nutrition standpoint, fast foods are often energy dense—high in fat and sugar—and low in micronutrients (except sodium), fiber, and phytochemicals.

You probably already know that supermarkets have the same snack foods and staple items (bread and milk) as convenience stores and usually offer these foods at lower prices. Furthermore, supermarkets have a much larger selection of foods, particularly more nutrient-dense raw or less processed foods, than convenience stores. It may be easier to run into a convenience store and load up on foods while you load up on gas than to shop in a supermarket. However, you pay extra for the convenience and your diet may suffer as a result of poor food choices.

A good way to save money is to buy foods in large quantities at "bulk" food stores or at smaller, "no frills," cash-only grocery stores. Although shopping at these places can reduce your food costs, food choices are usually more limited than the selection in supermarkets. It is important to recognize that buying food in bulk is a bargain only if you can use the item before it spoils.

How to Shop Wisely in Supermarkets

To lower your food costs, plan your meals and snacks before you shop for food. Prepare a shopping list to help avoid needless or impulse purchases and having to return to the store to buy forgotten items. Keep the grocery list in a convenient place, such as on the refrigerator, and jot down items as they become depleted.

When shopping for groceries, you will need to compare *unit costs* of similar food products. A "unit" of a packaged food item is usually indicated in ounces or pounds. Food packages and containers are available in different sizes and hold different amounts of food, which can make comparing costs of similar foods difficult. Using a small calculator to compare prices can be helpful. For example, a box of one brand of shredded wheat cereal contains 15.0 ounces of cereal and costs $3.49; a box of a different brand of shredded wheat that contains 11.5 ounces of cereal costs $3.29. Which box of cereal is lower in cost? To answer this question, determine the unit price of the cereal in each box by dividing the cost of the entire package by the number of units of food it contains.

Box #1

$3.49 entire box ÷ 15.0 ounces = approximately $.23/ounce

Box #2

$3.29 entire box ÷ 11.5 ounces = approximately $.29/ounce

In this situation, the larger box of cereal is a better buy, even though it costs more than the smaller box. Some supermarkets indicate unit prices on shelf tags, but the tags may be difficult to read or confusing.

Supermarkets offer a wide variety of prepared foods, including deli items, frozen entrées, fresh cut—up fruit packaged in single—serving plastic bags or bins, and rotis— serie chicken. Although these "fast foods" are convenient, food processing and packaging add to the cost of food. Such foods may contain unhealthy amounts of salt, solid fat, or sugar. To save money and improve your diet, rely less on prepared foods and more on "slow foods"—foods that require some of your time and effort to prepare. Figure 7.22 uses various forms of chicken to illustrate this point. A 2.5–lb rotisserie—cooked chicken costs $3.00/lb, but you can save over 80 cents per pound by purchasing a whole chicken (2.19/lb) and roasting it yourself. Instead of buying raw, skinless, boneless chicken breasts ($5.19/lb), buy raw split chicken breasts that have the bones and skin ($3.79/lb). Remove the skin and bones after the chicken breasts are cooked. You can use the cooked chicken immediately, freeze the meat in containers for a future meal, or chill the meat before chopping it to make chicken salad.

Eating more fruits and vegetables is the natural way to add micronutrients, fiber, and phytochemicals to your diet. Many supermarkets offer fresh fruit and vegetables that have been trimmed, cut up, and packed into containers. Before you reach for one of these items, compare its price with that of its raw counterpart. For example, a 2.2–oz, single—serving package of sliced apples sells for $1.25, and a pound of raw apples is priced at $1.99. In this case, buying the raw apples and slicing them yourself is a money—saving practice. To make this determination, you will need to cal— culate the unit price of each product (Fig. 7.23). An ounce of the packaged apples costs about 57 cents ($1.25 divided

(a)

(b)

Figure 7.23 **Comparing apples to apples.** The cost of a 2.2–oz package of apple slices (*a*) is almost five times the cost of the same amount of fresh, sliced raw apples (*b*).

by 2.2 oz/package). A pound of apples equals 16 ounces, so an ounce of these apples costs about 12 cents ($1.99 divided by 16). Thus, the prepackaged sliced apples cost almost five times more than the bulk raw apples.

Produce that is grown in the United States is usually less expensive when it is in season and more plentiful. For example, berries are plentiful in the spring and early sum— mer, tomatoes and melons in late summer, and apples in the fall. "Fresh" produce that is shipped long distances to supermarket suppliers is often picked before its peak ripe— ness. As a result, the fruits and vegetables may not taste as good or be as nutritious as locally grown produce. Pro— duce loses some of its vitamin C content when it is bruised or becomes wilted. Therefore, consider buying fresh pro— duce directly from local farmers, if possible. Although you still need to compare prices of farmers' market items with those of fresh produce sold in supermarkets, you may be able to find reasonably priced produce that is grown within 100 miles of your home at farmers' markets. Buying produce from local farmers helps support your community's econ— omy, too.

An alternative to buying produce directly from growers is to purchase frozen or canned fruits and vegetables. These products are often less expensive than their fresh counterparts.

| Rotisserie chicken $3.00/lb | Whole chicken $2.19/lb |
| Raw, skinless, boneless chicken breasts $5.19/lb | Raw, whole chicken breast $3.79/lb |

Figure 7.22 **Convenience—Is it worth it?** You may save money by purchasing a raw whole chicken and cutting it into parts or a whole chicken breast and removing the skin and bones.

Furthermore, produce that is destined to be frozen is generally harvested when ripe and frozen immediately, maximizing much of its vitamin content and fresh flavor.

While shopping for foods in supermarkets, you can save money if you

- use unit pricing to compare costs of similar packaged products.
- are wary of appealing offers that are not bargains. For example, items marked "3 for $1.00" or "10 for $10.00" can be confusing to consumers. It is important to understand that you do not need to buy the entire quantity. For example, if a store offers 3 kiwifruits for a dollar, and you cannot use 3 of them, buy one for 34 cents. That price is still a bargain compared to buying kiwifruits that are "2 for $1.00." Also, beware of offers such as "10 oranges for $10." Paying $1 for an orange is not a bargain! The same store may be selling a bag of 10 oranges for $5. At that price, each orange costs only 50 cents.
- package sizes can be misleading, so ignore the size of a package and compare net weights of package contents to determine the best value.
- compare the unit price of organic foods and similar conventionally produced items. If an organic food item is more expensive, consider purchasing the conventional product instead.
- compare unit prices of preportioned snack foods such as chips or cookies in 100–Calorie packages with prices of the typical, larger package–size products. Such preportioned snacks may be convenient and helpful if you are trying to control your calorie intake, but they are usually more costly per ounce than the same foods purchased in larger packages. Furthermore, people may eat more of the preportioned snack foods, because they think they are lower in calories than the same items packed in larger containers. Make your own preproportioned snacks. For example, buy a large package of oatmeal cookies and place two–cookie portions into reusable storage bags. When you want a snack, eat the two cookies.
- use coupons when purchasing brand–name items. However, be aware that many stores offer similar products, often referred to as "store brands," that are less expensive than the brand–name items. Although store brand items do not have name recognition, these products are usually just as nutritious as their corresponding brand–name items.
- limit your carbonated soft drink, commercially prepared coffee, and bottled water purchases. When you are thirsty, locate the nearest water fountain and have a drink for free!

- check "sell by," "best if used by," or "use by" dates on packages of perishable foods such as eggs and dairy products. Compared to canned and frozen foods, perishable foods lose their appealing sensory qualities, such as fresh taste and appearance, more rapidly during storage. The "sell by" date informs store employees about the length of time the product should be displayed for sale. Obviously, it is best to buy foods before the sell–by date. The "best if used by" or "use by" dates indicate the last day to use the product before it loses its best flavor and other appealing sensory qualities. The date does not indicate the last day to purchase the food because of safety concerns.[32] Also, read food product labels for storage information. Many products must be refrigerated after opening to delay spoilage. Chapter 12 provides more information about proper food storage practices.
- have at least one vegetarian meal a week.
- use more chicken, turkey, and fish. Red meats are among the most expensive protein sources.
- have a meal with canned, baked, broiled, or grilled fish as the primary source of animal protein at least once a week.
- incorporate canned fish, such as tuna, salmon, and sardines, in meals. Canned fish can be a less expensive choice than fresh fish, because there is less waste (skin and large bones).
- remember that any food product is not a good buy if the item spoils before you can use it.

For more ways to save money on food, read the "Food & Nutrition Tips" on page 248.

Canned fish, such as tuna, salmon, and sardines, can be a less expensive choice than meat or fresh fish.

Prepare a shopping list to help avoid needless or impluse purchases.

For fresh seasonings, grow your own herbs such as basil, oregano, parsley, and thyme.

Food & Nutrition tips

- Prepare a shopping list to help avoid needless or impulse purchases and having to return to the store to buy forgotten items. Keep the grocery list in a convenient place, such as on the refrigerator, and jot down items as they become depleted.

- Empty-calorie foods often look more appealing when your stomach is empty. To reduce the likelihood of buying such foods on impulse, avoid shopping for groceries when you are hungry.

- Be wary of buying food items that are displayed near or along checkout aisles. They are usually energy-dense foods and are not nutrient dense, such as candy bars and baked goods.

- Many perishable foods, such as margarine, shredded cheese, and fluid fat-free milk, can be frozen.

- If you drink coffee, buy a small coffeemaker, a can of ground coffee, and coffee filters to make the beverage. Consider carrying a small thermos of coffee in your backpack. It is much less expensive to make a cup of your own coffee than to buy one from a coffeehouse.

- Canned beans are often sold in large cans that may be cheaper per ounce than beans in smaller cans. If the larger-sized product is less expensive, buy it. After opening the large can of beans, remove the amount needed for the meal, and freeze the remainder in an air-tight container for a future meal.

- For fresh seasoning, grow your own herbs. Basil, oregano, parsley, cilantro, and thyme grow well in flower pots placed in a sunny area. Snip as many leaves as needed for recipes, while keeping the rest of the plants intact.

- Share potluck dinners with friends. Plan the menu and ask your friends to bring certain items, such as vegetable or fruit salads and whole-grain rolls or breads. Inexpensive entrees (the main food items on the menu) include spaghetti and meat sauce, chicken burritos, vegetarian chili, tuna and noodle casserole, and tacos made with tuna fish.

Concept **Checkpoint 7.10**

30. List at least five ways to save money while shopping for food.
31. You can purchase a 5-pound bag of frozen sliced peaches for $7.00 or 5 pounds of fresh peaches for $1.50 per pound. Considering your situation, which is the more economical way to buy peaches? Explain why.

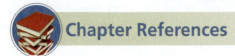

Chapter References

See Appendix H.

Summary

7.1 What Are Proteins?

- Proteins are organic compounds that contain nitrogen, the element cells need to make a wide array of important biological compounds with structural or metabolic functions in the body. Additionally, a relatively small amount of protein contributes to the body's energy needs.

- Proteins are comprised of amino acids. The typical amino acid has nitrogen-containing or amino, acid, and R groups. The diet must supply nine of the amino acids (essential amino acids), because the body cannot make them or make enough of them to meet its needs. Under normal conditions, cells can synthesize the remaining amino acids if the raw materials are available.

7.2 Proteins in Foods

- A high-quality or complete protein contains all essential amino acids in amounts that support growth in children Most animal proteins are high quality. A low-quality or incomplete protein lacks or contains inadequate amounts of one or more of the essential amino acids.

- Tryptophan, threonine, lysine, methionine, and cysteine are often the limiting amino acids in foods.

7.3 What Happens to Proteins in the Body?

- Human proteins are comprised of 20 different amino acids arranged in various combinations. Cells produce proteins by linking amino acids together in specific sequences that are dictated by instructions coded in DNA. Faulty DNA results in the wrong amino acids being inserted into peptide chains, causing genetic defects. If an essential amino acid is not available when protein synthesis occurs, proteins in muscles and organs can provide the essential amino acids. Otherwise, protein synthesis halts, and the amino acids in the unfinished peptide are removed and returned to the amino acid pool. Excess amino acids are metabolized for energy or converted into body fat.

- Protein turnover is the process of breaking down old or unneeded proteins into their component amino acids and recycling them to make new proteins. The body conserves nitrogen by recycling amino acids, but each day, it loses some protein and nitrogen. In positive nitrogen balance, the body retains more nitrogen than it loses; in negative nitrogen balance, the body loses more nitrogen than it retains.

- The protein requirement increases during pregnancy, breastfeeding, periods of growth, and recovery from serious illnesses, blood losses, and burns. The adult RDA for protein is 0.8 g/kg of body weight.

- Protein digestion begins in the stomach, where hydrochloric acid denatures food proteins and pepsin breaks proteins into polypeptides. In the small intestine, enzymes secreted by the pancreas and absorptive cells digest polypeptides primarily into di- and tripeptides. The absorptive cells convert the peptides into amino acids. The end-products of protein digestion, amino acids, travel to the liver. The liver uses the amino acids or releases them into the general circulation.

7.4 Protein Consumption Patterns

- The AMDR for adults is 10 to 35% of energy intake from protein. Total protein consumption as a percentage of daily calories has remained about the same since the early twentieth century, but Americans now eat more animal protein. People can reduce their intake of animal protein without sacrificing the protein quality of their diets.

7.5 Understanding Nutritional Labeling

- The Nutrition Facts panel on a packaged food product label provides information concerning the amount of protein in a serving of the food.

7.6 Proteins: Economical Considerations

- The average American consumes more protein than the RDA for the nutrient.

- In general, meat, fish, poultry, eggs, milk, and milk products contain high-quality proteins. When compared to animal foods, most plant foods provide low-quality protein. Quinoa and foods made from processed soybeans are good plant sources of essential amino acids.

7.7 Vegetarianism

- Vegetarian diets are based on plant foods and limit animal foods to some extent. Although vegetarians are generally healthier than people who eat Western diets, it is difficult to pinpoint diet as responsible for vegetarians' better health. If not properly planned, plant-based diets may not contain enough energy, high-quality protein, omega-3 fatty acids, vitamins B-12 and D, and zinc, iron, and calcium to meet a person's nutritional needs, especially children's needs.

7.8 Protein Adequacy

- High-protein diets are generally not recommended for healthy individuals.

- PEM affects people whose diets lack sufficient protein as well as energy; children are more likely to be affected by PEM than adults. In impoverished developing countries, PEM is a major cause of childhood deaths.

7.9 Food Allergies, Celiac Disease, and PKU

- A food allergy is an inflammatory response that occurs when the body's immune system reacts inappropriately to an allergen. Accurate diagnosis of a food allergy should be undertaken by an immunologist. Treatment involves avoidance of foods that contain the allergens.

- Celiac disease is an inherited condition that causes malabsorption of nutrients. People with the disease cannot eat foods that contain gluten, because the body's response to the protein damages villi in the small intestine. There is no cure for celiac disease, but people with the condition can be healthy as long as they avoid gluten-containing foods.

- Phenylketonuria (PKU) is a rare genetic metabolic disorder that occurs when cells cannot produce an enzyme that converts phenylalanine to other compounds. If PKU is not detected in early infancy, phenylalanine and its toxic by-products build up and damage tissues, including nerve cells in the brain. Treatment involves a special diet that contains limited amounts of phenylalanine and, in some cases, medication.

7.10 Nutrition Matters: Stretching Your Food Dollars

- In general, the less time a person spends preparing food, the more money he or she will spend by having someone else prepare the food. Convenience foods are often energy dense—high in solid fat and added sugar. A good way to save money is to buy foods in large quantities at "bulk" food stores, but buying food in bulk is a bargain only if the items can be used before they spoil.

Recipe for Healthy Living

Apricot Quinoa

The ancient Incas of South America cultivated quinoa and relied on the protein-rich vegetable as a dietary staple. Today, cooked quinoa is often added to vegetable salads or served as an accompaniment to chicken or pork. This quinoa recipe makes about two ½-cup servings. Each serving provides about 250 kcal, 7 g protein, 3 g fat, 6 g fiber, 3 mg iron, 2 mg zinc, and 57 mcg folate.

INGREDIENTS:

1 ⅓ cups water
½ cup quinoa
⅓ cup dried apricots, chopped
¼ tsp ground cinnamon
1 Tbsp maple syrup

PREPARATION STEPS:

1. Add water to a small saucepan and bring to a boil. Add quinoa to boiling water.

2. Cover saucepan and cook quinoa over medium heat until all the water is absorbed (about 12–15 minutes).

3. Remove from heat; fluff quinoa with fork; and stir chopped apricots into the quinoa.

4. Place quinoa into a bowl, drizzle with maple syrup, and sprinkle cinnamon on the quinoa.

5. If desired, garnish with fresh fruit. Serve warm.

 Further analyze this and other recipes through activities on Connect at www.mcgrawhillconnect.com.

11%   11%

78%

- Fat
- Protein
- Carbohydrate

	% of DV/serving
Calories*	13
Protein	15
Fat	5
Fiber	24
Iron	16
Folate	14
Zinc	24

*2000 daily total kcal

Personal Dietary Analysis

1. Refer to the 3-day food log from the "Personal Dietary Analysis" feature in Chapter 3. Calculate your average protein intake by adding the grams of protein eaten each day, dividing the total by 3, and rounding the figure to the nearest whole number.

Sample Calculation:

Day 1 $\underline{76}$ g

Day 2 $\underline{55}$ g

Day 3 $\underline{103}$ g

Total grams $\underline{234}$ g ÷ 3 days = $\underline{78}$ g of protein/day

Your Calculation:

Day 1 _____ g

Day 2 _____ g

Day 3 _____ g

Total grams _____ ÷ 3 days = _____ g/day

My average daily protein intake was _____ g.

2. The RDA for protein is based on body weight. Using the RDA of 0.8 g of protein/kg of body weight, calculate the amount of protein that you need to consume daily to meet the recommendation. To determine your body weight in kilograms, divide your weight (pounds) by 2.2, then multiply this number by 0.8 to obtain your RDA for protein. Then round the figure to the nearest whole number.

My weight in pounds _____ ÷ 2.2 = _____ kg

My weight in kg _____ × 0.8 = _____ g

My RDA for protein = _____ g

   a. Did your average intake of protein meet or exceed your RDA level that was calculated in step 1? _____ yes _____ no

   b. If your answer to 2a is yes, which foods contributed the most to your protein intake?

3. Review the log of your 3-day food intake. Calculate the average number of kilocalories that protein contributed to your diet each day during the 3-day period.

   a. Each gram of protein provides about 4 kcal; therefore, you must multiply the average number of grams of protein obtained in step 1 by 4 kcal to obtain the average number of kcal from protein.

Sample Calculation:

78 g/day × 4 kcal/g = 312 kcal from protein

Your Calculation:

_____ g/day × 4 kcal/g = _____ average number of kcal from protein

4. Determine your average energy intake over the 3-day period by adding the kilocalories for each day and dividing the sum by 3, and round to the nearest whole number.

Sample Calculation:

Day 1   <u>2500</u> kcal

Day 2   <u>3200</u> kcal

Day 3   <u>2750</u> kcal

Total kcal   <u>8450</u> ÷ 3 days = <u>2817</u> kcal/day (average caloric intake)

Your Calculation:

Day 1   _____ kcal

Day 2   _____ kcal

Day 3   _____ kcal

Total kcal   _____ ÷ 3 days = _____ kcal/day (average)

5. Determine the average percentage of energy that protein contributed to your diet by dividing the average kilocalories from protein obtained in step 3 by the average total daily energy intake obtained in step 4. Then round this figure to the nearest one-hundredth. Multiply this value by 100 (move the decimal point two places to the right, drop the decimal point, and add a percent symbol).

Sample Calculation:

<u>312</u> kcal from protein ÷ <u>2817</u> kcal intake = <u>0.11</u> (rounded)

0.11 × 100 = 11%

Your Calculation:

_____ kcal from protein ÷ _____ kcal intake = _____

_____ × 100 = _____ %

6. Did your average intake of protein meet the recommendation of 10 to 35% of total calories? If your average protein intake was below 10%, list at least five foods you could eat that would boost your intake.

 Complete the Personal Dietary Analysis activity online at www.mcgrawhillconnect.com

Critical Thinking

1. Have you used or are you currently using protein or amino acid supplements?

   _____ yes _____ no

   If you answered yes, explain why you use these supplements.

2. Are you a vegetarian? If so, describe your dietary practices (e.g., vegan or semivegetarian), and explain why you decided to become vegetarian. If you are not a vegetarian, explain why you would or would not consider this lifestyle.

3. Plan a day's meals and snacks for a healthy 132–pound (60 kg) adult lactoovovegetarian female who is not pregnant or breastfeeding. The menu should contain all essential amino acids but contain no animal foods other than eggs and foods from the dairy group. Your meal plan can range from 1800 to 2200 kcal, and it should include foods from the major food groups and follow the recommendations of the U.S. Department of Agriculture's MyPlate food guide.

4. Using only plant foods, plan a day's meals and snacks for a healthy 154–pound (70 kg) adult vegan male. The menu should supply at least 2200 kcal, follow the recommendations of MyPlate, and include foods from the major food groups (except for the dairy group, unless calcium–fortified soy milk is used).

5. A recipe for bean salad has the following main ingredients:

   1 cup kidney beans
   1 cup green beans
   1 cup butter beans
   1 cup black beans
   1 ½ cups wine vinegar
   ⅓ cup canola oil
   ¼ cup chopped onion

Explain why this recipe is not a complementary mixture of plant proteins. What plant foods could you add to the recipe to make it a complementary mixture?

Practice Test

Select the best answer.

1. A protein

   a. is comprised of glucose molecules.
   b. has nitrogen in its chemical structure.
   c. provides more energy per gram than carbohydrate.
   d. is a complex inorganic molecule.

2. Which of the following statements is false?

   a. Certain hormones are proteins.
   b. Nearly all enzymes are proteins.
   c. Proteins are part of triglycerides.
   d. The body uses amino acids to make antibodies.

3. Which of the following foods generally provide the least amount of protein per serving?

   a. fruits
   b. milk
   c. nuts
   d. seeds

4. Which of the following foods is not a source of complete protein?

   a. peanut butter
   b. cheese
   c. fish
   d. eggs

5. In cells, _____ controls the assembly of amino acids into proteins.

   a. PEU
   b. DNA
   c. IOM
   d. ATP

6. _____ is the process of removing nitrogen from an amino acid.

   a. Transamination
   b. Denaturation
   c. Hydrogenation
   d. Deamination

7. Which of the following physical states is (are) characterized by positive nitrogen balance?

 a. starvation
 b. illness
 c. puberty
 d. marasmus

8. What is the RDA for protein of a healthy adult woman who weighs 62 kg?

 a. 49.6 g
 b. 59.6 g
 c. 69.6 g
 d. 79.6 g

9. Which of the following foods is not a source of complementary protein?

 a. red beans and rice
 b. hummus on pita bread
 c. soynut butter on a bagel
 d. whole-wheat bread with fruit spread

10. A person following a vegan diet would eat

 a. eggs.
 b. cheese.
 c. nuts.
 d. fish.

11. A sign of marasmus is

 a. increased muscle growth.
 b. rapid weight gain.
 c. diabetes.
 d. wasting.

12. People with celiac disease should

 a. take amino acid supplements.
 b. limit their protein intake to 20 g per day.
 c. avoid foods that contain gluten.
 d. eliminate protein from plant sources.

13. Which of the following tips is a recommended way to reduce food costs?

 a. buying food in bulk, if it can be used before spoiling
 b. purchasing preportioned, packaged foods
 c. shopping at convenience stores, if the stores are within 5 miles of your home
 d. eating at fast-food outlets at least three times a week

Answers to Quiz Yourself

1. Animal foods such as meat and eggs are almost 100% protein. **False.** (p. 218)

2. Foods made from soybeans can be sources of high-quality protein. **True.** (p. 219)

3. Americans typically consume more protein from animal sources than from plant foods. **True.** (p. 228)

4. Registered dietitians generally recommend that healthy people take amino acid supplements to increase their protein intake. **False.** (p. 236)

5. People can nourish their hair by using shampoo that contains protein. **False.** (p. 223)

LEARNSMART
ADVANTAGE

Get the most out of your study of nutrition with McGraw-Hill's innovative suite of adaptive learning products including McGraw-Hill LearnSmart®, SmartBook®, LearnSmart Achieve®, and LearnSmart Prep®. Visit www.learnsmartadvantage.com.

Vitamins

Quiz Yourself

Can vitamins give you more energy or reduce your chances of developing heart disease or cancer? Which cooking methods can increase the loss of vitamins from foods? Which vitamins are added to cereal grains during enrichment? Test your knowledge of vitamins by taking the following quiz. The answers are on page 313.

1. Natural vitamins are better for you because they have more biological activity than synthetic vitamins.
   _____ T _____ F

2. Certain vitamins are toxic.
   _____ T _____ F

3. Vitamin E is an antioxidant.
   _____ T _____ F

4. Vitamins are a source of "quick" energy.
   _____ T _____ F

5. According to scientific research, taking large doses of vitamin C daily prevents the common cold. _____ T _____ F

8.1 Vitamins: Basic Concepts

Learning Outcomes

1 Explain why all vitamins have been discovered.

2 Define *vitamin* and explain how scientists determine whether a substance is a vitamin.

3 Classify vitamins according to whether they are fat soluble or water soluble.

4 Discuss ways to conserve the vitamin content of foods or increase vitamin bioavailability.

5 Explain the function of an antioxidant.

6 Define *enrichment* and *fortification.*

For centuries, taking lengthy ocean voyages was a dangerous venture, not just because of the threat of severe storms and pillaging pirates but also because of a terrifying and deadly disease called **scurvy.** The first signs and symptoms of scurvy—fatigue and *petechiae (peh–tee′–key–eye)*, pinpoint hemorrhages under the skin—occurred about 20 to 40 days after setting sail. As the disease progressed, the affected person's skin bruised easily; gums swelled, became spongy, and bled after being barely touched; teeth loosened and fell out. Not surprisingly, the person suffering from scurvy also became irritable and depressed. A particularly devastating sign of the disease was the opening up of old scars, exposing wounds that could become infected. Scurvy victims eventually died, generally from infections, brain hemorrhages, or heart complications.

In 1753, British physician James Lind published an article describing an experiment he had performed on 12 sailors suffering from scurvy. Lind divided the sick sailors into six pairs, and each pair received a different treatment. The six treatments were cider, vinegar, sulfuric acid, seawater, nutmeg, or oranges and lemons. Lind observed that the pair of sailors given the citrus fruit were the only ones to recover from scurvy. By today's standards, Lind's experiment was primitive, but as a result of his testing, Lind found the cure for scurvy: eating oranges and lemons. Eventually, food rations for British sailors included lemon juice to prevent the disease. The sailors earned the nickname "limeys" because at that time, people often referred to citrus fruits collectively as "limes."

Today, we know that scurvy results from a deficiency of vitamin C and that citrus fruits are among the richest dietary sources of the vitamin. Although Lind is often credited with having discovered the cure for scurvy, he did not suspect the disease resulted from the lack of something in the typical seafarer's diet. At that time, scientists were unaware that food contained vitamins. Lind thought scurvy was a digestive system disorder that could be treated with substances associated with warm climates.[1] In his experiment, Lind happened to administer citrus fruits to a pair of the sailors with scurvy because these fruits were associated with such climates.

In 1911, Polish chemist Casimir Funk discovered a substance in an extract made from rice bran that he thought would cure the disease beriberi. Funk called the compound a "vitamine" (*vita* = necessary for life; *amine* = a type of nitrogen–containing substance)

because of its chemical structure. The term *vitamine* was later modified to *vitamin*, when scientists determined that there were several kinds of these substances in foods and not all were amines. By the end of the twentieth century, scientists had added riboflavin, niacin, biotin, B–6, B–12, pantothenic acid, folate, ascorbic acid, A, D, E, and K to the list of vitamins. Humans also require *choline*, especially during *prenatal* (before birth) development. Like vitamin D, the body can make choline, but under certain conditions, the body does not synthesize enough to meet its needs.[2] Choline is considered to be a *vitamin–like* essential nutrient.

It is unlikely that any vitamins still need to be discovered. Why? Babies grow and thrive on infant formulas, synthetic liquid diets containing vitamins and other nutrients known to be essential for health. Additionally, very ill people who cannot eat solid food can be kept alive for years on liquid synthetic feedings that contain all known nutrients, including vitamins. If a vitamin remained undiscovered, infants and people who are unable to consume solid foods would not be able to survive on formula diets.

This chapter presents information about the 13 vitamins and choline, including physiological roles and major food sources. By reading this chapter, you will learn what can happen to the body when consumption of certain vitamins is too small or too great. Many Americans take vitamin supplements to prevent disease; the "Vitamins as Medicines" section of this chapter examines current scientific evidence concerning the usefulness of taking megadoses of certain vitamins. In general, a megadose is at least 10 times the recommended amount of the micronutrient.[3]

What Is a Vitamin?

vitamin complex organic molecule that regulates certain metabolic processes

What is a vitamin? A **vitamin** is a complex organic compound that regulates certain metabolic processes in the body. A vitamin meets the following criteria:

- The body cannot synthesize the compound or make enough to maintain good health.

- The compound naturally occurs in commonly eaten foods.

- Signs and symptoms of a health problem (*deficiency disorder*) eventually occur when the substance is missing from the diet.

- Good health is restored, if the deficiency disorder is treated early by supplying the missing substance.

Although vitamins are organic molecules in foods, they are distinctly different from carbohydrates, fats, and proteins. Foods generally contain much smaller amounts of vitamins than of macronutrients. A slice of whole–wheat bread, for example, weighs 28 grams. Of that weight, only about 0.005% (1.48 mg) is comprised of vitamins; carbohydrate, water, protein, fat, and minerals make up the remaining weight of the bread. Furthermore, the body requires vitamins in milligram or microgram amounts, but it needs grams of macronutrients.

In the past, amounts of most vitamins in foods, particularly fat–soluble vitamins, were often expressed in *International Units (IUs)*. Today, IUs have largely been replaced by more precise milligram or microgram measures. One microgram of vitamin D, for example, equals 40 IUs of the vitamin. Food composition tables and the information panels on food and supplement labels often still list IU values for fat–soluble vitamins.

38% Water

10% Protein

46% Carbohydrate

4% Fat
<1% Vitamins
<1% Minerals

A slice of bread weighs about 1 ounce (28 g). Vitamins comprise only about 0.005% (1.48 mg) of the weight of the bread.

Classifying Vitamins

Vitamins A, D, E, and K are **fat—soluble vitamins.** These vitamins are in the lipid portions of foods and tend to associate with lipids in the body. Thiamin, riboflavin, niacin, vitamin B—6, pantothenic acid, folate, biotin, vitamin B—12 (collectively known as the B vitamins), and vitamin C are **water—soluble vitamins.** Water—soluble vitamins dissolve in the watery components of food and the body. (Choline is also water soluble.) Table 8.1 presents the vitamins and provides some other names that may be used to identify them.

Why is it important to know the difference between fat— and water—soluble vitamins? The body generally has more difficulty eliminating excess fat—soluble vitamins because these nutrients do not dissolve in watery substances such as urine. As a result, the body stores extra fat—soluble vitamins, primarily in the liver and in body fat. Over time, these vitamins can accumulate and cause toxicity. On the other hand, the body stores only limited amounts of most water—soluble vitamins; vitamin B—12 is an exception. Furthermore, kidneys can filter excesses of water—soluble vitamins from the bloodstream and eliminate them in urine. Thus, water—soluble vitamins are generally not as toxic as fat—soluble vitamins.

Roles of Vitamins

Vitamins play numerous roles in the body, and each of these micronutrients gen—erally has more than one function (Fig. 8.1). Some vitamins, such as vitamin D, act as hormones; other vitamins, such as vitamin C and thiamin, participate in chemical reactions by accepting or donating electrons. In general, vitamins regulate a variety of body processes, including those involved in cell division and development as well as the growth and maintenance of tissues.

Advertisements for vitamins often promote the notion that the micronu—trients can "give" you energy. Vitamins, however, are not a source of energy, because cells do not metabolize them for energy. Although the body does not use vitamins directly for energy, many vitamins participate in the chemical reactions that release energy from glucose, fatty acids, and amino acids. The diagram in Appendix E presents a simplified view of energy metabolism and indicates vita—mins that are involved in the various steps of the process.

Most vitamins have more than one chemical form that functions in the body. For example, *retinol*, *retinal*, and *retinoic acid* are chemically related types of vitamin A that have roles in the body. Additionally, some vitamins have precursors (*provitamins*) that do not function as vitamins until the body converts them into active forms. For example, the plant pigment beta—carotene is a provitamin for vitamin A, and the amino acid tryptophan is a precursor for the B—vitamin niacin.

What Is an Antioxidant?

When many biochemical reactions take place, the compounds participating in the reactions lose or gain electrons. When an atom or molecule gains one or more electrons, it has been *reduced*. When an atom or molecule loses one or more electrons, it has been *oxidized*. An **oxidizing agent** is a substance that removes electrons from atoms or molecules. An oxidation reaction can form a **radical** (commonly referred to as a "free radical"), a substance with an unpaired electron. Radicals are highly reactive (chemically unstable), and they remove electrons from more stable mol—ecules, such as proteins, fatty acids, and DNA (Fig. 8.2). As a result, radicals can damage or destroy these molecules. If the loss of electrons is uncontrolled, a chain reaction can occur in which excessive oxidation takes place and affects many cells. Many medical researchers suspect excess oxidation is responsible for promoting

TABLE 8.1 Classifying Vitamins

Fat-Soluble Vitamins
A (retinol)
D
E (alpha-tocopherol, other tocopherols)
K

Water-Soluble Vitamins
Thiamin (thiamine, B-1)
Riboflavin (B-2)
Niacin (B-3, nicotinamide, nicotinic acid)
B-6 (pyridoxine)
B-12 (cobalamin, cobalamine)
Biotin (H)
Pantothenic acid (B-5)
Folate (folic acid)
C (ascorbic acid)

Vitamin-Like
Choline

fat-soluble vitamins vitamins A, D, E, and K

water-soluble vitamins thiamin, riboflavin, niacin, vitamin B-6, pantothenic acid, folate, biotin, vitamin B-12, and vitamin C

oxidizing agent substance that removes electrons from atoms or molecules

radical substance with an unpaired electron

Bone Health

Vitamin A

Vitamin D

Vitamin K

Vitamin C

Growth and Development

Vitamin A

Vitamin D

Choline

Energy Metabolism

Thiamin

Riboflavin

Niacin

Pantothenic acid

Biotin

Vitamin B-12

Vitamin B-6

Red Blood Cell Formation

Vitamin B-6

Vitamin B-12

Folate

Riboflavin (indirect)

Blood Clotting

Vitamin K

Immune Function

Vitamin A

Vitamin C

Vitamin D

Vitamin E

Amino Acid Metabolism

Vitamin B-6

Folate

Vitamin B-12

Vitamin C

Choline

Antioxidant Defense

Vitamin E

Vitamin C (likely)

Certain carotenoids

Figure 8.1 Functions of vitamins and related compounds. Groups of vitamins and related compounds (e.g., choline and certain carotenoids) work together to maintain good health.

chemical changes in cells that ultimately lead to heart attack, stroke, cancer, Alzheimer's disease, and even the aging process.

Some radical formation in the body is necessary and provides some benefits.[4] Radicals, for example, stimulate normal cell growth and division. Additionally, white blood cells generate radicals as part of their activities that destroy infec‒ tious agents. Under normal conditions, cells regulate oxidation reactions by using antioxidants such as vitamin E. **Antioxidants** protect cells by giving up electrons to radicals. When a chemically unstable substance accepts an electron, it can form a more stable structure that does not pull electrons away from other compounds. By sacrificing electrons, antioxidants protect molecules such as polyunsaturated fatty acids in the membrane or DNA in the nucleus from being oxidized (Fig. 8.3).

Sources of Vitamins

antioxidants substances that gives up electrons to radicals to protect cells

Plants, animals, fungi, and even bacteria supply natural forms of vitamins in our diets. In addition to foods, vitamin supplements are another source of these micro‒ nutrients. Although chemists can synthesize vitamins, certain types of bacteria

1. A radical acts as an "arrow" by hitting a vulnerable molecule, such as DNA.

2. The damaged molecule becomes the source of another radical that "strikes" another vulnerable molecule, in this case, a phospholipid.

3. The reaction repeats itself as another radical forms and attacks another vulnerable molecule, such as a protein.

Figure 8.2 What is a radical? A radical is a highly reactive substance because it has an unpaired electron. Radicals remove electrons from more stable molecules, such as DNA in the cell's nucleus.

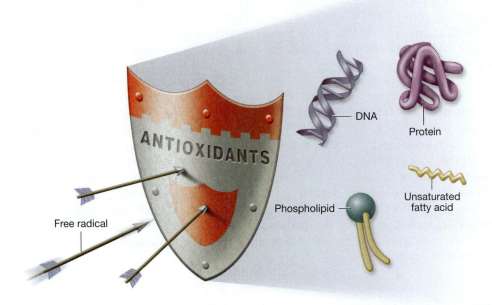

Figure 8.3 Antioxidant action. Antioxidants can protect the cell's plasma membrane and DNA from radicals.

Did You Know?

Rancidity results when fat in food, particularly the unsaturated fat, undergoes oxidation. Rancid fat makes the food smell and taste bad, and people usually refuse to eat it. To inhibit oxidation of fatty acids and increase a food's "shelf life," manufacturers add antioxidants such as BHT and BHA to the food during production.

and algae produce vitamins. These organisms can be grown in laboratory settings for the purpose of "harvesting" their vitamins to use in supplement production.[5]

Regardless of whether a particular vitamin is naturally in foods or syn—thesized in a laboratory, it generally has the same chemical structure and works equally well in the body—but there are exceptions. The natural form of vitamin E has more **biological activity,** that is, it produces more effects in the body, than synthetic vitamin E. On the other hand, *synthetic folic acid*, the type of folate that is added to flour and many ready—to—eat and cooked cereals, has almost twice the biological activity as the natural form of the vitamin.

biological activity describes vitamin's degree of potency or effects in the body

Many adult Americans take multivitamin supplements that contain two or more vitamins and may also supply one or more minerals (*multivitamin/ mineral supplement*). According to data collected in the Third National Health and Examination Survey in 2003–2006, 40% of adults reported regular use of a multivitamin–multimineral supplement that contained at least three vitamins.[6] Such products are often marketed as "one–a–days" or for a particular target audience, such as men, people with diabetes, athletes, or older adults.

It is not necessary to consume 100% of every vitamin each day. If you are healthy and usually follow a nutritionally adequate diet, your cells should contain a supply of vitamins that can last for several days and possibly even years, depending on the vitamin. Furthermore, bacteria that reside in your lower intestinal tract produce certain vitamins, particularly biotin and vitamin K, and you can absorb these micronutrients to some extent. Additionally, your body can synthesize vitamin D and niacin under certain conditions.

Vitamin Enrichment and Fortification

Cereal grains such as wheat, rice, and corn lose considerable amounts of their natural vitamin contents during milling (refinement). The federally regulated enrichment program specifies amounts of four B vitamins (thiamin, riboflavin, niacin, and folic acid) and the mineral iron that manufacturers must add to their refined wheat flour and certain other milled grain products. At present, health experts are considering whether vitamin B–12 should be included as an enrichment nutrient. Enrichment helps protect Americans from developing the deficiency diseases associated with the lack of these nutrients. However, enrichment does not replace the vitamin E, vitamin B–6, potassium, magnesium, several other micronutrients, and fiber that were naturally in the unrefined grains. This is the major reason dietitians and other nutrition experts promote regular consumption of whole–grain products, such as whole–wheat bread and brown rice.

Fortification involves the addition during manufacturing of one or more vitamins (and/or other nutrients) to a wide array of commonly eaten foods. The vitamins that are added may or may not be in the food naturally. For example, milk is often fortified with vitamins A and D, and many ready–to–eat cereals have additional vitamins baked into or sprayed on them before packaging.[7] In the United States, fortification and enrichment of foods have improved vitamin intakes of Americans. However, some food manufacturers add vitamins to foods and beverages, particularly flavored drinks, that would otherwise be considered "empty–calorie" items. Many nutrition experts are concerned that by substituting such human–made products for more natural foods and beverages, Americans may consume excessive amounts of a few vitamins while reducing their intake of others.

Vitamin Absorption

The small intestine is the primary site of vitamin absorption. However, the intestine does not absorb 100% of the vitamins in food. Vitamin absorption tends to increase when the body's needs for the micronutrients are also higher than usual. The body's requirements for vitamins generally increase during periods of growth, such as infancy and adolescence, and during pregnancy and breastfeeding.

Fat–soluble vitamins are chemically similar to lipids, and the vitamins are in fatty portions of food. Thus, processes that normally occur during fat digestion facilitate the absorption of fat–soluble vitamins. For example, bile enhances lipid as well as fat–soluble vitamin absorption. In the small intestine, the presence of fat stimulates the secretion of a hormone that causes the gallbladder to release bile. Therefore, adding a small amount of fat to low—fat foods, such as tossing raw vegetables with some salad dressing, adding a pat of soft margarine to steamed carrots, or stir—frying green beans in peanut oil, can enhance the intestinal tract's ability to absorb the fat—soluble vitamins in these foods. To review lipid digestion, see Chapter 6.

Diseases or conditions that affect the GI tract can reduce vitamin absorption and result in deficiencies of these micronutrients. People with the inherited disease *cystic fibrosis (sis'—tik fie—broe'—sis)* are unable to digest fat properly, because the disease causes blockages to form in ducts that convey pancreatic enzymes to the small intestine. As a result, cystic fibrosis reduces fat absorption, and people with the disease often develop deficiencies of fat—soluble vitamins. People who are unable to absorb vitamins may need to take large oral doses of vitamin supplements just to enable small amounts of the vitamins to be absorbed. In other cases, physicians inject vitamins into their patients' bodies, completely bypassing the need for the intestine to absorb the micronutrients.

Vitamin Deficiency and Toxicity Disorders

A diet that contains adequate amounts of a wide variety of foods, including minimally processed fruits, vegetables, and whole—grain breads and cereals, can help supply the vitamin needs of most healthy people. Vitamin deficiency disorders generally result from inadequate diets or conditions that increase the body's requirements for vitamins, such as reduced intestinal absorption or higher—than—normal excretion of the micronutrients. Today, severe vitamin deficiencies are uncommon in the United States, thanks in part to modern food preservation practices, food enrichment and fortification, and the year—round, widespread availability of fresh fruits and vegetables from other countries. Many Americans, however, consume considerably less than recommended amounts of certain vitamins, particularly E, D, and the vitamin—like compound choline.[8]

A few segments of the population have a high risk of vitamin deficiencies. These vulnerable people include alcoholics, older adults, and patients who are hospitalized for lengthy periods. Additionally, people who have anorexia nervosa, intestinal conditions that interfere with vitamin absorption, or rare metabolic defects that increase their vitamin requirements are more likely to develop vitamin deficiency disorders than people who do not have these conditions.

If your usual diet is nutritionally adequate but you occasionally have low intakes of vitamins, you are unlikely to develop vitamin deficiency diseases, because your cells store these micronutrients to some extent. The likelihood of developing a deficiency disease increases when a person's diet consistently lacks the vitamin. When this happens, the person's body stores or tissue levels of the vitamin become depleted, and the signs and symptoms of the nutrient's deficiency disease begin to occur. A person, for example, can become vitamin C–deficient after about a month of consuming a diet that provides little or no vitamin C.[9]

If you are considering taking vitamin supplements or are taking them already, you need to recognize that more is not necessarily better. When cells are saturated with a vitamin, they contain all they need and cannot accept additional amounts of the micronutrient. When this situation occurs, continuing to take the vitamin can produce a toxicity disorder, because exposure to the excess micro—nutrient or its by—products can damage cells.

Do you need to be concerned about developing a vitamin toxicity disorder? Probably not, unless you are taking excessive amounts (megadoses) of vitamin supplements or consuming large amounts of vitamin—fortified foods regularly. In their natural states, most commonly eaten foods do not contain toxic levels of vitamins. Taking a "one—a—day" type of multivitamin supplement regularly is unlikely to cause toxic effects in adults, because these products usually contain less than two times the Daily Values of each micronutrient component.

A farmers' market can be a source of locally grown fresh produce during the growing season.

Preserving the Vitamin Content of Foods

Regardless of whether you pick fruits and vegetables from your own garden or buy them from a farmers' market or supermarket, many kinds of produce, especially berries and leafy vegetables, are highly perishable. Therefore, these foods should be eaten as soon as they are harvested or purchased to ensure maximum vitamin retention. In many instances, unpackaged ("bulk") fresh fruits or vegetables that are sold in supermarkets do not have dates indicating when they should be used, and consumers have no way of knowing when the produce was harvested.

Fresh fruits and vegetables can lose substantial amounts of vitamins as a result of improper handling or lengthy storage conditions. Therefore, select fresh produce carefully when buying it in grocery stores. Avoid produce that is bruised, wilted, or shriveled, or shows signs of decay such as mold. If you are uncertain how to choose ripe fruits and vegetables, ask the person who manages the produce section of the store for advice.

Some vitamins, such as niacin and D, resist destruction by usual food storage conditions or preparation methods. Other vitamins—particularly vitamin C, thiamin, and folate—are easily destroyed or lost by improper food storage and cooking methods. Fresh produce is more likely to retain its natural vitamin content when stored at temperatures near freezing, in high humidity, and away from air. Therefore, you should keep most fresh fruits and vegetables in plastic packaging and chilled until you are ready to use them. Tomatoes, bananas, and garlic should be stored at room temperature. Although precut, packaged salad greens and other vegetables may be convenient to use, they are highly perishable and should be used soon after purchasing.

Exposure to excessive heat, alkaline substances, light, and air can destroy certain vitamins, especially vitamin C. To reduce such losses, trim, peel, and cut raw fruits and vegetables just before eating or serving them. The darker leaves of vegetable greens generally contain more vitamins than the inner, paler color leaves or stems. Therefore, lightly trim away the outer leaves of lettuce and cabbage, and keep edible peels intact; just remove rotten or shriveled parts.

Water-soluble vitamins can leach out of food and dissolve in the cooking water, which is often discarded. By cooking vegetables in small amounts of water and reusing that water for soups or sauces, you are likely to consume those water-soluble nutrients. When preparing produce for cooking, cut the food into large pieces to reduce the amount of surface area that will be exposed to heat, water, and other conditions that can increase vitamin losses. Whenever possible, cook fruits and vegetables in their skins, and if the skins are edible, eat them, too.

Quick cooking methods that involve little contact between produce and water, such as microwaving, steaming, and stir-frying, can conserve much of the vitamin content of the food. According to the Food and Drug Administration (FDA), microwave cooking does not reduce the nutrient content of foods any more than do conventional cooking methods.[10] Microwave cooking may help conserve more vitamins in food because the method cooks quickly and without the need to add much water.

To steam vegetables, place them in a steamer basket that fits inside a pot, add enough water to touch the bottom of the basket, cover the pot, and then heat the water until it boils (Fig. 8.4). As the steam gently cooks the vegetables, add more water, if necessary.

To stir-fry vegetables, heat a small amount of oil in a wok or pan that has deep sides, add small pieces of fresh vegetables, and stir the mixture, lightly coating the vegetables with oil (Fig. 8.5). Stir–fried vegetables should be cooked until they are barely tender to retain their nutrients as well as appealing textures, fl avors, and colors. The "Recipe for Healthy Living" feature of this chapter has a recipe for stir–fried vegetables.

Are fresh fruits and raw vegetables better sources of vitamins than canned or frozen versions? Sometimes they are. During the canning process, the heating of food can cause the destruction of certain vitamins. However, produce that is frozen immediately after being harvested and then properly stored can be just as nutritious as fresh produce. Frozen fruits and vegetables are often economical alternatives to fresh produce, but they need to be cooked without thawing to conserve much of their vitamin content. The thawing process causes some of the water that was naturally in the produce to drip out, taking water–soluble vitamins with it. If this water is discarded, vitamins in the fluid are lost. The following "Food & Nutrition Tips" box provides practical ways to preserve the vitamin content of food.

Food & Nutrition tips

- Eat fresh fruits and vegetables along with their edible peels or skins whenever possible.

- Cook fresh vegetables by microwaving, steaming, or stir-frying. Vegetables generally have high water content; therefore, add no water or just a small amount when microwaving vegetables.

- Do not overcook vegetables and minimize reheating, because prolonged heating reduces vitamin content.

- Do not add margarine or butter to vegetables during cooking, because fat-soluble vitamins and phytochemicals may enter the fat and be discarded when the fat is drained before serving. Fat in foods can enhance the body's absorption of fat-soluble vitamins; therefore, you can add some fat, such as olive oil or soft margarine, to vegetables after they are cooked.

- Store canned foods in a cool place. Canned foods can vary in the amount of nutrients they contain, largely because of differences in storage times and temperatures. If the can has been on the shelf for an extended period of time, the food's vitamin content may have deteriorated, and its taste and texture may be less than desirable. To get maximal nutritive value from canned vegetables, drain the liquid that is packed with the food and use it as a base for soups, sauces, or gravies. If the liquid is too salty, discard it.

Figure 8.4 Conserving vitamins. Steaming vegetables can conserve much of the vitamin content of the produce.

Concept **Checkpoint 8.1**

1. List at least three criteria used to designate a substance as a vitamin.
2. List three factors that distinguish vitamins from macronutrients.
3. Define the following terms: *provitamin, antioxidant,* and *radical.*
4. Explain the difference between enrichment and fortification.
5. Discuss at least five ways to preserve the vitamin content of fruits and vegetables during food preparation and storage.

Figure 8.5 Conserving vitamins. Stir-frying conserves vitamins by cooking vegetables quickly without adding water.

8.2 Fat-Soluble Vitamins

Learning Outcomes

1 List the four fat-soluble vitamins, and identify good food sources of each fat-soluble vitamin (or provitamin).

2 Discuss major functions of each fat-soluble vitamin.

3 Identify health problems associated with excesses and deficiencies of fat-soluble vitamins.

This section focuses on fat–soluble vitamins. Table 8.2 presents a summary of general information about all fat–soluble vitamins. Unless otherwise noted, RDA/AI values are for adults 19 to 50 years of age, excluding pregnant or breastfeeding women. Figure 8.6 indicates food groups of MyPlate that are good sources of fat–soluble vitamins.

TABLE 8.2   Summary of Fat-Soluble Vitamins

Vitamin	Major Functions in the Body	Adult RDA/AI (adult RDA = bold)	Major Dietary Sources	Major Deficiency Signs and Symptoms	Major Toxicity Signs and Symptoms
Vitamin A (preformed and provitamin A)	Normal vision and reproduction, cellular growth, and immune system function	**700–900 mcg RAE**	Preformed: liver, milk, fortified cereals Provitamin: yellow-orange and dark green fruits and vegetables	Night blindness, xerophthalmia, poor growth, dry skin, reduced immune system functioning	**Adult Upper Limit (UL) = 3,000 mcg/day** Nausea and vomiting, headaches, bone pain and fractures, hair loss, liver damage, interference with vitamin K absorption
Vitamin D	Absorption of calcium and phosphorus, maintenance of normal blood calcium, calcification of bone, maintenance of immune function	15–20 mcg	Vitamin D–fortified milk, fortified cereals, fish oils, fatty fish	Rickets in children, osteomalacia in adults: soft bones, depressed growth, and reduced immune system functioning	**Adult UL = 100 mcg/day** Poor growth, calcium deposits in soft tissues
Vitamin E	Antioxidant, maintenance of nervous and immune system functions	**15 mg** (alpha-tocopherol)	Vegetable oils and products made from these oils, certain fruits and vegetables, nuts and seeds, fortified cereals	Loss of muscular coordination, nerve damage, reduced immune system function	**Adult UL = 1000 mg/day** Excessive bleeding as a result of interfering with vitamin K metabolism
Vitamin K	Production of active blood-clotting factors	**90–120 mcg**	Green leafy vegetables, canola and soybean oils, and products made from these oils	Excessive bleeding	**Adult UL = undetermined** Unknown

Oils
- Vitamin E
- Vitamin D (cod liver oil, margarine)
- Vitamin A (margarine)
- Vitamin K (soybean oil)

Fruits
- Vitamin A precursors
- Vitamin E (mangoes)

Vegetables
- Vitamin A precursors
- Vitamin K
- Vitamin E

Dairy
- Vitamins A and D (if fortified)

Grains
- Vitamin E (wheat germ, whole grains, whole-grain or fortified ready-to-eat cereals)

Protein
- Vitamin E (nuts and seeds, sardines)
- Vitamin A (liver and eggs)
- Vitamin D (salmon, egg yolk, liver)

Figure 8.6 MyPlate and fat-soluble vitamins. This illustration highlights MyPlate food groups that are generally good sources of fat-soluble vitamins.

Vitamin A

Do you associate vitamin A with eating carrots and good vision? It is true that vitamin A is involved in the visual process and carrots contain vitamin A precursors. However, vitamin A can multitask: It has numerous functions in the body. Furthermore, carrots are not the only source of vitamin A precursors; many fruits and vegetables are rich sources of these compounds.

Vitamin A is actually a family of compounds that includes retinol. **Retinol (preformed vitamin A)** is the most active form of the vitamin in the body. Although retinol and the other forms of vitamin A are only in animal foods, plants contain hundreds of yellow–orange pigments called **carotenoids.** A few carotenoids are vitamin A precursors, because the body can use them to make some retinol. Amounts of vitamin A in food are often reported as micrograms of retinol activity equivalents (RAE). One RAE is approximately 1 mcg of retinol.

All cells in the body need vitamin A to develop and function properly. Vitamin A participates in the processes of cell production, growth and development, function, and maintenance. For example, the vitamin is necessary for the production, maturation, and maintenance of **epithelial cells,** cells that form protective tissues that line the body, including skin and linings of the digestive, respiratory, and reproductive tracts (Fig. 8.7). Certain epithelial cells secrete *mucus*, a sticky

retinol (preformed vitamin A) most active form of vitamin A in the body

carotenoids yellow-orange pigments in fruits and vegetables

epithelial cells cells that form protective tissues that line the body

Skin surface

Vitamin A

Plasma membrane

Nucleus

DNA

Epithelial cells of skin

Epithelial stem cell

Mature epithelial cell

Figure 8.7 Vitamin A and epithelial cells. Vitamin A is necessary for epithelial stem (unspecialized) cells to differentiate and mature properly.

Figure 8.8 **Vitamin A and vision.** The retina, the light-sensitive area inside each eye, contains *rods* and *cones,* specialized nerve cells that are essential for vision.

fluid that keeps the tissue moist and forms a barrier against many environmental pollutants and infectious agents. When the mucus-secreting epithelial cells do not have vitamin A, they deteriorate and no longer produce mucus. A lack of vitamin A can also reduce fertility, because the vitamin is required for maintaining the epithelial cells that line the reproductive tracts of men and women.

Vitamin A plays a role in regulating the activity of the immune system. Recall from Chapter 4 that the immune system helps protect the body from infections. Thus, vitamin A–deficient people are at greater risk of infections than those with adequate levels of the vitamin in their bodies.

Normal bone growth and development also require vitamin A. Although your bones do not appear to change their shape, they are constantly remodeled by processes that involve tearing down and rebuilding the tissues to meet the physical demands that you place on them each day. Vitamin A participates with other vitamins and minerals in the bone remodeling process.

What Is Night Blindness? Have you ever walked from a brightly lit theater lobby into the darkened movie auditorium and felt blinded for a few seconds? This is a normal visual response to the sudden and dramatic reduction in light intensity. The *retina*, the light-sensitive area inside each eye, contains *rods* and *cones*, specialized nerve cells that are essential for vision (Fig. 8.8). Rods enable you to adapt to poorly lit environments and see objects as shades of black. Cones are responsible for color vision and function in well-lit environments. Rods and cones need vitamin A, particularly retinol, to function properly.

Food & Nutrition tip

When preparing salads or other dishes, do not discard the edible dark green leaves of lettuce, cabbage, or broccoli. These darkly pigmented parts of the plants contribute more provitamin A carotenoids to your diet than the lighter-colored parts. Use them in salads or on sandwiches. In addition to carotenoids, many fruits and vegetables contain hundreds of other phytochemicals that may benefit your health. To obtain a variety of these compounds, include colorful vegetables and fruits in your meals and snacks.

Fruits and vegetables generally are good sources of antioxidants, including carotenoids such as beta-carotene and lycopene.

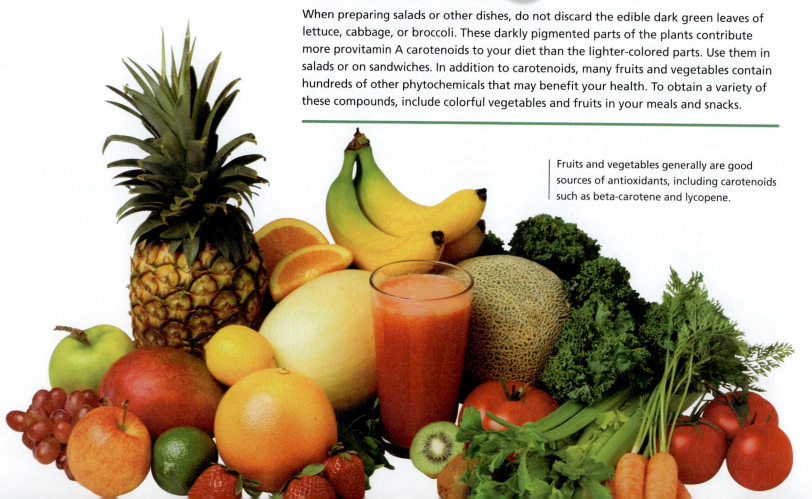

Figure 8.9 illustrates the visual cycle involving rods. Rods remove retinol from the bloodstream and convert it to retinal. In dark conditions, retinal binds to a protein called *opsin* to form **rhodopsin** (*visual purple*). Rhodopsin is necessary for vision in dim light. When you are in a dark environment and exposed to a small amount of light, such as moonlight, the light strikes your rods, activating rhodop—sin. Activation alters the shape of the retinal portion of rhodopsin and bleaches the compound. This process causes retinal to split away, reforming opsin. The trans—formation of rhodopsin to opsin stimulates the rod to send a nervous impulse to the brain that signals the visual processing areas to interpret what is seen. After splitting away from opsin, retinal can bind to the protein, forming rhodopsin again.

As a result of the visual process shown in Figure 8.9, some retinal is destroyed. To replace the retinal, rods remove some retinol (vitamin A) from the bloodstream and convert it to retinal. *Night blindness*, the inability to see in dim light, occurs if retinol is unavailable. Night blindness is an early sign of vitamin A deficiency. Although cone cells also need vitamin A to function, the inability to see certain colors (color blindness) is not the result of a vitamin A deficiency.

Food Sources of Vitamin A

Animal foods such as liver, butter, fish, fish oils, and eggs are good sources of preformed vitamin A. Some foods are fortified with the vitamin during processing. Vitamin A–fortified milk, yogurt, margarine, and cereals are important sources of

rhodopsin vitamin A–containing protein that is needed for vision in dim light

Food & Nutrition tip

Be wary of claims that taking vitamin A supplements will improve your vision so you will not need to wear eyeglasses or contact lenses. Vitamin A deficiency does not cause the kinds of visual defects that are correctable with glasses or contacts. Furthermore, large doses of vitamin A are toxic.

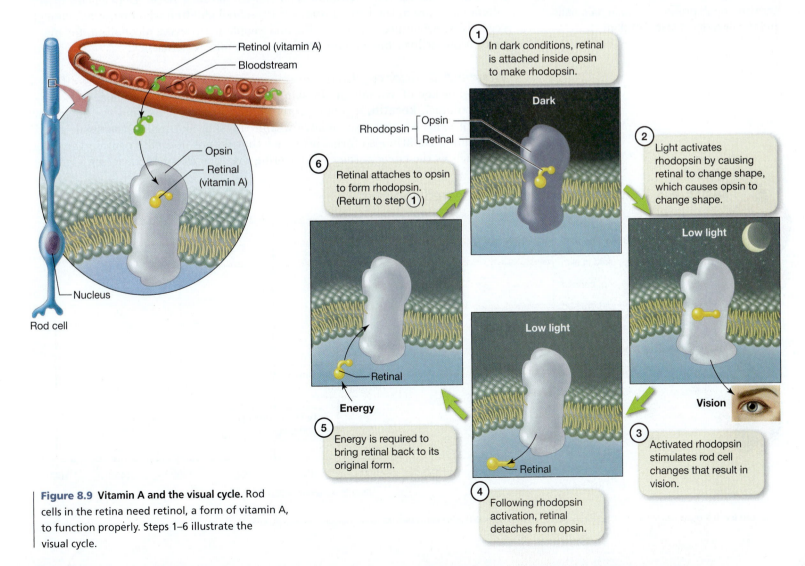

Figure 8.9 Vitamin A and the visual cycle. Rod cells in the retina need retinol, a form of vitamin A, to function properly. Steps 1–6 illustrate the visual cycle.

the nutrient for Americans. Carrots, spinach and other leafy greens, pumpkin, sweet potatoes, broccoli, mangoes, and cantaloupe are rich sources of **beta—carotene,** a carotenoid that the body can convert to vitamin A. However, the body obtains only 1 mcg of retinol from every 12 mcg of beta—carotene in a food.

In addition to beta—carotene, common carotenoids include lutein (*loo'—tee—en*), zeaxanthin (*zee—ah—zan'—thin*), and lycopene (*lie'—ko—peen*). Green, leafy vegetables, such as spinach and kale, have high concentrations of lutein and zeaxanthin. Tomato juice and other tomato products, including pizza sauce, contain considerable amounts of lycopene. Although lutein, zeaxanthin, and lycopene are carotenoids, the body does not convert them to vitamin A. Nevertheless, these plant pigments may function as beneficial antioxidants in the human body.

Darkly pigmented fruits and vegetables usually contain more beta—carotene and other provitamin A carotenoids than lightly colored produce. For example, carrots, sweet potatoes, mangoes, and peaches contain more beta—carotene than celery, white potatoes, apples, and bananas. Dark green fruits and vegetables also contain carotenoids, but their green pigment *chlorophyll* contents hide the yellow—orange pigments. Table 8.3 lists some foods that are sources of vitamin A and its precursors.

beta-carotene carotenoid that the body can convert to vitamin A

keratin tough protein found in hair, nails, and the outermost layers of skin

Dietary Adequacy

For adults, the RDA for vitamin A is 700 to 900 mcg RAE. Deficiencies of the vitamin are rare in the United States.[11] Preschool children who do not eat enough vegetables, urban poor, older adults, and people with severe alcoholism, fat mal—absorption, or liver diseases are at risk for vitamin A deficiency.

Vitamin A Deficiency   Epithelial cells are among the first to become affected by a deficiency of vitamin A. In skin, vitamin A–deficient epithelial cells pro—duce too much **keratin,** a tough protein found in hair, nails, and the outermost layers of skin. Keratin accumulates within the skin and makes the tissue rough and bumpy. Keratin also forms in tissues that do not normally contain the pro—tein, such as the *cornea*, the clear covering over the iris of the eye (see Fig. 8.8).

TABLE 8.3   Vitamin A Content of Selected Foods

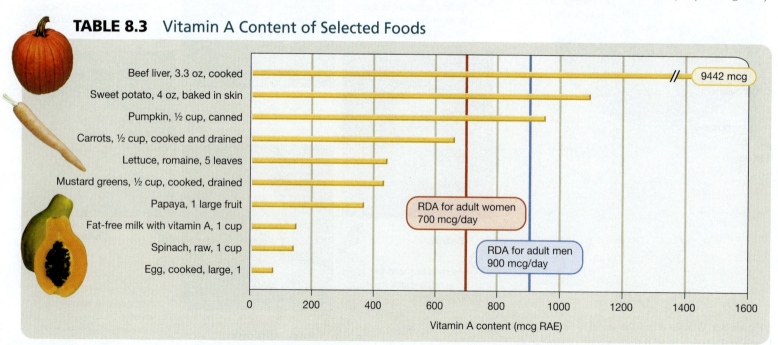

Source: Data from U.S. Department of Agriculture, Agricultural Research Service: *USDA national nutrient database for standard reference, Release 26,* 2013.

The cornea enables light to enter the eye. The epithelial cells that line the inner eyelids secrete mucus that helps keep the cornea moist and clean. In a person suffering from chronic vitamin A deficiency, these cells accumulate keratin, and the white of the eye develops "foamy" areas (Fig. 8.10). Eventually, the epithelial cells harden and stop producing mucus. This condition is called **xerophthalmia** (*zir–op–thal'–me–a*) or "dry eye." Corneas affected by xerophthalmia can be damaged easily by dirt and bacteria. Unless a person with xerophthalmia receives vitamin A, the condition eventually leads to blindness.

Each year, thousands of children in developing nations, especially in Africa and Southeast Asia, become blind because of severe vitamin A deficiency.[12] Vitamin deficiency also reduces the effectiveness of the immune system, and many children suffering from vitamin A deficiency die from infections such as measles. In countries where vitamin A deficiency is widespread, public health efforts are being taken to reduce the prevalence of the condition. Such efforts include educating people about the need to eat regionally grown foods that are rich in beta–carotene and giving vitamin A injections periodically to vulnerable populations. In some countries, governments encourage food manufacturers to fortify commonly eaten foods, such as sugar and margarine, with vitamin A.

Vitamin–A deficient women are more likely to die during pregnancy than pregnant women who are not lacking the vitamin.[11] Furthermore, infants who are born to vitamin A–deficient women are more likely to die than babies born to healthy women. However, pregnant women should not take vitamin A supplements to prevent birth defects without consulting with their physicians. When taken during pregnancy, excess vitamin A is a **teratogen,** an agent that causes birth defects.

Vitamin A Toxicity   The UL for vitamin A intake is 3000 mcg/day for adults. Excessive consumption of vitamin A can damage the liver, because the organ is the main site for vitamin A storage. Toxicity signs and symptoms include headache, nausea, vomiting, visual disturbances, hair loss, bone pain, and bone fractures.

Miscarriage and birth defects may result when excessive amounts of vitamin A are taken early in pregnancy. Women of childbearing age should limit their overall intake of vitamin A to about 100% of the Daily Value (5000 IU). In addition, women who may become pregnant or who are pregnant should restrict their intake of rich food sources of vitamin A, such as liver and fish liver oils.

Carotenemia (*kar'–et–eh–ne'–me–ah*), a condition characterized by yellowing of the skin, can result from eating too much beta–carotene–rich produce or taking too many beta–carotene supplements.[11] This condition occasionally develops in infants who eat a lot of baby foods that contain carrots, apricots, winter squash, or green beans. In most instances, carotenemia is harmless. The skin's natural color eventually returns to normal when the carotenoid–rich foods are no longer eaten.

Figure 8.10 **Early sign of xerophthalmia.** Vitamin A deficiency can cause drying of the surface of the eye. The white foamy areas are signs of such dryness. If untreated, this condition can lead to blindness.

xerophthalmia condition affecting the eyes that results from vitamin A deficiency

teratogen agent that causes birth defects

carotenemia yellowing of the skin that results from excess beta-carotene in the body

Did You Know?

In the early 1900s, teams of explorers raced to discover and explore the North and South Poles. Starvation was a major risk of embarking on such expeditions. Some explorers learned survival techniques from the Inuits, an Eskimo population who inhabit the Arctic region of North America. The Inuits warned the explorers to avoid eating polar bear and seal livers because severe illness and death could result. Unfortunately, many Western explorers did not know that their sled dogs were also not safe for human consumption.

From 1911 to 1913, Douglas Mawson and Xavier Mertz were on an ill-fated expedition to explore an area near the South Pole. As the two men struggled to return to their winter base camp, they had to eat their sled dogs, particularly the animals' livers, to avoid starvation. Both men suffered terribly from the diet; Mertz did not survive. Over 50 years later, scientists determined that sled dogs can accumulate large amounts of vitamin A in their livers without showing ill effects. However, eating just a few ounces of sled dog liver can be toxic for humans.

Figure 8.11 Rickets. A child suffering from rickets has soft bones that do not grow properly. The youngster's leg bones bow under the weight of carrying the upper part of the body.

rickets vitamin D deficiency disorder in children

Physicians may prescribe medications derived from vitamin A, such as isotretinoin, to treat severe acne and other skin disorders. Although these medications are less toxic than natural vitamin A, ingesting excessive amounts can produce harmful symptoms. Furthermore, vitamin A derivatives can cause miscarriage or severe birth defects in the offspring of women who use them during pregnancy. Therefore, women of childbearing age should avoid pregnancy while using these medications.

Vitamin D

By the 1700s, some people in parts of northern Europe had learned that exposing children to sunlight or giving the youngsters fish liver oil could prevent or treat **rickets.** Children with rickets have bones that are soft and can become misshapen. Leg bones, for example, bow under the weight of carrying the upper part of the body (Fig. 8.11). Additionally, the affected child's joints, rib cage, and hips (pelvis) become deformed, and the child may complain of muscle pain. In 1922, scientists discovered a fat−soluble factor in cod liver oil that was needed for proper bone health and preventing rickets. The scientists thought the factor that cured rickets was a vitamin, and they named the substance *vitamin D*. The fat−soluble factor in cod liver oil is still considered a vitamin, because rickets can be prevented and treated by taking vitamin D supplements or eating vitamin D−rich foods. However, vitamin D is actually a hormone.

The body can make vitamin D when skin cells are exposed to the sun's ultraviolet radiation (*UVB*, in particular), which explains why the nutrient is often called the "sunshine vitamin." The radiation converts a substance in skin that is derived from cholesterol into a prohormone (*vitamin D_3*). Vitamin D_3 circulates to the liver, where the substance is converted to the inactive compound *25−OH vitamin D*. Eventually, the kidneys convert 25−OH vitamin D into the active hormone we call "vitamin D" (Fig. 8.12).

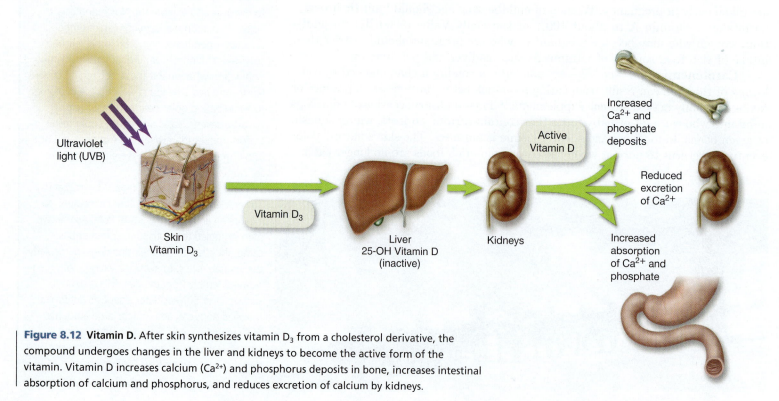

Figure 8.12 Vitamin D. After skin synthesizes vitamin D_3 from a cholesterol derivative, the compound undergoes changes in the liver and kidneys to become the active form of the vitamin. Vitamin D increases calcium (Ca^{2+}) and phosphorus deposits in bone, increases intestinal absorption of calcium and phosphorus, and reduces excretion of calcium by kidneys.

REAL PEOPLE | REAL STORIES

Amanda Croker

Amanda Croker, a junior majoring in East Asian Language and Culture at the University of Kansas, routinely tried to limit her sun exposure to avoid sunburn and the possibility of skin cancer in the future. "My skin is so light," Amanda says, "I even got a sunburn in Kansas in the middle of October, because I was outside for a couple hours!" She was unaware that her efforts to protect her skin were also limiting her body's ability to make vitamin D, "the sunshine vitamin."

"I'm taking a prescription dose of vitamin D, because my family doctor tested my blood and found out that I didn't have enough of the vitamin in my body, "Amanda says." She told me that people need sunlight to make vitamin D, but she said she wasn't surprised that I'm deficient, since I have red hair. I told her that I try to avoid being out in the sun for more than 30 minutes, because I 'crisp' when I get exposed to sun. Anyway, I don't notice that much of a difference now that I'm on the medication." Although Amanda does not "feel" different now, her bones eventually may have become soft and weak, if her doctor had not discovered that Amanda was vitamin D–deficient. Before the discovery and purification of vitamin D, children were given cod liver oil to prevent rickets, the vitamin's deficiency disease.

As a result of the treatment, Amanda's blood level of vitamin D became normal within a few weeks. Because few foods are good sources of vitamin D, she will need to take a daily supplement of the micronutrient, which is available without a prescription, for the rest of her life. By taking the supplement, she should be able to maintain a healthy blood level of the fat-soluble vitamin.

Why Is Vitamin D Necessary?

Vitamin D is necessary for the metabolism of the minerals calcium and phosphorus, and the production and maintenance of healthy bones. Vitamin D also stimulates small intestinal cells to absorb calcium and phosphorus from food. When vitamin D is lacking, the intestine absorbs only 10 to 15% of the calcium in foods; with the vitamin, intestinal absorption of dietary calcium increases to 30 to 80%.[13] Vitamin D also stimulates bone cells to form *calcium phosphate*, the major mineral compound in bone. Without adequate vitamin D, bone cells cannot deposit enough calcium and phosphorus to produce strong bones (see Fig. 8.12).

When blood calcium levels drop, vitamin D works with *parathyroid hormone (PTH)* to signal bones to release calcium. PTH also stimulates the kidneys to increase vitamin D production and decrease the elimination of calcium in urine. These actions help raise the level of calcium in blood to normal (Fig. 8.13). Removing too much calcium from bones can weaken them, but calcium is essential for normal heartbeat and other muscle contractions. If bones did not supply calcium for such vital functions, a person could experience serious, even fatal consequences.

Vitamin D has other roles in the body, including regulating neuromuscular and immune function and reducing inflammation.[14] Vitamin D is also involved in controlling cell growth, and as a result, the micronutrient may reduce the risk of certain cancers. However, more research is needed to clarify the vitamin's role in immune function and disease prevention.

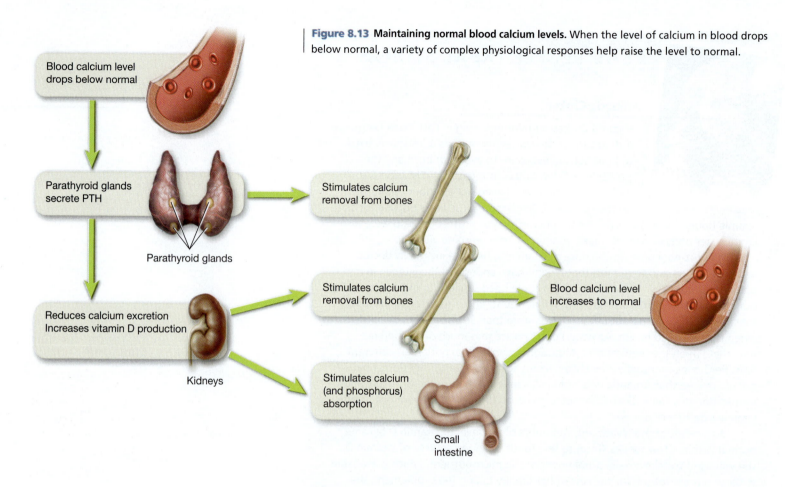

Figure 8.13 Maintaining normal blood calcium levels. When the level of calcium in blood drops below normal, a variety of complex physiological responses help raise the level to normal.

Sources of Vitamin D

Fish liver oils and fatty fish, especially salmon, herring, and catfish, are among the few foods that naturally contain vitamin D. Milk is routinely fortified with vitamin D, and some brands of ready−to−eat cereals, orange juice, and marga−rine have the vitamin added to them as well. Table 8.4 lists some food sources of

TABLE 8.4 Vitamin D Content of Selected Foods

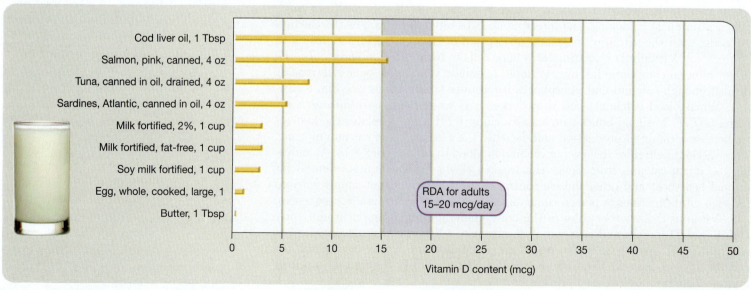

Source: Data from U.S. Department of Agriculture, Agricultural Research Service: *USDA national nutrient database for standard reference, Release 26,* 2013.

vitamin D. Food composition tables often list the vitamin D content of foods in International Units; 1 mcg of vitamin D equals 40 IU.

Vitamin D and Sunlight   Vitamin D is not widespread in food; therefore, your body depends on sun exposure to synthesize the vitamin. If you live south of the 37th parallel and are outdoors for about 5 to 30 minutes when sunlight is most intense (between 10 A.M. and 3 P.M.), you may obtain enough sun exposure to synthesize vitamin D most of the year.[14] The amount of time you need to spend in the sun to form adequate amounts of vitamin D depends primarily on your location, the time of day and year, and your age and skin color.

Earth's atmosphere blocks UV radiation. In North America, the 37th parallel extends from about southern Virginia through southern Missouri to San Francisco, California (Fig. 8.14). If you live north of the 37th parallel, the angle of the winter sun is such that the sun's rays must pass through more of the atmosphere than at other times of the year (Fig. 8.15). As a result, your skin cannot make sufficient amounts of provitamin D during the winter, and you may not have adequate vitamin D stored in your body to last until spring. You may need to take a supplement that contains 100% of the adult Daily Value for vitamin D (see Appendix B), especially from November through February. Clouds, shade, window glass, and air pollution are environmental factors that can also limit the amount of UV radiation that reaches your skin.

Skin contains *melanin*, the brown pigment that can reduce the skin's ability to produce vitamin D from sunlight. Darker skin contains more melanin than lighter skin. If you have dark skin, you may need to spend even more time in the sun to form adequate amounts of the vitamin. Otherwise, you should consider consuming foods that contain the vitamin or a vitamin D supplement regularly.

Although you may think tanned skin is attractive, tanning and severe sunburn increase the risk of developing wrinkles and skin cancer. Ultraviolet (UV) radiation is a major risk factor for skin cancer, including melanoma, the most deadly form of skin cancer. Dermatologists often advise people to apply sunscreens consistently before going outdoors. Using a sunscreen, however, limits skin's ability to synthesize prohormone vitamin D_3. When properly applied, a sunscreen with a *sun protection factor (SPF)* of 8 or more blocks sunlight that is needed to form the prohormone.[14] To allow your body to synthesize some vitamin D, you can expose your skin to the sun for about 15 minutes *before* applying a commercial sunscreen. Concerns about the risk of skin cancer have made it difficult for scientists to develop guidelines for the amount of sunlight exposure that is necessary to optimize vitamin D synthesis.

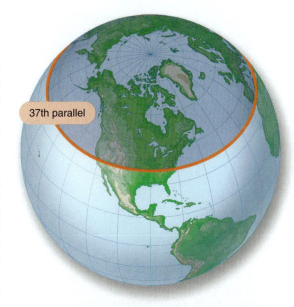

Figure 8.14 Latitude and vitamin D status. In North America, the 37th parallel extends from about southern Virginia through southern Missouri to San Francisco, California. If you live in North America south of the 37th parallel and are outdoors when sunlight is most intense during the day, you are likely to obtain enough sun exposure to synthesize vitamin D most of the year.

Did You ⟩ Know?

Information provided by tanning parlors may include claims that the tanning process is safe. Nevertheless, the ultraviolet radiation emitted by tanning beds increases the risk of wrinkles and skin cancer. Therefore, the use of tanning beds should be avoided.

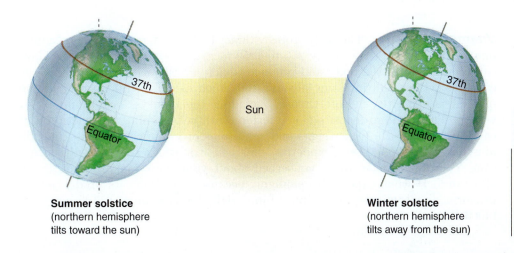

Summer solstice
(northern hemisphere tilts toward the sun)

Winter solstice
(northern hemisphere tilts away from the sun)

Figure 8.15 Seasonal variations in sunlight intensity. If you live north of the 37th parallel, the angle of the winter sun is such that the sun's rays must pass through more of the atmosphere than at other times of the year. As a result, skin tends to form less prohormone vitamin D in the winter.

Dietary Adequacy

For adults under 70 years of age, the RDA for vitamin D is 15 mcg/day. Many Americans do not consume enough vitamin D to meet the RDA.[8] According to the Dietary Guidelines, the vitamin is a "nutrient of public health concern." Younger people, however, generally have higher blood levels of the vitamin than older adults.

In the United States, a national effort to fortify milk with vitamin D began in the 1930s, and as a result, rickets became rare in this country. Although severe rickets is uncommon, public health officials are concerned about the recent increase in the number of cases reported among infants and toddlers. Breast milk contains insufficient amounts of vitamin D to prevent rickets. Infants who are most likely to develop rickets are breastfed, and they have dark skin, minimal sunlight exposure, and little or no vitamin D intake.[14] Exposing breastfed babies to sunlight reduces their risk of the disease, but as mentioned earlier, medical experts do not know how much sun exposure is necessary. Thus, breastfed infants should consume a supplement containing 10 mcg (400 IU) of vitamin D per day soon after birth. The adult form of rickets is called **osteomalacia** (*ahs'—tee—o—mah—lay'—she—a*). The bones of people with osteomalacia have normal amounts of *collagen*, the protein that provides structure for the skeleton, but they contain less—than—normal amounts of cal—cium. The bones are soft and weak, and break easily as a result. Muscle weak—ness is also a symptom of osteomalacia.

Adults who are confined indoors or almost fully covered during the day, such as for religious reasons, are at risk for osteomalacia (Fig. 8.16).[14] Osteomalacia is a risk for adults who have kidney, liver, or intestinal diseases, because these conditions may reduce both vitamin D production and calcium absorption. Exposing skin to sunlight, eating vitamin D–rich foods, or taking vitamin D supplements can help adults avoid vitamin D deficiency and osteomalacia.

As a person ages, production of prohormone vitamin D_3 in skin declines and conversion of the prohormone to active vitamin D in kidneys also decreases. As a result of these age—related changes, older adults are more likely to develop vitamin D deficiency than younger persons. Older adults are also at risk for bone fractures. An analysis of several studies indicated older adults who took 700 to 800 IUs of vitamin D per day had a lower risk of hip fractures than elderly persons who took 400 IUs of vitamin D per day. Thus, people over 50 years of age may benefit from using a daily vitamin D supplement.[15]

Although *osteoporosis* is usually associated with inadequate calcium intakes, a long—term vitamin D deficiency contributes to the condition because calcium absorption is reduced.[14] The calcium section of Chapter 9 provides more information about osteoporosis.

Vitamin D Toxicity The body stores vitamin D. Long—term ingestion of vita—min D supplements that supply 250 to 1250 mcg/day (10,000 to 50,000 IU/day) can accumulate in the body and produce toxicity.[14] When excess vitamin D is consumed, the small intestine absorbs too much calcium from foods and the mineral is deposited in soft tissues, including the kidneys, heart, and blood vessels. The calcium deposits can interfere with cells' ability to function and cause cellular death. Other signs and symptoms of vitamin D toxicity include muscular weakness, loss of appetite, diarrhea, vomiting, and mental confu—sion. You do not have to be concerned about your body making toxic levels of vitamin D when exposed to sunlight, because skin limits its production of prohormone vitamin D_3. The Upper Limit (UL) for vitamin D is 100 mcg/day (4000 IU/day).

osteomalacia adult rickets; condition characterized by poorly mineralized (soft) bones

Figure 8.16 Clothing and vitamin D status. Adults who are almost fully covered during the day, such as for religious reasons, are at risk for osteomalacia.

Vitamin E

Vitamin E has several forms, but only the *alpha–tocopherol (al'–fah toe–koff'– e–roll)* form is used by the body.[16] **Alpha–tocopherol** (*vitamin E*) is an antioxidant that protects polyunsaturated fatty acids in cell membranes from being damaged by radicals (Fig. 8.17). Such oxidative damage may be associated with the development of atherosclerosis, the process that occurs within arteries and contributes to heart attack and stroke; cancer; and premature cellular aging and death. Other roles for vitamin E include maintaining immune system function.

alpha-tocopherol vitamin E

Food Sources of Vitamin E

Rich food sources of vitamin E include sunflower seeds, almonds, and plant oils, especially sunflower, safflower, canola, and olive oils. Products made from vitamin E–rich plant oils, such as margarines and salad dressings, so supply the micronutrient. Other important dietary sources of the vitamin include fish, whole grains, nuts, seeds, and certain vegetables. Meats, processed grain products, and dairy products generally do not contain much vitamin E. Table 8.5 lists some common foods that are sources of the micronutrient.

Harvesting, processing, storage, and cooking methods influence the amount of vitamin E retained in food. During the milling process, most of the vitamin E that is in whole grains is lost, and it is not restored by enrichment. Furthermore, vitamin E is highly susceptible to destruction by exposure to oxygen, metals, and light, as well as high temperatures that occur when heating oil for deep–fat frying.

Dietary Adequacy

For adults, the RDA for vitamin E is 15 mg/day of alpha–tocopherol. Although many American adults do not consume recommended amounts of vitamin E,

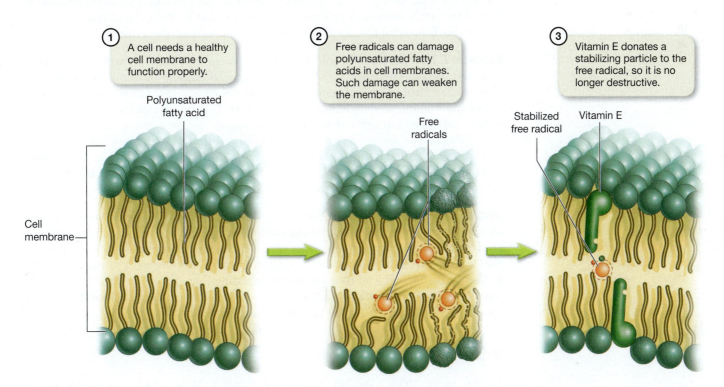

| **Figure 8.17 Vitamin E and the cell membrane.** Vitamin E protects unsaturated fatty acids in cell membranes from being damaged by radicals.

TABLE 8.5   Vitamin E Content of Selected Foods

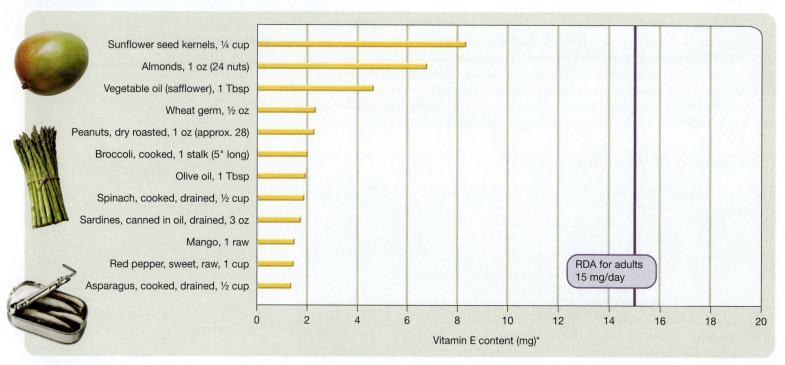

* As alpha-tocopherol.

Source: Data from U.S. Department of Agriculture, Agricultural Research Service: *USDA national nutrient database for standard reference, Release 26,* 2013.

vitamin E deficiency is rare.[16] A healthy body stores the vitamin in body fat, skeletal muscle, and the liver.

Amounts of vitamin E may be reported as a number of IUs. One mg of alpha–tocopherol is about 1.5 IU of the natural form of the vitamin. Synthetic vitamin E is used to fortify foods and produce supplements that contain the vitamin. One mg of vitamin E is equal to 2.22 IU of the synthetic form of the vitamin.[16]

Vitamin E Deficiency   People who have diseases that interfere with fat absorp– tion may become deficient in vitamin E, because dietary fat enhances intestinal absorption of the micronutrient. Vitamin E deficiency can reduce the function– ing of the immune system. Long–term vitamin E deficiency damages the nervous system and results in nerve damage, loss of neuromuscular control, and blindness.[16]

Infants who are born too early (premature infants) may have low vitamin E stores, because the vitamin is transferred from mother to fetus late in pregnancy. If premature infants develop signs of vitamin E deficiency, they can be given special infant formulas and supplements that provide the vitamin.

Vitamin E Toxicity   For healthy adults, the UL for vitamin E is 1000 mg/day of alpha–tocopherol. Consuming amounts of vitamin E in foods has not been associ– ated with any negative effects on health.[16] However, taking dietary supplements that supply excessive amounts of the vitamin may interfere with vitamin K's role in blood clotting and lead to uncontrolled bleeding (hemorrhage). Therefore, people who are taking medications that interfere with blood clotting ("blood thinners") should check with their physicians before using vitamin E supplements.

Vitamin K

In the early 1930s, Danish researcher Henrick Dam discovered a factor in alfalfa that played a role in blood clotting (coagulation). Dam named the factor vitamin "K" after *koagulation,* the Danish spelling of coagulation. Vitamin K is a family of compounds that includes *phylloquinone (fill—o—kwin'—own)* from plants and *menaquinones (men—eh—kwin'—owns)* in fish oils and meat. Bacteria that normally live in the large intestine also synthesize menaquinones that can be absorbed by the body. However, scientists have been unable to determine the extent to which bacteria contribute to the body's vitamin K supply.[17]

The presence of dietary fat, bile, and pancreatic juice help vitamin K be absorbed in the small intestine. Some vitamin K is stored in the liver, and some is incorporated in lipoproteins for transport in the bloodstream. The liver also breaks down vitamin K and eliminates the vitamin's by—products by adding them to bile.

Why Is Vitamin K Necessary?

Blood contains inactive clotting factors and cell fragments called *platelets* that are necessary for blood clotting to occur. When a blood vessel is cut, blood in the injured area undergoes a complex series of steps to form a clot that stops the bleeding (Fig. 8.18). A clot is comprised of strands of the protein *fibrin* that traps blood cells, forming a mesh. The liver synthesizes several blood—clotting factors, and the organ needs vitamin K to produce four of them, including *prothrombin*, properly. When vitamin K is unavailable, the blood does not clot effectively. Some people take the prescribed medication warfarin because their blood clots too easily. Vitamin K can interfere with warfarin's "blood—thinning" activity, so people who take the medication should not consume vitamin K supplements. Additionally, these patients should try to maintain consistent dietary intakes of the vitamin each day.

Vitamin K also helps bone—building cells produce *osteocalcin*, a protein needed for normal bone mineralization. Low blood levels of vitamin K are associated with the risk of *osteoporosis*, a condition characterized by bones with low mineral density. However, more research is needed to clarify the vitamin's role in bone health.

Food Sources of Vitamin K

Major food sources of vitamin K are green leafy vegetables such as kale, turnip greens, salad greens, cabbage, and spinach; broccoli; and green beans. Other reliable sources of the vitamin are soybean and canola oils, and products made from these oils, such as margarine and salad dressing. Table 8.6 lists some foods that are sources of the vitamin. The chemical structure of vitamin K is very stable and resists being destroyed by usual cooking methods.

Figure 8.18 Vitamin K and blood clotting. When a blood vessel is cut, blood in the injured area undergoes a series of steps to form a clot that stops the bleeding. The liver needs vitamin K to make prothrombin and three other blood-clotting factors.

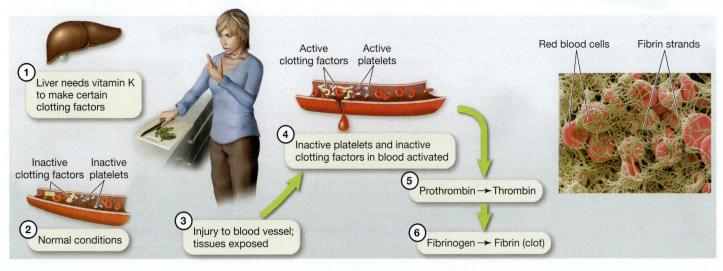

1. Liver needs vitamin K to make certain clotting factors

Inactive clotting factors   Inactive platelets

2. Normal conditions

3. Injury to blood vessel; tissues exposed

Active clotting factors   Active platelets

4. Inactive platelets and inactive clotting factors in blood activated

5. Prothrombin → Thrombin

6. Fibrinogen → Fibrin (clot)

Red blood cells   Fibrin strands

TABLE 8.6 Vitamin K Content of Selected Foods

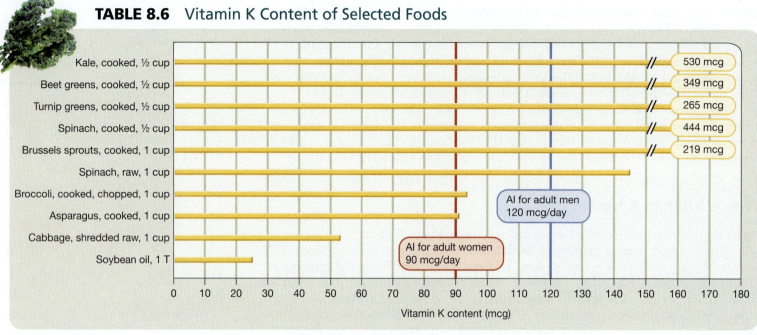

Food	Vitamin K content (mcg)
Kale, cooked, ½ cup	530 mcg
Beet greens, cooked, ½ cup	349 mcg
Turnip greens, cooked, ½ cup	265 mcg
Spinach, cooked, ½ cup	444 mcg
Brussels sprouts, cooked, 1 cup	219 mcg
Spinach, raw, 1 cup	
Broccoli, cooked, chopped, 1 cup	
Asparagus, cooked, 1 cup	
Cabbage, shredded raw, 1 cup	
Soybean oil, 1 T	

AI for adult men 120 mcg/day

AI for adult women 90 mcg/day

Vitamin K content (mcg)

Source: Data from U.S. Department of Agriculture, Agricultural Research Service: *USDA national nutrient database for standard reference, Release 26*, 2013.

Dietary Adequacy

No RDAs for vitamin K have been established, but AIs for the vitamin are 120 mcg/day for men and 90 mcg/day for women. The AIs can be met easily be eating a salad that contains 1 cup of leafy vegetables and 2 tablespoons of salad dressing made with soybean oil.

Vitamin K: Deficiency and Toxicity Although the body stores very little vitamin K, deficiencies among adults rarely occur.[17] Vitamin K deficiency, however, can develop in people who have liver diseases or conditions that impair fat absorption, such as cystic fibrosis. Additionally, long-term antibiotic therapy can reduce the number of bacteria in the colon that synthesize vitamin K and, as a result, contribute to a deficiency of the nutrient. The most reliable sign of vitamin K deficiency is an increase in the time it takes for blood to clot.

Babies are generally born with low vitamin K stores, and a deficiency of the vitamin can occur soon after birth. Vitamin K–deficient infants are at risk of serious bleeding because their bodies are unable to make certain blood–clotting factors. To prevent vitamin K deficiency from developing during infancy, new-borns generally receive a single injection of vitamin K.

Ingesting amounts of natural forms of vitamin K that exceed the AIs has not been reported to be harmful to humans. However, synthetic forms of mena-dione ("vitamin K_3") are toxic.[17]

| Brussels sprouts are a good source of vitamin K.

Concept **Checkpoint 8.2**

6. Prepare a table for fat-soluble vitamins. For each vitamin, indicate its major function in the body, major food sources, deficiency disorder (if it has a specific name), and major signs and symptoms of the deficiency disorder. If the vitamin is known to be toxic, also indicate major toxicity signs and symptoms. Check your table against the information provided in Table 8.2.

8.3 Water-Soluble Vitamins

Learning Outcomes

1 List the water-soluble vitamins, and identify good food sources of each vitamin (or its precursor).

2 Discuss major functions of each water-soluble vitamin.

3 Identify health problems associated with excesses and deficiencies of water-soluble vitamins.

In the body, most water–soluble vitamins function as components of specific coenzymes. A **coenzyme** is a *cofactor*, an ion or small molecule that inter–acts with enzymes and, as a result, regulates a chemical reaction. To synthesize a coenzyme, cells combine one of the B vitamins with a nitrogen–containing, nonprotein compound (Fig. 8.19). When activated by the coenzyme, the enzyme enables the reaction to occur (see Fig. 8.19).

Many of the chemical reactions involved in the metabolism of carbohydrates, fats, and amino acids involve coenzymes that contain B vitamins. Thiamin, riboflavin, niacin, vitamin B–6, and pantothenic acid function as part of coenzymes involved in energy metabolism. Coenzymes containing these vitamins are also necessary for synthesizing glucose, amino acids, and certain lipids.

Foods contain B vitamins in their coenzyme forms. Health–food stores often sell supplements that contain coenzymes, but buying these products is a waste of money. In the small intestine, coenzymes in food or supplements are not absorbed intact. The compounds undergo digestion to release their B vitamin components. The small intestine absorbs many of the B vitamins that were in foods and supplements, and the micronutrients eventually enter the general cir–culation. Cells then remove the free vitamins from the bloodstream and use them to rebuild coenzymes.

This section of the chapter focuses on the water–soluble vitamins: thiamin, riboflavin, niacin, B–6, folate, B–12, biotin, pantothenic acid, and C; as well as the vitamin–like nutrient choline. Table 8.7 provides a summary of general information about all the water–soluble vitamins and choline. Unless otherwise noted, RDA/AI values are for adults 19 to 50 years of age, excluding pregnant or breastfeeding women. Figure 8.20 indicates food groups that are good sources of water–soluble vitamins.

Thiamin

In the body, thiamin is used to make a coenzyme that participates in chemical reactions involved in the release of energy from carbohydrates. Additionally, the thiamin–containing coenzyme plays a role in the metabolism of certain amino acids, and the coenzyme may be necessary for the synthesis of neurotransmitters. A neurotransmitter is a chemical produced by a nerve cell that enables the cell to communicate to other nerve cells.

Food Sources of Thiamin

Foods that contribute thiamin to American diets include whole–grain and enriched breads and cereals, pork, legumes, and orange juice. Brewer's yeast is a rich source of thiamin, but most Americans do not eat the product. Table 8.8 lists some common foods that are good sources of thiamin. Overcooking and cooking food in alkaline solutions, such as water to which some baking soda has been added to brighten the color of green vegetables, can destroy thiamin.

① A coenzyme is a small molecule that helps an enzyme function. To make a coenzyme, cells combine an inactive compound with a B vitamin.

Inactive compound
B vitamin
Coenzyme

② Some enzymes cannot function unless they bind to a specific coenzyme.

Inactive enzyme
Coenzyme

③ When the coenzyme binds to the enzyme, the enzyme is activated and can bind to a molecule that needs to be changed ("molecule B").

Activated enzyme
Molecule B

④ Now, the active enzyme can split molecule B into compound 1 and compound 2. Other coenzymes activate enzymes that build substances your body needs.

Compound 1
Compound 2

| **Figure 8.19 Coenzymes and their function.**

coenzyme small molecule that interacts with enzymes, enabling the enzymes to function

TABLE 8.7 Summary of Water-Soluble Vitamins and Choline

Vitamin	Major Functions in the Body	Adult RDA/AI (adult RDA = bold)	Major Dietary Sources	Major Deficiency Signs and Symptoms	Major Toxicity Signs and Symptoms
Thiamin	Part of coenzyme needed for carbohydrate metabolism and the metabolism of certain amino acids; may help neurotransmitter production	**1.1–1.2 mg**	Pork, wheat germ, enriched breads and cereals, brewer's yeast	Beriberi and Wernicke-Korsakoff syndrome: Weakness, abnormal nervous system functioning	None (Upper limit [UL] not determined)
Riboflavin	Part of coenzymes needed for carbohydrate, amino acid, and lipid metabolism	**1.1–1.3 mg**	Milk, yogurt, and other milk products; enriched breads and cereals; liver	Inflammation of the mouth and tongue, eye disorders	None (UL not determined)
Niacin	Part of coenzymes needed for energy metabolism	**14–16 mg**	Enriched breads and cereals, beef, liver, tuna, salmon, poultry, pork, mushrooms	Pellagra: • Diarrhea • Dermatitis • Dementia • Death	**Adult UL = 35 mg/ day** Flushing of facial skin, itchy skin, nausea and vomiting, liver damage
Pantothenic acid	Part of the coenzyme that is needed for synthesizing fat and releasing energy from macronutrients	5 mg	Beef and chicken liver, sunflower seeds, mushrooms, yogurt, soy milk, fortified cereals	Rarely occurs	Unknown (UL not determined)
Biotin	Cofactor needed for synthesizing glucose and fatty acids	30 mcg	Liver, eggs, peanuts, salmon, pork, mushrooms, sunflower seeds	Rarely occurs: Skin rash, hair loss, convulsions, and other neurological disorders; developmental delays in infants	Unknown (UL not determined)
Vitamin B-6	Part of coenzyme needed for amino acid metabolism, involved in neurotransmitter and hemoglobin synthesis	**1.3–1.7 mg**	Meat, fish, and poultry; potatoes, bananas, spinach, sweet red peppers, broccoli	Dermatitis, anemia, depression, confusion, and neurological disorders such as convulsions	**Adult UL = 100 mg/ day** Nerve destruction
Folate	Part of coenzyme needed for DNA synthesis and conversion of cysteine to methionine, preventing homocysteine accumulation	**400 mcg DFE**	Dark green, leafy vegetables, liver, legumes, asparagus, broccoli, orange juice, enriched breads and cereals (folic acid)	Megaloblastic anemia, diarrhea, neural tube defects in embryos	**Adult UL = 1000 mcg/ day** May stimulate cancer cell growth
Vitamin B-12	Part of coenzymes needed for various cellular processes, including folate metabolism; maintenance of myelin sheaths	**2.4 mcg**	Animal foods, fortified cereals, fortified soy milk	Pernicious anemia: Megaloblastic anemia and nerve damage resulting in paralysis and death	None (UL not determined)
Ascorbic acid (vitamin C)	Connective tissue synthesis and maintenance; antioxidant; synthesis of neurotransmitters and certain hormones; immune system functioning	**75–90 mg** (nonsmokers)	Peppers, citrus fruits, papaya, broccoli, cabbage, berries	Scurvy: Poor wound healing, pinpoint hemorrhages, bleeding gums, bruises, depression	**Adult UL = 2000 mg/ day** Diarrhea and GI tract discomfort
Choline	Neurotransmitter and phospholipid synthesis; methionine metabolism	425–550 mg	Widely distributed in foods and human biosynthesis (production)	Liver damage	Fishy body odor and reduced blood pressure

Figure 8.20 MyPlate: Water-soluble vitamins and choline. This illustration highlights MyPlate food groups that generally are good sources of water-soluble vitamins and choline.

Dairy
- Riboflavin
- Choline
- Vitamin B-12
- Pantothenic acid

Fruits
- Folate
- Vitamin C

Grains
- Thiamin
- Folic acid
- Riboflavin
- Other B vitamins (whole-grain and fortified cereals)
- Niacin

ChooseMyPlate.gov

Vegetables
- Folate
- Vitamin C

Protein
- Thiamin
- Vitamin B-6
- Riboflavin
- Vitamin B-12
- Niacin
- Choline
- Biotin
- Pantothenic acid

Dietary Adequacy

The adult RDA for thiamin is 1.2 mg/day and 1.1 mg/day for men and women, respectively. There are no reports of toxicity from consuming high amounts of thiamin from food or supplements,[18] probably because the excess vitamin is readily excreted in urine. Thus, no UL has been established for thiamin.

The thiamin deficiency disease is called **beriberi.** People suffering from beriberi are very weak and have poor muscular coordination (Fig. 8.21). The severe lack of thiamin also negatively affects the functioning of the cardiovascular, digestive, and nervous systems.

beriberi thiamin deficiency disease

TABLE 8.8 Thiamin Content of Selected Foods

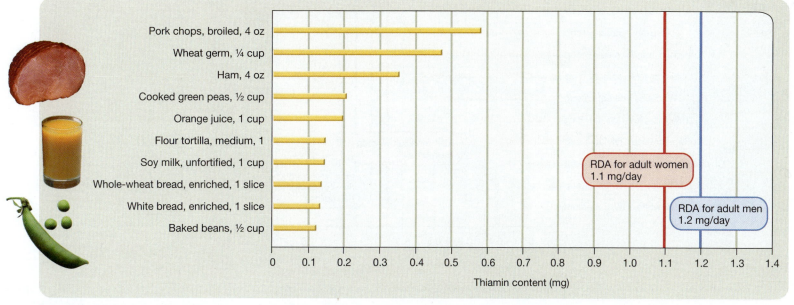

	Thiamin content (mg)
Pork chops, broiled, 4 oz	
Wheat germ, ¼ cup	
Ham, 4 oz	
Cooked green peas, ½ cup	
Orange juice, 1 cup	
Flour tortilla, medium, 1	
Soy milk, unfortified, 1 cup	
Whole-wheat bread, enriched, 1 slice	
White bread, enriched, 1 slice	
Baked beans, ½ cup	

RDA for adult women 1.1 mg/day

RDA for adult men 1.2 mg/day

0 0.1 0.2 0.3 0.4 0.5 0.6 0.7 0.8 0.9 1.0 1.1 1.2 1.3 1.4
Thiamin content (mg)

Source: Data from U.S. Department of Agriculture, Agricultural Research Service: *USDA national nutrient database for standard reference, Release 26,* 2013.

Figure 8.21 Beriberi. The woman sitting in the chair has a form of beriberi called "wet beriberi." Her signs include cardiovascular abnormalities that result in severe "pitting" edema in her lower legs.

Wernicke-Korsakoff syndrome
degenerative brain disorder resulting from thiamin deficiency that occurs primarily among alcoholics

In the United States, the degenerative brain disorder associated with thia−min deficiency is called **Wernicke–Korsakoff syndrome** (*vear'−nih−key kor'−sah−koff*). Most cases of Wernicke–Korsakoff syndrome occur in alcoholics, because alcohol reduces thiamin absorption and increases the vitamin's excretion. People with alcoholism also tend to have poor eating habits that contribute to deficiencies of thiamin and other vitamins. Signs of Wernicke–Korsakoff syn−drome include abnormal eye movements, staggering gait, and distorted thought processes. Treatment involves avoiding alcohol and obtaining thiamin injections. Without prompt treatment, people with Wernicke–Korsakoff syndrome can become disabled permanently or die.

Riboflavin

Riboflavin is a component of two coenzymes that play key roles in metabolism of carbohydrates, lipids, and amino acids. Milk, yogurt, and other milk products; enriched cereals; and liver are among the best sources of riboflavin. Mushrooms, broccoli, asparagus, and spinach and other green leafy vegetables also contain substantial amounts of the vitamin. Table 8.9 lists these and other food sources of riboflavin. Riboflavin's chemical structure is fairly stable, but exposure to light causes the vitamin to break down rapidly. Therefore, riboflavin−rich foods, such as milk and milk products, should not be packaged or stored in clear glass containers.

Dietary Adequacy

The RDA for riboflavin is 1.1 mg/day for women and 1.3 mg/day for men. The typical riboflavin intake of North Americans is about 1.5 mg/day for women and 2.1 mg/day for men.[18] In the United States, riboflavin deficiency rarely occurs, because many commonly eaten foods contain riboflavin (see Table 8.9). However, people who do not consume milk, milk products, or enriched breads and cereals may develop mild cases of riboflavin deficiency. A symptom of mild ribofla−vin deficiency is to become fatigued easily. Riboflavin is rapidly eliminated in urine, so consuming large amounts of the vitamin does not appear to cause side effects.[18] Thus, no UL has been established for riboflavin.

TABLE 8.9 Riboflavin Content of Selected Foods

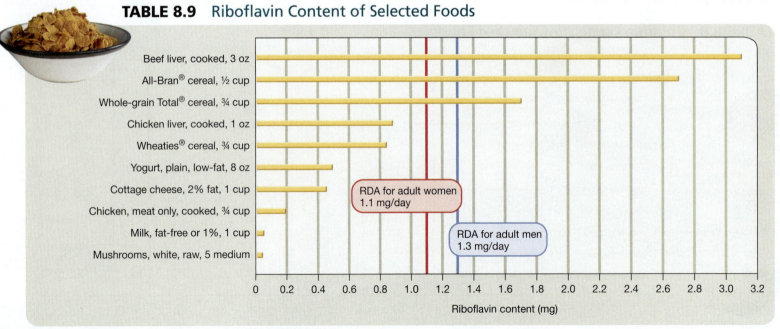

Source: Data from U.S. Department of Agriculture, Agricultural Research Service: *USDA national nutrient database for standard reference, Release 26,* 2013.

TABLE 8.10   Niacin Content of Selected Foods

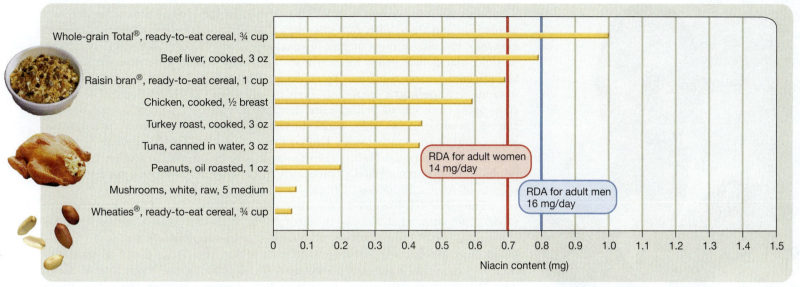

Source: Data from U.S. Department of Agriculture, Agricultural Research Service: *USDA national nutrient database for standard reference, Release 26,* 2013.

Niacin

The body uses niacin to synthesize two coenzymes that participate in at least 200 reactions, including those involved in the release of energy from macronutrients. Major food sources of niacin include enriched cereals, beef liver, tuna, salmon, poultry, pork, and mushrooms (Table 8.10). The chemical structure of niacin is very heat stable, so food retains much of its niacin content during usual prepa—ration and cooking methods.

When diets supply plenty of protein—rich foods, the human body can syn—thesize niacin from a precursor, the amino acid tryptophan. It takes about 60 mg of tryptophan to yield about 1 mg of niacin. For example, eggs and milk lack niacin, but they are rich sources of tryptophan that can be converted to the B vitamin.

The niacin content of corn is considerably higher than that of most other vegetables, but the B vitamin is tightly bound to a protein that resists digestion. Thus, people who eat corn as their staple food are prone to develop pellagra. The traditional Mexican diet is corn based, but pellagra was not a widespread disease in Mexico when it was a major health concern in other parts of the world. Why? The Mexican practice of soaking corn kernels in lime water before using them to prepare tortillas helps free the nia—cin, enhancing its ability to be absorbed. In the United States, corn products such as hominy and grits are sources of niacin because they have been treated with lime before cooking.

The traditional Mexican practice of soaking corn kernels in lime water before using them to prepare tortillas helps free the niacin, enhancing its ability to be absorbed.

Figure 8.22 Pellagra. This person with pellagra shows one of the classic signs of the niacin deficiency disease: dermatitis, particularly on parts of the body exposed to sun.

pellagra niacin deficiency disease

hemoglobin iron-containing protein in red blood cells that transports oxygen

anemia disorder characterized by too few red blood cells and poor oxygen transport in blood

Dietary Adequacy

The adult RDA for niacin is 14 to 16 mg/day. In the United States, people with alcoholism and those with rare disorders that disrupt tryptophan metabolism are generally the only groups at risk of niacin deficiency. Early signs and symptoms of mild niacin deficiency include poor appetite, weight loss, and weakness. If the affected person continues to consume a niacin–deficient diet, the condition worsens and **pellagra** (*peh–lah'–gra* or *peh–lay'–gra*) develops. The classic signs and symptoms of pellagra are dermatitis, diarrhea, dementia, and death— the "4 Ds of pellagra" (Fig. 8.22). In the early twentieth century, pellagra was widespread in the southeastern United States (see the "Did You Know?" box on page 36 of Chapter 2). Today, the disease is rare in Western societies, but it still occurs among impoverished populations in developing countries, particularly in regions of Africa, India, and China.

The adult UL for niacin (nicotinic acid) is 35 mg/day. There have been no reports indicating that the niacin naturally in foods can cause toxicity.[18] Physicians may prescribe megadoses of nicotinic acid supplements to treat elevated blood cholesterol levels. However, patients taking such high doses of the vitamin may experience side effects such as facial flushing and even liver damage. The "Vitamins as Medicines" section of this chapter discusses the use of niacin supplements to reduce cholesterol levels.

Vitamin B-6

The body requires vitamin B–6 to make a coenzyme needed for amino acid metabolism, including the conversion of the amino acid tryptophan to niacin and transamination reactions that form nonessential amino acids (see Fig. 7.11). The coenzyme that contains vitamin B–6 also helps convert a toxic amino acid, homocysteine, to cysteine, a nonessential amino acid.

During red blood cell production, the coenzyme participates in the synthesis of heme. Heme is the iron–containing portion of **hemoglobin,** the protein in RBCs that transports oxygen. If vitamin B–6 is unavailable for heme synthesis, a type of anemia develops. **Anemia** is a disorder characterized by too few red blood cells and poor oxygen transport in blood. Vitamin B–6 is also involved in the synthesis of *neurotransmitters*, chemicals that nerves produce to transmit messages.

Food Sources of Vitamin B-6

Liver, meat, fish, and poultry are among the best dietary sources of vitamin B–6. Additionally, potatoes, bananas, spinach, sweet red peppers, and broccoli are good sources of vitamin B–6. During the refining process, the vitamin B–6 that is naturally in grains is lost, and the nutrient is not added back to the grain products during enrichment. However, many ready–to–eat and cooked cereals have been fortified with the vitamin. Table 8.11 lists some foods that are major sources of vitamin B–6. During cooking, excessive heat can cause major losses of the vitamin.

Dietary Adequacy

The adult RDAs for vitamin B–6 range from 1.3 to 1.7 mg/day. In the United States, the average adult consumes more than the RDA of the vitamin. Therefore, cases of vitamin B–6 deficiency are rare, but they can result from alcoholism or genetic conditions that affect vitamin B−6 metabolism. Signs and symptoms of vitamin B−6 deficiency include dermatitis, anemia, convulsions, depression, and confusion.

The adult UL for vitamin B−6 is 100 mg/day. Unlike most B vitamins, megadoses of vitamin B−6 are toxic.[19] The "Vitamins as Medicines" section of this chapter provides information about vitamin B−6 toxicity.

Folate

"Folate" is the name for a group of related compounds that includes **folic acid.** Folic acid refers specifically to the synthetic form of the vitamin found in sup−plements and added to fortify foods. In the body, cells convert all forms of folate to a group of folate−containing coenzymes collectively called **tetrahydrofolic** ($te'−tra−hi−drow−foe−lik$) **acid** or simply **THFA.** THFA accepts a single−carbon group, such as CH_3, from one compound and transfers it to another sub−stance. As a result, THFA participates in many chemical reactions involved in DNA synthesis and amino acid metabolism. As cells prepare to divide, they need THFA to make DNA.

Certain roles of folate and vitamin B−12 are interrelated. THFA can trans−fer a CH_3 group to vitamin B−12, which, in turn, transfers the CH_3 group to homocysteine, forming methionine (Fig. 8.23). This process recycles methionine. When vitamin B−12 is unavailable, folate cannot be used, and a deficiency of the vitamin occurs, even though dietary intakes of folate are adequate.

Meat, fish, and poultry are among the best dietary sources of vitamin B-6.

Food Sources of Folate

Leafy vegetables, liver, legumes, asparagus, broccoli, and orange juice are good sources of naturally occurring folate. The synthetic folic acid that is used to for−tify or enrich food is better absorbed than naturally occurring forms of folate.

folic acid form of folate

tetrahydrofolic acid (THFA) folate coenzyme

TABLE 8.11 Vitamin B-6 Content of Selected Foods

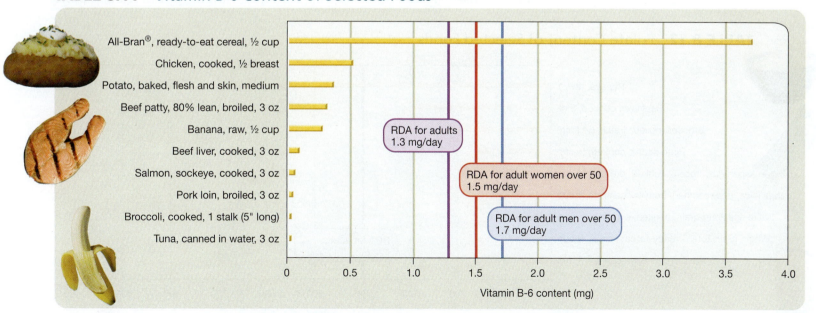

Source: Data from U.S. Department of Agriculture, Agricultural Research Service: *USDA national nutrient database for standard reference, Release 26,* 2013.

Figure 8.23 Folate and vitamin B-12: Working together. This diagram shows how folate (THFA) works with vitamin B-12 to transfer a methyl group (CH₃).

Thus, enriched grain products and fortified cereals are among the richest sources of folate in the American diet. Enriched grain products currently supply U.S. adults with about 200 mcg folic acid/day—half the RDA.[8]

The folate content of foods may be reported as micrograms of *dietary folate equivalents (DFEs)*. DFE units account for differences in the body's ability to absorb folic acid and natural forms of folate. Table 8.12 lists the folate content of selected foods in micrograms of DFE.

Folate is extremely susceptible to destruction by heat, oxidation, and ultra–violet light. Food processing and preparation can destroy 50 to 90% of the folate in food. By eating fresh fruits and raw or lightly cooked vegetables, you are likely to obtain most of the foods' folate content.

Dietary Adequacy

The adult RDA for folate is 400 mcg (DFE)/day. The diets of most Americans provide adequate amounts of folate.[20] The risk of folate deficiency is highest in alcoholics, women of childbearing age, pregnant women, and people with disor–ders of the intestinal tract that reduce the vitamin's absorption.[20]

Folate deficiency usually results from nutritionally inadequate diets, but excess alcohol consumption and use of certain medications can negatively affect the body's ability to absorb and use folate, resulting in deficiencies of the vitamin. Initially, folate deficiency affects cells that rapidly divide, such as red blood cells

TABLE 8.12   Folate Content of Selected Foods

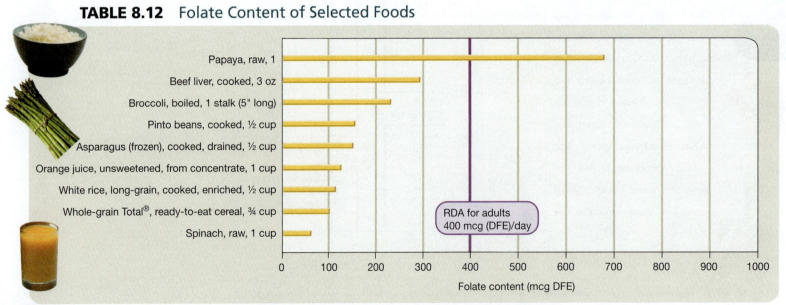

Source: Data from U.S. Department of Agriculture, Agricultural Research Service: *USDA national nutrient database for standard reference, Release 26,* 2013.

(RBCs). Mature RBCs do not have nuclei, and they live for only about 4 months. Thus, the body must replace old or worn—out RBCs constantly. To keep up with their rapid rate of cell division, the precursor cells that mature into RBCs must actively synthesize DNA. Without folate, RBC precursor cells that reside in bone marrow enlarge, but they cannot divide normally, because they are unable to form new DNA. Bone marrow releases some of the abnormal RBCs into the bloodstream before they mature (Fig. 8.24). This condition, called megaloblastic (*mega =* large; *blast* = immature cell) anemia, is characterized by large, immature RBCs (*megaloblasts*) that still have nuclei and do not carry normal amounts of oxygen.

Because many of folate's metabolic roles are related to those of vitamin B−12, diets that lack either vitamin produce a number of identical deficiency signs and symptoms. For example, being deficient in folate or vitamin B−12 can cause megaloblastic anemia. Therefore, a person with this type of anemia needs further analysis of his or her blood to determine which vitamin is lacking.

Although the folate naturally in foods does not appear to be toxic, the UL for the synthetic form of the vitamin (folic acid) is 1000 mcg/day. The UL was established because taking folic acid supplements can cure not only the anemia that occurs in folate deficiency but also the anemia that is a sign of vitamin B−12 deficiency. Folic acid supplementation, however, does not prevent the serious

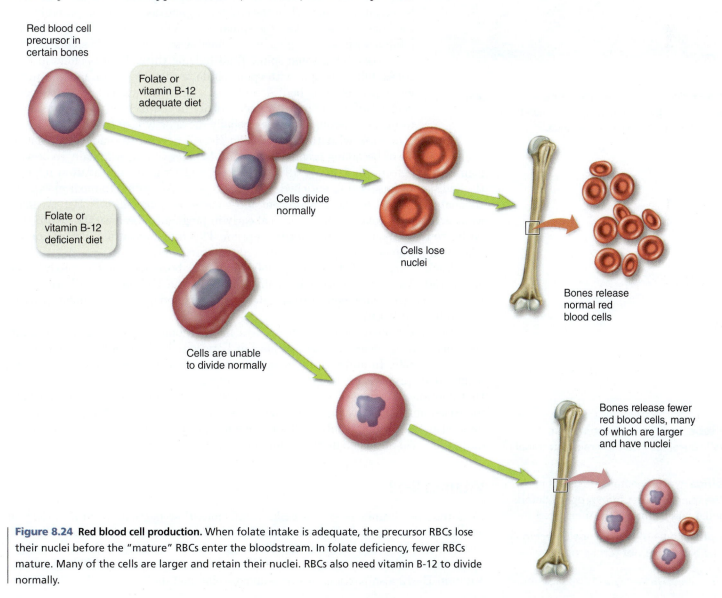

Red blood cell precursor in certain bones

Folate or vitamin B-12 adequate diet

Folate or vitamin B-12 deficient diet

Cells divide normally

Cells lose nuclei

Bones release normal red blood cells

Cells are unable to divide normally

Bones release fewer red blood cells, many of which are larger and have nuclei

Figure 8.24 Red blood cell production. When folate intake is adequate, the precursor RBCs lose their nuclei before the "mature" RBCs enter the bloodstream. In folate deficiency, fewer RBCs mature. Many of the cells are larger and retain their nuclei. RBCs also need vitamin B-12 to divide normally.

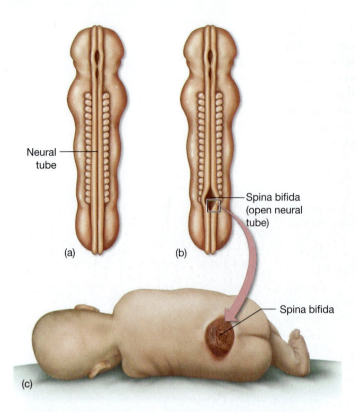

Figure 8.25 **Neural tube.** (*a*) Normal neural tube in an early embryo. (*b*) Spina bifida (abnormal neural tube) in an early embryo. (*c*) Infant with severe spina bifida.

nervous system damage that accompanies the B−12 deficiency. Furthermore, some medical experts are concerned that taking folic acid supplements and consuming foods that contain the micronutrient may cause excess folic acid to accumulate in blood and produce negative health effects as a result. Thus, more research is needed to determine whether ingesting too much folic acid poses health risks.

Neural Tube Defects   A woman's diet before and during pregnancy provides the raw materials for her developing offspring's needs, as well as her body's needs. Not surprisingly, recommendations for intakes of many nutrients increase during pregnancy. A pregnant woman has an increased requirement for folate, because DNA synthesis and cell division take place at a rapid pace during embryonic development.

During the first few weeks after conception, the **neural tube** forms in the human embryo (Fig. 8.25a). This tube eventually develops into the brain and spinal cord. Pregnant women who suffer from folate deficiency have high risk of giving birth to infants with neural tube defects. The two most common neural tube defects are **spina bifida** (*spy'−na bif'−eh−dah*) and **anencephaly** (*an−en−sef'−ah−lee*). Spina bifida occurs when the embryo's spine does not form properly, and the bones fail to enclose the spinal cord. As you can see in Figure 8.25c, infants with severe spina bifida have a section of their spinal cord or a sac containing some spinal fluid bulging through an opening in their backs. Often, people with spina bifida are unable to use muscles in the lower part of their bodies, and as a result, they cannot walk independently. Infants born with anencephaly have much of their brain malformed or missing, and they usually die shortly after birth.

In 1992, officials with the U.S. Public Health Service recommended that all women capable of becoming pregnant consume 400 mcg of folic acid daily to prevent neural tube defects. In January 1998, the Food and Drug Administration required the addition of folic acid to enriched flour and cereals. According to medical experts, adequate folic acid intake can prevent most cases of spina bifida.[21] For pregnant women, adequate folate status is critical early in pregnancy, because the neural tube begins to form about 21 days after conception. This developmental milestone occurs when many women are not even aware they are pregnant.

Each year, about 1 in every 4800 babies is born with anencephaly[22] and about 1500 babies are born with spina bifida in the United States.[23] However, the prevalence of these neural tube defects has declined since enrichment of foods with folic acid began.

Because women of childbearing age may become pregnant at some point, they need to be aware of the association between the lack of folate and neural tube defects. In addition to including folate−rich foods in their diets, young women can prepare for pregnancy by taking a daily multivitamin supplement that contains 400 mcg of synthetic folic acid.[21] Although folic acid intakes have increased among Americans since the United States began enriching grain products with the vitamin, only 40% of women who are of childbearing age take a daily folic acid supplement that supplies at least 400 mcg.[24]

Vitamin B-12

Cells require vitamin B−12 to make coenzymes that participate in a variety of cellular processes, including the transfer of CH_3 groups in the metabolism of folate (see Fig. 8.23). Vitamin B−12 is also needed to convert folate to coenzyme forms that are needed for metabolic reactions, including DNA synthesis. Vitamin B−12 also participates in homocysteine metabolism.

neural tube embryonic structure that eventually develops into the brain and spinal cord

spina bifida type of neural tube defect in which the spine does not form properly before birth, and it fails to enclose the spinal cord

anencephaly type of neural tube defect in which the brain does not form properly or is missing

There is one vital function of vitamin B–12 that does not involve folate: maintaining the *myelin sheaths* that wrap around parts of certain nerve cells, insulating them. Myelin enables the nerves to communicate effectively. Without vitamin B–12, segments of myelin sheath gradually undergo destruction that can lead to paralysis. If a person who is vitamin B–12 deficient does not obtain treatment with the vitamin, he or she could die as a result of the deficiency.

Absorbing the vitamin B–12 that is naturally in food requires a complex series of steps that are unique for a vitamin (Fig. 8.26). Natural vitamin B–12 is bound to animal protein that prevents its absorption. When the food enters the stomach, the vitamin is released from the protein, primarily by the actions of hydrochloric acid (HCl) in gastric juice. Synthetic vitamin B–12 in dietary supplements or fortified foods is not bound to food protein, so it does not need stomach acid to release the protein.

In the small intestine, vitamin B–12 binds to **intrinsic factor (IF),** a com‐ pound produced by certain stomach cells. Eventually, the vitamin B–12/intrinsic factor complex reaches the ileum of the small intestine, where the vitamin com‐ plex is absorbed. Within the absorptive cells, vitamin B–12 is separated from intrinsic factor and attached to transport molecules. The transport molecules enter the bloodstream and travel to the liver via the hepatic portal vein. The liver removes vitamin B–12 from many of the carrier molecules and stores about 50% of the vitamin. A healthy liver has enough vitamin B–12 reserves to last 5 to 10 years.[25] Therefore, a healthy person who decides to follow a diet that com‐ pletely lacks vitamin B–12 is not likely to experience signs and symptoms of the vitamin's deficiency disorder for as long as 10 years.

intrinsic factor (IF) substance produced in the stomach that facilitates intestinal absorption of vitamin B-12

Food Sources of Vitamin B-12

Plants do not make vitamin B–12; therefore, we rely almost entirely on animal foods to supply the vitamin naturally. Major sources of vitamin B–12 in the typical American diet are meat, milk and milk products, poultry, fish, shellfish, and eggs. Although liver is not a popular food, it is one of the richest sources of vitamin B–12. Many soy products, such as soy milk, and ready–to–eat cereals are fortified with synthetic vitamin B–12. Table 8.13 lists some foods that provide vitamin B–12.

Dietary Adequacy

The adult RDA for vitamin B–12 is 2.4 mcg/day. Most Americans consume more than the RDA.[26] No UL has been established for vitamin B–12, because no adverse effects have been observed with excess intake from food or dietary supplements.

Vitamin B-12 Deficiency   Vitamin B–12 deficiency is characterized by nerve damage and megaloblastic RBCs. Other common signs and symptoms of the deficiency include muscle weakness, sore mouth, smooth and shiny tongue, memory loss, confusion, difficulty walking and maintaining balance, and numb‐ ness and tingling sensations, particularly in the lower extremities. Most cases of vitamin B–12 deficiency result from problems that interfere with intestinal absorption of the vitamin (cobalamin) in foods (*food–cobalamin malabsorption*) and not from inadequate intakes.[25]

Vitamin B–12 deficiency is common among older adults. As people age, HCl production in their stomachs declines. Thus, many older adults have food–cobalamin malabsorption because they are unable to release vitamin B–12 from animal protein.[26] People with this condition can develop vitamin B–12 deficiency disorder despite consuming diets that contain the vitamin. In addition to advanced age, chronic alcoholism, gastric bypass surgeries for weight reduc‐ tion, and certain medications, particularly those that reduce stomach acid secre‐ tion, can contribute to food–cobalamin malabsorption. People with this form of

B-12 bound to animal protein

B-12 **P**

① B-12 bound to animal protein is swallowed and enters the stomach.

② Hydrochloric acid (HCl) separates B-12 from animal protein.

③ Stomach secretes IF.

④ B-12 and IF exit the stomach.

⑤ B-12 binds to IF in duodenum, forming IF/B-12 complex.

⑥ IF/B-12 complex enters ileal cell. IF separates from B-12, and the vitamin binds to a carrier molecule for transport in the blood stream.

Duodenum

Ileum

Absorptive cell in wall of ileum

B-12 carrier molecule

To bloodstream

Figure 8.26 Natural vitamin B-12 absorption. Absorbing natural vitamin B-12 from food requires a complex series of steps.

TABLE 8.13   Vitamin B-12 Content of Selected Foods

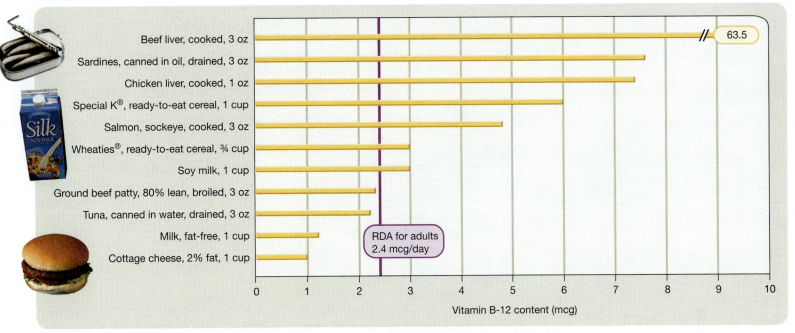

Source: Data from U.S. Department of Agriculture, Agricultural Research Service: *USDA national nutrient database for standard reference, Release 26,* 2013.

malabsorption produce intrinsic factor, so they can absorb synthetic forms of the vitamin in dietary supplements that contain B−12.

About 1 to 2% of older adults have an autoimmune disorder that causes inflammation and destruction of the cells in the stomach that produce intrinsic factor.[26] (An autoimmune disorder results when a person's immune system attacks his or her own cells.) In these cases, diets may supply adequate amounts of vitamin B−12, but the lack of intrinsic factor prevents most of the micronutrient from being absorbed. Eventually, people who lack intrinsic factor develop a disease called **pernicious** ("deadly") **anemia.** As its name implies, pernicious anemia can lead to vitamin B−12 deficiency and death. Treatment involves bypassing the need for intrinsic factor and intestinal absorption, usually by providing routine vitamin B−12 injections. Furthermore, taking large doses of vitamin B−12 floods the intestinal tract with the vitamin and enables a small amount to be absorbed without the need for intrinsic factor.

In addition to advanced age, family history is a risk factor for pernicious anemia. Therefore, it is a good idea to have your blood tested for signs of vitamin B−12 deficiency as you grow older, and especially if you have a close relative with pernicious anemia.

Vegans ("total" vegetarians) avoid eating animal products. Plant foods supply little vitamin B−12, so vegans need to be concerned about their intakes of the nutrient (see the "Vegetarianism" section of Chapter 7). People who eat few or no animal products should consume foods that have been fortified with vitamin B−12, such as fortified soy milk and cereals, or take supplements that supply the vitamin. Vegan women who breastfeed their babies need to be aware that their breast milk may contain inadequate amounts of vitamin B−12. Babies who consume only vitamin B−12–deficient breast milk are likely to develop megaloblastic anemia and serious nervous system problems, including diminished brain growth and spinal cord damage. The signs and symptoms of the deficiency are likely to occur during the first few months of life, particularly when the infants' mothers did not supplement their diets with vitamin B−12 during pregnancy. Providing vitamin B−12 to the deficient babies promptly can prevent permanent damage to the children's nervous systems.[27]

pernicious anemia condition caused by the lack of intrinsic factor and characterized by vitamin B-12 deficiency, nerve damage, and megaloblastic RBCs

Pantothenic Acid

Pantothenic acid is a component of *coenzyme A*, which is critical for energy metabolism and fatty acid production in the body. Pantothenic acid is so wide—spread in foods that a nutritional deficiency is unlikely to occur among healthy people who eat varied diets. Rich sources of pantothenic acid include cereals that have been fortified with the vitamin, beef and chicken liver, sunflower seeds, mushrooms, peas, and soy milk.

Most Americans consume adequate amounts of pantothenic acid, and as a result, deficiencies of the vitamin are rare. When scientists experimentally cause pantothenic deficiency in human subjects, they note signs and symptoms that include headache, fatigue, impaired muscle coordination, and GI tract dis—turbances. People who abuse alcohol may develop pantothenic acid and other B—vitamin deficiencies, particularly if their diets are lacking other nutrients as well. At this time, scientists have not set an UL for the vitamin, because there have been no reports of toxicity from taking high doses.

Biotin

In its coenzyme form, biotin participates in chemical reactions that add carbon dioxide to other compounds. By doing so, the vitamin promotes the synthesis of glucose and fatty acids and the breakdown of certain amino acids. Severe defi—ciencies of biotin rarely occur because intestinal bacteria produce some biotin, and the vitamin is in a wide variety of foods. Liver, eggs, peanuts, salmon, pork, mushrooms, and sunflower seeds are good sources of biotin. The typical diet of American adults provides adequate amounts of the micronutrient.

Conditions that reduce intestinal bacteria's biotin production, such as sur—gical removal of a large part of the colon or taking antibiotics for many months, can contribute to a biotin deficiency. Signs and symptoms of biotin deficiency include skin rash, hair loss, convulsions, and some other nervous system disor—ders. Because reports of biotin toxicity are lacking, nutrition scientists have not set an UL for the micronutrient.

Vitamin C

Most animals do not need dietary sources of vitamin C (**ascorbic acid**) because they can synthesize all the vitamin they need. Humans and guinea pigs are among the few species that are unable to make vitamin C, and for these animals, the micronutrient is essential.

ascorbic acid vitamin C

Vitamin C absorption occurs in the small intestine. As intakes of the vitamin increase, the amount absorbed decreases. The small intestine, for example, absorbs 50% or less of the vitamin when intakes are 1 g or more/day. Additionally, the kidneys increase their excretion of the vitamin in response to high intakes. There—fore, taking megadoses of vitamin C may be wasteful, because such high amounts of the vitamin are not well absorbed and excesses are eliminated in urine.

Functions of Vitamin C

Vitamin C does not function as part of a coenzyme as do B vitamins, but the vitamin serves as a nutrient cofactor that facilitates certain chemical reac—tions. Vitamin C performs a variety of important cellular functions, primarily by donating electrons to other compounds. In the body, vitamin C has widespread physiological roles; the following sections describe some of the micronutrient's most well—understood functions.

Swollen gums that bleed easily are a sign of scurvy.

Collagen Synthesis Vitamin C participates in reactions that form and maintain collagen. **Collagen** is a fibrous protein that gives strength to *connective tissue*. Connective tissues, such as bone, cartilage, and tendons, connect and support other structures in the body. During collagen formation, vitamin C helps create numerous cross—connections between the amino acids in collagen that greatly strengthen the connective tissue (Fig. 8.27). If vitamin C is unavailable, the body forms weak connective tissue and is unable to maintain existing collagen. Some of the more obvious signs of scurvy, such as swollen gums that bleed easily, teeth that loosen and fall out of their sockets, skin that bruises easily, and old scars that open, are primarily the result of poorly formed and maintained collagen.

Antioxidant Activity Results of some experiments indicate that vitamin C can act as an antioxidant by donating electrons to radicals. Vitamin C also may donate electrons to another antioxidant—vitamin E. Thus, vitamin C recycles vitamin E so it can regain its antioxidant function. Scientists, however, do not know the extent of vitamin C's antioxidant abilities in the human body. Taking excessive amounts of vitamin C may be harmful, because in high doses, the vitamin has **prooxidant** effects. A prooxidant promotes radical production.

Other Roles of Vitamin C in the Body Vitamin C plays a role in the body's immune function, and the vitamin is necessary for the synthesis of bile and certain neurotransmitters. Vitamin C is also involved in the production of various hormones, including the "stress hormone" cortisol; adolsterone, a hormone involved in blood pressure regulation; and thyroxin, the thyroid hormone that regulates energy metabolism.

Food Sources of Vitamin C

Plant foods are the best dietary sources of vitamin C. Peppers, citrus fruit, papaya, broccoli, and berries contain relatively high amounts of the micronutrient (Table 8.14). Potatoes and vitamin C–fortified fruit drinks and cereals also supply vitamin C. Most animal foods are not sources of the micronutrient.

Vitamin C is very unstable in the presence of heat, oxygen, light, alkaline conditions, and the minerals iron and copper. Storing vitamin C–rich foods in cool conditions, such as in the refrigerator, will help preserve the micronutrient. Because vitamin C is easily lost during cooking, eat raw fruits and vegetables whenever possible.

collagen fibrous protein that gives strength to connective tissue

prooxidant substance that promotes free radical production

MY DIVERSE PLATE

Guava

Guava is a tropical fruit that is available in many varieties. Although guavas can be eaten fresh, the fruit is often used to make sauces, jellies, and juices. Guavas are an excellent source of fiber and vitamin C. The white or pink flesh of a guava contains more vitamin C than an orange.

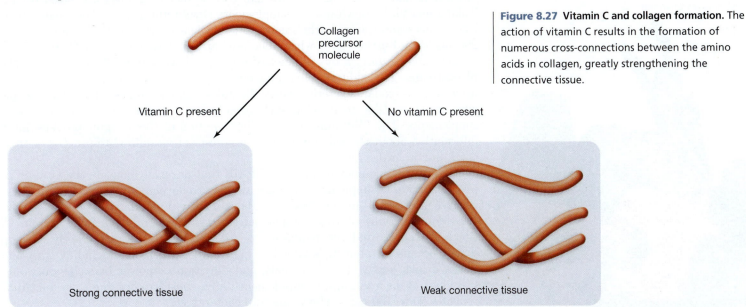

Figure 8.27 Vitamin C and collagen formation. The action of vitamin C results in the formation of numerous cross-connections between the amino acids in collagen, greatly strengthening the connective tissue.

Collagen precursor molecule

Vitamin C present

No vitamin C present

Strong connective tissue

Weak connective tissue

TABLE 8.14   Vitamin C Content of Selected Foods

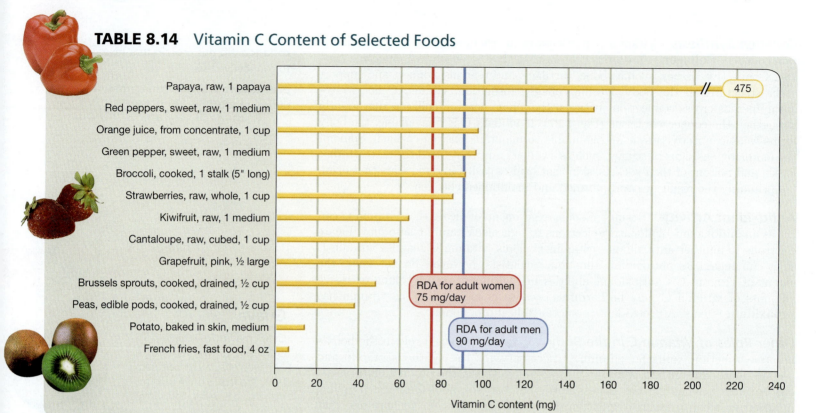

Food	Vitamin C content (mg)
Papaya, raw, 1 papaya	475
Red peppers, sweet, raw, 1 medium	
Orange juice, from concentrate, 1 cup	
Green pepper, sweet, raw, 1 medium	
Broccoli, cooked, 1 stalk (5" long)	
Strawberries, raw, whole, 1 cup	
Kiwifruit, raw, 1 medium	
Cantaloupe, raw, cubed, 1 cup	
Grapefruit, pink, ½ large	
Brussels sprouts, cooked, drained, ½ cup	
Peas, edible pods, cooked, drained, ½ cup	
Potato, baked in skin, medium	
French fries, fast food, 4 oz	

RDA for adult women 75 mg/day

RDA for adult men 90 mg/day

Source: Data from U.S. Department of Agriculture, Agricultural Research Service: *USDA national nutrient database for standard reference, Release 26,* 2013.

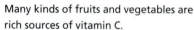

Many kinds of fruits and vegetables are rich sources of vitamin C.

Dietary Adequacy

The adult RDA for vitamin C is 75 and 90 mg/day for women and men, respectively. Cigarette smokers need to add an extra 35 mg/day to their RDA, because exposure to cigarette smoke increases radical formation in their lungs.[4] By including vitamin C–rich fruits and vegetables in their diets, healthy people can obtain adequate amounts of vitamin C.

The adult UL for vitamin C is 2000 mg/day. When people exceed this amount of the vitamin, gastrointestinal upsets, including diarrhea, often occur.[4] Taking megadoses of vitamin C supplements is wasteful, because the small intestine reduces absorption of the micronutrient when intakes of the vitamin exceed 200 mg/day. Furthermore, when cells are saturated with vitamin C, the excess vitamin and *oxalate*, a by–product of breaking down vitamin C, circulate in the bloodstream. The kidneys filter and eliminate these unnecessary substances in urine. Excess oxalate excretion raises the risk of kidney stones.[9] Therefore, people who are susceptible to develop such stones should avoid consuming vitamin C supplements. The "Vitamins as Medicines" section of this chapter provides more information about the value of taking megadoses of vitamin C to prevent or treat colds and other disorders.

Even if you do not regularly eat foods that naturally contain the vitamin or take a vitamin C supplement, you are unlikely to develop a vitamin C deficiency, because most people require less than 10 mg of the vitamin daily to prevent scurvy. A 6–ounce serving of fresh orange juice provides about 60 mg of vitamin C, which is well beyond the requirement. Additionally, Americans rarely develop scurvy because vitamin C is added to many processed foods, including fruit and sports drinks, ready–to–eat cereals, and nutrition or power bars. If you would still like to take a vitamin C supplement daily, consider choosing a product that provides 50 to 100 mg of the vitamin in each tablet.

Choline

The body needs choline to produce phospholipids in cell membranes and acetyl–choline, a neurotransmitter associated with learning and memory, muscle control, and many other nervous system functions. Additionally, the liver uses choline to synthesize a part of a phospholipid (see Chapter 6). Choline is widely distributed in foods. Liver, eggs, beef, and pork are among the richest sources of the nutri–ent. The source of choline in egg yolk is the phospholipid lecithin (see Chapter 6).

The adult AI for choline is 425 to 550 mg/day. The typical American diet provides about 320 mg of choline per day.[8] Although the amount of choline that Americans consume is often less than the AI for the micronutrient, the body can make choline from serine, an amino acid. It is possible, however, that the body cannot produce enough choline to meet the amount that is required, especially during some life stages. Choline deficiency can cause liver damage.

Concept **Checkpoint 8.3**

7. Prepare a table for water-soluble vitamins and choline. For each of these micronutients, indicate its major function in the body, major food sources, deficiency disorder (if it has a specific name), and major signs and symptoms of the deficiency disorder. If the micronutrient is known to be toxic, also indicate major toxicity signs and symptoms. Check your table against the information provided in Table 8.7.

8.4 Vitamins as Medicines

Learning Outcome

1 Evaluate the use of vitamin supplements with respect to their potential health benefits and hazards.

Are you among the millions of Americans who take vitamin supplements? If your answer is yes, why do you use them? Many people take multiple vitamin/mineral supplements as an "insurance policy" in case their diets are not nutri–tionally adequate. Other people use specific vitamin supplements because they think the practice will result in optimal health. Vitamin supplements are effective for treating people with specific vitamin deficiency diseases, metabolic defects that increase vitamin requirements, and a few other medical conditions. However, scientific evidence generally does not support claims that megadoses of vitamins can prevent or treat everything from gray hair to lung cancer.

How did vitamins earn the reputation of being cure–alls? The fact that a very small amount of a vitamin can prevent or cure the vitamin's deficiency disease provides the foundation for beliefs that these micronutrients are useful for preventing or treating serious chronic diseases. Furthermore, many people think that vitamins are helpful and safe in any amount. When ingested in high doses, however, vitamins and related compounds such as carotenoids often have druglike effects in the body. In some cases, these physiological responses are beneficial, but in other instances, vitamin excesses cause unpleasant and even dangerous side effects. Therefore, people should be just as cautious about using megadoses of vitamins as they need to be when taking medications. This section of

Vitamin C supplements that contain "ester" forms of the vitamin do not provide any advantage over "regular" vitamin C supplements. The ester forms of the supplements are usually more expensive, too.

Chapter 8 focuses on some current scientific evidence regarding the useful—ness and safety of using large doses of vitamins and related compounds as medications.

Niacin as Medicine?

In Chapter 6, we discussed the association between elevated blood levels of LDL cholesterol and increased risk of cardiovascular disease (CVD), the number one killer of Americans. Heart disease and stroke are the major forms of CVD. Prescription forms of niacin have been used to treat elevated LDL cholesterol levels. However, results of recent studies indicate that such niacin therapy is neither safe nor effective.[28]

Vitamin B-6 as Medicine?

Popular sources of nutrition information often recommend large doses of vitamin B−6 to treat *premenstrual syndrome (PMS)*, a condition that many women experience a few days before their menstrual period begins. However, stud—ies investigating the value of vitamin B−6 supplementation for relieving PMS do not provide strong support for the use of the micronutrient to treat the disorder.[19]

Unlike most other B vitamins, vitamin B−6 is toxic in high doses, caus—ing severe sensory nerve damage when taken in doses that exceed the UL for extended periods. Signs and symptoms of vitamin B−6 toxicity include walk—ing difficulties and numbness of the hands and feet. The nerve damage usually resolves when affected people stop ingesting megadoses of vitamin B−6.

Folic Acid, B-6, and B-12 as Medicine?

Deficiencies of folic acid, vitamin B−6, and vitamin B−12 are associated with elevated blood levels of homocysteine. High homocysteine levels may be a bio—chemical marker (an indicator in the body) or a risk factor for cardiovascu—lar disease. However, results of research do not provide evidence that lowering homocysteine levels by taking these B vitamins reduces the risk of heart disease.[19] More research is needed to determine whether healthy people can reduce their risk of heart disease and other forms of CVD by using folic acid, B−6, and B−12 supplements for long periods.

Elevated blood homocysteine levels may also be a marker or risk factor for Alzheimer's disease (AD). Alzheimer's disease is characterized by a gradual pro—gressive decline in cognitive functioning, including memory and decision—making skills. There is no cure or effective treatment for the disease. Studies to determine whether folic acid, vitamin B−6, and vitamin B−12 can improve cognitive func—tioning have provided disappointing results.[19] As is often the case, more research is needed to determine whether using supplements that contain these micronutri—ents can reduce the risk of cognitive decline or slow the progression of AD.

Vitamin C as Medicine?

In 1970, Nobel Prize–winning American chemist Dr. Linus Pauling (1901–1994) published *Vitamin C and the Common Cold*. This bestselling book established the popular belief that megadoses of vitamin C could prevent colds. As a result of Pauling's claim, many Americans take megadoses of the micronutrient when they notice the first cold symptoms.

In the years that followed the publication of *Vitamin C and the Common Cold*, Pauling became more convinced of vitamin C's health benefits. He claimed large doses of vitamin C could battle a variety of diseases, including influenza, cancer, and CVD. He even believed the vitamin could slow the aging process. Despite Pauling's impressive credentials in chemistry, conventional nutrition scientists have approached his ideas about vitamin C's health benefits with caution and skepticism.

Can taking vitamin C protect you against infection by cold viruses? The evidence collected from several scientific studies indicates that routine vitamin C supplementation (200 mg or more of the vitamin daily) does not prevent colds in the general population.[9] However, taking such large doses of the vitamin may reduce the duration of cold symptoms by a day or so. Additionally, vitamin C may reduce the severity of cold symptoms because the micronutrient acts like an antihistamine when taken in very large doses.[4]

Beyond the Common Cold

When LDL cholesterol is oxidized, it is more likely to contribute to atherosclerosis than nonoxidized LDL cholesterol (see Chapter 6). As an antioxidant, vitamin C may reduce the oxidation of LDL cholesterol, lowering the risk of CVD. Studies to determine whether vitamin C can help prevent CVD have not provided consistent evidence that the micronutrient reduces the risk of CVD or dying from the condition.[9] Atherosclerosis takes years and probably decades to result in heart attack, strokes, and other forms of CVD. Thus, more research is needed to determine whether long-term vitamin C supplementation can reduce the risk of this leading killer of Americans.

According to findings of epidemiological studies, people who consume diets containing high amounts of vitamin C–rich fruits and vegetables have lower risk of cancer than people who do not eat much of these foods. Although there is some encouraging scientific evidence that vitamin C may be useful in treating cancer, high doses of the vitamin may interfere with certain cancer-fighting treatments, lowering their effectiveness.[9] The "Nutrition Matters" section in this chapter provides more information concerning the role of diet in cancer development and prevention.

It is important to note that complex chronic diseases such as CVD, Alzheimer's disease, and cancer generally do not have simple causes. Inherited factors as well as lifestyle practices other than diet—smoking, obesity, and lack of physical activity—contribute to the development of these diseases. Therefore, it is unlikely that people will be able to prevent or treat cancer simply by taking vitamin C (or any other supplement).

Vitamin E as Medicine?

Major studies fail to show that high intakes of vitamin E consistently reduce the risk of CVD, cancer, and mild cognitive impairment, a condition characterized by declining thought-processing abilities that can progress to Alzheimer's disease.[16] Furthermore, use of vitamin E supplements has been associated with an increased risk of prostate cancer (men) and hemorrhagic stroke. More clinical research is needed to determine whether combinations of vitamin E and other antioxidant nutrients can prevent or slow the development of chronic diseases, such as CVD, cancer, and Alzheimer's disease.

Did scientists *prove* vitamin E supplements are useless or "bad"? No. Vitamin E has several forms, and it is possible that the alpha-tocopherol form of vitamin E that is typically in supplements does not have any beneficial druglike effects on the body. The dosage of vitamin E and the length of time the supplements are administered during clinical tests may provide other reasons why research findings do not always support epidemiological observations. To detect positive effects on health, scientists may need to test higher doses of the vitamin than have been studied in the past. Additionally, studies that last longer may be necessary; the health benefits of vitamin E supplementation may take several years to become evident.

Vitamin A and Carotenoids as Medicine?

Findings of observational studies suggest an association between eating diets rich in fruits and vegetables and lower risk of certain cancers, heart disease, and *age—related macular degeneration*; see the following section, "Dietary Supplements and AMD". Such diets provide plenty of beta—carotene and other antioxidant carotenoids. Scientists have conducted numerous large—scale studies to determine whether carotenoid supplements provide health benefits. The following sections summarize research findings regarding the health effects of taking these supplements.

Cancer

Results of clinical studies have not provided support for taking vitamin A or beta—carotene supplements to reduce the risk of cancer.[11] In two major studies, smokers who took beta—carotene supplements were *more* likely to die of lung cancer than smokers who took placebos.[11] Nevertheless, more research is needed to determine whether other carotenoids, such as lycopene and *beta—cryptoxanthin (bay'—ta krip—toe—zan'—thin)*, protect against various forms of cancer.

Dietary Supplements and AMD

In the United States, age—related macular degeneration (AMD) is one of the leading causes of blindness among older adults.[11] The disease is associated with changes in the *macula*, the region within the eye that provides the most detailed central vision (Fig. 8.28). When the macula is damaged, objects appear to be distorted, as in the grid shown in Figure 8.29 (right side). Major risk factors for AMD are genetics, smoking, and advanced age, but diet also plays a role in the development of the condition.

The macula contains the carotenoids lutein and zeaxanthin. In the Age—Related Eye Disease Study (AREDS), patients who already had AMD

Figure 8.28 **The macula.** The macula is the region within the eye that provides the most detailed central vision.

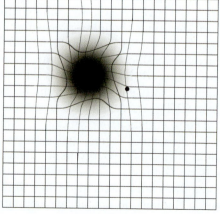

Figure 8.29 **Visual effect of macular degeneration.** When shown a grid comprised of straight lines, people with normal vision see the grid on the left. However, people with age-related macular degeneration (AMD) would see distorted gridlines, as shown in the right illustration.

took dietary supplements that contained relatively high amounts of vitamins C and E, beta–carotene, and the minerals copper and zinc.[11] The combination of these substances slowed the progression of vision loss associated with advanced macular degeneration. However, there was no clear scientific evidence that taking antioxidant supplements *prevents* healthy people from developing AMD. Additionally, the long–term use of these supplements could be harmful.

Some Final Thoughts

According to a report issued by the U.S. Preventive Services Task Force, people do not need to be discouraged from taking vitamin supplements unless there is strong evidence to indicate the practice is harmful, as in the case of smokers who use beta–carotene supplements.[29] Nevertheless, the Task Force report states, "... taking vitamins does not replace the need to eat a healthy diet." Although the health benefits of vitamin supplementation are often uncertain, there is more consistent evidence that a diet high in fruits, vegetables, and legumes has important benefits. It is possible that other constituents besides vitamins may account for the benefits of such diets.

Consuming a wide variety of vitamins, antioxidants, and phytochemicals in their natural states and concentrations (in foods) may be the most effective way to lower your risk of CVD, cancer, and many other serious chronic diseases. Why? These substances probably work together to enhance health, and isolating them from their natural sources or synthesizing and concentrating them into supplements may reduce their usefulness and increase their risks.[30] Therefore, dietitians recommend that adults eat a variety of fruits and vegetables each day rather than take antioxidant or phytochemical supplements.

Nutrition experts tend to emphasize the importance of combining a nutritious diet with regular exercise for achieving and maintaining good health. However, an overwhelming amount of scientific evidence links tobacco use to several forms of cancer, heart disease, AMD, and other serious chronic conditions. If you smoke tobacco, quitting may have a greater beneficial impact on your long–term health than improving your diet or increasing your physical activity level while still continuing tobacco use.

Concept **Checkpoint 8.4**

8. Explain why people should be careful about taking megadoses of vitamin supplements.
9. List three side effects from taking megadoses of nicotinic acid.
10. Explain why people should avoid taking high doses of vitamin B-6.
11. A friend of yours takes 1000 mg of vitamin C daily, because she thinks the vitamin prevents colds, heart attacks, and Alzheimer's disease. After reading section 8.4, what would you tell your friend about her vitamin C use?
12. Dorothy is 85 years of age. She has excellent vision, but she takes megadoses of vitamins C and E, because she thinks these vitamins prevent macular degeneration. Based on the information in section 8.4, what would you tell Dorothy about her vitamin C and vitamin E use?

8.5 Nutrition Matters: Diet and Cancer

Learning Outcomes

1 Define the following terms: *metastasize, carcinogen,* and *malignant tumor.*

2 Identify common cancer sites and causes of cancer deaths for Americans.

3 Identify lifestyle practices associated with increased risk of certain cancers.

4 Identify foods that may increase risk of cancer.

5 Discuss some practical steps that people can take to reduce their risk of cancer.

For many people, no diagnosis evokes more fear than that of *cancer*. Although modern medical technologies have enabled physicians to make great progress in treating many types of cancer successfully, the disease is still the second-leading cause of death in the United States. According to the American Cancer Society, one in four Americans dies as a result of cancer.[31]

In 2014, the three leading sites of new cancer cases (excluding common types of skin cancer) for American men were prostate, lung, and colon and rectal (colorectal) cancers. The three leading sites of new cancer cases in American women were breast, lung, and colorectal cancers. As shown in Figure 8.30, lung cancer is responsible for more cancer deaths than prostate (males), breast (females), and colorectal cancers. There is good news: A significant number of cancer deaths are preventable.

Figure 8.30 Leading cancer sites and deaths. This figure indicates leading sites of cancer deaths and percentages of cancer deaths according to 2014 estimates.
Source: American Cancer Society: *Cancer facts & figures 2014.* www.cancer.org. Accessed: July 2, 2014

This section focuses on the roles of diet and exercise in the development, progression, and possible prevention of certain cancers. For more information about cancer,

| **Figure 8.31 Cancer development and progression.**

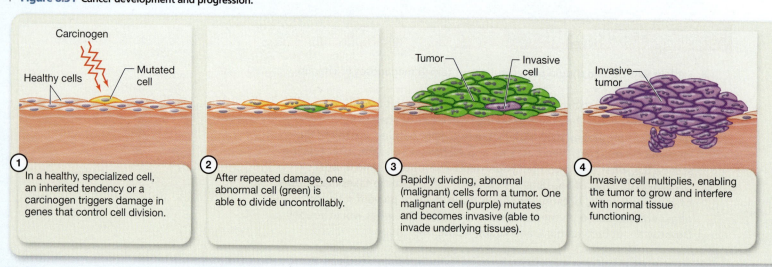

1 In a healthy, specialized cell, an inherited tendency or a carcinogen triggers damage in genes that control cell division.

2 After repeated damage, one abnormal cell (green) is able to divide uncontrollably.

3 Rapidly dividing, abnormal (malignant) cells form a tumor. One malignant cell (purple) mutates and becomes invasive (able to invade underlying tissues).

4 Invasive cell multiplies, enabling the tumor to grow and interfere with normal tissue functioning.

including specific forms of cancer, visit the American Cancer Society's website at www.cancer.org or the National Cancer Institute's website at www.cancer.gov.

What Is Cancer?

Cancer is the term for a group of chronic diseases characterized by cells that have undergone damage to certain genes (*mutations*). Genes are portions of DNA that code for the production of specific proteins (see Chapter 7). DNA dictates cellular growth, division, and eventual death. The rate at which healthy cells develop, grow, divide, and die occurs in a controlled fashion. As a normal body cell develops and matures, it acquires specialized functions. Examples include the ability of muscle cells to contract and that of certain stomach cells to secrete hydrochloric acid.

Cancerous (*malignant*) cells are literally "out of control": They divide repeatedly and frequently, and they do not die. If genes that regulate cellular growth, division, and death mutate, abnormal cell development, rapid cell growth, and unchecked cell division can result. When a cell becomes malignant, it does not perform the specialized functions of the cells from which it was derived. A cancerous liver cell, for example, does not remove toxins from the bloodstream or store nutrients properly.

As a result of their rapid growth rate, many types of cancer cells form masses, called **malignant tumors.** Malignant cells often break away from the tumor. These cells can move to and invade other parts of the body. When cancer spreads to other tissues, the disease has **metastasized** (*meh–tass'–tah–sized*).

Some cells multiply excessively and form *benign* (*bih-nine'*) masses or tumors as a result. A benign tumor is not cancerous, because the tumor's cells do not destroy nearby tissues or metastasize. Benign tumors are usually harmless. In some cases, however, a benign tumor grows large enough to interfere with the functioning of healthy structures, such as a blood vessel or brain tissue. When this occurs, the tumor needs to be treated to reduce its size or remove it.

A **carcinogen** (*car–sin'–o–jin*) is an environmental factor, such as radiation, tobacco smoke, or a virus, that triggers cancer. Carcinogens can irritate tissues, causing an inflammatory response by the body. Over time, the inflammation may result in cancer development. Some carcinogens damage DNA, causing mutations to genes that control certain cell behaviors. Over time, repeated exposures to various carcinogens take their toll on cells, making malignant cells more likely to develop. In fact, it is not unusual for cancerous cells to develop during a person's lifetime. However, a healthy immune system identifies the malignant cells and destroys them before they multiply uncontrollably. Nutrient deficiencies, the aging process, and environmental insults, such as exposure to radiation and certain chemicals, reduce the effectiveness of the immune system. As a result, cancer cells are able to divide unchecked and eventually metastasize. Figure 8.31 illustrates major steps in the development and behavior of most cancerous cells.

Because of their rapid growth and frequent cell divisions, malignant cells require more nutrients than normal cells. To supply enough nutrients to meet their needs, cancerous tumors stimulate the body to form blood vessels that divert blood away from healthy cells and into the tumor (see Fig. 8.31). Much of the severe body wasting that usually accompanies advanced cases of cancer happens because healthy tissues are unable to obtain adequate supplies of nutrients, and they die.

malignant tumor mass of cancerous cells

metastasized spread to other tissues

carcinogen factor that triggers cancer

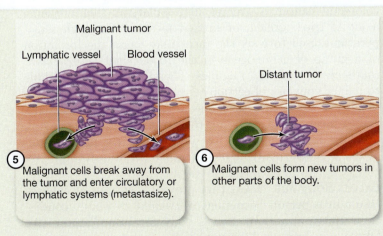

5 Malignant cells break away from the tumor and enter circulatory or lymphatic systems (metastasize).

6 Malignant cells form new tumors in other parts of the body.

7 Tumor stimulates development of its own blood supply, depriving the rest of the body of nourishment.

Regular health checkups and various screening methods can detect cancer in its early stages, when many forms can be effectively treated. Screening methods include using a special scope to view the inside of the lower gastrointestinal tract to detect colorectal cancer (*colonoscopy*). Conventional medical treatments for cancer typically involve surgical removal of cancerous tissue; chemotherapy, medications that are toxic to cancer cells or limit their growth; and radiation that kills cancer cells. Early diagnosis of cancer is very important. Once cancer metastasizes, it is far more difficult to treat.

What Causes Cells to Become Cancerous?

Why do many smokers develop lung cancer and some not develop it? Why do some women have breast cancer and others remain free of the disease? Medical researchers have discovered several risk factors for many forms of the disease, including the following:

- Aging (most cancers occur in people over 55 years of age)
- Having a family history of cancer
- Using tobacco
- Being exposed to some forms of radiation
- Being exposed to certain environmental substances, such as irritants
- Having certain viral and bacterial infections
- Having elevated levels of certain hormones
- Consuming alcohol and certain foods
- Being physically inactive and having excess body fat[31]

People can lower their risk of cancer by avoiding known carcinogens, especially tobacco smoke. Approximately one of every three cancer deaths is associated with smoking tobacco.[31] Mouth, larynx ("voicebox"), esophageal, stomach, pancreatic, kidney, and bladder cancers are also associated with tobacco use. In 2014, experts with the American Cancer Society estimated that over 176,000 Americans would die as a result of tobacco use.[31]

Cancer causation is a complex process. Therefore, it may be impossible to pinpoint a single cause of a patient's cancer. Individuals differ widely in their genetic makeups, lifestyle practices, environmental exposures, and nutritional states. Some forms of the disease are likely to be inherited, but lifestyle factors, including diet, contribute to most cases of cancer.[31] Poor diet, physical inactivity, and excess body fat are responsible for 25 to 33% of new cases of cancer that occur in the United States.[31] The following sections examine relationships between dietary factors and the risk of cancer.

The Role of Diet in Cancer Development

Rates of specific cancers vary widely among different populations. Men and women living in Asian countries, for example, have lower risks of prostate and breast cancer,

respectively, than men and women living in Western countries. After Asian men and women migrate to Western countries, their risks of prostate and breast cancer increase and eventually become similar to the risks of their adopted country's native population. Such findings provide epidemiological evidence of associations between cancer and certain lifestyle choices.

According to results of observational and experimental studies, certain substances in foods and beverages promote cancer development. Alcohol, for example, is a carcinogen. People who consume alcoholic drinks daily have higher than average risks of cancers of the mouth, throat, esophagus, larynx, colorectum (men), liver, female breast, and possibly pancreas.[31] The risk rises as the amount of alcohol consumed increases and when cigarette smoking is combined with drinking. To reduce your risk of cancer, avoid alcoholic beverages or drink in moderation: no more than one standard drink per day for women and no more than two standard drinks per day for men. (A *standard* alcoholic drink is 1.5 oz of liquor, 12 oz of regular beer, and 5 oz of wine.)

Certain molds that can grow on nuts or grains produce a chemical called *aflatoxin* (ah'–fla–tox'–in). Consuming foods that are contaminated with these molds increases the risk of liver cancer. Although liver cancer is not common among Americans, populations that consume peanuts and grains that have been stored improperly have high rates of this type of cancer. Chapter 12 discusses toxic molds and ways to protect the food supply from them and other foodborne health threats.

Diets that contain large amounts of processed meats and/or red meat (defined as beef, pork, and lamb) are associated with increased risk of colorectal, pancreatic, and prostate cancer.[31] Processed meat ("deli" meat) has sodium nitrate and sodium nitrite added to it during production. Under certain conditions, these chemicals form *nitrosamine* (ni–tros'–ah–menes), which are carcinogens. Eating high amounts of smoked or salt–preserved (*pickled*) foods, such as salted fish, may increase the risk of stomach cancer.[32]

According to findings of some studies, the risk of colorectal cancer is greater in populations that consume a lot of fried, grilled, or broiled meats.[33] The high temperatures used to cook the meat may cause the formation of a group of carcinogens in the food called *heterocyclic* (het'–eh–ro–si'–klic) amines. Therefore, you may be able to reduce your risk of certain cancers by limiting your intake of grilled meats and avoiding charred parts of charcoal–grilled meats. Also, covering the grate with aluminum foil, poking a few holes in the foil, and placing the meat on top of it will reduce charring of the meat.

Excess Body Fat Diets that provide a surplus of calories result in a person becoming overweight or obese, conditions characterized by excess body fat (see Chapter 10). Obese people have higher risks of cancers of the colon, breast (in postmenopausal women), uterus, kidney, and

TABLE 8.15
Possible Diet-Related Carcinogens

Possibly Carcinogenic	Common Dietary Sources	Possible or Known Action
Aflatoxin	Moldy nuts and grains	Can cause liver cancer
Arsenic	Natural contaminant in drinking water	May increase risk of bladder cancer
Alcohol	Alcoholic beverages	Unclear, but may increase certain hormone levels or the body's breakdown of alcohol may result in carcinogens
Excess calorie intake	All macronutrients	Excess calorie intake is linked to obesity.
Heterocyclic amines	Foods exposed to high temperature, especially grilled meat that has charred areas	Formation of heterocyclic amines that alter DNA of colon cells
Sodium nitrate and nitrite	Cured meats, such as deli meats, hot dogs, and bacon	Formation of nitrosamines
Trans fat	Partially hydrogenated fats used to make shortening, "stick" margarines, and baked goods	Unclear whether trans fats are carcinogenic, but they may alter the normal balance of fatty acids in the colorectum

esophagus than people who have healthy amounts of body fat.[31] Excess body fat may also increase the risk of other forms of cancer. The reasons for the relationship between excess body fat and cancer development are unclear. However, overweight and obese people often have elevated insulin, estrogen, and testosterone levels. Excesses of these and possibly other hormones may stimulate the production of cell factors that promote malignant cell development and growth. In some cases, cancer triggers are easier to identify. For example, overweight and obesity are associated with the increased risk of esophageal cancer. Excess abdominal fat contributes to the reflux of stomach acid into the esophagus by restricting the ability of the stomach to expand during meals. As a result, the gastroesophageal sphincter is unable to keep the stomach's contents from moving into the esophagus. (See Chapter 4 "Nutrition Matters.") Chronic exposure to stomach acid irritates the lining of the esophagus, making cancerous cells more likely to develop in the affected area.

Table 8.15 indicates dietary factors that may be associated with increased risk of various cancers. Currently, there is no scientific evidence that consuming artificial sweeteners, such as aspartame; coffee; fluoridated water; genetically modified foods; or foods preserved by radiation (*irradiated foods*) causes cancer.[33] However, physical activity and some dietary practices may *reduce* the risk of cancer.

Nutrition and Physical Activity Cancer Prevention

Consuming a nutritious diet that contains adequate fluids and a variety of foods, especially plant foods, may prevent or delay the development of certain cancers. Drinking enough water and other nonalcoholic fluids may reduce the risk of bladder cancer, because water dilutes carcinogens that may be present in urine.[34] Adequate fluid intake also encourages frequent urination, which reduces the time that carcinogens remain in contact with the walls of the bladder.

High intakes of fruits and vegetables may reduce the risk of cancer.[33] Fruits and vegetables are rich sources of vitamin C as well as carotenoids and other phytochemicals that may have antioxidant activity in the body. Antioxidants protect DNA from free radical damage, preventing potentially cancer–causing mutations from occurring. Although research is ongoing, results of scientific studies generally do not provide evidence that taking dietary supplements that contain antioxidants reduces the risk of cancer.[33] Some medical experts are concerned that taking antioxidant supplements may *increase* the risk of lung and prostate cancers, especially among smokers and men with family histories of prostate cancer.

Many plant foods naturally contain chemicals that reduce carcinogens' ability to damage DNA. Other phytochemicals inhibit tumor growth by being toxic to cancer cells, interfering with their ability to form supportive blood vessels, or creating conditions that make it difficult for cancer cells to flourish. For example, broccoli, cabbage, Brussels sprouts, and other *cruciferous (crew–siff'–er–us)* vegetables; and *turmeric (tur'–mur–ik)*, a spice found in curry powder, contain substances that are toxic to cancer cells. Medical researchers do not know whether taking supplements that contain phytochemicals offers the same benefits as consuming the chemicals in their natural forms. Currently, much of the evidence about the cancer–protective benefits of specific plant–based chemicals is from laboratory experiments on animals or cell cultures. Testing the chemicals in clinical settings is necessary to determine whether the results observed in laboratories also occur in people. Thus, more research is needed to support the use of phytochemicals to prevent or treat cancer.

Reducing the Risk Although medical researchers are studying the cancer–fighting potential of various chemicals naturally in food, no major breakthroughs have occurred. Avoiding obesity by establishing healthy eating and physical activity habits, especially early in life, may reduce the risk of cancer. According to results of epidemiological studies, people who exercise regularly have lower risks of certain cancers, including colon and breast cancer. Regular physical activity may reduce the risk by helping to control weight, improving immune system functioning, and enhancing the body's regulation of various hormones. Following the American Cancer Society's recommendations does not guarantee zero risk of cancer. As mentioned earlier in this "Nutrition Matters" section, an individual's cancer risk is ultimately determined by the complex interaction of numerous factors, not just diet and physical activity. However, people may be able to reduce their risk of many types of cancer significantly by improving their dietary choices and increasing their physical activity.

At this point, the best course of action is to take steps to prevent cancer. According to the American Cancer Society, people can change their diets to reduce their risk of cancer by:

- limiting alcohol consumption;
- achieving and maintaining a healthy weight;
- adopting a physically active lifestyle;
- eating a healthy diet that limits intakes of red and processed meats and emphasizes intakes of plant foods, including fruits, vegetables, and whole grains.[33]

Concept **Checkpoint 8.5**

13. Which form of cancer is the leading cause of cancer deaths in the United States?
14. Margaret's breast cancer metastasized to her lungs. Define *metastasize*.
15. List three dietary factors that may contribute to cancer.
16. List three steps people can take to reduce their risk of cancer.

Chapter References

See Appendix H.

Summary

8.1 Vitamins: Basic Concepts

- Vitamins are organic compounds that the body cannot synthesize or make enough of to maintain good health; that naturally occur in commonly eaten foods; that cause deficiency disease when they are missing from diets; and that restore good health when added back to the diet.

- Vitamins play numerous roles in the body, and each vitamin generally has more than one function. In general, vitamins regulate a variety of body processes, including those involved in cell division and development as well as the growth and maintenance of tissues. Vitamins are not a source of energy. Some vitamins have precursors that do not function as vitamins until the body converts them into active forms.

- An oxidation reaction can form a radical. Radicals damage or destroy molecules by removing electrons from them. Cells normally regulate oxidation reactions by using antioxidants such as vitamin E.

- Vitamins A, D, E, and K are fat-soluble vitamins; thiamin, riboflavin, niacin, vitamin B-6, pantothenic acid, folate, biotin, vitamin B-12, and vitamin C are water-soluble vitamins. The body stores extra fat-soluble vitamins. Over time, these vitamins can accumulate and cause toxicity. Water-soluble vitamins are generally not as toxic as fat-soluble vitamins.

- The enrichment program specifies amounts of thiamin, riboflavin, niacin, and folic acid and the mineral iron that manufacturers must add to their refined wheat flour and certain other milled grain products. Fortification involves the addition of one or more vitamins (and/or other nutrients) to a wide array of commonly eaten foods during manufacturing. The vitamins that are added may or may not be in the food naturally.

- Vitamin deficiency disorders generally result from inadequate diets or conditions that increase the body's requirements for vitamins, such as reduced intestinal absorption or higher-than-normal excretion of the micronutrients. Severe vitamin deficiencies are uncommon in the United States. The chances of developing a vitamin deficiency disease increase when the diet consistently lacks the micronutrient and levels of the nutrient in the body become depleted.

- Most commonly eaten foods do not contain toxic levels of vitamins. Vitamin toxicity is most likely to occur in people who take megadoses of vitamin supplements or consume large amounts of vitamin-fortified foods regularly.

8.2 Fat-Soluble Vitamins

- Vitamin A is involved in vision, immune function, and cell development. The vitamin A precursor, beta-carotene, functions as an antioxidant. Dietary sources of preformed vitamin A include liver, fish, and fish oils; provitamin A carotenoids are especially plentiful in dark green and orange fruits and vegetables. Excess vitamin A can be quite toxic and cause birth defects when taken during pregnancy.

- Vitamin D is both a hormone and a vitamin. Exposure to sunlight enables human skin to synthesize a precursor of the vitamin from a cholesterol-like substance. The body can convert this substance to the active form of the vitamin. A few foods, including fatty fish and fortified milk, are dietary sources of the vitamin. Vitamin D helps regulate the level of blood calcium by increasing calcium absorption from the intestine. Infants and children who do not obtain enough vitamin D may develop rickets, and adults with inadequate amounts of the vitamin in their bodies may develop osteomalacia. Older people and breastfed infants often need a supplemental source of the vitamin. Excess intakes of vitamin D can cause the body to deposit calcium in soft tissues.

- Vitamin E functions primarily as an antioxidant. By donating electrons to electron-seeking compounds, vitamin E neutralizes them. Plant oils and products made from these oils are generally rich sources of vitamin E.

8.3 Water-Soluble Vitamins

- Thiamin, riboflavin, and niacin play key roles as part of coenzymes in energy-yielding reactions. These water-soluble vitamins help cells metabolize carbohydrates, fats, and proteins. Enriched grain products are common sources of all three of the vitamins. Beriberi is the severe thiamin deficiency disease; pellagra results from a severe lack of niacin. Excess intakes of niacin can cause toxicity.

- Vitamin B-6 is involved in protein metabolism, especially in synthesizing nonessential amino acids. The vitamin also participates in the synthesis of neurotransmitters and the metabolism of homocysteine. Healthy people can obtain enough vitamin B-6 by eating a varied diet that contains animal foods and rich plant sources of the micronutrient. High doses of vitamin B-6 should be avoided because the vitamin can cause nervous system damage.

- Folate plays important roles in DNA synthesis and homocysteine metabolism. Rich food sources of folate are leafy vegetables, organ meats, and orange juice. Signs of folate deficiency include megaloblastic anemia. Pregnancy increases the body's needs for folate; a deficiency during the first month of pregnancy can result in neural tube defects in offspring. Women of childbearing age can meet the RDA for the vitamin by taking dietary supplements that contain synthetic folic acid. Excess folate in the diet can mask a vitamin B-12 deficiency.

- The body needs vitamin B-12 to metabolize folate and homocysteine, and maintain the insulation surrounding nerves. Although vitamin B-12 does not occur naturally in plant foods, the vitamin is in animal foods and products that have been fortified with the micronutrient. Vitamin B-12 deficiency is more common in older adults. As people age, they produce less HCl, which can result in B-12 deficiency even though adequate amounts of the micronutrient are consumed in foods. Loss of intrinsic factor production in the stomach also causes vitamin B-12 deficiency and a condition called pernicious anemia.

- The body uses vitamin C to synthesize and maintain collagen, a major protein in connective tissue. Vitamin C also functions as an antioxidant. Fresh fruits and vegetables, especially citrus fruits, are generally good sources of the micronutrient. Because vitamin C is readily lost in cooking, diets should emphasize fresh or lightly cooked fruits and vegetables. Smoking increases the body's requirement for vitamin C. Scurvy is the vitamin C deficiency disease. Excess vitamin C may cause diarrhea and increase the risk of kidney stones in some people.

8.4 Vitamins as Medicines

- Although the health benefits of vitamin supplementation remain uncertain, there is consistent epidemiological evidence that a diet high in fruits, vegetables, and legumes may lower the risk of CVD, cancer, and other serious chronic disease. Consuming a wide variety of vitamins, antioxidants, and phytochemicals in their natural states and concentrations (in foods) may be the most effective way to achieve good health. Therefore, people should consume a variety of fruits and vegetables daily rather than take vitamin or antioxidant supplements.

8.5 Nutrition Matters: Diet and Cancer

- Cancer occurs when genes that regulate cellular growth, division, and death mutate, resulting in abnormal cell development, rapid cell growth, and unchecked cell division. Maintaining a healthy body weight, exercising regularly, consuming diets that supply plenty of fruits and vegetables, limiting intakes of red and/or processed meats, and avoiding tobacco smoke and excess alcohol may reduce the risk of cancer.

Recipe for Healthy Living

Stir-Fried Vegetable Medley

"Eat your vegetables!" Does this order bring back some not-so-fond dinnertime memories? If you are like many Americans, cooked vegetables were not high on your list of favorite foods when you were a child. Corn on the cob was fun to eat, but you may have picked at your peas and carrots, and refused to eat broccoli unless it was smothered in a gooey cheese sauce. You probably drew a "line in the sand" when offered Brussels sprouts. Now that you have read Chapter 8, you should appreciate the nutritional contribution that a wide variety of colorful vegetables can make to your diet. Your parents told the truth when they said, "Vegetables are good for you."

This vegetable medley can be the foundation of a vegetarian meal or a colorful accompaniment to main dishes. You don't need to use all the vegetables in the recipe; feel free to improvise, especially when certain fresh vegetables are in season and plentiful. If you use fresh vegetables, wash them in cool water and drain on paper towels before cutting them into bite-size pieces. If you use frozen vegetables, add them directly to the hot oil, without thawing them first. Be careful because ice from the vegetables can cause hot oil to spatter.

Your goal is to heat the vegetables in a small amount of hot oil only until they are still colorful and crisp—about 4 to 8 minutes. Add the quicker-cooking vegetables (for example, mushrooms) last, so they don't overcook. Use a slotted spoon to drain oil from vegetables and serve immediately.

This recipe (without rice or noodles) makes about four ½-cup servings. Each serving supplies approximately 107 kcal, 3 g protein, 7 g fat, 3 g fiber, 45 mg vitamin C, and 43 mcg folate.

INGREDIENTS:

1 Tbsp low-sodium soy sauce
2 Tbsp water
1 Tbsp brown sugar
⅛ tsp ground black pepper
2 Tbsp vegetable oil
1 large garlic clove, minced
½ cup onions, sliced
1 cup asparagus, cut into 2"-long pieces
½ cup broccoli, small pieces
½ cup carrots, sliced into "coins"
½ medium green pepper, cut in 2" strips, about ¼" wide
½ medium sweet red pepper, cut in 2" strips, about ¼" wide
6 button mushrooms, crosscut into quarters

PREPARATION STEPS:

1. In a small dish, prepare mixture of soy sauce, water, and brown sugar. Set aside.
2. Heat oil in a wok or large deep frying pan over medium-high heat. Add garlic and onions. Stir.
3. When onions and garlic are translucent, add asparagus, broccoli, carrots, peppers, and mushrooms. Stir mixture constantly to coat vegetables with oil.
4. Add soy sauce, water, and brown sugar mixture.
5. Add zucchini. Sprinkle black pepper over vegetables.
6. Do not overcook. If the mixture seems too dry, add another tablespoon of water.
7. Serve immediately over cooked rice or noodles.

Further analyze this and other recipes through activities on Connect at www.mcgrawhillconnect.com.

Personal Dietary Analysis

Using the DRIs

1. Refer to your 1- or 3-day food log from the "Personal Dietary Analysis" feature in Chapter 3.

   a. Find the RDA values for vitamins under your life stage/sex group category in the DRI tables (see Tables A through F at the end of this book). Write those values under the "My RDA " column in the table on the following page.

   b. Review your personal dietary assessment. Find your 3-day average intakes of vitamins A, E, C, D, folate, B-12, thiamin, riboflavin, and niacin. Write those values under the "My Average Intake" column of the table.

   c. Calculate the percentage of the RDA you consumed for each vitamin by dividing your intake by the RDA amount and multiplying the figure you obtain by 100. For example, if your average intake of vitamin C were 100 mg/day, and your RDA for the vitamin were 75 mg/day, you would divide 100 mg by 75 mg to obtain 1.25. To multiply this figure by 100, simply move the decimal point two places to the right, and replace the decimal point with a percentage sign (125%). Thus, your average daily intake of vitamin C was 125% of the RDA. Place the percentages for each vitamin under the "% of My RDA" column.

   d. Under the ">, <, or =" column, indicate whether your average daily intake was greater than (>), less than (<), or equal to (=) the RDA.

2. Use the information you calculated in the first part of this activity to answer the following questions:

   a. Which of your average vitamin intakes equaled or exceeded the RDA value?

   b. Which of your average vitamin intakes was below the RDA value?

   c. What foods would you eat to increase your intake of the vitamins that were less than the RDA levels? (Review sources of certain vitamins in Chapter 8.)

   d. Turn in your completed table and answers to your instructor.

Personal Dietary Analysis: Vitamins

Vitamin	My RDA	My Average Intake	% of My RDA	>, <, or =
A				
E				
C				
D				
Folate				
B-12				
Thiamin				
Riboflavin				
Niacin				

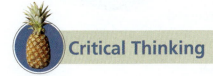

Complete this Personal Dietary Analysis activity online at www.mcgrawhillconnect.com.

Critical Thinking

1. Choose a vitamin and type the nutrient's name in the search box of an Internet browser. Locate three sites that sell products containing the vitamin. Review the pages of each site, making notes about claims, prices, and the kinds of links provided. Then write a three-to five-page report that describes and compares the information you found at the sites. In your paper, discuss any claims made on behalf of these products that you consider false or misleading. Include the URLs for the sites mentioned in your report.

2. Choose three different websites that sell vitamin supplements. Choose three different products and compare prices for the same product at the different websites. Then compare prices of the vitamins from these sites with the prices you would pay at a local supermarket, discount department store, or drugstore. Make sure to compare products with the same chemical composition (single vitamin, for example) and that have the same amount of the vitamin in each dose. Write a one-page report about your findings.

3. While watching an infomercial on TV, you hear a so-called nutrition expert make claims for a substance that he or she claims to be a vitamin. What questions would you ask the expert to ascertain whether the substance truly is a vitamin?

4. One of your friends takes megadoses of vitamin A, C, B-6, and E because she thinks they help her stay healthy. What would you tell her about taking such large doses of these vitamins?

5. According to MyPlate, a person who needs 2000 kcal/day should consume 2 cups of fruit and 2.5 cups of vegetables daily. Plan a day's meals and snacks that provide these amounts of fruits and vegetables. In your plan, incorporate foods you like to eat. For information concerning how much of a certain form of fruit or type of vegetable equals 1 cup, visit http://www.choosemyplate.gov/MyPlate and click on the "Fruits" and then the "Vegetables" tabs.

Practice Test

Select the best answer.

1. Megadoses of vitamins
   a. are safe to take, if the vitamins are water soluble.
   b. prevent certain chronic diseases.
   c. are available naturally from a wide variety of foods.
   d. may be toxic.

2. Vitamins
   a. are metabolized to yield energy.
   b. occur in gram amounts in foods.
   c. are organic molecules.
   d. are macronutrients.

3. People who are unable to absorb fat are likely to develop a _____ deficiency.
   a. vitamin A
   b. folate
   c. vitamin B–12
   d. riboflavin

4. Enriched grain products have specific amounts of _____ added during processing.
   a. vitamin C
   b. vitamin A
   c. vitamin B–12
   d. thiamin

5. The vitamin content of a vegetable can be affected by
   a. soil composition.
   b. the vegetable's maturity when harvested.
   c. sunlight exposure.
   d. All of the above are correct.

6. Which of the following foods is not a rich source of pro–vitamin A?
   a. beef
   b. carrots
   c. squash
   d. sweet potato

7. Children who lack vitamin D can develop
   a. pellagra.
   b. rickets.
   c. beriberi.
   d. scurvy.

8. During pregnancy, excess _____ intake is known to be teratogenic.
   a. vitamin A
   b. biotin
   c. vitamin K
   d. folate

9. Lack of vitamin _____ causes scurvy.
   a. A
   b. C
   c. D
   d. K

10. Vitamin K can be produced by
    a. skin exposure to ultraviolet radiation.
    b. hydrolysis of seawater.
    c. intestinal bacteria.
    d. conversion of lactic acid into lactate.

11. Diets that lack niacin can lead to
    a. rickets.
    b. beriberi.
    c. pellagra.
    d. pernicious anemia.

12. To reduce the likelihood of giving birth to babies with neural tube defects, women of childbearing age should obtain adequate

    a. folate.
    b. biotin.
    c. cellulose.
    d. niacin.

13. Major food sources of vitamin B−12 include

    a. enriched grain products.
    b. meat and milk products.
    c. fruit and vegetables.
    d. nuts and seeds.

14. Which of the following statements is false?

    a. Intrinsic factor is needed for vitamin B−12 absorption.
    b. Vitamin B−12 deficiency is common among elderly persons.
    c. Patients with pernicious anemia are treated with high doses of folic acid.
    d. If untreated, pernicious anemia can be deadly.

15. Which of the following foods is a rich source of vitamin C?

    a. whole milk
    b. egg white
    c. hamburger patty
    d. green pepper

16. Which of the following practices may reduce your risk of cancer?

    a. eating fruits and vegetables
    b. eating grilled meats regularly
    c. smoking no more than 10 cigarettes daily
    d. consuming two to three standard alcoholic drinks daily

LEARNSMART®
ADVANTAGE

Get the most out of your study of nutrition with McGraw-Hill's innovative suite of adaptive learning products including McGraw-Hill LearnSmart®, SmartBook®, LearnSmart Achieve®, and LearnSmart Prep®. Visit www.learnsmartadvantage.com.

Answers to Quiz Yourself

1. Natural vitamins are better for you because they have more biological activity than synthetic vitamins. **False.** (p. 261)

2. Certain vitamins are toxic. **True.** (p. 259)

3. Vitamin E is an antioxidant. **True.** (p. 277)

4. Vitamins are a source of "quick" energy. **False.** (p. 259)

5. According to scientific research, taking large doses of vitamin C daily prevents the common cold. **False.** (p. 299)

CHAPTER 9

Water and Minerals

Quiz Yourself

Can water be toxic when consumed in excess? What is osteoporosis? Which foods are rich sources of iron? Test your knowledge of water and minerals by taking the following quiz. The answers are on page 369.

1. Your body constantly loses water through insensible perspiration, a form of water loss that is not the same as sweat. _____T _____ F

2. Ounce per ounce, cottage cheese contains more calcium than plain yogurt. _____ T _____ F

3. Potassium, sodium, and chloride ions are involved in fluid balance. _____ T _____ F

4. Selenium is an essential mineral. _____ T _____ F

5. In general, plants are good sources of iron because the plant pigment chlorophyll contains iron. _____ T _____ F

connect | NUTRITION   www.mcgrawhillconnect.com

A wealth of proven resources are available on Connect® Nutrition including McGraw-Hill LearnSmart®, SmartBook®, NutritionCalc Plus, and many other dynamic learning tools. Ask your instructor about Connect!

9.1 Introducing Water and Minerals

Learning Outcomes

1 Explain what can happen when dehydration occurs.

2 Classify mineral nutrients as major, trace, or possible essential minerals.

3 Explain the difference between a major mineral and a trace mineral.

In late August 1997, a 19—year—old student wrestler who weighed 233 pounds attended a university in North Carolina. The young man was anxious to lose enough weight to qualify for the 195—pound weight class when the collegiate wrestling season began later that semester. By November 6, the wrestler had lost 23 pounds, but the first tournament was to be held in 2 days and he was still 15 pounds too heavy. To lose ("cut") the extra weight, he engaged in an intense, almost nonstop training session. In a 12—hour period that spanned November 6 and 7, the wrestler restricted his water and food intake severely. Addition—ally, he wore a special suit made from a rubberized material that was *vapor impermeable*, and he even covered it with a cotton warm—up outfit. By wearing this combination of clothing, the young man perspired profusely. Sweating can cause the body to lose a significant amount of "water weight"; however, sweat—ing can also cause **dehydration** (body water depletion), especially when a person restricts his or her fluid intake. Severe dehydration is a life—threatening condition that requires urgent medical care.

At 3 P.M. on November 6, the college wrestler began exercising vigorously in a hot environment. By 11:30 P.M. that night, he had lost 9 pounds. After resting for about 2 hours, the young man resumed his exercise regimen in a desperate effort to lose the remaining 6 pounds. Around 2:45 A.M. on November 7, he had to discontinue exercising: he was extremely fatigued and unable to communicate. An hour later, he stopped breathing and his heart ceased beating. Attempts to revive him were unsuccessful. **Hyperthermia** (very high body temperature) is likely to have contributed to his death.[1]

The rapid weight—loss practices that resulted in the death of the young wrestler were prohibited by National Collegiate Athletic Association (NCAA) regulations. However, many wrestlers were determined to lose enough weight prior to a meet so they could gain a competitive edge by wrestling in weight categories that were lower than their preseason weights. Today, NCAA rules prohibit wrestlers from losing weight rapidly by any means, including restrict—ing food and fluid intakes excessively. Failure to follow the NCAA's wrestling guidelines can result in suspension from competition.

We often take water for granted, but this simple molecule is highly essen—tial. You can survive for weeks, even months, if your diet lacks carbohydrates, lipids, proteins, and vitamins. But if you do not have any water, your life will end within a week or two.

Many of water's functions involve certain minerals. About 15 min—eral elements have known functions in the body and are necessary for human health. The body requires these particular micronutrients in milligram or microgram amounts. The essential minerals are classified into two groups: **major minerals** and **trace minerals** (Table 9.1). If we require 100 mg or more of a mineral per day, the mineral is classified as a major mineral; otherwise, the micronutrient is a trace mineral. The body also contains very small amounts of

dehydration body water depletion

hyperthermia very high body temperature

major minerals essential mineral elements required in amounts of 100 mg or more per day

trace minerals essential mineral elements required in amounts that are less than 100 mg per day

315

TABLE 9.1 Minerals with Known or Possible Roles in the Body*

Major Mineral	Trace Mineral	Possible Essential Mineral
Calcium (Ca)	Chromium (Cr)	Arsenic (As)
Chloride (Cl⁻)	Fluoride (F⁻)**	Boron (B)
Magnesium (Mg)	Copper (Cu)	Lithium (Li)
Phosphorus (P)	Iodine (I)	Nickel (Ni)
Potassium (K)	Iron (Fe)	Silicon (Si)
Sodium (Na)	Manganese (Mn)	Vanadium (V)
Sulfur (S)	Molybdenum (Mo)	
	Selenium (Se)	
	Zinc (Zn)	

* Chemical symbol is shown in parentheses next to mineral's name.

** Although fluoride is not essential, the mineral plays an important role in strengthening teeth and bones.

other minerals, such as nickel and arsenic. The essential nature of this particular group of minerals has not been fully determined, so we will refer to them as "possible essential minerals" (see Table 9.1).

The mineral nutrients are key components of body structures and play vital roles in metabolism, water balance, muscle movement, and various physiological processes. Mineral deficiencies can cause serious health problems and, in severe cases, death. In this chapter, we will focus on water first and then discuss mineral nutrients, some of which are of major concern for public health officials in the United States and other parts of the world.

Concept **Checkpoint 9.1**

1. What is the difference between a major mineral and a trace mineral?
2. List at least five trace minerals.
3. List at least five major minerals.

9.2 Water

Learning Outcomes

1 Discuss the functions of water in the body as well as typical sources of intake and loss.

2 Identify foods that have high and low water contents.

3 Discuss how the body maintains its water balance.

4 Explain why dehydration and water intoxication can be life-threatening conditions.

Compared to other nutrients, water is so unusual, it is in a class by itself. Water is a simple compound: A molecule of water is comprised of two hydrogen atoms and one oxygen atom (H_2O). Water does not need to be digested, and it is easily absorbed by the intestinal tract.

Depending on a person's age, sex, and body composition, 50 to 75% of his or her body is water weight. Lean muscle tissue contains more water (about 73%) than fat tissue (about 20%). On average, young adult men have more lean tissue than young women. Approximately 60% of an average young man's body weight is water; the average young adult woman's body has more fat and, therefore, slightly less water than an average young man's body. A person's percentage of body weight that is water declines from birth to old age.[2]

Water is a major solvent; many substances, including glucose, dissolve in water. Water often participates directly in chemical reactions, such as those involved in digesting food. Water's other physiological roles include transporting substances, removing waste products, lubricating tissues, and regulating body temperature and acid–base balance (proper blood pH). Furthermore, water is a major component of blood, saliva, sweat, tears, mucus, and the fluid in joints. Table 9.2 lists roles of water in the body. Although water has numerous functions in the body, this unique nutrient does not provide energy.

Membrane Transport

One reason why water is such a vital nutrient is its role in helping cells obtain materials from their environment and eliminate wastes. To understand some of water's functions in the body, it is necessary to understand how water–soluble substances can become distributed when they are in water. In some instances, substances move by **simple diffusion,** that is, they move from where they are highly concentrated to where they are less concentrated (Fig. 9.1). For example, simple diffusion occurs when a sugar cube is dropped into a cup of hot tea. As the cube dissolves, the concentration of sugar molecules around the cube becomes higher than the concentration of sugar molecules near the surface of the tea. However, the sugar molecules spontaneously diffuse throughout the tea, and eventually, the concentration of sugar molecules and water molecules becomes evenly distributed within the beverage.

TABLE 9.2 Functions of Water in the Body

Water
is a solvent
is a major component of blood, saliva, sweat, tears, mucus, joint fluid
removes wastes
helps transport substances
lubricates tissues
regulates body temperature
helps digest foods
participates in many chemical reactions
helps maintain proper blood pH

Did You Know?

The layer of fat that is under the skin (*subcutaneous fat*) interferes with the transfer of heat to the skin. This explains why overweight people who are in warm conditions are more uncomfortable and perspire more than slender people.

Figure 9.1 Simple diffusion. Simple diffusion can occur when there is a greater concentration of a substance in one region than in another. In this example, the dye is more concentrated on the left side of the container than on the right side. Eventually, the dye molecules diffuse (move) from where they are more concentrated to where they are less concentrated. The diffusion stops when the dye molecules are equally distributed throughout the container.

simple diffusion movement of substances from a region of higher to lower concentration

Simple diffusion also occurs when there is a greater concentration of substances on one side of a *selectively permeable membrane* than on the other. A **selectively permeable membrane** is a barrier that allows the passage of certain substances and prevents the movement of other substances through it. **Osmosis** is the diffusion of a solvent, such as water, through a selectively permeable membrane, such as the plasma membrane of a human cell. The concentration of substances dissolved in the water, such as glucose, influences osmosis. Water moves from a region that has less material dissolved in it (dilute) to a region that has more material dissolved in it (Fig. 9.2). The diffusion stops when the concentrations of the material on either side of the plasma membrane are equal.

To survive, a human cell carefully controls the passage of substances through its plasma membrane. Some materials, such as oxygen and carbon dioxide, easily pass through the cell's plasma membrane by simple diffusion. Large molecules, such as proteins, may be unable to pass through the cell's membrane, unless there are special carrier molecules to help them enter the cell. Chapter 4 discussed other ways cells can obtain substances from their environment.

Body Water Distribution

The body has two major fluid compartments: intracellular water and extracellular water (Fig. 9.3). **Intracellular water** is inside cells. **Extracellular water** surrounds cells (tissue fluid) or is the fluid portion of blood (*plasma*). About two-thirds of the body's water is in the intracellular compartment.

The body maintains the balance of compartmental fluids and proper **hydration,** water status, primarily by controlling concentrations of ions in each compartment. Recall from Chapter 4 that ions are elements or small molecules that have electrical charges. Ions that conduct electricity, such as sodium and potassium ions, are called *electrolytes*. Table 9.3 lists several mineral ions that function in the body.

Maintenance of intracellular water volume depends to a large extent on the intracellular concentration of potassium and phosphate ions. On the other hand, maintenance of extracellular water volume depends primarily on the extracellular concentration of sodium and chloride ions. Changes in the normal

selectively permeable membrane barrier that allows the passage of certain substances and prevents the movement of other substances

osmosis diffusion of a solvent, such as water, through a selectively permeable membrane

intracellular water water that is inside cells

extracellular water water that surrounds cells or is in liquid portion of blood

hydration water status

Figure 9.2 Osmosis. Osmosis is the diffusion of a solvent, such as water, through a selectively permeable membrane. Water moves from a compartment that is less concentrated to a compartment that has more material dissolved in it.

Selectively permeable membrane

Side A   Side B

Time

Start   **30 minutes later**

Figure 9.3 **Fluid compartments in the body.** Intracellular water is inside cells; extracellular water surrounds cells (tissue fluid) or is the fluid in blood (*plasma*). Water is exchanged between plasma and tissue fluid (green arrows) as well as between tissue and intracellular fluids (black arrows).

concentrations of these ions can cause water to shift out of one compartment and move into the other. For example, if extracellular fluid has fewer than normal sodium ions, water moves from the extracellular compartment into cells. When this occurs, the cells swell and can burst (Fig. 9.4a). On the other hand, if extra-cellular fluid has an excess of sodium ions, water moves out of cells. As a result, the cells shrink and die because they lack enough intracellular fluid to function (Fig. 9.4b). Recall from Chapter 7 that edema occurs when an excessive amount of water moves into the space surrounding cells (see Fig. 7.1). To function normally, the body must maintain intracellular and extracellular water volumes within certain limits.

TABLE 9.3   Some Common Ions (Minerals)

Sodium (Na^+)
Calcium (Ca^{2+})
Potassium (K^+)
Magnesium (Mg^{2+})
Chloride (Cl^-)
Phosphate (PO_4^{3-})
Sulfate (SO_4^{2-})

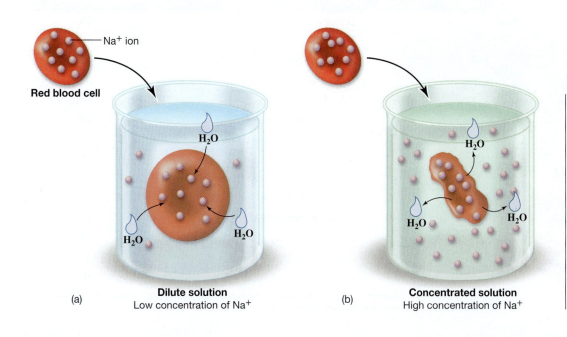

(a) Dilute solution Low concentration of Na^+

(b) Concentrated solution High concentration of Na^+

Figure 9.4 **Maintaining proper hydration.** Cells, such as red blood cells, need to maintain their fluid balance. The cell in beaker (*a*) is placed in a solution that contains few sodium ions (Na^+) in relation to the concentration of Na^+ in the cell. As a result, water moves from the solution and into the red blood cell. The cell can swell and burst. The solution in beaker (*b*) has an excess of sodium ions (Na^+) compared to the concentration of Na^+ inside the cell. Water moves out of the red blood cell placed in beaker (*b*). As a result, the cell shrinks, and can die.

Sources of Water

How much water is necessary to drink for good health? Contrary to popular belief, there is no "rule of thumb" recommendation that specifies how many glasses of water to consume each day.[3] Factors such as environmental temperatures, health conditions, physical activities, and dietary choices influence individual water requirements. Thus, total water intakes vary widely. **Total water intake** refers to water ingested by consuming beverages and foods.

The Adequate Intake (AI) for *total* water intake is approximately 11 cups (2.7 L) for young women and approximately 15.5 cups (3.7 L) for young men.[4] These amounts do not need to be consumed in the form of water. Other sources of water include fruit juice, milk, soup, coffee, tea, soft drinks, and flavored bottled water. Most solid foods also contain some water. Fruits and vegetables appear to be solid, but they generally contain 60 to 95% water weight. Table 9.4 lists some commonly consumed foods and their water content by weight. About 80% of our total water intake is from water and other beverages; food supplies the remaining amount of our water intake.[4]

In addition to the water in beverages and foods, a considerable amount of water enters the digestive tract daily through secretions from the mouth, stomach, intestine, pancreas, and gallbladder. The intestinal tract absorbs most of this water, too. Each day, only about 0.4 to 0.8 cup (approximately 100 to 200 ml) of the water that enters the digestive tract is not absorbed. The body eventually eliminates the unabsorbed water in feces.

Cells also form some water as a by-product of metabolism ("metabolic water"). **Metabolic water** also contributes to the body's fluid balance.

The Essential Balancing Act

An average healthy adult consumes and produces approximately 2.6 quarts (2500 ml) of water daily (Fig. 9.5).[2] The body eliminates about 2.6 quarts of water in urine, exhaled air, feces, and perspiration (see Fig. 9.5). Thus, a healthy person's average daily water input equals his or her average daily losses (output).

total water intake water in beverages and foods

metabolic water water formed by cells as a metabolic by-product

TABLE 9.4 How Much Water Is in That Food or Beverage?

Food	Water % by Weight
Lettuce	95
Tomato	95
Watermelon	91
Milk, 1% fat	90
Apple, with skin	86
Avocado (Florida)	79
Potato, white, baked with skin	75
Banana	75
Chicken, white meat, roasted	65
Ground beef, 80% lean, broiled	56
Bread, whole wheat	39
Margarine, stick	16
Crackers, saltines	5
Vegetable oil	0

Source: Data from U.S. Department of Agriculture, Agricultural Research Service, USDA Nutrient Data Laboratory: *USDA national nutrient database for standard reference, Release 26, 2013.*

Metabolic water 200 ml	Food 700 ml	Drink 1600 ml

Intake
2500 ml/day

Output
2500 ml/day

Expired air 300 ml	Insensible perspiration 400 ml	Sweat 100 ml	Urine 1500 ml	Feces 200 ml

Figure 9.5 Daily water balance. An average healthy adult consumes and produces approximately 2500 ml of water and eliminates about 2500 ml of water daily. Thus, a healthy person's average daily water input equals his or her average daily losses.

Various factors influence a person's fluid input and output. Environmental factors such as temperature, humidity, and altitude can affect body water losses. Physiological conditions, especially fever, vomiting, and diarrhea, as well as life—style practices, such as exercise habits and sodium and alcohol intakes, can also alter the body's fluid balance.

Perspiration is body water that is secreted by sweat glands in skin. When perspiration reaches the skin's surface, it evaporates into the air. This process helps cool the body and maintain its normal temperature. *Insensible perspiration* is body water that diffuses through the layers of skin or is exhaled from the lungs instead of being secreted by sweat glands.[3] People are usually unaware that their bodies are constantly losing water in this manner; hence, the term *insensible* perspiration.

Kidneys and Hydration

The kidneys are the major regulator of the body's water content and ion concen—trations. In a healthy person, the kidneys maintain proper hydration by filtering excess ions from blood as it flows through the kidney's tissues. When the kidneys remove ions such as sodium, water follows and becomes the main component of urine. If you drink more watery fluids than your body needs, your kidneys excrete the excess water in urine.

Kidneys also remove drugs and metabolic waste products, such as urea, from the bloodstream. Sometimes, minerals and waste products settle out of urine and collect into crystals. If the crystals enlarge and form a hard mass, the object is called a kidney stone (Fig. 9.6). Kidney stones often contain the mineral calcium.[2] As a kidney stone moves out of the kidney and enters the tube leading to the bladder, it may cause considerable pain and bloody urine until it passes out of the body. Dehydration increases the likelihood of forming kidney stones.

Water Conservation

As mentioned in the opener of this chapter, body water depletion is called dehy—dration. Dehydration can be a life—threatening condition. When you are hot and perspiring heavily, your kidneys try to conserve as much water as possible to

Figure 9.6 Kidney stones. Some people form kidney stones. Although small enough to fit on a fingertip, such stones can be quite painful when they move from the kidneys and are eliminated in urine.

Figure 9.7 Effects of antidiuretic hormone and adolsterone on kidneys. In response to dehydration, the posterior pituitary gland in the brain secretes antidiuretic hormone (ADH), which signals the kidneys to conserve water. Additionally, the adrenal glands secrete the hormone aldosterone. Aldosterone reduces urinary excretion of sodium. When the kidneys retain sodium, they return the mineral to the general circulation.

antidiuretic hormone (ADH) hormone that participates in water conservation

aldosterone hormone that participates in sodium and water conservation

diuretic substance that increases urine production

avoid dehydration. **Antidiuretic hormone (ADH)** and **aldosterone** ($al-dahs'-te-rown$) are two hormones that participate in the body's efforts to maintain fluid balance. In response to dehydration, the posterior pituitary gland in the brain releases antidiuretic hormone. Antidiuretic hormone stimulates the kidneys to conserve water. Additionally, the adrenal glands secrete aldosterone. Aldosterone signals kidneys to reduce the elimination of sodium in urine and, as a result, the kidneys return the mineral and water to the general circulation. The diagram in Figure 9.7 summarizes the effects of antidiuretic hormone and aldosterone on the kidneys.

The simplest way to determine if you are consuming enough water is to notice the amount of urine you eliminate. When your fluid intake is adequate, your kidneys will produce enough urine to maintain fluid balance. If you consume more fluid than needed, your kidneys will eliminate the excess, and you will produce plenty of urine. On the other hand, if you limit your fluid intake or have high fluid losses such as in sweat, you will produce small amounts of urine.

In addition to urine volume, the color of urine may be a useful indicator of hydration status. Straw–colored (light yellow) urine can indicate adequate hydration, whereas dark–colored urine may be a sign of dehydration. However, the color of urine is not always a reliable guide for judging a person's hydration status.[5] It is important to recognize that having urinary tract infections or ingesting certain medications, foods, and dietary supplements, especially those containing the B–vitamin riboflavin, can alter urine's color.

What Is a Diuretic?   Caffeine is a **diuretic,** a substance that increases urine production. Coffee, tea, energy drinks, and soft drinks often contain caffeine or caffeine–related compounds. However, the water consumed in caffeinated beverages is not completely lost in urine, so drinking these fluids may still contribute to meeting your water needs.[4]

Alcohol is also a diuretic. Normally, antidiuretic hormone signals the kidneys to conserve water. Alcohol, however, inhibits ADH secretion from the pituitary gland in the brain, enabling the kidneys to eliminate more urine than normal. Alcohol consumption actually results in urinary water losses that are greater than the volume of fluid consumed. Therefore, alcohol contributes to dehydration.

Scientists do not know what causes a "hangover," the headache and overall discomfort that occurs a few hours after drinking too much alcohol. Dehydration, the body's immune response, and *congeners* may be responsible for the unpleasant, delayed side effects of excess alcohol consumption.[6] Congeners are substances in alcoholic drinks that contribute to the taste and color of the beverages. (Beer and vodka have lower congener contents than red wine and whiskey.) Alcoholic drinks with high congener contents tend to produce more severe hangovers than drinks with lower contents of these substances.

Dehydration

Despite the body's mechanisms to balance its water content, some fluid is constantly being lost, primarily via the skin and lungs. If a person does not consume enough fluids to replace that water, dehydration can occur. Rapid weight loss is a sign of dehydration. Every 16 ounces (about 0.5 L) of water that the body loses represents a pound of body weight. If you lose 1 to 2% of your usual body weight in fluids, you will feel fatigued and thirsty. If you weigh 150 pounds, for example, and your weight drops 3 pounds after exercising in hot conditions, you have lost 2% of your body weight, primarily as water weight.

As the loss of body water approaches 4% of body weight, muscles lose considerable amounts of strength and endurance. By the time body weight is reduced by 7 to 10% as a result of body fluid losses, severe weakness results. At a 20% reduction of body weight, coma and death are likely.

Thirst is the primary regulator of fluid intake.[2] The thirst response alerts you to the need to replenish water that was lost by sweating and other means. The majority of healthy people meet their AI for water by letting thirst be their guide.[4] Thirst stimulates people to drink fluids *before* severe dehydration occurs. However, people who are dehydrated and older than 60 years of age do not sense thirst as accurately as younger adults.[7] Furthermore, older adults may be more susceptible to developing dehydration than younger persons, because as kidneys age, they become less able to conserve water when fluid intakes are low. Therefore, it may be necessary to remind older adults to drink more watery fluids, especially when they are physically active or in warm conditions. Nevertheless, healthy elderly persons are generally able to maintain adequate hydration.[7]

People who are sick, especially children with fever, vomiting, diarrhea, and increased perspiration, may need to be given special solutions of water and electrolytes to prevent dehydration. Athletes and other people who work or exercise outdoors, especially in hot conditions, also need to stay properly hydrated to avoid dehydration and heat-related illnesses such as heat exhaustion. Chapter 11 provides information about heat-related illnesses.

People who work or exercise outdoors, especially in hot conditions, need to stay hydrated to avoid dehydration and heat-related illnesses.

Did You Know?

A massive earthquake struck the island nation of Haiti on January 12, 2010, devastating a region that included the island's highly populated major city, Port-au-Prince. As a result of the earthquake, many Haitians had no access to drinkable water. People can survive for a few days in such conditions before dehydration contributes to their deaths.

Can Too Much Water Be Toxic?

There is no Upper Limit (UL) for water. **Water intoxication,** however, can occur when an excessive amount of water is consumed in a short time period or the kidneys have difficulty filtering water from blood. The excess water dilutes the sodium concentration of blood, disrupting water balance. As a result of the imbalance, too much water moves into cells, including brain cells. Signs and symptoms of water intoxication may include dizziness, headache, confusion, inability to

water intoxication condition that occurs when too much water is consumed in a short time period or the kidneys have difficulty filtering water from blood

Marathon runners who consume large amounts of plain water in an effort to keep hydrated during competition may be at risk of water intoxication.

Cheese is a good source of calcium, phosphorus, and sodium.

coordinate muscular movements, bizarre behavior, and seizures.[8] If the condition is not detected early and treated effectively, coma and death can result.

Healthy people rarely drink enough water to become intoxicated. However, water intoxication can develop in people with disorders that interfere with the kidney's ability to excrete water normally. Marathon runners who consume large amounts of plain water in an effort to keep hydrated during competition may be at risk of water intoxication. Chapter 11 discusses the importance of proper hydration for athletes.

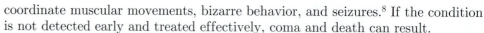

Concept **Checkpoint 9.2**

4. List at least five different functions of water in the body.
5. Define osmosis.
6. Which ions are found primarily in extracellular water? Which ions are found primarily in intracellular water?
7. Discuss ways the body obtains and loses water.
8. What can happen to cells if the body is unable to regulate its water balance?
9. How do antidiuretic hormone and aldosterone help maintain fluid balance in the body?
10. How much water do healthy young men and women need to consume daily (AI values)?
11. What is a diuretic? Identify two diuretics commonly consumed by Americans.
12. List at least three signs and symptoms of dehydration.
13. List at least three signs and symptoms of water intoxication.

9.3 Minerals: Basic Concepts

Learning Outcomes

1. Identify general functions of minerals in the body.
2. Discuss factors that influence the body's ability to absorb and use minerals.
3. Describe factors that can affect retention of minerals during food preparation.

Minerals, such as iron and calcium, are a group of elements in Earth's rocks, soils, and natural water sources. Plants, animals, and other living things cannot synthesize minerals. Plants obtain the minerals they need from soil or fertilizer; animals generally obtain minerals when they consume plants and other animals or substances that contain these elements. About 15 mineral elements have known functions in the body and are necessary for human health.

Several minerals, including lead and mercury, are often found in the human body, but they are environmental contaminants that have no known functions. The body can eliminate most minerals in urine. However, exposure to excessive amounts of minerals can cause toxicity.

Unlike vitamins, minerals are indestructible. Because minerals cannot be destroyed, heating a food or exposing it to most other environmental conditions will not affect the food's mineral content. However, minerals are water soluble, and they can leach out of a food and into cooking water. By using the cooking water to make soups or sauces, you can obtain minerals from the food that would otherwise be discarded.

Why Are Minerals Necessary?

Essential minerals have diverse roles in the body (Fig. 9.8). Some minerals form inorganic structural components of tissues, such as calcium and phosphorus in bones and teeth. Minerals may also function as inorganic ions, substances that have negative or positive charges (see Chapter 4). For example, calcium ions (Ca^{2+}) participate in blood clotting and sodium ions (Na^+) help maintain fluid balance. Phosphate ions participate in acid–base balance. Some ions, such as magnesium (Mg^{2+}) and copper (Cu^{2+}), are cofactors. A **cofactor** is an ion or molecule that activates certain chemical reactions. Many minerals are components of various enzymes, hormones, or other organic molecules, such as cobalt in vitamin B–12, iron in hemoglobin, and sulfur in the amino acids methionine and cysteine. Although cells cannot metabolize minerals for energy, certain minerals are involved in chemical reactions that release energy from macronutrients.

In some instances, the digestive tract absorbs more minerals than the body needs, but the excess is excreted, primarily in urine or feces. In other instances, the body stores the extra minerals in the liver, bones, or other tissues. Toxicity signs and symptoms occur when minerals accumulate in the body to such an extent that they interfere with the functioning of cells. Under normal conditions, the human body does not store large quantities of most minerals, and it loses small amounts of these essential elements every day. Therefore, people should choose their diets carefully so their bodies can maintain an adequate supply of minerals.

cofactor ion or molecule that activates certain chemical reactions

Figure 9.8 Minerals and their functions. Groups of minerals work together to maintain good health.

Bone Health

Calcium
Phosphorus
Iron
Zinc
Copper
Manganese
Fluoride
Magnesium

Fluid Balance

Sodium
Potassium
Chloride
Phosphorus
Magnesium

Blood Clotting

Calcium

Transmission of Nerve Impulses

Sodium
Potassium
Chloride
Calcium

Red Blood Cell Formation

Iron
Copper

Muscle Contraction and Relaxation

Sodium
Potassium
Calcium
Magnesium

Cellular Metabolism

Iron
Calcium
Phosphorus
Magnesium
Zinc
Chromium
Iodide
Copper
Manganese

Antioxidant Defense

Selenium
Zinc
Copper
Manganese

Growth and Development

Calcium
Phosphorus
Zinc

Sources of Minerals

Although most foods contain small amounts of minerals, Figure 9.9 indicates food groups from MyPlate that are generally rich sources of various minerals. The digestive tract, however, does not absorb 100% of the minerals in foods or dietary supplements. The body's ability to absorb and use minerals (*bioavailability*) depends on many factors. A major factor is the body's need for the mineral. In general, requirements increase during periods of growth, such as infancy and puberty, and during pregnancy and breastfeeding. During these critical life stages, the bioavailability of minerals also tends to increase to help meet the body's demand.

Compared to plant foods, animal foods tend to be more reliable sources of minerals, such as iron and calcium. Why? Animal products often have higher concentrations of these minerals. Additionally, plant foods can contain substances that reduce the bioavailability of minerals, particularly calcium, zinc, and iron. On the other hand, plants supply more magnesium and manganese than animal foods.

In general, the more processing a plant food undergoes, the lower its natural mineral content. Cereal grains, for example, naturally contain selenium, zinc, copper, and some other minerals, but these micronutrients are lost during refinement. Iron is the only mineral added to grains during enrichment. To obtain a variety of minerals, include some whole-grain products in your diet each day. By following the recommendations of MyPlate (see Chapter 3) and eating a variety of plant and animal foods, you are likely to obtain adequate amounts of all essential minerals.

Figure 9.9 MyPlate: Good sources of minerals. Each MyPlate food group contributes minerals to the diet.

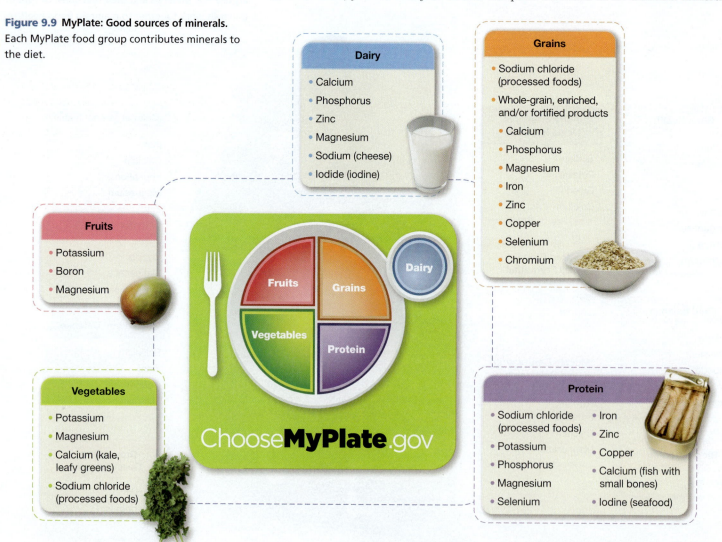

Dairy
- Calcium
- Phosphorus
- Zinc
- Magnesium
- Sodium (cheese)
- Iodide (iodine)

Grains
- Sodium chloride (processed foods)
- Whole-grain, enriched, and/or fortified products
- Calcium
- Phosphorus
- Magnesium
- Iron
- Zinc
- Copper
- Selenium
- Chromium

Fruits
- Potassium
- Boron
- Magnesium

Vegetables
- Potassium
- Magnesium
- Calcium (kale, leafy greens)
- Sodium chloride (processed foods)

Protein
- Sodium chloride (processed foods)
- Potassium
- Phosphorus
- Magnesium
- Selenium
- Iron
- Zinc
- Copper
- Calcium (fish with small bones)
- Iodine (seafood)

ChooseMyPlate.gov

To estimate the mineral contents of packaged foods, you can check the panels on food labels. Daily Values have been established for several mineral nutrients (see Appendix B).

Other Sources of Minerals

The tap water in your community may be a source of minerals that you may have overlooked. Fluoride is often added to public water supplies. Although fluoride is not essential for life, the mineral strengthens bones and teeth when consumed in adequate amounts. "Hard" water naturally contains a variety of minerals, including calcium, magnesium, sulfur, iron, and zinc. Water with high mineral content often tastes and smells unpleasant. Many people drink bottled water as a substitute for tap water because they think bottled water tastes better and it is safer. To learn more about bottled water, read the "Nutrition Matters" section at the end of this chapter.

Dietary supplements are another source of minerals. A daily multiple vitamin and mineral supplement is generally safe for healthy people, because a dose of this type of supplement does not provide high amounts of minerals. However, people need to be careful when taking dietary supplements that contain individual min-erals, such as iron or selenium. Many minerals have a narrow range of safe intake; therefore, it is easy to consume a toxic amount, especially by taking supplements that contain only a particular mineral (Fig. 9.10). Additionally, an excess of one mineral can interfere with the absorption or metabolism of other minerals. For example, the presence of a large amount of zinc in the intestinal tract decreases copper absorption. Single–mineral supplements are usually unnecessary unless they are prescribed to treat a specific medical condition, such as iron deficiency.

Figure 9.10 Mineral intake. Many minerals have a narrow range of safe intake. As a result, it is relatively easy to consume a toxic amount, especially by taking supplements that only contain a particular mineral.

Concept **Checkpoint 9.3**

14. List at least three different functions of minerals in the body, and provide an example of a mineral that performs each function.
15. Explain how foods that are naturally good sources of minerals can become poor sources of those minerals by the time you eat them.
16. Discuss factors that influence mineral absorption in the digestive tract.
17. In the United States, which mineral is added to grain products as part of the enrichment program?

9.4 Major Minerals

Learning Outcomes

1 List key functions and good food sources of the major mineral nutrients.

2 Discuss deficiency and toxicity disorders associated with the major minerals.

3 Discuss hypertension and osteoporosis, including risk factors.

4 Discuss ways to improve intakes of major minerals without relying on dietary supplements.

This section focuses on the major minerals. Table 9.5 summarizes nutrition–related information about these micronutrients. Unless otherwise noted, RDA/AI values are for adults, excluding pregnant or breastfeeding women. For more information about Dietary Reference Intake values for minerals, see the last pages of this textbook.

TABLE 9.5   Summary of Major Minerals

Mineral	Major Functions in the Body	Adult RDA/AI (adult RDA = bold)	Major Dietary Sources	Major Deficiency Signs and Symptoms	Major Toxicity Signs and Symptoms
Calcium (Ca)	• Structural component of bones and teeth • Blood clotting • Transmission of nerve impulses • Muscle contraction • Regulation of metabolism	**1000–1200** mg	Milk and milk products, canned fish, tofu made with calcium sulfate, leafy vegetables, calcium-fortified foods such as orange juice	• Increased risk of osteoporosis • May increase risk of hypertension	UL = 2.0 to 2.5 g/day • Intakes > 2.5 g/day may cause kidney stones and interfere with absorption of other minerals.
Sodium (Na)	• Maintenance of proper fluid balance • Transmission of nerve impulses • Muscle contraction • Transport of certain substances into cells	1500 mg (19–50 years of age)	Table salt; luncheon meats; processed and canned foods; pretzels, chips, and other snack foods; condiments; sauces	• Muscle cramps	UL = 2300 mg/day • Contributes to hypertension in susceptible individuals • Increases urinary calcium losses
Potassium (K)	• Maintenance of proper fluid balance • Transmission of nerve impulses	4700 mg	Fruits, vegetables, milk, meat, legumes, whole grains	• Irregular heartbeat • Muscle cramps	No UL has been determined. • Slowing of heart rate that can result in death
Magnesium (Mg)	• Strengthens bone • Cofactor for certain enzymes • Heart and nerve functioning	Men: **400–420 mg** Women: **310–320 mg**	Wheat bran, green vegetables, nuts, chocolate, legumes	• Muscle weakness and pain • Poor heart function	UL = 350 mg/day (medication-related) • Diarrhea
Phosphorus (P)	• Structural component of bones and teeth • Maintenance of acid-base balance • Component of DNA, phospholipids, and other organic compounds	**700 mg**	Dairy products, processed foods, soft drinks, fish, baked goods, meat	• None reported	UL = 4 g/day • Poor bone mineralization
Chloride (Cl⁻)	• Maintenance of proper fluid balance • Production of stomach acid • Maintenance of acid-base balance	2300 mg (19–50 years of age)	Processed foods, salty snacks, table salt	• Convulsions (observed in infants)	UL = 3600 mg/day • Hypertension (because of the association with sodium in sodium chloride [table salt])
Sulfur (S)	• Component of organic compounds such as certain amino acids and vitamins	None	Protein-rich foods	• None reported	• Unlikely from dietary sources

Calcium (Ca)

Calcium is the most plentiful mineral element in the human body. All cells need calcium, but more than 99% of the body's calcium is in an inorganic compound that forms the structural component of bones and teeth. The remaining calcium is in muscle tissue and extracellular fluid.

Why Is Calcium Necessary?

Although the body needs calcium to form bones and teeth, the mineral is vital to all cells. Calcium is involved in muscle contraction, blood clot formation, nerve impulse transmission, and cell metabolism. Additionally, calcium may play important roles in maintaining healthy blood pressure and functioning of the immune system.

Maintaining Normal Blood Calcium Levels   The body has complex hormonal systems to maintain calcium homeostasis. The thyroid and parathyroid glands help regulate blood calcium levels (Fig. 9.11). In response to falling blood calcium levels, the parathyroid glands secrete **parathyroid hormone (PTH),** which signals special bone cells called **osteoclasts** to tear down bone tissue. This process releases calcium from bones so the mineral can enter the bloodstream. PTH also works with vitamin D to increase intestinal calcium absorption and reduce calcium excretion in urine (see Fig. 8.13).

When the level of calcium in blood is too high, the thyroid gland secretes the hormone **calcitonin** (*cal'–sih–toe'–nin*). Calcitonin signals another type of bone cell **(osteoblasts)** to remove excess calcium from blood and build bone tissue. All these physiological responses help maintain your blood calcium level within the normal range.

Did You Know?

Bone remodeling occurs throughout life, and as a result of this process, most of your skeleton is replaced about every 10 years.[9]

parathyroid hormone (PTH) hormone secreted by parathyroid glands when blood calcium levels are too low

osteoclasts bone cells that tear down bone tissue

calcitonin hormone secreted by the thyroid gland when blood calcium levels are too high

osteoblasts bone cells that add bone to where the tissue is needed

Thyroid

Larynx
"voice box"

Thyroid
gland

Trachea
"windpipe"

Pharynx

Posterior of
thyroid gland

Parathyroid
glands

Esophagus

Trachea
"windpipe"

Anterior (front) view   **Posterior (back) view**

Figure 9.11 **Thyroid and parathyroid glands.** Four parathyroid glands are imbedded in the back (posterior) of the thyroid.

Bone Development and Maintenance   Although your bones do not appear to change shape, they are being remodeled continually in response to the physical stresses placed on them. The remodeling process involves breaking down bone where there is little stress and building bone where there is more stress. For example, if you begin to play tennis regularly and hold the racket in your right hand, osteoblasts in the bones of your right arm build bone tissue where it is needed to help support the muscular activity. As a result, the bones in that arm become denser than the bones in your left arm. Bones that are denser have greater bone mass. As a result, they are stronger and less likely to fracture than less dense bones. Figure 9.12 shows x–rays of bone tissue. By just looking at the photos, can you tell which bone is denser and has greater mass?

Figure 9.12 **Bone tissue.** Normal spine tissue is on the left; the spine tissue on the right is from a person with osteoporosis.

MY DIVERSE PLATE

Bok Choy (Pak Choi or Chinese Cabbage)

Bok choy is a cruciferous vegetable that is typically used in Asian cookery. Cruciferous vegetables contain phytochemicals that may have cancer-fighting activity. The leaves and stalks are steamed or sautéed with other vegetables. Bok choy is a good source of minerals, especially iron, calcium, and potassium; the vegetable also contains high amounts of vitamin C.

Sources of Calcium

Table 9.6 includes some foods that are among the richest sources of calcium. Milk products, such as fluid milk, yogurt, and cheese, provide about 75% of the calcium in American diets.[10] Moreover, the calcium in milk products is well absorbed and used by the body. Not all products made from milk are rich sources of calcium. Cottage cheese, for example, does not supply as much calcium as the milk from which it is made, because the milk loses about half of its calcium content when it is processed to make cottage cheese (see Table 9.6). Although butter, sour cream, and cream cheese are made from whole milk, people generally do not eat enough of these high−fat foods to contribute much calcium to their diets.

Certain foods from plants contain calcium, but the foods also contain *phytic* (fi′−tik) *acid* or *oxalic* (awk−sal′−ik) *acid*, naturally occurring substances that interfere with calcium absorption. Phytic acid is a compound in whole grains and in certain seeds and beans. Spinach, collard greens, and sweet potatoes have high amounts of oxalic acid. In fact, rhubarb leaves are toxic because they contain such high amounts of the chemical.

Good plant sources of calcium include broccoli and leafy greens, especially kale, collard, turnip, bok choy, and mustard greens. Nevertheless, the calcium in plant foods is generally not as bioavailable as the calcium in milk and milk products. For example, 1 cup of fat−free milk supplies almost 300 mg of calcium, and about 30% of the calcium in milk is bioavailable.[11] A cup of raw spinach supplies 30 mg of calcium, but only about 13% of that amount is bioavailable. Figure 9.13 shows approximately how much cooked spinach, broccoli, and kale a person would need to eat to obtain about the same amount of calcium that is in 1 cup of fat−free milk.[12]

TABLE 9.6 Calcium Content of Selected Foods

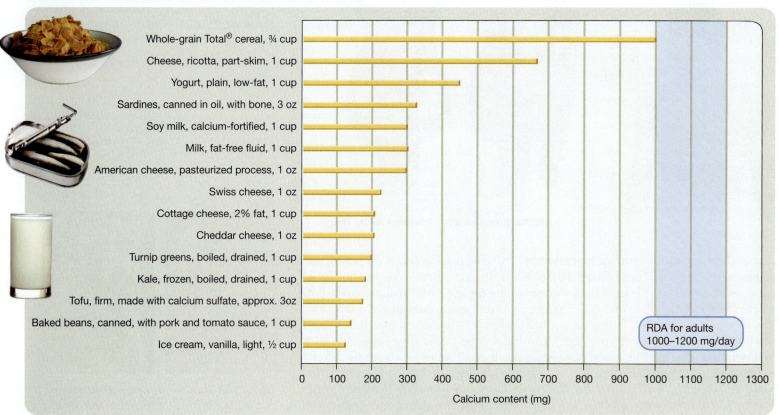

Source: Data from U.S. Department of Agriculture, Agricultural Research Service: *USDA national nutrient database for standard reference, Release 26,* 2013.

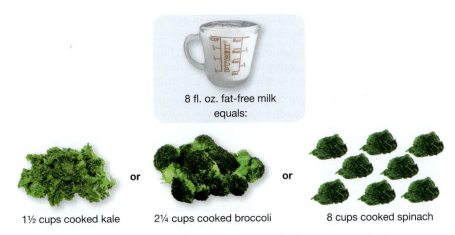

8 fl. oz. fat-free milk equals:

1½ cups cooked kale   **or**   2¼ cups cooked broccoli   **or**   8 cups cooked spinach

Figure 9.13 Calcium bioavailability of various foods. To obtain approximately the same amount of calcium that is in 8 fluid ounces of fat-free milk, you would need to consume the amounts of the foods shown.

Calcium is added to a variety of foods, including fortified orange juice, margarine, soy milk, cereals, and breakfast bars. Another source of calcium is soybean curd (tofu) that is made with calcium sulfate. Figure 9.14 indicates food groups from MyPlate that are good sources of calcium.

Calcium Supplements Many adults find it difficult to consume enough milk products and other calcium–rich foods to achieve adequate intakes of the mineral. Thus, taking calcium supplements or antacids that contain calcium has become a common practice, especially among older adults. If you choose to take a cal–cium supplement, consider products that include vitamin D, because the vitamin

Did You Know?

Certain brands of antacids contain calcium carbonate. These products can be an inexpensive way of obtaining some calcium. An antacid pill that contains 750 mg of calcium carbonate provides 300 mg of elemental calcium. To avoid calcium toxicity, consumers should avoid taking too many calcium-containing antacids.

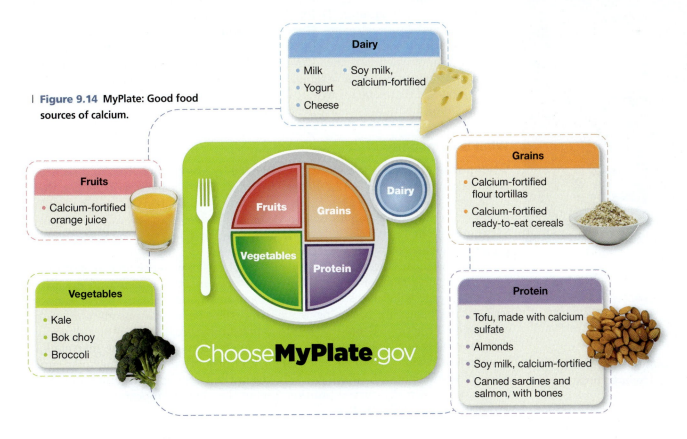

| **Figure 9.14** MyPlate: Good food sources of calcium.

Dairy
- Milk
- Yogurt
- Cheese
- Soy milk, calcium-fortified

Grains
- Calcium-fortified flour tortillas
- Calcium-fortified ready-to-eat cereals

Fruits
- Calcium-fortified orange juice

Vegetables
- Kale
- Bok choy
- Broccoli

Protein
- Tofu, made with calcium sulfate
- Almonds
- Soy milk, calcium-fortified
- Canned sardines and salmon, with bones

ChooseMyPlate.gov

Each of the following foods contains about the same amount of calcium that is in 1 cup of fat-free milk (approximately 300 mg):

   1.5 cups low-fat (2% milk) cottage cheese

   1 oz processed cheese (American cheese)

   ⅔ cup plain, low-fat yogurt

   1.5 oz natural cheese (e.g., cheddar or Swiss)

   1 cup calcium-fortified soy milk

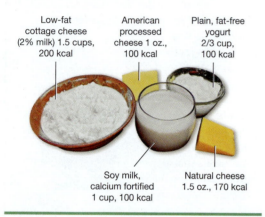

Low-fat cottage cheese (2% milk) 1.5 cups, 200 kcal

American processed cheese 1 oz., 100 kcal

Plain, fat-free yogurt 2/3 cup, 100 kcal

Soy milk, calcium fortified 1 cup, 100 kcal

Natural cheese 1.5 oz., 170 kcal

| **Figure 9.15** Osteoporosis.

hypercalcemia condition characterized by higher-than-normal concentration of calcium in blood

osteoporosis chronic disease characterized by loss of bone mass and reduced bone structure

enhances calcium absorption. Taking only 500 mg of calcium at a time and ingesting the supplement with meals will also improve the mineral's absorption. Dietary supplements, including calcium supplements, may have a "seal of approval" displayed on the label. A seal of approval indicates that the supplement was properly manufactured, contains the ingredients that are listed on the label, and does not contain harmful levels of contaminants. However, seals of approval are not a guarantee that products are safe or effective.[13]

Dietary Adequacy

The adult RDA for calcium ranges from 1000 to 1200 mg/day. In the United States, average calcium intakes were 1146 mg/day for men and almost 900 mg/day for women in 2009–2010.[14] Thus, women consumed less than the RDA for calcium, whereas most men had intakes that were close to the RDA. Total vegetarians (vegans) and people who are lactose-intolerant are at risk of calcium deficiency, because they often avoid consuming milk and milk products, the most reliable dietary sources of calcium. According to the Dietary Guidelines, calcium is a "nutrient of public health concern" (see Chapter 3).

Healthy adults absorb about 30% of the calcium in foods, but this percentage varies, depending on the type of food.[10] During stages of life when the body needs extra calcium—such as infancy and pregnancy—absorption can be as high as 60%. Vitamin D enhances calcium absorption.

Older people, especially women, do not absorb calcium as well as younger people. Thus, recommendations for calcium intakes are higher for people over 70 years of age than for younger adults. In addition to advanced age, other factors that reduce calcium absorption include vitamin D deficiency and diarrhea.

Calcium Toxicity   The Upper Level (UL) for calcium is 2000 to 2500 mg/day. Normally, the small intestine prevents too much calcium from being absorbed. However, taking too many calcium-containing antacids or supplements, or drinking too much vitamin D-fortified milk can result in excessive calcium absorption and hypercalcemia. **Hypercalcemia** (*hyper* = excess; *calcemia* = calcium in the blood) is a condition characterized by a higher-than-normal concentration of calcium in blood. Signs and symptoms of hypercalcemia include bone pain, muscle weakness, fatigue, and people with hypercalcemia can develop kidney stones. Treatment for hypercalcemia may include avoiding vitamin D and calcium supplements to reduce calcium absorption.

What Is Osteoporosis?

Osteoporosis is a chronic disease characterized by loss of bone mass and reduced bone structure (see Fig. 9.12). People with osteoporosis have weak bones that are susceptible to fractures. In the United States, osteoporosis is a major public health problem. More than 10 million Americans have osteoporosis, and another 34 million are at risk of the disease because they have loss of bone mass.[10] Most people with osteoporosis are older adult women.

Each year, an estimated 1.5 million Americans experience an osteoporosis-related fracture. Half of women and up to one-fourth of men who are over 50 years of age will have such a fracture at some point.[15] Many people do not realize their bones are becoming weaker and they have osteoporosis until they experience a fracture. People with osteoporosis may break a bone by falling, or they may experience spontaneous fractures, in which the fragile bone shatters for no apparent reason. Osteoporosis-related fractures often involve the spine, hip, wrist, or ankle bones. In severe cases, bones in the upper spine fracture and then heal in an abnormally curved position, giving the obvious appearance associated with osteoporosis (Fig. 9.15).

Fractures, especially hip fractures, can be devastating events for the elderly. One in five older Americans who experiences a broken hip dies within 1 year of the injury.[16]

What Causes Osteoporosis? Several factors, including smoking and lack of physical activity, contribute to bone loss and osteoporosis (Table 9.7). Note that some of the factors cannot be modified, but other factors can be changed to pre—vent or delay the development of the disease.

By 25 years of age, most healthy young men and women have acquired all of their adult bone mass.[16] Regardless of one's sex, loss of bone tissue begins in mid—adulthood. In men, bone loss is slow and steady beginning around age 30. In women, however, the rate of bone loss increases significantly after *meno—pause*, that is, after menstrual cycles have ceased. At this time of life, women have the highest risk of osteoporosis. Why? The sex hormones **testosterone** and **estrogen** are needed for normal bone development and maintenance. In women of childbearing age, ovaries are the primary source of estrogen. After menopause, a woman's ovaries no longer produce estrogen, and as a result, her rate of bone loss exceeds the rate of bone replacement. Because estrogen is so important to maintaining strong bones, young adult women should see a physician if they have signs of estrogen deficiency, such as irregular menstrual cycles.

A simple way to monitor bone mass is by tracking height. Losing an inch or more of adult height may be the first sign that a person has experienced fractures of the spine due to osteoporosis.[17] If osteoporosis is suspected, a person can undergo special painless x—ray testing to determine the extent of bone loss. Individuals with a family history of osteoporosis, men who have low testosterone levels, and women who are postmenopausal should ask their physician if testing to determine bone mineral density is necessary. Treatment for osteporosis may include certain medications, calcium and vitamin D supplements, and regular physical activity.[18]

Reducing the Risk of Osteoporosis Efforts to reduce the risk of osteoporosis should begin early in life. Proper diet and regular exercise are especially important from early childhood through late adolescence, because the body actively builds bone during these life stages. By following the recommendations of MyPlate, most

testosterone hormone needed for normal bone development and maintenance

estrogen hormone that plays a role in normal bone development and maintenance

TABLE 9.7 Risk Factors for Osteoporosis

Factors People Cannot Change:
Being a woman
Growing older
Having white or Asian ancestry (confers the highest risk)
Having a family history of osteoporosis
Having a small, thin-boned body frame

Factors People Can Change:
Having low estrogen levels in women, low testosterone levels in men
Having anorexia nervosa
Following long-term diets that contain inadequate amounts of calcium and vitamin D
Being physically inactive
Smoking cigarettes
Consuming excessive alcohol

Modified from http://www.niams.nih.gov/Health_Info/Bone/Osteoporosis/overview.asp

Certain leafy vegetables, such as bok choy and collard greens, contain calcium that is bioavailable.

Food & Nutrition tips

The following suggestions can add more calcium to your diet:

• Sprinkle grated low-fat cheeses on top of salads, bean or pasta dishes, and cooked vegetables.

• If you do not like the taste of plain fat-free milk, try adding a small amount of flavored syrup to the beverage. Two teaspoons of "lite" chocolate syrup add 50 kcal and some trace minerals to the milk.

• For a snack, melt a slice of low-fat cheese on half a whole-wheat bagel, whole-wheat crackers, or a slice of rye bread.

• If a recipe calls for water, substitute fat-free milk for water, if it is appropriate. For example, use fat-free milk when making cooked oatmeal or pancake batter.

• Add ¼ cup nonfat milk powder to 1 pound of raw ground meat when preparing hamburgers, meat-balls, or meatloaf.

• Make homemade smoothies by blending plain low-fat yogurt with fresh or frozen fruit and fat-reduced ice cream or sherbet (see "Recipe for Healthy Living" at the end of this chapter).

people can obtain adequate amounts of calcium from foods. Exposing skin to sun—light can stimulate the body's ability to form vitamin D, but some people will need to take calcium and vitamin D supplements.

Exercise training, especially performing weight—bearing activities, increases bone mass, because contracting muscles keep tension (physical stress) on bones.[19] Table 9.8 lists examples of weight—bearing and non—weight—bearing activities. Regardless of one's age, regular physical activity that includes weight—bearing muscular movements provides numerous benefits to health, such as improving balance and reducing the likelihood of falling.

Everyone needs to be concerned about his or her risk of osteoporosis and focus on maximizing bone mass while he or she is young. The interac—tive osteoporosis risk test at the International Osteoporosis Foundation's website

These older adults are performing tai chi, an activity that can improve balance and may reduce the likelihood of falling.

TABLE 9.8 Examples of Weight-Bearing and Non-Weight-Bearing Activities

Weight-bearing	Non-weight-bearing
Low-impact aerobics	Lying in bed
Basketball	Swimming
Running or jogging	Water aerobics
Walking	Cycling
Jumping rope	Traveling in reduced-gravity situations (e.g., space flight)
Dancing	
Hiking	
Stair climbing	
Strength training with weights	
Tennis and other racket sports	

(www.iofbonehealth.org/iof–one–minute–osteoporosis–risk–test) can help you determine whether you or someone you know is at risk for the disease.

Sodium (Na)

Salt is the primary source of sodium in American diets. The chemical commonly called "table salt" or simply "salt" is actually *sodium chloride*, a compound comprised of two minerals, sodium and chloride. A teaspoon of table salt supplies 2325 mg of sodium. (Unless otherwise noted, we will refer to sodium chloride simply as "salt" or "table salt.") The human digestive tract absorbs almost all of the sodium that is in foods and beverages.

Why Is Sodium Necessary?

As mentioned in the "Water" section of this chapter, sodium plays a major role in maintaining normal fluid balance. The mineral is also necessary for the transmission of impulses by nerves, for transporting small substances such as glucose and amino acids into cells, and for functioning of muscles.

Sources of Sodium

Most uncooked vegetables, raw meats, and grain products are naturally low in sodium. Thus, most of the sodium Americans consume is from the salt that is added to food during processing (including canning), during preparation, or at the table. As a food additive, salt enhances flavors and can prevent the growth of microorganisms responsible for food spoilage. Other food additives that contain sodium include sodium nitrate, sodium citrate, and *monosodium glutamate* (*MSG*), a seasoning that is often added to foods served in Chinese restaurants.

Salted snack foods, French fries, canned and dried soups, sauces and gravies, hot dogs and "deli" meats, cheeses, and pickled foods are high in sodium (Table 9.9). If you frequently eat these foods, your sodium intake is probably higher than recommended.

Dietary Adequacy

Humans require only about 180 mg of sodium per day, but the AI for adults under 51 years of age is 1500 mg/day. The AI for sodium does not apply for people who perspire heavily, such as marathon runners, or people who work in extremely hot conditions.[4] Sweat contains small amounts of sodium, chloride, and some other minerals. People who perspire extensively can lose large amounts of these minerals in their sweat.

Sodium Deficiency The typical North American's diet supplies far more sodium than the AI amount, and as a result, the average person is unlikely to become sodium deficient. A healthy body is able to regulate its sodium concentration effectively, but sodium depletion can occur in certain situations. A person who loses more than 2 to 3% of body weight as a result of excessive sweating is at risk of sodium depletion. In most cases, drinking fluids and simply eating some salty foods or adding salt to foods is usually effective for restoring the body's sodium content. However, endurance athletes may need to consume sports drinks during competition to avoid dehydration and sodium depletion. Salt tablets are generally not recommended for sodium replacement. Sodium depletion also can result from diarrhea or vomiting, especially in infants. In these cases, it is necessary to obtain medical care promptly to replace the lost fluids and electrolytes, because infants can develop dehydration rapidly.

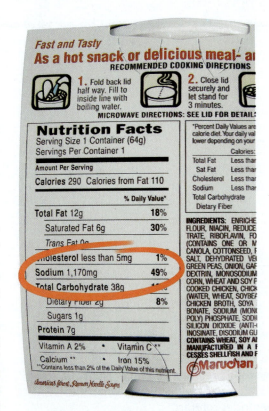

This dried soup product is high in sodium.

TABLE 9.9 Sodium Content of Selected Foods/Food Additives

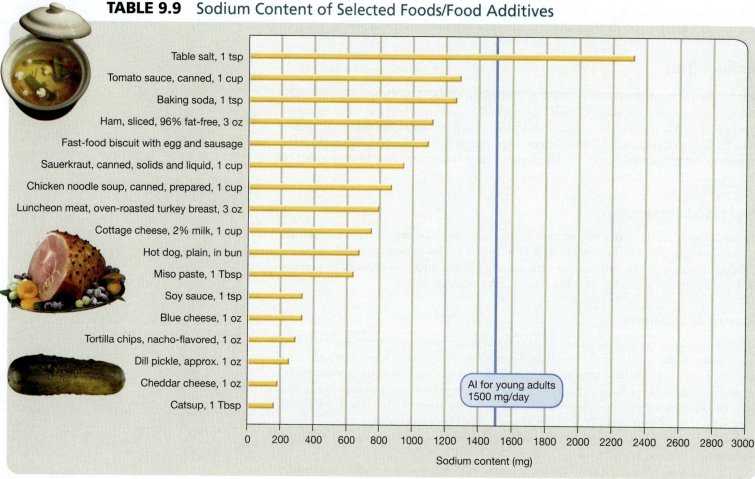

Food	Sodium content (mg)
Table salt, 1 tsp	~2325
Tomato sauce, canned, 1 cup	~1280
Baking soda, 1 tsp	~1260
Ham, sliced, 96% fat-free, 3 oz	~1130
Fast-food biscuit with egg and sausage	~1120
Sauerkraut, canned, solids and liquid, 1 cup	~940
Chicken noodle soup, canned, prepared, 1 cup	~870
Luncheon meat, oven-roasted turkey breast, 3 oz	~800
Cottage cheese, 2% milk, 1 cup	~760
Hot dog, plain, in bun	~680
Miso paste, 1 Tbsp	~640
Soy sauce, 1 tsp	~335
Blue cheese, 1 oz	~330
Tortilla chips, nacho-flavored, 1 oz	~280
Dill pickle, approx. 1 oz	~240
Cheddar cheese, 1 oz	~175
Catsup, 1 Tbsp	~155

AI for young adults 1500 mg/day

Source: Data from U.S. Department of Agriculture, Agricultural Research Service: *USDA national nutrient database for standard reference, Release 26*, 2013.

Sodium Toxicity The adult UL for sodium is 2300 mg/day. On average, Americans consumed more than 3400 mg of sodium per day in 2009–2010.[14] According to the results of numerous studies, high salt (sodium chloride) intakes are associated with increased risk of hypertension.[20] The Dietary Guidelines recommend limiting sodium intake to less than 2300 mg/day. To evaluate your sodium intake, take the "Sodium Intake Assessment" on the following page.

Sodium and Hypertension Hypertension, a condition characterized by persistently elevated blood pressure, is a serious public health problem in the United States. Compared to people with normal blood pressure, hypertensive individuals have greater risk of cardiovascular disease (CVD), especially heart disease and stroke, as well as kidney failure and damage to other organs. Approximately one-third of adult Americans have hypertension.[21] Children can also develop hypertension. An estimated 3 to 5% of American children have chronically elevated blood pressure levels.[22] Hypertension is often called the "silent killer," because high blood pressure generally does not cause symptoms until the affected person's organs and blood vessels have been damaged.

The best way to detect hypertension is to have regular blood pressure screenings. When you have your blood pressure determined, two measurements are actually taken. The first measurement is the **systolic pressure,** which is the maximum blood pressure within an artery. This value occurs when the ventricles, the heart's pumping chambers, contract. The second measurement is the

systolic pressure maximum blood pressure within an artery that occurs when the ventricles contract

Sodium Intake Assessment

For each question, place a check in the column that best describes your sodium intake habits. How often do you . . .	Rarely	Occasionally	Often	Daily
1. Eat cured or processed meats ("deli" meats), such as bacon, sausage, hot dogs, ham, and other luncheon meats?				
2. Eat canned or frozen vegetables with sauce?				
3. Eat commercially prepared meals, main dishes, or canned or dehydrated soups?				
4. Eat processed cheeses, such as cheese spreads?				
5. Eat salted nuts, popcorn, pretzels, corn chips, or potato chips?				
6. Add salt to cooking water for vegetables, rice, or pasta?				
7. Add salt, seasoning mixes, salad dressings, or condiments—such as soy sauce, steak sauce, pickles, and catsup—to foods during preparation or at the table?				
8. Salt your food before tasting it?				
9. Ignore reading the Nutrition Facts panel for sodium content when buying foods?				
10. Choose menu items that are salty or with sauces when dining out?				

Scoring: The more checks you put in the "often" or "daily" columns, the higher your dietary sodium intake is.

Adapted from USDA: *Home and Garden Bulletin*, No. 232–6, April 1986.

diastolic pressure, which measures the pressure in an artery when the ventricles relax between contractions. The systolic value is always higher than the diastolic value. For adults, healthy blood pressure readings are less than 120/80 millimeters of mercury (mm Hg). After having your blood pressure measured, ask the clinician for your systolic and diastolic readings and keep a record of the values.

A person who is under physical or emotional stress can expect his or her blood pressure to rise temporarily. However, persistent systolic blood pressure readings of 120 mm Hg to 139 mm Hg and diastolic readings of 80 mm Hg to 89 mm Hg are signs of **prehypertension.** People with prehypertension are more likely to develop hypertension than people with normal blood pressure. If a person's blood pressure persists at systolic values that are greater than or equal to ($\geq$) 140 mm Hg and diastolic values that are $\geq$ 90 mm Hg, he or she has hypertension. Table 9.10 presents categories for blood pressure levels in adults.

diastolic pressure pressure in an artery that occurs when the ventricles relax between contractions

prehypertension persistent systolic blood pressure readings of 120 mm Hg to 139 mm Hg and diastolic readings of 80 mm Hg to 89 mm Hg

TABLE 9.10 Categories for Blood Pressure Levels in Adults (Ages 18 Years and Older)

Category*	Blood Pressure Level (mm Hg)	
	Systolic	Diastolic
Normal	< 120 and	< 80
Prehypertension	120 to 139 or	80 to 89
Hypertension	$\geq$ 140 or	$\geq$ 90

*When systolic and diastolic blood pressures fall into different categories, the higher category should be used to classify blood pressure level. For example, a person with a blood pressure of 160/80 mm Hg would be classified as having hypertension. In people who are older than 50 years, elevated systolic values are a more significant risk factor for heart disease and stroke than elevated diastolic readings.

Source: National Heart, Lung, and Blood Institute: *Your guide to lowering high blood pressure: Categories for blood pressure levels in adults.* ND. http://www.nhlbi.nih.gov/hbp/detect/categ.htm. Accessed January 12, 2014

What Causes Hypertension?   Most cases of hypertension do not have simple causes, but advanced age, African–American ancestry, obesity, physical inactivity, smoking cigarettes, and excess alcohol and sodium intakes are among the major risk factors for the condition (Table 9.11). Blood pressure usually increases as a person ages, probably in part because plaque builds up in arteries (atherosclerosis) and interferes with the normal functioning of the blood vessels. Healthy arteries are flexible tubes that expand with each heartbeat and recoil in between beats. Atherosclerotic arteries are less flexible and cannot expand as much as healthy arteries. As a result, the heart must work harder to pump blood through the stiff arteries and blood pressure becomes chronically elevated.

Obesity, a condition characterized by excessive amounts of body fat, is a major risk factor for hypertension. Physical inactivity is another leading risk factor related to hypertension. Obesity and physical inactivity are modifiable risk factors. By exercising and losing some excess fat, obese people who have hyper–tension may experience reductions in their blood pressure.[23]

Excessive alcohol intake increases the risk of hypertension. To reduce their chances of developing high blood pressure, people should avoid alcohol or limit their consumption to two or fewer drinks/day (men) and only one drink/day (women and older adults). Other important risk factors for hypertension include having diabetes and using tobacco.

Finally, a high–sodium diet is associated with increased risk of hyperten–sion.[21] Many medical researchers think some people are genetically "sodium sen–sitive." A person who is sodium sensitive is more likely to develop hypertension as a result of consuming a high–sodium diet than an individual who lacks this sensitivity.

As mentioned earlier, the Dietary Guidelines recommend consuming less than 2300 mg of sodium daily. One teaspoon of salt contains about 2300 mg of sodium. Members of high–risk populations, African–Americans, for example—may need to limit their sodium intake to less than this amount. People who are being treated for hypertension should check with their physician for advice concerning an acceptable sodium intake.

If you want to lower your sodium intake, try gradually reducing your use of salt and consumption of salty foods. By doing so, you will eventually become accustomed to the taste of less salty food. To replace salt as a seasoning, try using garlic, citrus juice, and herbs and spices to enhance the taste of foods. Furthermore, avoid buying seasonings with added salt, such as "garlic salt" or "onion salt," and check the ingredient list to purchase seasonings without added salt (garlic *powder* or onion *powder*) instead.

Information about a packaged food's sodium content is a mandatory com–ponent of the Nutrition Facts panel. If you take the time to read labels, you can find foods that have little or no salt added to them during processing. For

TABLE 9.11   Major Risk Factors for Hypertension

Family history
Advanced age
African-American ancestry
Obesity
Physical inactivity
Consuming excess sodium
Cigarette smoking
Consuming excess alcohol
Type 2 diabetes

Food & Nutrition tip

To reduce your sodium intake, consider taking these actions:

• Prepare homemade meals and snacks as much as possible so you have control over your salt intake.

• Do not add salt while preparing foods, even though instructions tell you to "add salt."

• Taste your food *before* salting it. Adjust to eating foods with less salt in them.

• Do not keep a salt shaker on your table.

• Read the Nutrition Facts panels before purchasing packaged foods to determine sodium contents of the items.

• When ordering items in restaurants, request that no salt be added to your food while it is being prepared.

example, an ounce of salted peanuts provides 230 mg of sodium; the same amount of unsalted peanuts has only 2 mg of sodium. The "Food & Nutrition Tip" feature on this page provides some suggestions for reducing your salt (sodium) intake.

Even if your blood pressure is normal now, it is important to have regular blood pressure checks as you grow older, because the risk of hypertension increases with age. Young adults, however, are not immune to hypertension. Justin Steinbruegge, the college student featured in "Real People, Real Stories" on page 340, was 18 when he found out he had hypertension. When was the last time you had your blood pressure measured? What were the systolic and diastolic values?

Treatment for hypertension usually includes taking certain medications, following dietary modifications, and making some other lifestyle changes (Table 9.12). The *Dietary Approaches to Stop Hypertension (DASH)* diet

By reading the label, you can find foods that have high amounts of added sodium. A serving of these chips provides about 10% of the maximum recommended amount of sodium for a day.

TABLE 9.12 Practical Steps to Reduce Your Risk of Hypertension

• Follow the dietary recommendations of MyPlate concerning fruit, vegetable, and low-fat milk intakes. Furthermore, consider using fresh fruit and nuts to replace some empty calories in your daily meals and snacks. (See Chapter 3 for more information about empty calories.)

• Reduce your consumption of salty foods and have your blood pressure checked regularly.

• Attain and maintain a healthy body weight.

• Incorporate more physical activity into your daily schedule. For example, walk more often and use steps instead of elevators or escalators.

• If you drink alcohol, consume alcoholic beverages in moderation—no more than two drinks/day for men and one drink/day for women and older adults.

• Avoid using tobacco products.

is low in sodium, total fat, and saturated fat, and high in fruits, vegetables, whole grains, and fat–free or low–fat dairy products. Research indicates that people can lower their blood pressure and reduce their risk of CVD by following the DASH diet, losing excess body fat, and increasing their physical activity level.[24] To obtain more information about this diet and some low–sodium recipes, visit the National Heart, Lung, and Blood Institute's website: http://www.nhlbi.nih.gov/health/health–topics/topics/dash .

Potassium (K)

Potassium is the primary positively charged ion in the intracellular fluid. In fact, most of the body's potassium is in cells. Like sodium, potassium plays a key role in maintaining proper fluid balance. Unlike sodium, potassium is associated with lower, rather than higher, blood pressure values. Potassium is also necessary for transmitting nerve impulses, contracting muscles, and maintaining normal

REAL PEOPLE | REAL STORIES

Justin Steinbruegge

In the spring of his senior year of high school, Justin Steinbruegge was surprised to learn that he had hypertension. "It was a huge shock. I had no signs or symptoms of hypertension. I didn't even know what hypertension was," says Justin. To manage his high blood pressure, he took medication prescribed by his physician, but he had difficulty controlling his sodium intake. "Eating pizzas and salty snacks seemed to keep my blood pressure on a never-ending roller coaster ride," he says.

"When I was 23, I enrolled in a police academy. Four months prior to entering the academy, I started an exercise program, and by the time classes began, I was running 35 or more miles a week. I thought I was in fantastic shape," says Justin, "but I was training too much, and my diet was horrible—loaded with too many processed foods and not enough fresh fruits, vegetables, and meats. I was ignorant about the importance of proper nutrition to good health."

After finishing at the top of his class at the police academy, Justin focused on improving his health. "I developed a healthy combination of diet and exercise that I continue to follow," he says. "I avoid eating out, and I try to cook everything myself. I eat mainly fresh meats, cheeses, nuts, fruits, and vegetables. I drink only water—no juice, soda, or alcohol.

"Exercise is also a necessary part of my healthy lifestyle... I work out 6 days a week, and I include lifting free weights, rowing, light running, and yoga in my exercise routine. I am able to maintain my weight between 165 to 175 pounds, and my body fat never goes above 13%," says Justin, who is is 6 feet, 1 inch tall. "My journey to achieving good health has become a rewarding experience. Now, I don't need to take blood pressure medicine."

kidney function. Potassium–rich diets, such as the DASH diet, may lower blood pressure.[25] A natural way to counteract high sodium intakes is to consume foods naturally rich in potassium and low in sodium, such as fruits.

Sources of Potassium

Overall, fresh fruits, fruit juice, and vegetables are good dietary sources of potassium. Milk, whole grains, dried beans, and meats are also major contributors of potassium to American diets. Table 9.13 lists foods that are among the richest sources of this mineral. Figure 9.16 indicates food groups that are naturally good sources of potassium.

Dietary Adequacy

The adult AI for potassium is 4700 mg per day. On average, Americans consume only about 2640 mg of potassium per day.[14] Because Americans tend to consume lower than recommended amounts of potassium, the mineral is a "nutrient of public health concern." People can raise their potassium intakes by following the DASH diet.

The body is unable to conserve potassium as well as sodium; therefore, the risk of potassium deficiency is greater than that of sodium deficiency. Individuals

TABLE 9.13 Potassium Content of Selected Foods

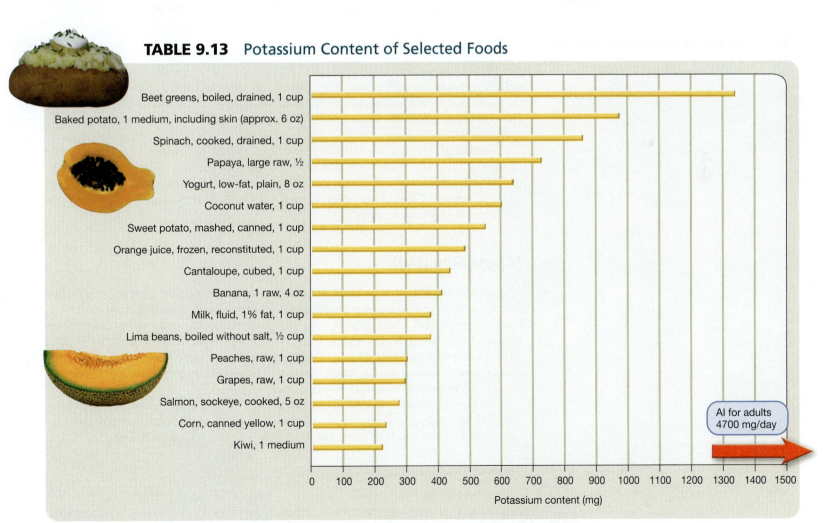

Source: Data from U.S. Department of Agriculture, Agricultural Research Service: *USDA national nutrient database for standard reference, Release 26,* 2013.

| Figure 9.16 **MyPlate: Good sources of potassium.**

suffering from excessive sweating, vomiting, diarrhea, or kidney diseases that increase potassium excretion are at risk for potassium depletion. Symptoms of the condition generally include loss of appetite, muscle cramps, confusion, and constipation.

Although there is no UL for potassium, taking potassium supplements can upset the GI tract. Moreover, if a person's kidneys are not able to eliminate the excess potassium, the mineral accumulates in the blood and can cause the heart to stop beating. To avoid toxicity, do not take potassium supplements unless you are under a physician's care.

Magnesium (Mg)

Magnesium participates in more than 300 chemical reactions in the body.[27] The essential mineral also helps regulate normal muscle and nerve function as well as blood pressure and blood glucose levels. Additionally, the body needs magnesium to maintain strong bones and a healthy immune system. Following diets that supply adequate amounts of magnesium may enhance bone health and reduce the risk of heart disease, stroke, and diabetes.[27] However, more research is needed to clarify the mineral's role in these diseases.

Normally, people absorb about 30 to 40% of the magnesium in their diets. The kidneys regulate blood concentrations of magnesium and can reduce urinary losses of the mineral when the body's level of magnesium is low.

Sources of Magnesium

Magnesium is in chlorophyll, the green pigment in plants. Therefore, it is not surprising that plant foods, such as spinach, green leafy vegetables, whole grains, beans, nuts, seeds, and chocolate, are the richest sources of magnesium. Animal products, such as milk and meats, also supply some magnesium. Table 9.14 lists some commonly eaten foods that supply magnesium. Refined grains are generally low in magnesium, because the magnesium-rich bran and germ are removed during processing. Figure 9.17 indicates food groups that are naturally good sources of magnesium.

Other sources of magnesium are "hard" tap water and dietary supplements. However, amounts of magnesium in tap water can vary considerably. Moreover, the body does not absorb the form of magnesium (magnesium oxide) in multivitamin/mineral supplements very well. Nevertheless, hard water and magnesium supplements can still contribute to meeting a person's magnesium needs.

Dietary Adequacy

Adult RDAs for magnesium range from 310 to 420 mg/day. Many people in the United States do not consume recommended amounts of magnesium.[14] Despite this, cases of magnesium deficiency rarely occur among healthy members of the population.[27] Nevertheless, alcoholics, people with poorly controlled diabetes, or persons who use certain medications (diuretics) that increase urinary excretion of magnesium have high risk of magnesium deficiency. Older adults are also at risk of magnesium deficiency because their bodies absorb less of the mineral and urinary losses increase with advancing age.

In humans, mild magnesium deficiency can cause irritability, weakness, loss of appetite, and muscle twitching. Signs and symptoms of severe magnesium deficiency often include rapid heartbeat, inability to relax muscles, disorientation, and hallucinations. Chronic magnesium deficiency may increase the risk of osteoporosis, because the deficiency lowers the level of calcium in blood.

TABLE 9.14 Magnesium Content of Selected Foods

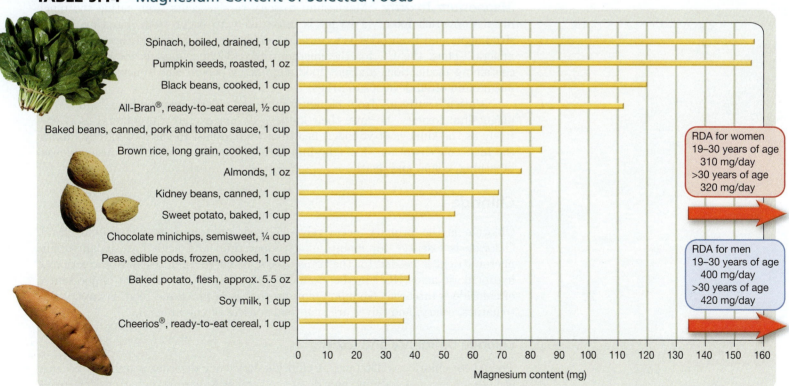

Source: Data from U.S. Department of Agriculture, Agricultural Research Service: *USDA national nutrient database for standard reference, Release 26,* 2013.

| **Figure 9.17** MyPlate: Good sources of magnesium.

Magnesium Toxicity Magnesium toxicity rarely occurs from eating too much magnesium—rich food.[27] Toxicity is more likely to occur from ingesting excessive magnesium from laxatives, antacids, or dietary supplements that contain the mineral. Thus, the UL for the micronutrient (350 mg/day) is for magnesium—containing medications and not food sources. A person who consumes too much magnesium often develops diarrhea.

Patients suffering from kidney failure and elderly persons have high risk of magnesium toxicity, because their kidneys do not excrete the mineral as effectively as the kidneys of younger, healthier individuals. In cases of kidney failure, the high concentration of magnesium in blood causes weakness, nausea, slowed breathing, coma, and death.

Chloride

Chloride is the primary negatively—charged ion found in extracellular fluid. Chloride is essential for maintaining proper fluid and acid—base balance. The micronutrient is needed for the transmission of nerve impulses and production of hydrochloric acid (HCl) in the stomach. For most Americans, the major source of chloride is table salt (sodium chloride) that is in processed food. Seaweed, rye, tomatoes, celery, and olives are rich food sources of the mineral.

Chloride Deficiency and Toxicity

The AI for chloride is 2300 mg. A chloride deficiency disorder is unlikely because of high amounts of sodium chloride in the typical American diet. However, deficiencies may be seen in cases of extreme vomiting, diarrhea, and/or sweating, as well as with diuretic use. Fatigue and loss of appetite are common symptoms of chloride deficiency.

The UL for chloride is 3600 mg/day. Elevated blood chloride levels may result from excessive sodium chloride intake. As in cases of excess sodium inges—tion, consuming too much chloride can contribute to hypertension.

Sulfur

Sulfur is a component of several organic compounds, including the amino acids methionine and cysteine, and the vitamins biotin and thiamin. Sulfur is essential for the activity of many enzymes and as part of antioxidant molecules. Protein—rich foods are among the best food sources of sulfur. Some foods and beverages, including many wines, are also sources of sulfur (*sulfites*). In the United States, cases of sulfur deficiency are rare but can occur in people who have severe protein deficiency. Sulfur toxicity is unlikely from dietary sources. Thus, there is no AI, RDA, or UL established for sulfur.

Consuming too much chloride can contribute to hypertension.

Concept **Checkpoint 9.4**

18. What is osteoporosis, and why is it a major public health concern in the United States?
19. Identify at least four major risk factors for osteoporosis. Which risk factors can be modified to reduce the risk of osteoporosis?
20. What is prehypertension? What is hypertension? What are major risk factors for hypertension?
21. What is the DASH diet? Aside from making dietary modifications, what other life-style changes can people with hypertension make to lower their blood pressure?
22. Prepare a table for the major minerals that includes information about each mineral's major roles in the body, primary food sources, and signs and symptoms of the mineral's deficiency as well as toxicity disorders. Check your table against the information provided in Table 9.5.

9.5 Trace Minerals

Learning Outcomes

1 List key functions and good food sources of trace minerals.

2 Discuss deficiency and toxicity disorders associated with the trace minerals.

Although the body requires trace minerals in very small amounts, obtaining ade—quate amounts of these important nutrients can be difficult. Iron, for example, is one of Earth's most plentiful metals, but the total amount of iron in the human body is quite small, averaging only about 0.006% of a person's body weight.[2] Table 9.15 summarizes nutrition—related information about iron and other trace minerals. Unless otherwise noted, RDA/AI values are for adults, excluding preg—nant or breastfeeding women.

TABLE 9.15 Summary of Trace Minerals

Mineral	Major Functions in the Body	Adult RDA/AI* (adult RDA = bold)	Major Dietary Sources	Major Deficiency Signs and Symptoms	Major Toxicity Signs and Symptoms
Iron (Fe)	• Component of hemoglobin and myoglobin that carries oxygen • Energy generation • Immune system function	Women: **18 mg** Men: **8 mg**	Meat and other animal foods, except milk; whole-grain and enriched breads and cereals; fortified cereals	• Fatigue upon exertion • Small, pale red blood cells • Low hemoglobin levels • Poor immune system function • Growth and developmental retardation in infants	UL = 45 mg/day • Intestinal upset • Organ damage • Death
Zinc (Zn)	• Component of numerous enzymes	Women: **8 mg** Men: **11 mg**	Seafood, meat, whole grains	• Skin rash • Diarrhea • Depressed sense of taste and smell • Hair loss • Poor growth and physical development	UL = 40 mg/day • Intestinal upset • Depressed immune system function • Supplement use can reduce copper absorption.
Copper (Cu)	• Promotes iron metabolism • Component of antioxidant enzymes • Component of enzymes involved in connective tissue synthesis	900 mcg	Liver, cocoa, legumes, whole grains, shellfish	• Anemia • Reduced immune system function • Poor growth and development	UL = 10,000 mcg/day • Vomiting • Abnormal nervous system function • Liver damage
Selenium (Se)	• Component of an antioxidant system	55 mcg	Meat, eggs, fish, seafood, whole grains	• Muscle pain and weakness • Form of heart disease	UL = 400 mcg/day • Nausea • Vomiting • Hair loss • Weakness • Liver damage
Iodine (I)	• Component of thyroid hormones	150 mcg	Iodized salt, saltwater fish, dairy products	• Goiter • Cretinism (intellectual impairment and poor growth in infants of women who were iodine deficient during pregnancy)	UL = 1100 mcg/day • Reduced thyroid gland function
Fluoride (F⁻)	• Increases resistance of tooth enamel to cavity formation • Stimulates bone formation	Women: 3 mg Men: 4 mg	Fluoridated water, tea, seaweed	• No true deficiency, but increased risk of tooth decay	UL = 10 mg/day • Stomach upset • Staining of teeth during development • Bone deterioration
Chromium (Cr)	• Enhances insulin action	Women: 20–25 mcg Men: 30–35 mcg	Egg yolks, whole grains, pork, nuts, mushrooms	• Blood glucose level remains elevated after meals	• Unknown but currently under scientific investigation • May interact with certain medications
Manganese (Mn)	• Cofactor for certain enzymes, including some involved in carbohydrate metabolism	Women: 1.8 mg Men: 2.3 mg	Nuts, oats, beans, tea	• None in humans	UL = 11 mg/day • Abnormal nervous system function
Molybdenum (Mo)	• Component of certain coenzymes	45 mcg	Liver, peas, beans, cereal products, leafy vegetables, low-fat milk	• None in healthy humans	UL = 2000 mcg/day • Rarely occurs from usual dietary sources • Overdoses of dietary supplements containing molybdenum may cause joint pain; side, lower back, or stomach pain; swelling of feet or lower legs.

* Values are for adults, excluding pregnant or breastfeeding women.

Iron (Fe)

Do you think of "iron" when you think of "strength"? Associating iron with strength makes sense, because muscular strength and endurance are reduced when the body lacks iron. Iron is a component of hemoglobin and *myoglobin* (*my'−o−glow−bin*). **Hemoglobin** is the iron−containing protein in red blood cells that transports oxygen to tissues and some carbon dioxide away from tissues. Hemo−globin is also responsible for the red color of oxygenated blood. **Myoglobin** is the iron−containing protein in muscle cells that controls oxygen uptake from red blood cells. Oxygen is critical for energy metabolism. Cells also contain iron in **cytochromes** (*sigh'−toe−crowms*), a group of proteins that are necessary for certain chemical reactions involved in the release of energy from macronutrients. If the body does not have enough iron to make hemoglobin, myoglobin, and the cytochromes, cells cannot obtain the energy they need to perform work. Thus, fatigue is a major symptom of iron deficiency. Iron also plays roles in immune system function and brain development.

Sources of Iron

Beef, fish, and poultry ("meat") contain more iron than most plant foods. Some of the iron in meat is present as hemoglobin and myoglobin. These forms of iron are collectively referred to as **heme iron.** The remaining iron in meat, as well as all the iron in vegetables, grains, and supplements, is **nonheme iron.**

The intestinal tract absorbs more of the heme iron than nonheme iron in foods.[28] Some plant foods, such as spinach, contain nonheme iron, but oxalic acid in spinach binds to the mineral, reducing its absorption. Other naturally occur−ring compounds that reduce iron absorption include phytic acid in whole grains, tannins in tea, and substances that are chemically related to tannins in coffee.

Meat is the major source of iron in the typical American diet. Other impor−tant sources of iron are fortified cereals and products made from enriched flour, such as breads and rolls. Dairy products are poor sources of iron. Figure 9.18 indicates food groups that are good sources of iron. Table 9.16 lists some foods that are among the richest sources of iron.

hemoglobin iron-containing protein in red blood cells that transports oxygen to tissues and some carbon dioxide away from tissues

myoglobin iron-containing protein in muscle cells that controls oxygen uptake from red blood cells

cytochromes group of proteins involved in the release of energy from macronutrients

heme iron form of iron in hemoglobin and myoglobin

nonheme iron form of iron that is primarily in vegetables, grains, meats, and supplements

Figure 9.18 MyPlate: Good sources of iron.

Fruits
- Peaches
- Prune juice
- Dried apricots

Vegetables
- Spinach
- Peas
- Potatoes
- Green beans
- Broccoli

Grains
- Whole grains
- Enriched grains
- Wheat germ
- Oatmeal

Protein
- Beef
- Tofu
- Beans
- Seafood
- Organ meats

ChooseMyPlate.gov

TABLE 9.16   Iron Content of Selected Foods

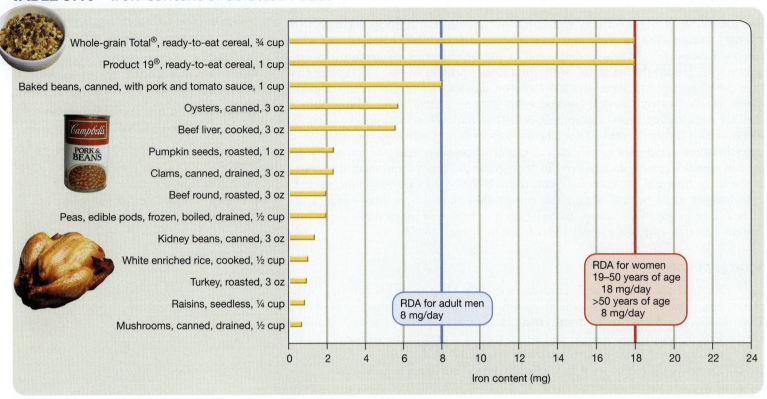

Source: Data from U.S. Department of Agriculture, Agricultural Research Service: *USDA national nutrient database for standard reference, Release 26,* 2013.

Regulating Iron   Under normal conditions, the body regulates iron absorption and conservation. The digestive tract absorbs only 5 to 15% of the iron in foods. However, the intestinal tract can absorb more iron when the body's need for the trace mineral increases. Despite iron enrichment and fortification, only about 5% of the iron added to grain products is absorbed.[28] The liver, the body's main site for iron storage, incorporates the trace mineral into the protein ferritin (*fer'—ih—tin*) until it is needed.

After red blood cells die, the body breaks them down and conserves most of the iron that was in hemoglobin. By doing so, the body can recycle the trace mineral to make hemoglobin for new red blood cells. Nonetheless, some iron is lost each day via the GI tract, urine, and skin. Any form of bleeding, including menstruation, also contributes to iron losses. Replacing the iron is essential to good health.

Dietary Adequacy

For adult men, the RDA for iron is 8 mg per day; for adult women between 19 and 50 years of age, the RDA for iron is 18 mg/day. The average daily intake for American men is 17.5 mg, whereas the average daily intake for American women is about 13.0 mg/ day.[14] Thus, women between 19 and 50 years of age are more likely than men to have inadequate iron intakes.

Iron Deficiency–Related Disorders Low blood iron levels usually result from losing blood, consuming diets that lack iron, or being unable to absorb dietary iron. In cases of **iron deficiency,** the body's iron stores are low but not low enough to result in severe health problems. Nevertheless, iron deficiency can still have wide–spread negative effects on the body, including interfering with normal growth, behavior, immune system function, cardiac function, and energy metabolism.[29] Furthermore, iron deficiency can lead to iron deficiency anemia.

Anemia occurs when oxygen transport in blood is impaired, generally because there are not enough red blood cells to carry the oxygen or the red blood cells do not contain enough hemoglobin (Fig. 9.19). If oxygen is lacking, cells cannot release considerable amounts of energy from macronutrients, so symp–toms of iron deficiency anemia include lack of energy and difficulty concentrating on mental activities. Furthermore, the heart of a person suffering from anemia has to work harder to circulate oxygen–poor blood throughout the body. Over time, anemia can cause rapid or irregular heartbeat, chest pain, an enlarged heart, and even heart failure. Table 9.17 lists common signs and symptoms of iron deficiency anemia.

There are many different kinds of anemia, but iron deficiency anemia is the most common form. According to the World Health Organization (WHO), over 30% of the world's population suffers from anemia, and many cases of the condition are due to iron deficiency.[30] In the United States, iron deficiency is the most common nutritional deficiency and the leading cause of anemia.[31]

Substantial blood loss is a common cause of iron deficiency anemia. Such losses of blood often result from serious intestinal diseases, severe physical inju–ries, and excessive menstrual bleeding. Diseases that reduce red blood cell for–mation or increase red blood cell destruction also cause anemia. It is important to note that some types of anemia are the result of genetic defects and not dietary deficiencies. Blood testing can determine which kind of anemia a person has developed, so the condition can be treated properly.

Women of childbearing age generally lose some iron during menstruation. Women with heavy menstrual blood losses are especially prone to iron deficiency anemia. Although pregnant women do not have to contend with menstrual blood losses, they still need to be concerned about their iron intake. According to the Dietary Guidelines, iron is a "nutrient of public health concern" for women who are pregnant or able to become pregnant The "Food & Nutrition Tips" feature on page 350 suggests practical ways to increase dietary sources of iron.

iron deficiency condition characterized by low body stores of iron

TABLE 9.17 Signs and Symptoms of Iron Deficiency Anemia

Pale skin
Fatigue and weakness
Irritability
Difficulty concentrating and thinking
Brittle nails
Headache

Source: U.S. Library of Medicine (Medline), National Institutes of Health: Iron deficiency anemia. *Medline plus.* www.nlm.nih.gov/medlineplus/ency/article/000584.htm. Accessed January 5, 2014

(a)

(b)

Figure 9.19 Iron-deficient red blood cells. (*a*) Normal red blood cells. (*b*) Iron-deficient red blood cells. Arrow points to a deficient cell.

During pregnancy, a woman's need for iron increases as her blood supply expands and new tissues are added to both her body and that of her fetus. Pregnant women who suffer from iron deficiency anemia have higher risk of dying during pregnancy than healthy pregnant women. Anemic pregnant women are also more likely to give birth to premature or low—birth—weight infants. Premature babies are born before the 37th week of pregnancy; normally, pregnancies last about 40 weeks from the date of the mother's last menstrual period. A low—birth—weight baby weighs less than 5½ pounds at birth. Compared to healthy newborns, premature or low—birth—weight infants are more likely to die during their first year of life.

Because of their rapid growth rates, infants and toddlers have higher needs for iron than older children. Furthermore, iron appears to be necessary for normal nervous system functioning, including brain development. Iron—deficient infants can experience delays in the development of normal motor and mental functions.

Consuming too much milk may play a role in the development of iron deficiency in children. Milk is a poor source of iron. Thus, children who drink excessive amounts of milk may not have the appetite to eat foods that are more reliable iron sources. The calcium that is in milk may interfere with iron absorption when the beverage is consumed with foods that contain the mineral.[33] To reduce the risk of iron deficiency, children should be encouraged to eat more iron—rich foods, such as meat, products made from soybeans, and iron—fortified cereals.

Total vegetarians have a higher risk of iron deficiency–related disorders than people who eat meat, because meat provides heme iron. Combining a small amount of meat with plant foods improves the bioavailability of the plant's nonheme iron. Vegetarians, however, may reject recipes that include any meat, especially red meats. Some plant foods contain high amounts of oxalic acid and phytic acid, substances that can depress iron absorption. On the other hand, vegetarian diets usually are rich in vitamin C, a factor that increases nonheme iron absorption. Thus, vegetarians should consume vitamin C–rich foods along with plant foods, especially those that contain appreciable amounts of iron, such as spinach, lentils, and soybeans. Eating iron—fortified ready—to—eat cereals can

Food & Nutrition tips

The following suggestions can add more iron to your diet:

• Eat lean meat, poultry, or fish with plant sources of iron.

• Combine soybeans with tomatoes or tomato sauce.

• Add orange segments or chopped tomatoes to spinach salads or cooked spinach.

• Add chopped onions and green peppers to peas or beans.

• Serve sweet potatoes with fresh orange segments or dried apricots.

• Add raspberries, strawberries, raisins, or dried apricots to cereal.

• Drink orange juice when eating peanut butter or soy nut butter sandwiches.

• Consume watermelon, dried plums, dried apricots, or raisins for snacks.

also be helpful for vegetarians, even though the form of iron used to fortify cereals is not as well absorbed as heme iron. Finally, vegetarians can take a multivitamin and mineral supplement that contains iron to ensure their iron and other mineral intakes are adequate.

Treatment for iron deficiency anemia generally includes iron supplements and the addition of iron—rich foods to the diet. It is also important to find and treat factors that may be causing the deficiency, such as intestinal bleeding.

Iron Toxicity The UL for iron is 45 mg/day. Although not having enough iron in the body interferes with normal growth, development, and functioning, ingesting too much iron poses the risk of toxicity. Between 1988 and 1997, 29 American children under 6 years of age died as a result of accidentally taking too many iron—containing dietary supplements.[34] Early signs of acute iron poisoning include vomiting and diarrhea that may progress to coma and death.

In 1997, the U.S. Food and Drug Administration (FDA) required a warning statement on the packaging of iron supplements to reduce the number of iron poisoning cases among young children. The agency also required unit—dose packaging of oral iron supplements that contained 30 mg of iron or more per dose. The individually wrapped supplements were designed to make it difficult for young children to ingest large quantities of the supplements at a time. After these rules were instituted, only one child died from iron poisoning between 1998 and 2002.[34] In 2003, however, a federal court ruled that the FDA did not have the legal authority to require special unit—dose packaging of iron supplements. The agency, however, could continue to require warning statements on supplement labels.

Iron Overload: Hereditary Hemochromatosis *Iron overload* is a condition characterized by excess iron in the body. Iron overload occurs when toxic amounts of iron supplements are ingested, but the condition also results from certain genetic diseases.[35] **Hereditary hemochromatosis** (*he'—mo—crow'—ma—toe—sis*) is the most common type of iron overload disease.[35] People who have hereditary hemochromatosis (HH) absorb too much iron. The body has no way to eliminate the excess iron, so the mineral accumulates in tissues and can cause joint pain, abnormal bronze skin color, and damage to the liver, heart, adrenal glands, and pancreas.

HH most often affects people who have northern European ancestors. In the United States, about 5 of every 1000 non—Hispanic white Americans are susceptible to developing the disease.[35] Men are more likely to be diagnosed with HH than women. Additionally, men tend to develop health problems from the excess iron at a younger age than women with the condition.

Joint pain is the most common complaint of people suffering from HH. Other common signs and symptoms of the disorder include fatigue, lack of energy, abdominal pain, loss of sex drive, and heart problems. Even though people with HH begin accumulating iron early in life, they often do not report any signs and symptoms of the disease until they are over 30 years of age. Testing is available to determine the presence of the genes that are responsible for the disease.

Many people who have HH experience vague symptoms or no symptoms at all. If the disease is not detected early and treated effectively, the organ damage resulting from the condition can be deadly. Treatment usually includes visiting a clinic periodically to have blood removed. This process stimulates the tissues that produce red blood cells to use storage iron for hemoglobin production. People with HH should avoid taking dietary supplements that contain iron.

Did You Know?

Cooking utensils may be a source of dietary iron. When acidic foods, such as tomato sauce, are cooked in cast-iron cookware, some iron migrates from the cookware and enters the food. Replacing the heavy iron cookware with lighter stainless steel and aluminum pots and pans can reduce the amount of iron in diets.

hereditary hemochromatosis most common type of iron overload disease

Zinc (Zn)

In 1958, physician Ananda Prasad was working in Iran when he examined a 21–year–old man with dwarfism, intellectual disability, iron deficiency anemia, and underdeveloped sexual organs.[36] Prasad noted that the young man ate unleavened ("flat") bread almost exclusively. After examining other patients in Iran and Egypt with similar health problems and dietary practices, Prasad hypothesized that diet was responsible for the condition. Eventually, medical researchers determined that Prasad's patients had severe zinc deficiencies. After these patients were given zinc supplements, they began to grow and develop normally. Prasad later determined that girls also experienced stunted growth and delays in sexual maturation as a result of zinc deficiency.[37]

In the regions where the men who were zinc deficient lived, the typical diet was comprised primarily of unleavened whole–wheat bread and little animal protein. Unleavened whole–wheat bread is naturally high in phytic acid and fiber, substances that decrease zinc bioavailability. In places where people use yeast to leaven (raise) bread dough, severe zinc deficiency is less likely to occur. Yeast reduces the binding effects of phytic acid and fiber, making zinc more bio–available. Consuming zinc–rich sources of animal protein, such as meat and milk, also reduces the likelihood of zinc deficiency.

Other factors that influence the bioavailability of zinc include the body's need for the mineral and the presence of large amounts of certain other metals. During times when a healthy body needs zinc, the small intestine absorbs more. However, the presence of excess copper or iron in the small intestine interferes with zinc absorption. Thus, iron supplements should be taken between meals instead of with them.[38]

Why Is Zinc Necessary?

Zinc is a component of about a hundred enzymes.[38] Zinc is necessary for wound healing, the sense of taste and smell, DNA synthesis, healthy skin, proper functioning of the immune system (Fig. 9.20). Zinc is also essential for growth and development during pregnancy, childhood, and adolescence.

Figure 9.20 Sign of zinc deficiency in a baby. Zinc is necessary for healthy skin and normal physical growth. This child has a type of dermatitis that is a sign of zinc deficiency.

Sources of Zinc

Zinc is widespread in foods (Table 9.18). Red meat and poultry products supply most of the zinc in the typical American diet. Figure 9.21 indicates MyPlate food groups that have foods that are good sources of zinc.

Dietary Adequacy

Adult RDAs for zinc range from 8 mg to 11 mg/day. In the United States, the average adult consumes adequate amounts of zinc.[14] Thus, zinc deficiency is not a widespread problem in the United States. However, alcoholics have high risk of zinc deficiency, because alcohol reduces zinc absorption and increases excretion of the mineral in urine. Making matters worse, many people who suffer from alcoholism do not consume nutritious diets. Vegetarians need more zinc than people who eat meat, because the GI tract does not absorb zinc from plant foods as well as from animal foods.[38] Older adults are at risk of zinc deficiency because they often consume foods that do not provide adequate amounts of the trace mineral.

Although breast milk contains zinc, the milk does not supply enough of the trace mineral for infants who are older than 6 months of age. To increase the likelihood that their diets contain enough zinc, breastfed babies who are between 6 and 12 months of age need to consume foods that contain the trace mineral, such as zinc–fortified infant cereal.

TABLE 9.18   Zinc Content of Selected Foods

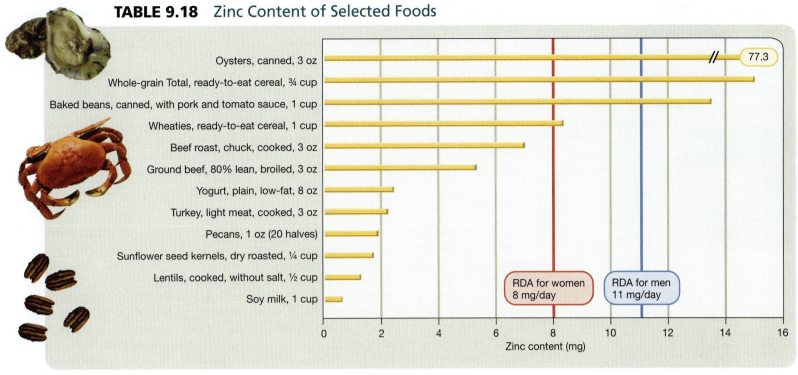

Food	Zinc content (mg)
Oysters, canned, 3 oz	77.3
Whole-grain Total, ready-to-eat cereal, ¾ cup	
Baked beans, canned, with pork and tomato sauce, 1 cup	
Wheaties, ready-to-eat cereal, 1 cup	
Beef roast, chuck, cooked, 3 oz	
Ground beef, 80% lean, broiled, 3 oz	
Yogurt, plain, low-fat, 8 oz	
Turkey, light meat, cooked, 3 oz	
Pecans, 1 oz (20 halves)	
Sunflower seed kernels, dry roasted, ¼ cup	
Lentils, cooked, without salt, ½ cup	
Soy milk, 1 cup	

RDA for women 8 mg/day

RDA for men 11 mg/day

Source: Data from U.S. Department of Agriculture, Agricultural Research Service: *USDA national nutrient database for standard reference, Release 26,* 2013.

In children and adolescents, zinc deficiency can cause growth retardation and delayed sexual maturation. Adult men who are zinc deficient may experience sexual dysfunction, particularly the inability to attain an erection. Other signs of zinc deficiency include loss of appetite, diarrhea, hair loss, dermatitis, poor wound healing, impaired sense of taste, and mental slowness.[38]

Zinc Toxicity   The UL for zinc is 40 mg/day. Zinc intakes that exceed the UL can reduce beneficial HDL cholesterol levels in blood. Ingesting more than 100 mg

| **Figure 9.21** **MyPlate: Good food sources of zinc.**

of zinc per day can also result in diarrhea, cramps, nausea, vomiting, and depressed immune system function. Additionally, megadoses of zinc may interfere with copper absorption and metabolism. Therefore, people should avoid high intakes of zinc, unless they are under a physician's supervision.

In 2009, the FDA warned the public about using two *intranasal* ("within the nose") forms of a nonprescription, zinc-containing product. The agency had received several reports that the alternative medical treatment for the common cold may result in loss of sense of smell.[38] In response to FDA actions, the manufacturer voluntarily removed the product from the marketplace. Results of studies do not provide consistent evidence that zinc helps reduce the severity or duration of colds, but more research is needed to clarify whether cold products that contain zinc may be beneficial.

Copper

The body uses copper to make several enzymes that act as antioxidants. The mineral is also involved in iron metabolism, immune function, and collagen production. A wide variety of foods contain copper, but the foods listed in Table 9.19 are among the richest sources of the micronutrient.

The adult RDA for copper is 0.9 mg/day, and Americans typically consume more than this amount.[14] Consuming high amounts of iron or zinc can interfere with the intestinal tract's ability to absorb copper, so taking these supplements may cause copper deficiency. People with chronic digestive system diseases may also develop copper deficiency, because their bodies' ability to absorb the mineral is depressed. A deficiency of copper can lead to anemia, impaired functioning of the immune and nervous systems, abnormal skin pigmentation, and poor growth (children).

TABLE 9.19 Copper Content of Selected Foods

Food	mg
Beef liver, 3 oz, cooked	12.40
Crab meat, ½ cup, canned	1.10
Cashews, 1 oz, dry roasted	0.63
Mushrooms, ½ cup, white, cooked, drained	0.40
Soybeans, ½ cup, mature, boiled, drained	0.35
Chocolate, ¼ cup, semisweet	0.30
Baked beans, ½ cup, canned, with pork and tomato sauce	0.27
Sunflower seeds, 1 oz, dry roasted	0.26

RDA adults = 0.9 mg/day

Source: Data from U.S. Department of Agriculture, Agricultural Research Service: *USDA national nutrient database for standard reference, Release 25, 2013.*

Iodine (Iodide)

During World War I, physicians noted that men drafted into the U.S. military from the Great Lakes region were far more likely to have goiter (*goy'-ter*) than men from some other areas of the country. Goiter is an enlargement of the thyroid gland that is not the result of cancer (Fig. 9.22). Goiters often occur among populations living in areas that have iodine-depleted soil. In general, these regions are inland and far from an ocean. If people in these communities limit their diets to locally produced foods, they might not have enough iodine in their diets.

Iodine (I_2) is poisonous, but most ingested iodine loses an electron to become the iodide ion (I^-) in the digestive tract.[28] Iodide is the form of iodine that the body uses. Most of the iodide in an adult's body is located in the thyroid gland. Under normal conditions, the kidneys filter and eliminate excess iodide from blood.

| **Figure 9.22** Goiter.

From 1917 to 1922, researchers in Ohio conducted an experiment on a group of girls in which one group of the children received doses of iodine, whereas the other group (the control group) did not receive the trace mineral. The results of the study indicated iodine was nearly 100% effective in preventing goiter in the healthy children. Moreover, the majority of the girls who already had goiters when they received the iodine experienced a reduction in the size of their thyroid glands by the end of the study.[39] In 1924, iodide was added to table salt in the United States, and as a result, cases of goiter caused by iodine deficiency rarely occur in this country. Today, use of iodized salt is the major method of prevent—ing iodine deficiencies in developed nations, but inadequate iodine intake and goiters are still common in central Asia and central Africa.

Why Is Iodine Necessary?

People require iodine for normal thyroid function and for the production of two thyroid hormones, collectively referred to as **thyroid hormone.** Thyroid hormone controls the rate of cell metabolism, that is, the rate at which cells obtain energy. The thyroid gland traps iodide from the bloodstream and accumulates the element for thyroid hormone synthesis. If a person's iodine intake is too low, the pituitary gland in the brain releases a hormone that causes the thyroid gland to enlarge. As a result, the larger thyroid gland tries to remove as much iodide as possible from the bloodstream. It is important to note that an enlarged thyroid gland can also be a sign of some diseases and conditions that are not related to iodine intake.

Sources of Iodine

Major sources of iodine include saltwater fish; seafood; seaweed; some plants, especially the leaves of plants grown near oceans; and iodized salt. A half tea—spoon of iodine—fortified salt supplies the adult RDA for iodine. Iodide forti—fication of salt is voluntary in the United States, so not all salt has the trace mineral added to it. Other dietary sources of iodine include food additives that contain the mineral, such as certain dough conditioners and food dyes. Table 9.20 lists some foods that are good sources of iodine.

Did You Know?

The sea salt that is usually sold in supermarkets is not a good source of iodine and other minerals because it has undergone processing. Some stores sell "unrefined" or "natural" sea salt that contains much of its natural mineral content, including iodine.[40] Consumers, however, need to avoid excess sodium from all sources, including sea salt.

thyroid hormone hormone that regulates the body's metabolic rate

TABLE 9.20   Iodine Content of Selected Foods

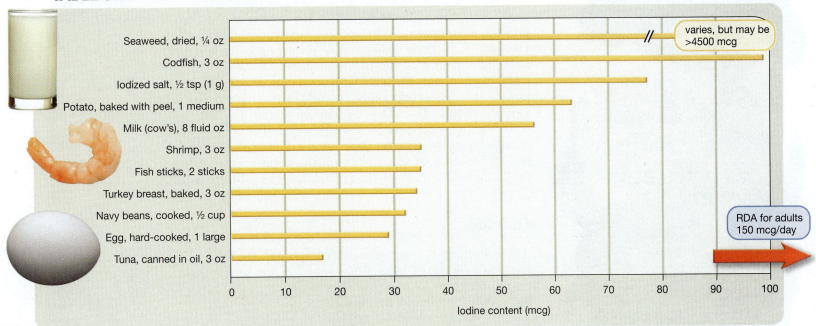

Source: Data from Higdon, J: Iodine. Micronutrient Information Center, Linus Pauling Institute, Oregon State University. Updated 2010. http://lpi.oregonstate.edu/infocenter/minerals/iodine/Accessed October 12, 2011

goitrogens compounds that inhibit iodide metabolism by the thyroid gland

cretinism condition affecting infants of women who were iodine deficient during pregnancy

Dietary Adequacy

The adult RDA for iodine is 150 mcg/day. Most Americans have adequate iodine intakes.[40] As many Americans, particularly older adults, try to reduce their risk of hypertension by using less salt, iodine intakes may decline to marginal or inadequate levels.

Iodine Deficiency   In cases of iodine deficiency, the thyroid gland produces insufficient amounts of thyroid hormone and goiter develops. As a result of the lack of thyroid hormone, iodine–deficient people generally have low metabolic rates and elevated blood cholesterol levels. Other signs and symptoms of iodine deficiency include fatigue, difficulty concentrating on mental tasks, weight gain, intolerance of cold temperatures, constipation, and dry skin.

Throughout the world, millions of people are at risk of iodine deficiency. Pregnant women who are iodine deficient have high risk of stillbirths (giving birth to a dead infant) or low–birth–weight babies. During fetal life, thyroid hormone is crucial for normal brain development. Thus, infants of iodine–deficient women are likely to be born with a condition called **cretinism** ($kre'-tin-ih-zim$). Babies with cretinism have permanent brain damage, reduced intellectual func-tioning, and growth retardation. Worldwide, iodine deficiency is the most com-mon cause of preventable intellectual disability.[40] Pregnant women can reduce the risk of giving birth to infants with cretinism by consuming adequate amounts of iodine throughout pregnancy.

Iodine deficiency is a serious threat to health in places where soils are iodine deficient and commonly eaten foods are not fortified with the trace mineral, such as regions of Latin America, India, Southeast Asia, and Africa. Currently, inter-national health organizations are engaging in efforts to eliminate iodine deficiency, primarily by promoting the use of iodized salt or iodide–fortified vegetable oils.

Iodide Toxicity   The UL for iodine is 1.1 mg/day. Over time, consuming very high amounts of iodine can cause thyroid gland enlargement and reduced produc-tion of thyroid hormone. These side effects are the same as those that occur when diets are deficient in iodine. Excess iodine is also associated with an increased risk of a form of thyroid cancer.[40]

Nuclear power plant accidents, such as the one that occurred after a major earthquake struck Japan in 2011, may release radioactive iodine (iodine–131) into the environment. When people are exposed to radioactive iodine, the ele-ment can enter their bodies and be picked up by their thyroid glands. Exposure to a high amount of the radiation increases the risk of thyroid cancer, espe-cially in children.[40] People who have iodine deficiency are more likely to accu-mulate the radioactive iodine in their thyroid glands than people who are not iodine deficient. To reduce the risk of thyroid cancer, people who are exposed to radioactive iodine can take supplements that contain 16 to 130 mg of potas-sium iodide, depending on their age, until the risk of extreme radiation exposure ends.[40] The thyroid gland picks up the potassium iodide, which helps block the thyroid gland's uptake of the radioactive form of the element.

Fluoride

Although fluoride is not an essential nutrient, the mineral strengthens bones and teeth when ingested in small amounts. In the some parts of the United States, well water contains high amounts of the trace mineral. To ensure that people living in other sections of the country obtain healthful amounts of fluoride, the mineral is often added to public water supplies, toothpastes, and dental rinses. Tea naturally contains fluoride.

Long—term consumption of too much fluoride can cause *fluorosis*. In cases of skeletal fluorosis, excess fluoride builds up in bones, causing joint stiffness and bone pain. Skeletal fluorosis rarely occurs in the United States. Dental fluorosis often affects young children who drink well water that contains high amounts of fluoride, but it also can occur in children who routinely swallow toothpaste and dental rinses. Children with severe fluorosis develop permanently stained teeth that do not resist decay as do healthy teeth (Fig. 9.23). Parents should teach their children to place a pea—sized amount of toothpaste on their brush, rinse with water, and spit out the excess fluid.

| **Figure 9.23** Dental fluorosis.

Selenium (Se)

Selenium is widespread in Earth's crust, but soils can vary widely in their content of the essential trace mineral. Areas of the western United States, including parts of Colorado and South Dakota, have unusually high concentrations of selenium in soil. Certain types of plants that grow in these places accumulate toxic levels of the mineral. Livestock that graze on the selenium—rich plants often ingest poi—sonous amounts of the trace mineral. In horses and cattle, selenium toxicity can cause hair and weight loss, malformed hooves that can separate from the animals' feet, muscle weakness and loss of muscular function (paralysis), and death.

Why Is Selenium Necessary?

In the body, selenium functions as a component of several proteins referred to as selenoproteins (*sell'—in—oh—pro'—teens*). Many selenoproteins are antioxidants. Other selenoproteins are necessary for the normal functioning of the immune system and thyroid gland.

Sources of Selenium

Although the selenium content of foods varies, nuts, whole—grain products, sea—food, and meats are generally rich sources of the trace mineral (Table 9.21). Because Brazil nuts can have very high selenium contents, people should not eat these nuts regularly.

| Brazil nuts have high selenium contents.

Dietary Adequacy

Most Americans' diets meet the RDA for selenium. In the United States, sele—nium deficiency is uncommon, but the condition may occur in people who have serious digestive tract conditions that interfere with the mineral's absorption. Selenium deficiency reduces thyroid gland activity and can lead to goiter. The deficiency also depresses immune system function and may contribute to the development of heart disease and cancer. In parts of China where the soil lacks selenium and the population consumes locally produced foods, diets typically contain inadequate amounts of selenium. Certain types of cancer and a form of heart disease are common in these areas of China. There is not enough scientific evidence, however, to support the use of selenium supplements to prevent or treat cancer or CVD.[41]

Selenium Toxicity   The UL for selenium is 400 mcg/day. In the United States, selenium toxicity (selenosis) (*sell'—in—o'—sis*) is rare. Chronic sel—enosis, however, can occur from drinking well water that naturally contains too much selenium. Selenium toxicity can develop by taking megadoses of dietary supplements. In humans, signs and symptoms of chronic selenosis include brittle fingernails, loss of hair and nails, garlicky body odor, nausea, vomiting, and fatigue.

TABLE 9.21   Selenium Content of Selected Foods

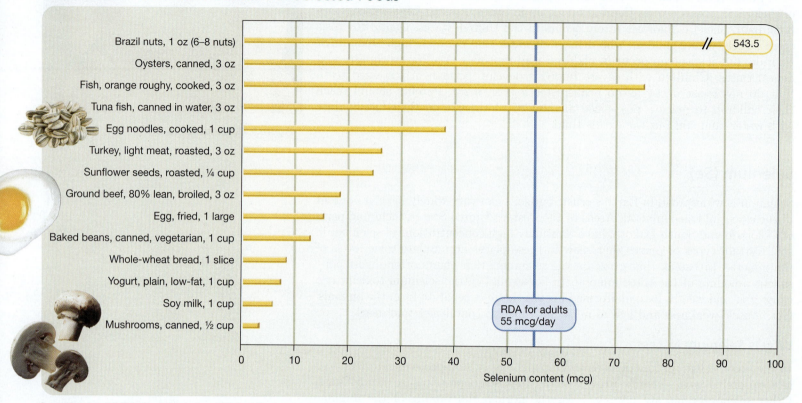

Food	Selenium content (mcg)
Brazil nuts, 1 oz (6–8 nuts)	543.5
Oysters, canned, 3 oz	~95
Fish, orange roughy, cooked, 3 oz	~75
Tuna fish, canned in water, 3 oz	~60
Egg noodles, cooked, 1 cup	~38
Turkey, light meat, roasted, 3 oz	~26
Sunflower seeds, roasted, ¼ cup	~24
Ground beef, 80% lean, broiled, 3 oz	~19
Egg, fried, 1 large	~15
Baked beans, canned, vegetarian, 1 cup	~13
Whole-wheat bread, 1 slice	~9
Yogurt, plain, low-fat, 1 cup	~7
Soy milk, 1 cup	~6
Mushrooms, canned, ½ cup	~3

RDA for adults 55 mcg/day

Source: Data from U.S. Department of Agriculture, Agricultural Research Service: *USDA national nutrient database for standard reference, Release 26,* 2013.

Chromium (Cr)

The importance of chromium as an essential trace mineral in human diets has been recognized only for about the past 40 years. The results of scientific stud—ies suggest that chromium plays an important role in maintaining proper car—bohydrate and lipid metabolism. The concentration of chromium in the body is generally low, because the digestive tract absorbs only about 0.4 to 2.5% of the chromium in foods; the remainder is excreted in the feces.[42] Vitamin C and the B—vitamin niacin enhance the intestinal tract's ability to absorb chromium.[42]

Why Is Chromium Necessary?

Most cells require the hormone insulin to obtain glucose from the blood—stream. Chromium may enhance insulin's action on cell membranes and, in a way, help to "hold the door open" for glucose's entry into the cells. Can people who have diabetes experience better blood glucose regulation by taking chro—mium supplements? A review of scientific research indicated mixed results when people took chromium supplements to improve their blood glucose levels. In some of the studies, chromium supplements were helpful for people with diabetes, but the results of other studies indicated no such benefits.

Sources of Chromium

Although chromium is widely distributed in foods, most foods contain less than 2 mcg of the mineral per serving.[42] Information regarding the chromium content of various foods is difficult to find, because most reliable food composition tables do not include this trace mineral. In general, meat, whole—grain products, yeast,

| Whole grains are good sources of chromium.

fruits, and vegetables are good sources of chromium. Like selenium, the amount of chromium in plant foods reflects the chromium content of soils where crops are grown.

Dietary Adequacy

The adult AIs for chromium are 25 mcg/day for young women and 35 mcg/day for young men. Well—balanced diets typically contain these amounts of chromium. On average, American adults consume diets that meet or exceed their AIs for chromium.[42]

Chromium Deficiency   Signs of chromium deficiency are impaired glucose tolerance and elevated blood cholesterol and triglyceride levels. The mechanism by which chromium influences cholesterol metabolism is not known but may involve enzymes that control the body's cholesterol production. Cases of chromium deficiency have been reported in people maintained on special—formula diets that did not contain chromium, as well as in severely malnourished children.

Chromium Toxicity   The form of chromium that is naturally in foods has not been shown to produce toxicity, so no UL has been set for the trace mineral. The long—term safety of taking various chromium supplements is unknown.[42] Therefore, taking supplemental chromium may be risky.

Manganese

Manganese is an important component and activator of many enzymes in the body. These manganese—dependent enzymes play a role in wound healing, metabolism, bone and cartilage formation, and antioxidant function.[43] Some experts suspect that the trace mineral may play a role in preventing osteoporosis, diabetes, and epilepsy. Food sources of manganese include leafy vegetables, whole grains, nuts, and tea. Small amounts of manganese are in natural sources of water.

Manganese deficiency rarely occurs in humans. Results of animal studies indicate that manganese deficiency interferes with reproduction, impairs growth, alters carbohydrate and lipid metabolism, and causes skeletal abnormalities.[43] Although a small amount of manganese is essential, too much is highly toxic. Overconsumption of manganese, which can occur from drinking water that is contaminated with the mineral, causes a nervous system disorder that is similar to Parkinson's disease. Cases of manganese toxicity from food consumption have not been reported.[43]

Molybdenum

Molybdenum is a cofactor that is needed for the functioning of four enzymes:

- Aldehyde oxidase
- Mitochondrial amidoxime
- Sulfite oxidase
- Xanthine oxidase

Legumes, grains, and nuts are excellent sources of molybdenum. There have been no reports of molybdenum deficiency in healthy persons, and excesses of the trace mineral generally have low toxicity.[44]

Concept **Checkpoint 9.5**

23. What is the difference between iron deficiency and iron deficiency anemia? What are the signs and symptoms of iron deficiency anemia? Which members of the population are most at risk of iron deficiency?
24. What is hemochromatosis? Identify at least three signs or symptoms of hemochromatosis. How is the condition treated?
25. Describe signs and symptoms of zinc deficiency in humans.
26. What is a goiter? What is cretinism? How can cretinism be prevented?
27. Which foods are rich sources of selenium?
28. What is the major role of chromium in the body?
29. Prepare a table for trace minerals that includes information about each trace mineral's major role or roles in the body, food sources, and signs and symptoms of the mineral's deficiency as well as toxicity disorders. Check your table against the information provided in Table 9.15.

9.6 Minerals with Possible Physiological Roles

Learning Outcome

1 List six possible essential minerals and their possible roles in the body.

A few minerals, including nickel, arsenic, and silicon, are found in small amounts in the body, but their roles in the body are unclear. At present, this group of minerals is not classified as essential nutrients. Table 9.22 summarizes the possible functions, suggested human intakes, and food sources of six minerals that may be essential to humans. Although there are reports of severe illness and deaths resulting from environmental exposure to high amounts of these minerals, foods generally do not contain toxic amounts of them.

TABLE 9.22 Summary of Six Possible Essential Minerals

Mineral	Possible Functions	Suggested Daily Human Intakes	Dietary Sources
Arsenic (As)	No clear biological function in humans but may play a role in methionine metabolism, growth, and reproduction (animal studies)	No UL has been established; however, arsenic is highly toxic	Fish, grains, cereals
Boron (B)	No clear biological function in humans but may be involved in steroid hormone metabolism	1–13 mg (UL: 20 mg/day)	Fruit, leafy vegetables, peanuts, beans, wine
Lithium (Li)	Reproduction; maintenance of appropriate mood	1000 mcg (No UL has been established)	Water supply, grains, vegetables
Nickel (Ni)	Amino acid and fatty acid metabolism	25–35 mcg (UL: 1 mg/day)	Chocolate, nuts, beans, whole grains
Silicon (Si)	Connective tissue, including bone formation	25–30 mg (Insufficient data to determine UL)	Root vegetables, whole grains
Vanadium (V)	Glucose metabolism; tooth and bone mineralization	10 mcg (UL: 1.8 mg/day)	Shellfish, mushrooms, black pepper, parsley, dill

Sources: Data from Food and Nutrition Board, Institute of Medicine: *Dietary Reference Intakes for vitamin A, vitamin K, arsenic, boron, chromium, copper, iodine, iron, manganese, molybdenum, nickel, silicon, vanadium, and zinc.* Washington, DC: Standing Committee on the Scientific Evaluation of Dietary Reference Intakes. National Academy Press, 2006. Schrauzer, GN: Lithium: Occurrence, dietary intakes, nutritional essentiality. *Journal of the American College of Nutrition*, 21(1):14, 2002.

Concept **Checkpoint 9.6**

30. Identify at least four minerals that are classified as possible essential minerals.
31. Prepare a table for arsenic, boron, lithium, nickel, silicon, and vanadium that includes information about each mineral's possible function and major food sources. Check your table against the information provided in Table 9.22.

9.7 Nutrition Matters: Bottled Water Versus Tap Water

Learning Outcomes

1 Identify natural sources of water.

2 Explain the roles of the FDA and EPA in regulating water safety in the United States.

3 Discuss the pros and cons of drinking bottled water.

4 Explain health risks associated with BPA.

Today, preparing for a class often involves bringing into the classroom a notebook, something to write with, and a bottle of cold water. Even many college instructors keep a bottle of water nearby as they lecture. Not long ago, most Americans got their water from a faucet ("tap water"). Now, millions of Americans are turning away from the tap and choosing to drink bottled water instead. If you prefer drinking bottled water over tap water, you are part of a growing trend. According to data provided by the Beverage Market Corporation, each American consumed, on average, about 31 gallons of bottled water in 2012.[45] Sales revenues for bottled water were about $12 billion in 2012.[45]

Why do so many Americans drink bottled water when tap water is much less costly? Among adults, taste, convenience, and health concerns were major reasons they chose bottled water over other beverages. For most Americans, however, bottled water is usually unnecessary and expensive, as it is often very similar to tap water. Consumers need to be aware that the water in some bottled water products actually comes from a municipal water supply. However, when public water supplies are disrupted by hurricanes, tornadoes, or earthquakes, drinking bottled water may be a consumer's only option. What is bottled water? Is it safe to drink?

The Environmental Protection Agency (EPA) regulates the sanitation of public water supplies in the United States. Another federal agency, the FDA, regulates bottled water products that are marketed for interstate commerce. Neither agency "certifies" bottled water.[46]

The FDA requires bottled water producers to:

- process, bottle, hold and transport bottled water under sanitary conditions;
- protect water sources from bacteria, chemicals, and other contaminants;
- use quality control processes to ensure the bacteriological and chemical safety of the water; and
- sample and test both the source of water and the final product for contaminants.[47]

Bottled water is sealed in containers and has no added ingredients other than a substance that prevents the growth of microbes, such as bacteria. Bottled water may have fluoride added, but amounts must meet FDA guidelines. If bottled water manufacturers add flavorings or other ingredients to their products, the name of the product must indicate the added ingredients; "Bottled Water with Cherry Flavor," for example. These drinks are often called "flavored water beverages." Flavored waters may simply contain additives that make the beverage taste good, but a growing number of flavored waters also have added nutrients other than sugars, such as sodium, potassium, and amino acids. The beverage's label must identify the additives in the list of ingredients.

The FDA uses place of origin to classify some bottled waters. "Artesian well water," for example, must come from a well that taps an *aquifer*, a body of water found between porous layers of rock, sand, and earth. Table 9.23 lists common types of water used for bottling purposes and their FDA definitions.

Safety standards for bottled water are similar to those established by the EPA for tap water. According to FDA guidelines, bottled water manufacturers are responsible for producing safe products. Production procedures for bottled water must follow manufacturing regulations established and enforced by the FDA. Additionally, the FDA inspects water bottling facilities regularly.

Because of FDA regulations and oversight, consumers can be assured that their supply of bottled water is safe.

TABLE 9.23
FDA Definitions for Classifying Some Types of Water

Water	Definition
Artesian water	Water from a well that taps a confined aquifer
Mineral water	Water containing not less than 250 ppm (parts per million) total dissolved solids and originates from a geologically and physically protected underground water source. No minerals may be added to mineral water.
Purified water	Water produced by distillation, deionization, reverse osmosis, or other suitable processes. The water must meet the definition of "purified water" in the *U.S. Pharmacopeia*.
Sparkling bottled water	Treated water that contains the same amount of carbon dioxide it had when it emerged from its source
Spring water	Water from an underground formation from which the water flows naturally to the surface of the Earth at an identified location.

Source: Data from U.S. Food and Drug Administration: *Food facts.* http://www.fda.gov/food/foodborneillnesscontaminants/buystoreservesafefood/ucm046894.htm

Figure 9.24 BPA and epoxy resins. The epoxy resin that is used to coat the inside of cans contains BPA.

Additionally, most Americans can trust the safety of their tap water because the vast majority of municipal water systems in the United States are regulated by the *Safe Drinking Water Act (SDWA)*. As a result of this law, most tap water undergoes a thorough purification process and is constantly tested for safety. If such testing indicates the water supply may pose a threat to public health, consumers are warned through media, and a "boil order"—requirement to boil water for 10 minutes to kill harmful microorganisms—may be issued.

Although bottled water is safe to drink, the plastic used to contain it may have toxic effects on health. *Bisphenol (biss'−feen−ol) A*, which is also called *BPA*, is a chemical used to make polycarbonate plastics and epoxy resins. Polycarbonate plastics are in many consumer products that come in contact with foods and beverages, including some water bottles and baby bottles. The epoxy resin that contains BPA is used to coat the inside of certain food cans. The coating prevents the can's metal from coming in contact with and being damaged by the food (Fig. 9.24). However, BPA can leach from polycarbonate plastic containers or epoxy resin–coated cans and enter the food or beverage stored within them.

In recent years, consumers have raised questions about the safety of BPA, especially in products used by infants and children. Scientists are studying BPA to determine the extent to which the chemical can affect human health. Concern over the safety of BPA has encouraged some manufacturers to discontinue using the chemical in their products. Plastic containers that are marked with recycle codes 1, 2, 4, 5, and 6 most likely do not contain BPA. Some plastics that are marked with recycle codes 3 or 7 may be made with BPA (Fig. 9.25).[48] To reduce exposure to BPA, consider taking these actions:

- Avoid heating foods in polycarbonate plastic containers.
- Avoid plastic containers that have the symbol shown in Figure 9.25.
- Do not wash polycarbonate containers in the dishwasher or with harsh detergents.
- Reduce intake of foods in cans lined with epoxy resins.

- Cook or store foods and beverages in glass, porcelain, or stainless steel containers.
- Avoid using polycarbonate dishware, cups, or eating utensils for serving foods (especially hot foods or liquids).
- Avoid using old plastic baby bottles and toys that may contain BPA.

Figure 9.25 Where's the BPA? This symbol indicates that the plastic used to make this water bottle may contain BPA.

Concept **Checkpoint 9.7**

32. According to the FDA, what is the difference between "sparkling water" and "spring water"?

33. List three ways to reduce your exposure to BPA.

Chapter References

See Appendix H.

Summary

9.1 Introducing Water and Minerals

- Dehydration can be deadly. A mineral nutrient can be classified as a major, trace, or possible essential mineral.

9.2 Water

- Water is a simple compound that does not undergo digestion. In the body, water is a major solvent that often participates directly in chemical reactions. Water's other physiological roles include transporting substances, removing waste products, lubricating tissues, and regulating body temperature and acid-base balance. Water does not provide energy for the body.

- The body maintains a balance between intracellular and extracellular fluids primarily by controlling concentrations of ions in each fluid compartment. If the normal concentrations of these ions change too much, water shifts out of a compartment, and cells shrink or swell as a result.

- Total water intake includes water from beverages and foods. Most of the water that enters the digestive tract is absorbed. Metabolic water is another source of water for the body.

- The body loses water in urine, perspiration, exhaled air, feces, and insensible perspiration. A healthy person's average daily total water input equals his or her average output. Environmental factors, physiological conditions, and lifestyle practices can alter the body's fluid balance. The kidneys are the major regulator of the body's water content and mineral ion concentrations.

- The AI for total water intake is 2.7 L for young women and 3.7 L for young men. These amounts do not need to be consumed in the form of fluids, because most solid foods and metabolic water contribute some water to the body. Thirst is the primary regulator of fluid intake.

9.3 Minerals: Basic Concepts

- Some minerals function as inorganic ions, cofactors, or structural components of tissues; other minerals are components of various enzymes, hormones, or other organic molecules. Cells cannot metabolize minerals for energy. The body, however, needs certain minerals to catalyze specific chemical reactions that release energy from macronutrients. Excessive amounts of minerals in the body can disrupt normal cell functioning, causing toxicity. Most foods contain small amounts of minerals. When the body's needs for minerals increase, the bioavailability of minerals generally increases to meet the demand.

9.4 Major Minerals

- Calcium is a major structural component of bones and teeth, and the mineral is necessary for blood clotting, muscle contraction, nerve transmission, and cell metabolism. Calcium absorption depends on vitamin D. Milk and milk products are rich calcium sources. Although people, especially women, are at risk of developing osteoporosis as they age, various lifestyle modifications help reduce this risk.

- Sodium, the major positively charged ion found outside cells, is vital for maintaining fluid balance and transmitting nerve impulses. The typical American diet provides high amounts of sodium, primarily from processed and canned foods. Diets high in sodium are associated with increased risk of hypertension.

- Hypertensive individuals have greater risk of CVD, kidney failure, and damage to other organs than people with normal blood pressures. Advanced age, African-American ancestry, obesity, physical inactivity, cigarette smoking, and excess alcohol and sodium intakes are major risk factors for hypertension. Treatment for hypertension usually includes following dietary modifications and making some other lifestyle changes.

- Potassium, the major positively charged ion found inside cells, has functions that are similar to those of sodium. Potassium-rich diets may lower blood pressure. Plant foods, meat, and milk are good sources of potassium.

- Magnesium is a cofactor for numerous chemical reactions and is needed for nerve and heart function. Plant foods are good sources of magnesium.

9.5 Trace Minerals

- Iron is a critical component of hemoglobin, myoglobin, and cytochromes. Hemoglobin in red blood cells transports oxygen from the lungs to the tissues. Iron deficiency can result in iron deficiency anemia. Iron absorption depends on the body's need for the mineral and the form of iron in food. Heme iron is better absorbed than nonheme iron.

- Women of childbearing age have higher needs for iron than men because of menstrual blood loss. Throughout the world, iron deficiency–related disorders are common. People who have hereditary hemochromatosis develop iron toxicity, because they absorb too much iron.

- Zinc functions as a cofactor that activates many enzymes. Zinc is involved in growth and development, antioxidant activity, immune function, and taste. Zinc deficiency can result in growth failure and decreased immune function. Iodine is needed to make thyroid hormone. When the diet lacks iodine, the thyroid gland enlarges, forming a goiter. Cretinism can occur in infants born to women who were iodine deficient during pregnancy. Iodine deficiency is rare in the United States because table salt is often fortified with iodide.

- Selenium functions as a component of selenoproteins, many of which are antioxidants. Other selenoproteins are involved in the normal functioning of the immune system and thyroid gland. Meat, fish, nuts, whole grains, and seeds are good sources of selenium. Chromium enhances the action of insulin. Chromium is found in meats and whole grains. More research is needed to determine the effects of taking chromium supplements.

9.6 Minerals with Possible Physiological Roles

- A few minerals, including nickel and silicon, are found in very small amounts in the body, but their roles in the body are unclear. At present, these particular minerals are not classified as essential nutrients.

9.7 Nutrition Matters: Bottled Water Versus Tap Water

- In the United States, bottled water is usually unnecessary and expensive, and it is often derived from a municipal water supply. The Environmental Protection Agency regulates the sanitation of public water supplies in the United States. The Food and Drug Administration regulates bottled water products that are marketed for interstate commerce. Although more research is needed to clarify the role of BPA in health, it is wise to avoid products that contain the chemical.

Recipe for Healthy Living

Easy Orange-Strawberry Smoothie

When made with fat-free milk or low-fat yogurt, smoothies are a tasty, low-fat, calcium- and potassium-rich snack. They are also easy to prepare: This recipe takes less than 10 minutes to make. For variety, substitute a banana, a mango, or raspberries for the strawberries, or use lime sherbet instead of orange sherbet. Experimenting with different fruits and flavored sherbets makes it easy to individualize smoothies, depending on your preferences and the fruit that's available. You'll need a sturdy blender to combine the ingredients.

The following recipe makes about three 8-fluid-ounce servings. Each serving supplies approximately 214 kcal, 9 g protein, 2 g fat, 290 mg calcium, 607 mg potassium, 125 mg sodium, 1.6 mg zinc, and 6 mcg selenium.

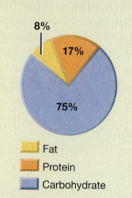

INGREDIENTS:

¼ cup frozen orange juice concentrate, calcium fortified
1 cup orange sherbet
1 ½ cups low-fat, plain yogurt
1 cup fresh strawberries, washed with leafy "caps" removed
  (can substitute frozen strawberries)
2 ice cubes

PREPARATION STEPS:

1. Place all ingredients, except ice cubes, in blender.

2. Blend until smooth. Add ice cubes and blend again, until ice is crushed.

3. Serve.

4. Refrigerate or freeze unused portion in a covered container. Partially thaw frozen smoothie before blending again.

ChooseMyPlate.gov

8%
17%
75%

- Fat
- Protein
- Carbohydrate

NUTRITION

Further analyze this and other recipes through activities on Connect at www.mcgrawhillconnect.com.

Calories* 11
Protein 18
Fat 5
Calcium 29
Sodium 5
Potassium 17
Selenium 9
Zinc 11

% of DV/serving

*2000 daily total kcal

Personal Dietary Analysis

Using the DRIs

1. Refer to your 3-day food log from the "Personal Dietary Analysis" feature in Chapter 3.

   a. Find the RDA/AI values for minerals under your life stage/sex group category in the DRI tables (see the last pages of this book). Write those values under the "My RDA/AI" column in the table below.

   b. Review your personal dietary assessment. Find your 3-day average intakes of iron, calcium, zinc, sodium, potassium, and magnesium. Write those values under the "My Average Intake" column of the table.

   c. Calculate the percentage of the RDA/AI you consumed for each mineral by dividing your intake by the RDA/AI amount and multiplying the figure you obtain by 100. For example, if your average intake of iron was 9 mg/day, and your RDA for the mineral is 18 mg/day, you would divide 18 mg by 9 mg to obtain .50. To multiply this figure by 100, simply move the decimal point two places to the right, and replace the decimal point with a percentage sign (50%). Thus, your average daily intake of iron was 50% of the RDA. Place the percentages for each mineral under the "% of My RDA/AI" column.

   d. Under the ">, <, or =" column, indicate whether your average daily intake was greater than (>), less than (<), or equal to (=) the RDA/AI.

2. Use the information you calculated in the first part of this activity to answer the following questions:

   a. Which of your average mineral intakes equaled or exceeded the RDA/AI?

   b. Which of your average mineral intakes was below the RDA/AI?

   c. What foods would you eat to increase your intake of the minerals that were less than the RDA/AI levels? (Review sources of the minerals in this chapter.)

   d. Turn in your completed table and answers to your instructor.

Personal Dietary Analysis: Minerals

Mineral	My RDA/AI	My Average Intake	% of My RDA/AI	>, <, or =
Iron				
Calcium				
Zinc				
Sodium				
Potassium				
Magnesium				

Complete the Personal Dietary Analysis activity online at www.mcgrawhillconnect.com.

Critical Thinking

1. Before the advent of refrigeration, salting meat was a common way of preventing microbes from spoiling the food. Explain why salting was effective as a means of food preservation.

2. A friend of yours refuses to drink tap water because she thinks it is contaminated. She drinks only bottled water or well water. If she asked you to explain why you drink tap water, what would you tell her?

3. A group of food manufacturers is considering fortifying some of their products with iron, chromium, boron, and iodide. Explain why you think they should or should not fortify the foods with each of these minerals.

4. What advice would you give a total vegetarian (vegan) concerning his need for calcium, iron, potassium, magnesium, and zinc?

5. Consider your family history and lifestyle to determine whether you are at risk of osteoporosis. If you are at risk, what steps can you take at this point in your life to reduce your chances of developing this disease?

6. Consider your family history and lifestyle to determine whether you are at risk of hypertension. If you are at risk, what steps can you take at this point in your life to reduce your chances of developing this disease?

7. In a televised interview, a person claiming to be a doctor recommends taking megadoses of zinc, iron, and selenium supplements to enhance muscular strength and endurance. Discuss why you would or would not follow this person's advice.

Practice Test

Select the best answer.

1. Which of the following statements is false?
   a. Lean tissue contains more water than fat tissue.
   b. Water is a major solvent.
   c. Generally, young women have more body water than young men.
   d. Water does not provide energy.

2. If the extracellular fluid has an excess of sodium ions,
   a. sodium ions move into cells.
   b. intracellular fluid moves to the outside of cells.
   c. phosphate and calcium ions are eliminated in feces.
   d. blood levels of arsenic and oxalate increase.

3. Which of the following foods has the lowest percentage of water?
   a. tomatoes
   b. oranges
   c. whole-grain bread
   d. vegetable oil

4. In the United States, table salt is often fortified with
   a. iron.
   b. selenium.
   c. potassium.
   d. iodide.

5. Which of the following foods is not a good source of calcium?
   a. butter
   b. American cheese
   c. canned sardines
   d. kale

6. Henry is concerned about his risk of osteoporosis. Which of the following characteristics is a modifiable risk factor for this chronic condition?
   a. family history
   b. racial/ethnic background
   c. physical activity level
   d. age

7. The primary source of sodium in the typical American diet is

   a. bottled water.
   b. unprocessed food.
   c. fruit.
   d. salt.

8. Which of the following populations has the highest risk of hypertension?

   a. people with African–American ancestry
   b. young, physically active Asian men
   c. Hispanic women who do not drink alcohol
   d. young adults who consume high amounts of fruit

9. Sources of heme iron include

   a. fortified grain products.
   b. beef.
   c. spinach.
   d. cast–iron cookware.

10. Worldwide, the most common nutrient deficiency dis–order is _____ deficiency.

    a. iodine
    b. cobalt
    c. iron
    d. calcium

11. Which of the following statements is false?

    a. Iodine is necessary for normal thyroid function.
    b. In the United States, milk is usually fortified with iodide.
    c. Having too much or too little iodine in the diet can cause the thyroid gland to enlarge.
    d. Saltwater fish and other seafood are sources of iodine.

12. Which of the following statements is true?

    a. Safety standards for bottled water are similar to those for tap water.
    b. Most brands of water bottled in the United States contain unsafe amounts of arsenic and lead.
    c. The EPA inspects and certifies water bottling facilities at least three times a year.
    d. The majority of Americans should drink bottled water because water from municipal systems is unsafe.

LEARNSMART
ADVANTAGE

Get the most out of your study of nutrition with McGraw-Hill's innovative suite of adaptive learning products including McGraw-Hill LearnSmart®, SmartBook®, LearnSmart Achieve®, and LearnSmart Prep®. Visit www.learnsmartadvantage.com.

CHAPTER 10

Energy Balance and Weight Control

Quiz Yourself

What is the difference between overweight and obesity? Why do most people gain body fat as they age? How can you tell whether a person is following a "fad" diet or a diet that is likely to be safe and effective? Are there any medications or dietary supplements that help people lose weight? Test your knowledge of energy balance and weight management concepts by taking the following quiz. The answers are on page 423.

1. You can determine whether you have an unhealthy amount of body fat simply by measuring your waistline.
_____ T _____ F

2. The safest way to lose a lot of weight and keep it off is to follow a low-carbohydrate, high-fat diet, such as the Atkins diet.
_____ T _____ F

3. As people age, their muscle cells turn into fat cells. _____ T _____ F

4. When a person consumes more protein than needed, the excess can be converted to fat and stored in fat cells.
_____ T _____ F

5. Cellulite is a unique type of fat that can be eliminated by taking certain dietary supplements. _____ T _____ F

10.1 The Obesity Epidemic

Learning Outcomes

1 Explain the difference between overweight and obesity.

2 Discuss how the prevalence of obesity in the United States changed between 1988–1994 and 2009–2010.

In the United States, overweight and obesity are widespread nutritional problems that have reached epidemic proportions (Fig. 10.1). According to the National Heart, Lung, and Blood Institute, **overweight** refers to having extra body weight that is contributed by bone, muscle, body fat, and/or body water.[1] A professional basketball player, for example, may be "overweight" because of his muscular body build—not because he has excess body fat. **Obesity** is a condition characterized by excessive and unhealthy amounts of body fat. Unless noted otherwise, we will use the term *overweight* to describe people who have too much body fat but are not obese.

It is important to recognize that some body fat is essential for good health. However, people who are overweight or obese ("overfat") have a greater risk for serious chronic health conditions and diseases than people who have healthy body weights.

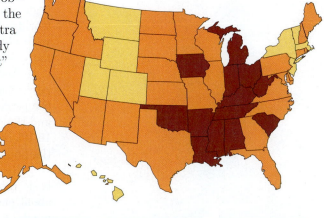

| 20%–<25% | 25%–<30% | 30%–<35% | ≥35% |

Figure 10.1 Obesity map of the United States, 2013. Source: Adapted from Centers for Disease Control and Prevention. http://www.cdc.gov/obesity/data/prevalence-maps.html Accessed September 5, 2014

Prevalence of Overweight and Obesity

To determine whether a person's weight is healthy, overweight, or obese, medical experts generally use the **body mass index (BMI).** BMI is a numerical value based on the relationship between body weight and risk of chronic health problems associated with excess body fat. According to data collected from a national survey, almost 69% of American adults over the age of 20 were either overweight or obese in 2009–2010.[2] One-third of Americans were overweight and more than one-third of them were obese.[3] As shown in Table 10.1, the percent of obese adults increased by almost 60% between 1988–1994 and 2009–2010.[4] People who are classified as being obese can be further categorized into a subgroup of individuals who are "extremely obese." In 2009–2010, over 6% of Americans were classified as being extremely obese. This percentage more than doubled since 1988–1994. The most recent data from 2009–2010, however, indicate that the increase in cases of obesity among American adults may be slowing or leveling off.[2]

TABLE 10.1 Prevalence of Overweight, Obesity, and Extreme Obesity Among Adults: United States, Trends 1988–1994 through 2009–2010

Weight Status	1988–1994	2009–2010
Overweight	33.1%	33.0%
Obese	22.9%	35.7%
• *Extremely Obese*	3.0%	6.3%

Source of data: Fryar CD and others: National Center for Health Statistics: *Prevalence of overweight, obesity, and extreme obesity among adults: United States, trends 1960–62 through 2009–2010.* Last updated September 13, 2012. http://www.cdc.gov/nchs/data/hestat/obesity_adult_09_10/obesity_adult_09_10.htm

overweight having extra weight from bone, muscle, body fat, and/or body water

obesity condition characterized by excessive and unhealthy amounts of body fat

body mass index (BMI) numerical value of relationship between body weight and risk of certain chronic health problems associated with excess body fat

Compared to non–Hispanic white adults, overweight and obesity are more common among non–Hispanic black and Mexican–American adults, particularly among non–Hispanic black women.[2] According to experts at the Centers for Disease Control and Prevention (CDC), cultural, behavioral, and environmental factors may be largely responsible for racial/ethnic differences in obesity rates.

The prevalence of obesity among American children and adolescents has also risen sharply over the past two decades. However, the most recent data comparing the prevalence of childhood and adolescent obesity from 2007–2008 to 2009–2010 showed no change.[5] Public health experts are very concerned about the high prevalence of obesity among children, because these youngsters are more likely to mature into obese adults than are children who are not obese. See Chapter 13 for a discussion of childhood obesity.

Overweight and obesity rates are also rising rapidly throughout the world ("globesity"). In 2008, the World Health Organization (WHO) estimated that worldwide, more than 1 *billion* adults were overweight and 500 million adults were obese.[6] Throughout the world, overweight and obesity are responsible for more deaths than underweight.[6]

According to national target goals established in *Healthy People 2020*, the percentage of obese adults should decline to 30.5% by 2020.[7] Furthermore, the percentage of obese children aged 6 through 11 years should decline to 15.7% and the percentage of obese youth aged 12 through 19 years of age should drop to 16.1% by 2020. Based on current trends concerning rising rates of obesity within the population, these goals may be unrealistic.

Regardless of whether a person wants to maintain, lose, or gain weight, the basic principles of energy balance apply. By reading this chapter, you will learn about energy balance, body composition, health consequences linked to having too much or too little body fat, and factors that contribute to unwanted weight gain. This chapter also provides practical tips for helping you achieve or maintain a healthy body weight through sensible eating and physical activity practices. Concern about body size can result in unhealthy eating practices. The "Nutrition Matters" feature discusses eating disorders, including anorexia nervosa and bulimia nervosa.

Concept **Checkpoint 10.1**

1. Calvin is overweight, but he has a healthy percentage of body fat. Explain why this situation can occur.

2. What percentage of adult Americans were obese in 2009–2010?

10.2 Body Composition

Learning Outcomes

1. List the components of the two major body compartments.
2. Discuss the difference between subcutaneous fat and visceral fat.
3. Describe the various ways body fat is measured and the pros and cons of each method.
4. Explain why it is important to have healthy amounts of body fat.

fat-free mass body compartment that is comprised of body water, mineral-rich tissues, and protein-rich tissues

total body fat essential fat and adipose tissue

The body is composed of two major compartments: **fat–free mass** (lean tissues) and **total body fat**. (Some scientists who study body composition divide the body into four compartments: body water, bone mineral, fat–free mass, and total body fat.)[8] Fat—free mass is comprised of body water; mineral—rich tissues such as bones and teeth; and protein—rich tissues, including muscles and organs. Total body fat includes "essential fat" and *adipose tissue*. Essential fat is in cell membranes, certain bones, and nervous tissue. Essential fat is vital for survival. Adipose tissue contains adipose cells that are specialized for storing energy in the form of triglycerides (see Fig. 6.13). Overweight and obese people have excessive amounts of fat stored in their adipose tissue.

Adipose Tissue

When food is plentiful, adipose cells remove excess fat from the bloodstream for storage. As the amount of fat stored in adipose cells increases, the size of each cell expands, and the body gains weight. At one time, scientists thought the body could only produce fat cells during periods of rapid growth, such as childhood. However, the body can also develop more fat cells when overeating occurs in adulthood, especially in cases of extreme obesity.[9] Once fat cells form, scientists think the cells remain, unless they die or are surgically removed.

When the body needs energy, adipose (fat) cells release fat for other cells to use as fuel. As each adipose cell loses some fat, it becomes smaller. If adipose cells continue to release fat, the body eventually loses weight as a result. In addition to storing and releasing fat, adipose cells secrete numerous proteins, some of which have roles in regulating food intake, glucose metabolism, and immune responses.[10]

Subcutaneous Fat and Visceral Fat

Subcutaneous (*sub* = under; *cutaneous* [*qu—tay'—nee—us*] = skin) tissue holds skin in place over underlying tissues such as muscles. Subcutaneous tissue also contains adipose cells. When subcutaneous tissue has more adipose cells than other kinds of cells, it is referred to as *subcutaneous fat*.[12] Subcutaneous fat helps insulate the body against cold temperatures and protects muscles and bones from bumps and bruises. Subcutaneous fat is unevenly distributed. This layer of fat is thicker in certain regions of men's and women's bodies, especially in the abdominal area, thighs, and buttocks (Fig. 10.2).

Key

= areas of thicker subcutaneous fat distribution

Figure 10.2 Uneven subcutaneous fat distribution. Subcutaneous fat is unevenly distributed. Thicker deposits occur in various regions of men's and women's bodies, especially in the abdomen, thighs, and buttocks.

Figure 10.3 What is visceral fat? Visceral fat forms a protective structure that is under abdominal muscles and hangs over the stomach and intestines.

In addition to subcutaneous fat, the body has *visceral* (*viss′–eh–rol*) fat. Visceral fat also contains adipose cells, but this type of body fat forms a protective structure that is under the abdominal muscles and hangs over the stomach and intestines (Fig. 10.3). Although there are some racial differences, women generally have more subcutaneous fat than men, whereas men tend to have more visceral fat than women.[14] Excessive amounts of visceral fat and/or subcutaneous abdominal fat result in what is commonly called a "beer belly" or the "middle–age spread."

Visceral fat makes substances that cause inflammation in the body. These inflammatory factors may increase risks of type 2 diabetes and cardiovascular disease (CVD). Section 10.5 discusses an easy way to determine whether you have too much visceral fat.

Measuring Body Fat

When you weigh yourself on a scale, you cannot determine whether your weight is healthy. Why? It is healthier to have more fat–free tissue than fat tissue, but the scale does not distinguish between these two major components of your body. Information concerning your body's composition, especially its *percentage* of fat, can help you predict your risk of obesity–related diseases.

There is no direct way to measure a living person's percentage of body fat. Nevertheless, scientists can use indirect methods of measuring body fat, such as "underwater weighing," dual–energy x–ray absorptiometry, air displacement, bioelectrical impedance, and skinfold thicknesses. The following sections describe these methods of assessing body composition, including their advantages and disadvantages.

Figure 10.4 Underwater weighing.

underwater weighing technique of estimating body composition that involves comparing weight on land to weight when completely submerged in a tank of water

Underwater Weighing

Underwater weighing involves comparing a person's weight "on land" to his or her weight when completely submerged in a tank of water (Fig. 10.4). Lean tissue is denser than water; fat tissue is not as dense as water. Thus, a person

Figure 10.5 Dual-energy x-ray absorptiometry (DXA). Although DXA is a highly accurate way to estimate body fat content, the equipment is very expensive and not widely available outside of clinical settings.

who has more body fat will weigh less when under water than a person who has more lean tissue. The underwater weighing method can be an accurate way of assessing body composition. However, the method is not a convenient, easy, inexpensive, or practical way to estimate body fat, because it requires special testing facilities.

Dual-Energy X-Ray Absorptiometry (DXA)

Dual–energy x–ray absorptiometry (DXA) involves the use of multiple low–energy x–rays to scan the entire body. The method provides a detailed "picture" of internal structures, including fat deposits (Fig. 10.5). During the scanning process, the equipment emits a dose of radiation that is lower than that used for a chest x–ray. Although DXA is a highly accurate way to estimate body fat content, the equipment is very expensive and not widely available outside of clinical settings.

Air Displacement

The **air displacement** method assesses the volume of a person's body, which can be used to calculate his or her body composition. After being weighed on a very precise scale, the subject sits in the chamber of a device called the BOD POD (Fig. 10.6). This device measures the volume of air in the chamber with the person in it and compares the value with the volume of air that was in the chamber when it was unoccupied. The person's volume is the volume of air that was displaced after the subject entered the chamber. Air displacement measurements provide highly

Figure 10.6 BOD POD.

dual-energy x-ray absorptiometry (DXA) technique of estimating body composition that involves scanning the body with multiple low-energy x-rays

air displacement method of estimating body composition by determining body volume accurate estimates of body fat content, but the measuring device is expensive and not practical for most consumers to use.

Bioelectrical Impedance

Bioelectrical impedance is a quick way to estimate body fat content. This method is based on the principle that water and electrolytes conduct electricity. Body fat resists the flow of electricity, because fat tissue contains less water and electrolytes than lean tissue. The bioelectrical impedance device sends a painless, low-energy electrical current via wires connected to electrodes placed on the subject's skin (Fig. 10.7). Within a few minutes, the device converts information about the body's electrical resistance into an estimate of total body fat. The method can be accurate, as long as the subject's hydration status is normal. Dehydration results in an overestimation of total body fat. Consumers can purchase a bioelectrical impedance device that resembles a bathroom scale, but scientific data about the machine's accuracy is lacking.

Figure 10.7 **Bioelectrical impedance.** The use of a device that measures bioelectrical impedance is a quick and painless way to estimate body fat content.

Skinfold Thickness

A common technique for estimating total body fat involves taking **skinfold thickness measurements** at multiple body sites, such as over the triceps muscle of the arm (Fig. 10.8). The width of a skinfold indicates the depth of the subcutaneous fat at that site. To perform the measurements, a trained person pinches a section of the subject's skin, gently pulls it away from underlying muscle tissue, and uses special calipers to measure the thickness of the fat. After taking the measurements, the values are incorporated into a mathematical formula that provides an estimate of the subject's amount of body fat.

Skinfold thickness measurements are relatively easy and inexpensive to perform, but the method's accuracy largely depends on the skill of the person performing the measurements. Also, the technique may underestimate total body fat when used on overfat subjects. However, by combining data collected from skinfold, waist and hip circumference, and body frame (skeletal joint) measurements, researchers can obtain more reliable estimates of an individual's total body fat.

Figure 10.8 **Measuring skinfold thickness.** Body fat content can be estimated by measuring skinfold thicknesses using a skinfold caliper.

bioelectrical impedance technique of estimating body composition in which a device measures the conduction of a weak electrical current through the body

skinfold thickness measurements technique of estimating body composition in which calipers are used to measure the width of skinfolds at multiple body sites

How Much Body Fat Is Too Much?

Some body fat is essential for good health, but too much adipose tissue, especially visceral fat, can interfere with the body's ability to function normally. Percentages of body fat can be used to develop weight classifications for adults. According to one such classification system, a man is overweight when his body is 22 to 25% fat; a woman is overweight when her body is 32 to 37% fat (Table 10.2).[15] It is important to note that the average healthy young woman has more body fat than the average healthy young man, because she needs the extra fat for hormonal and reproductive purposes.

Adults tend to gain adipose tissue as they age, but for elderly persons, some additional fat does not necessarily contribute to serious health problems. The extra fat may provide some health benefits, such as providing an energy reserve for a very ill person who cannot eat. Furthermore, the extra padding of fat may protect a person from being injured by falling.

TABLE 10.2 Adult Body Weight Classification by Percentage of Body Fat

Classification	Body Fat (%)	
	Men	Women
Healthy	13 to 21%	23 to 31%
Overweight	22 to 25%	32 to 37%
Obese	26 to 31%	38 to 42%
Extremely obese	32% or more	43% or more

Source: Adapted from Food and Nutrition Board: *Dietary Reference Intakes for energy, carbohydrate, fiber, fat, fatty acids, cholesterol, protein, and amino acids (macronutrients).* Table 5.5, page 126, 2005. http://www.nap.edu/catalog.php?record_id=10490 . Accessed: July 1, 2014

10.3 Energy for Living

Learning Outcomes

1 Define *basal metabolism*.

2 Use the "rule of thumb" method to estimate a person's daily basal metabolic energy needs.

3 Discuss the four major ways the body uses energy.

4 Describe factors that influence the basal metabolic rate.

Regardless of what you are doing—eating, watching television, studying, exercising, even sleeping—your body needs a constant supply of energy to function. **Energy** is defined as the capacity to perform work. There are several forms of energy, but heat, mechanical, chemical, and even electrical energy occur in living things. The total amount of energy is *constant*; that is, the amount remains the same, because energy cannot be created or destroyed. Nevertheless, the various forms of energy can be stored, released, moved, or transformed from one kind to another. The following sections discuss how human cells obtain and use energy.

Energy Intake

Just as a car engine uses a mixture of gasoline, ethanol, and oxygen to run properly, your body uses a mixture of *biological fuels* and oxygen to do its work. For humans, biological fuels are foods and beverages that contain macronutrients (**energy intake**). For some individuals, nonnutrient alcohol (ethanol) also provides energy. Under normal conditions, our cells metabolize primarily glucose and fatty acids, but small amounts of amino acids are also used for energy.

Cells release the energy stored in biological fuels by breaking bonds within the compounds' molecules. The energy that is released can be captured and stored in special compounds, such as **adenosine triphosphate (ATP),** until it is needed. Cells obtain only about 40% of the energy that was in macronutrients by forming ATP. Cells release the remaining energy as heat. Figure 10.9 summarizes events that result in macronutrient storage or breakdown for energy. The diagram in Appendix C summarizes the complex chemical pathways that most cells use to generate ATP from the metabolism of glucose, fat, and amino acids.

energy capacity to perform work

energy intake calories from foods and beverages that contain macronutrients and alcohol

adenosine triphosphate (ATP) molecule that stores energy

energy output calories cells use to carry out their activities

basal metabolism minimal number of kilocalories the body uses to support vital activities after fasting and resting for 12 hours

resting metabolic rate (RMR) body's rate of energy use a few hours after resting and eating

Energy Output

Energy output (*energy expenditure*) refers to the energy (calories) cells use to carry out their activities. For example, muscle cells need energy to contract, liver cells use energy to convert toxic compounds to safer substances, and intestinal cells need energy to absorb certain nutrients. The following sections discuss the major ways the body uses food energy.

Basal and Resting Metabolism

Metabolism refers to all chemical changes, or reactions, that constantly occur in living cells. Anabolic reactions require energy to occur; catabolic reactions release energy. **Basal metabolism** is the minimal number of calories the body uses for vital physiological activities after fasting and resting for 12 hours. Basal metabolic processes include breathing, circulating blood, and maintaining constant liver, brain, and kidney functions. Basal metabolism does not encompass energy needed for skeletal muscle movements (physical activity), digestion of food, and absorption and processing of nutrients. For the typical active person, basal metabolism accounts for about 60 to 75% of the body's total energy use.[8]

The **resting metabolic rate (RMR)** refers to the body's rate of energy use a few hours after resting and eating. A person's RMR is slightly higher than his or her BMR (basal metabolism rate). Although there is a difference between the BMR and the RMR, researchers often use the terms interchangeably in their publications.

Thyroid hormone, secreted by the thyroid gland, regulates metabolism (see Fig. 9.11). A person who has an overactive thyroid gland produces too much thyroid hormone. As a result, this person has a higher-than-normal metabolic rate. Signs and symptoms of excess thyroid hormone production (*hyperthyroidism*) include feeling warm, sweaty, nervous, and restless; having rapid heart rate and

Figure 10.9 What happens to macronutrients? (*a*) After being absorbed, macronutrients are used for energy or stored as glycogen or fat. (*b*) When energy is needed to fuel cells, macronutrients are released from storage and metabolized to synthesize ATP.

① In muscle, excess glucose is stored as glycogen.

Blood vessel

Glucose

② In the liver, excess glucose is stored as glycogen or converted to triglycerides and released into the bloodstream.

Triglycerides

③ Triglycerides may be stored in adipose cells.

Amino acids

④ Amino acids are picked up by all cells to be used for protein synthesis. In the liver, excess amino acids may be converted to glucose or triglycerides.

Energy (ATP)

⑤ A portion of the absorbed glucose, triglycerides, and amino acids are used for energy.

(a)

chronic diarrhea; fatigue; and losing weight despite having an increased appetite. You might think that hyperthyroidism is the key to treating unwanted weight gain, but the condition can have serious side effects, such as elevated blood pressure and heart failure. A person who suffers from *hypothyroidism* does not produce enough thyroid hormone, and as a result, he or she has a lower–than–normal metabolic rate. This individual typically complains of feeling cold, lacking energy and interest in usual activities, being constipated, and gaining weight easily. Treatment for a hypoactive thyroid gland generally includes medication that contains a form of thyroid hormone.

Factors That Influence the Metabolic Rate In addition to thyroid hormone, numerous factors can increase or decrease basal metabolic rates (Fig. 10.10). Thus, metabolic rates vary among individuals. Factors that influence basal metabolism include:

- *Body composition* Lean body mass is the major factor that influences the metabolic rate.[15] Muscle tissue, a component of lean body mass, is more metabolically active than fat tissue. In general, a person who has more muscle mass will have a higher metabolic rate than someone with less muscle tissue.

- *Sex* Males generally have higher metabolic rates than women because they tend to have more lean body mass.

- *Body surface area* A tall, slender person who weighs 150 pounds has a higher metabolic rate than a shorter person who also weighs 150 pounds. Why? The body constantly loses energy in the form of heat that moves to the skin's surface and then into the environment. Because the taller person's body

Blood vessel

Glucose

Fatty acids

Glycerol

Amino acids

① Glycogen is broken down to supply glucose.

② Fat cells break down triglycerides into fatty acids and glycerol.

③ Proteins are broken down into amino acids, some of which the liver uses to make glucose.

④ Nervous system cell:

Glucose → Energy (ATP)

Other cells:

Fatty acids → Energy (ATP)

(b)

Factors That Increase BMR

- Increased muscle mass
- Body temperature (Fever increases metabolism.)
- Excess thyroid hormone
- Periods of growth (e.g., pregnancy)
- Greater body surface area (tall height)
- Lactation (milk production for breastfeeding)
- Exercise and exercise recovery
- Stimulant drugs (e.g., caffeine)
- Stress

Factors That Decrease BMR

- Decreased muscle mass
- Starvation or very-low-calorie diets
- Low thyroid hormone
- Aging
- Lower body surface area (short height)

| **Figure 10.10** Factors that influence the metabolic rate.

has more surface area than the shorter person's body, the taller individual has to generate more heat energy to replace that which is lost.

- *Age* Basal metabolism declines as one grows older, primarily due to the loss of fat–free tissues such as muscle. After 20 years of age, a woman's BMR declines about 2% and a man's BMR about 3% per decade.[16] Therefore, the average adult needs about 150 fewer daily kilocalories per decade as he or she ages. As many adults grow older, they think their muscles have "turned into" fat. A muscle cell, however, cannot transform itself into a fat cell. During the aging process, lean tissue mass shrinks, as cells from muscle, bone, and organs die and are not replaced. Fat cells, however, can continue to develop throughout life, especially when a person overeats consistently. When adipose tissue expands in size, it can fill in spaces formerly occupied by muscle and organ tissues. Regular exercise helps build and preserve lean body mass, and to some extent, people can maintain a higher metabolic rate by being physically active as they grow older.

- *Calorie intake* Calorie intake also affects the metabolic rate. The body conserves energy use when calorie intakes are very low or lacking altogether. To enhance the rate of weight loss, an overfat person should reduce caloric intake while maintaining a normal metabolic rate. Because very–low–calorie diets reduce the metabolic rate, such diets are not generally recommended for weight loss.

The following factors increase the metabolic rate:

- *Fever*

- *Stimulant drugs* (caffeine, for example)

- *Pregnancy*

- *Milk production in a female who has given birth*

- *Recovery after exercise*

Calculating Metabolic Energy Needs The basal metabolic rate is fairly con–stant from day to day.[17] Thus, a young adult can estimate his or her daily meta–bolic rate by following a "rule of thumb" formula:

$$\text{Formula for men} = 1.0 \text{ kcal/kg/hr}$$
$$\text{Formula for women} = 0.9 \text{ kcal/kg/hr}$$

To estimate the number of calories you need for your basal metabolism, first convert your weight in pounds to kilograms by dividing your weight by 2.2. (A kilogram is approximately 2.2 pounds.)

_____ lb ÷ 2.2 lb = _____ kg

Then, depending on your sex, use one of the following formulas:

_____ kg × 0.9 (women) = _____ kcal/hr
_____ kg × 1.0 (men) = _____ kcal/hr

Finally, use this hourly basal metabolic rate to estimate your basal metabolic rate for an entire day by multiplying the hourly value by 24.

_____ kcal/hr × 24 hr = _____ kcal/day

These calculations only provide a rough estimate of your daily metabolic rate. To estimate your Estimated Energy Requirement (EER) for a 24–hour period, you need to add kilocalories used for physical and other activities to your BMR figure.

Energy for Physical Activity

thermic effect of food (TEF) energy used to digest foods and beverages as well as absorb and further process the macronutrients

Physical activity, voluntary skeletal muscle movement, increases energy expenditure above basal energy needs. The number of kilocalories expended for a particular physical activity depends largely on the type of activity, how long it is performed (duration), the degree of effort (intensity) used while performing the activity, and the weight of the person. A heavy person expends more kilocalories when performing the same activity, for the same duration, and at the same intensity than a lighter person. Why? The muscles of the heavier person must work harder to move the larger body.

To estimate your energy needs for physical activity, visit https://www.supertracker.usda.gov/ and click on "Physical Activity Tracker." Table 10.3 lists various physical activities and the approximate number of kilocalories an individual who weighs 150 pounds expends while performing each activity for a minute. For example, a 150-pound person who walks for 30 minutes (3.5 mph) burns approximately 153 kcal during the walk (30 × 5.1).

The number of calories you need for physical activity can vary widely, depending on how active you are each day. Because you can control the type, intensity, and duration of your physical activities, you can manipulate your energy output to increase, decrease, or maintain your weight.

Thermic Effect of Food (TEF)

The body needs a relatively small amount of energy to digest foods and beverages as well as to absorb and further process the macronutrients. The energy used for these tasks, generally 5 to 10% of total caloric intake, is referred to as the **thermic effect of food (TEF).** For example, if your energy intake was 3000 kcal/day, TEF would account for 150 to 300 kcal.

TABLE 10.3 Approximate Energy Expenditures of Selected Physical Activities (150-pound person)

Physical Activity	Approximate kcal/min.
Sitting and playing cards	1.9
Bowling	4.1
Walking (3.5 mph)	5.1
Bicycling (10 mph)	6.4
Canoeing (4 mph)	6.7
Dancing (active)	6.8
Hiking (with pack, 3 mph)	6.8
Walking (4.5 mph)	7.1
Tennis (singles, recreational)	7.5
Weight training	7.8
Touch football (vigorous)	8.3
Aerobic dancing	9.0
Swimming (vigorous breaststroke)	9.6
Running/jogging, steady pace (5.5 mph)	10.0
Bicycling (15 mph)	10.9
Karate	12.8

Source: Williams M: *Nutrition for health, fitness, and sport.* 9th ed. New York: McGraw-Hill, 2010.

nonexercise activity thermogenesis (NEAT) involuntary skeletal muscular activities such as fidgeting

Nonexercise Activity Thermogenesis (NEAT)

Nonexercise activity thermogenesis (*thermo* = heat; *genesis* = production) or **NEAT** refers to *involuntary* skeletal muscle activity, that is, physical activity that a person does not consciously control. NEAT activities include shivering, fidgeting, maintaining muscle tone, and maintaining body posture when not lying down. Some people may expend as much as 700 kcal daily as NEAT.[18] It is possible that some individuals resist weight gain from overeating because they have higher−than−average energy expenditures for NEAT. Nevertheless, the contribution of NEAT to overall calorie needs is fairly small for most people.

Putting It All Together

To estimate your daily energy expenditure, you could add the kilocalories you burned for basal metabolism, physical activity, TEF, and NEAT in a day. However, an easier method is to use one of the formulas published by the Food and Nutrition Board of the Institute of Medicine (FNB).[15] The following formulas are for men and women who are 19 years of age or older.

Men

$$\text{Estimated Energy Requirement (EER)} = 662 - (9.53 \times \text{AGE}) + \text{PA} \times (15.91 \times \text{WT} + 539.6 \times \text{HT})$$

Women

$$\text{Estimated Energy Requirement (EER)} = 354 - (6.91 \times \text{AGE}) + \text{PA} \times (9.36 \times \text{WT} + 726 \times \text{HT})$$

The variables in the formulas are:

$$\textbf{AGE} = \text{age in years}$$
$$\textbf{PA} = \text{physical activity estimate (Table 10.4)}$$
$$\textbf{WT} = \text{weight in kg (lb} \div 2.2)$$
$$\textbf{HT} = \text{height in meters (inches} \div 39.4)$$

To practice using the formula, consider a 24−year−old woman who is 5−feet, 5−inches (65 inches) tall, weighs 145 pounds, and has a low level of physical activity. With this information, you can determine the missing values for the formula.

This young woman's age is **24** and her value for physical activity level (PA) is **1.12.** To convert her weight in pounds to kilograms, divide her weight by 2.2.

$$145 \div 2.2 = 65.9 \text{ kg}$$

To convert her height to meters, divide her height (inches) by 39.4.

$$65.0 \div 39.4 = 1.65 \text{ meters (rounded value)}$$

TABLE 10.4 Physical Activity Level Estimates

Activity Level	PA (Men)	PA (Women)
Sedentary (no exercise)	1.00	1.00
Low activity (for example, walking the equivalent of 2 miles/day at 3 to 4 mph)	1.11	1.12
Active (for example, walking the equivalent of 7 miles/day at 3 to 4 mph)	1.25	1.27
Very active (for example, walking the equivalent of 17 miles/day at 3 to 4 mph)	1.48	1.45

Source of data: Food and Nutrition Board, National Institute of Medicine: *Dietary Reference Intakes for energy, carbohydrate, fiber, fat, fatty acids, cholesterol, protein, and amino acids (macronutrients).* Washington, DC: National Academies Press, 2005.

Now we can "plug" these values into the formula for a woman.

Estimated Energy Requirement (EER) $= 354 - (6.91 \times 24) +$
$\mathbf{1.12} \times (9.36 \times \mathbf{65.9} + 726 \times \mathbf{1.65})$

To solve the equation, move from left to right, but do the math in the paren—theses first.

$$EER = 354 - (6.91 \times 24)$$
$$EER = 354 - 165.84$$
$$354 - 165.84 = 188.16$$
$$EER = 188.16 + 1.12 \times (9.36 \times 65.9 + 726 \times 1.65)$$

Now, do the math in the remaining parentheses on the right.
Multiply the first two numbers in the parentheses together:

$$9.36 \times 65.9 = 616.82$$

Multiply the next two numbers together:

$$726 \times 1.65 = 1197.9$$

Add the two products together:

$$616.82 + 1197.9 = 1814.72$$

Plug this value into the formula and multiply

$$1.12 \times 1814.72 = 2032.49$$

And add the left and right sides of the formula together:

$$EER = 188.16 + 2032.49 = 2220.65$$
$$\mathbf{EER = approx.\ 2221\ kcal/day}$$

To estimate your EER, complete the "Personal Dietary Analysis" activity at the end of this chapter.

Concept **Checkpoint 10.3**

12. Using the "rule of thumb" formula, estimate the daily basal metabolic energy needs of a woman who weighs 185 pounds.
13. List the four major ways the body uses energy (energy output).
14. For most people, which form of energy expenditure uses the most energy on a daily basis?
15. Discuss at least five factors that influence basal metabolic rate.
16. Of the four major ways the body uses energy, which one is most easily altered?
17. Explain the differences between TEF and energy needs for physical activity.
18. What is NEAT? List at least three ways the body expends energy by NEAT.

10.4 Energy Balance

Learning Outcomes

1 Explain the concept of energy balance.

2 Compare states of positive and negative energy balance.

Understanding the concept of *energy balance* is critical to understanding why most people gain, lose, or maintain weight. Your body is in a state of **energy equilibrium** and "balanced" when your calorie intake from food and beverages equals your calorie output for basal metabolism, physical activity, TEF, and NEAT (Fig. 10.11). By maintaining a balanced energy state, your weight will remain relatively stable over time.

energy equilibrium calorie intake equals calorie output

Figure 10.11 Energy balance. Your energy state is in equilibrium and "balanced" when your calorie intake from food and beverages equals your calorie output for basal metabolism, physical activity, TEF, and NEAT.

negative energy balance calorie intake is less than calorie output

positive energy balance calorie intake is greater than calorie output

If your calorie intake is lower than your calorie output, you are in **negative energy balance.** In this state, your body needs more calories to carry out its activities than your diet is supplying. Therefore, your body metabolizes stored fat for energy. Weight loss results from being in a negative energy state. Over time, you will notice your clothes have become baggy as your adipose tissue shrinks.

If your calorie intake from macronutrients (and alcohol) is greater than your calorie output, you are in a state of **positive energy balance.** In this state, your body stores excess dietary fat in adipose cells. Additionally, the body converts surplus dietary carbohydrate, protein, and alcohol to fat and stores that fat in adipose cells. Weight gain results from being in a positive energy state, and eventually, you will notice that your clothes seem to have shrunk.

Positive energy balance is necessary for pregnant women, because extra calories are needed to add new tissues that support the pregnancy. Positive energy balance also occurs during periods of growth, such as during fetal development, infancy, childhood, and adolescence. Over time, however, even a small positive energy balance can cause anyone's weight to increase, regardless of his or her age. Maintenance of energy balance—matching calorie intake to calorie output over the long term—is critical for controlling body weight (Fig. 10.12).

Concept **Checkpoint 10.4**

19. What happens to a person's body weight when he or she is in a state of positive energy balance?
20. When is it desirable for a person to be in a positive energy balance state?
21. When is a person in a negative energy balance state?

Energy Balance (Equilibrium)

Intake: 3000 kcal   Output: 3000 kcal   Weight change: No change

Positive Energy Balance

Intake: 4000 kcal   Output: 2000 kcal   Weight change: Increase

Negative Energy Balance

Intake: 2000 kcal   Output: 3000 kcal   Weight change: Decrease

Figure 10.12 **The body's possible energy states.** This figure presents three possible energy states.

10.5 Classifying Overweight and Obesity

Learning Outcomes

1 Use the formula to calculate BMI, and classify a person's BMI as underweight, healthy, overweight, obese, or extremely obese.

2 Discuss serious health problems that are associated with having too much body fat and being obese in particular.

3 Compare "apple" to "pear" body shapes in terms of fat distribution and effects on health.

4 Explain how to measure waist circumference and the usefulness of this information in regard to a person's health.

At one time, people referred to height/weight tables to determine whether their body weights were "ideal" or "desirable." Today, medical experts use the body

TABLE 10.5 Adult Weight Status Categories (BMI)

BMI	Weight Status
Below 18.5	Underweight
18.5 to 24.9	Healthy
25.0 to 29.9	Overweight
30.0 to 39.9	Obese
40 and above	Extremely obese

Source: National Heart, Lung, and Blood Institute: *The practical guide: Identification, evaluation, and treatment of overweight and obesity in adults*. NIH Publication 00-4084, 2000. www.nhlbi.nih.gov/guidelines/obesity/prctgd_c.pdf Accessed January 20, 2014

mass index (BMI) to judge whether an adult's weight is healthy. As mentioned in the chapter opener, BMI is a numerical value based on the relationship between body weight and risk of chronic health problems associated with excess body fat.[15]

Table 10.5 presents adult weight classifications based on BMI ranges. Healthy BMIs range from 18.5 to 24.9. *Overweight* adults have BMIs that range from 25.0 to 29.9; *obese* adults have BMIs that range from 30.0 to 39.9. People whose BMIs are 40 or higher are classified as *extremely obese*. Extremely obese people are far more likely to develop the serious chronic diseases associated with excess body fat and to die prematurely than people who have BMIs that range from 18.5 to 30.0.

Muscle is denser than fat; therefore, many muscular people may have BMIs in the overweight range, yet have healthy percentages of body fat. For example, a muscular person with a BMI of 25.0 is more likely to be healthy than a sedentary (physically inactive) person who also has a BMI of 25.0. The BMI may under–estimate body fat in people who have lost muscle tissue as a result of aging or illness.[20] Therefore, BMIs should not be applied to highly muscular individuals, people who are elderly, or chronically ill persons. However, sedentary people with BMIs of 30 or higher generally have excess body fat.

How Can I Calculate My BMI?

To calculate your BMI, you can use the following formula:

$$\frac{\text{weight (lb)}}{[\text{height (in)}]^2} \times 703$$

For example, a person who weighs 140 pounds and is 5–feet, 3–inches (63 inches) tall has a BMI of approximately 24.8. This person's BMI is almost at the upper limit of the healthy range.

$$\text{Calculation: } [140 \div (63)^2] \times 703$$

$$(140 \div 3969) \times 703 =$$

$$0.03527 \times 703 = 24.8$$

People with BMIs of 40 or higher are extremely obese.

Excess Body Fat: Effects on Health

People with BMIs greater than 25 have increased risks of type 2 diabetes, hyper–tension, and CVD. Many types of cancer, including cancers of the gallblad–der, pancreas, cervix, uterus, breast (postmenopausal women), colon, rectum, and kidney, are more common in obese people. Furthermore, obese patients have high risk of experiencing serious complications during and after surgery. Such patients often require more anesthesia and their incisions are more likely to become infected than surgical patients whose weights are within the healthy range. Compared to people with healthy BMIs, obese people are more likely to die prematurely from all causes.[21]

Overweight and obese people are more likely to develop osteoarthritis, a painful chronic condition that affects joints and interferes with the person's abil–ity to move. Obese people typically have difficulty carrying out routine daily activities, especially those that require walking, carrying, kneeling, and stooping. Additionally, obese people are more likely to suffer from chronic heartburn as well as *sleep apnea*, a condition that causes breathing to stop periodically during sleep.

Obese men and women are more likely to have fertility problems than peo–ple with healthy BMIs. *Polycystic ovary disease* often affects obese women and can reduce the women's chances of becoming pregnant. During pregnancy, obese women have high risk of *gestational diabetes* and a form of hypertension that can be deadly. Additionally, obese pregnant women are at greater risk for still—births or giving birth to babies with birth defects than are pregnant women who have lower BMIs.

A person's mental health and self—esteem can be negatively affected by his or her "weight problem." Many Americans admire slim and muscular body builds over overfat body shapes. Thus, overfat people often suffer from poor self—images because they think their bodies are unattractive. The general public often views obesity as a condition that results from lack of willpower and the inability to "push oneself away from the table." Thus, many overfat people also deal with the negative attitude (stigma) that many people have toward them. People who are not overfat often characterize obese persons as lazy, stupid, and sloppy.[22] The stigma of obesity can result in discriminatory practices that limit an obese person's chances for career opportunities and access to adequate health care. It is not surprising that depression tends to accompany obesity. Table 10.6 lists these and other major health problems associated with excessive body fat.

Body Fat Distribution: Effects on Health

The results of medical research suggest that the distribution of excess body fat has a closer association with obesity—related diseases than does the percentage of total body fat. Some people, especially women, tend to store extra subcutaneous fat below the waist, primarily in the buttocks and thighs (Fig. 10.13a). Having this particular pattern of fat distribution (a "pear shape") adds stress to hip and knee joints that must carry the extra weight, but the pattern is not associated with increased risk of more serious chronic diseases such as type 2 diabetes.

Men and African—American women tend to store extra visceral fat in the abdominal or central region of their bodies.[23] **Central—body obesity** is characterized by a large amount of visceral fat ("spare tire") that spreads beyond buttocks and thighs. A person with central—body obesity is sometimes described as having an "apple" body shape (see Fig. 10.13b). People with central—body obesity have higher risks of cardiovascular disease and type 2 diabetes ("diabesity") than people who have waists that do not extend beyond their hips.[24]

(a) Lower-body fat distribution (pear shape) (b) Central-body fat distribution (apple shape)

Figure 10.13 Body fat distribution: Typical differences. Some people, especially women, tend to store extra subcutaneous fat below the waist (*a*). Men and African-American women tend to store extra visceral fat in the central region of their bodies (*b*).

TABLE 10.6   Health Problems Associated with Excess Body Fat

Overweight and obesity increase the risk of:	
Cardiovascular disease (CVD)	Chronic low back pain
Hypertension	Loss of mobility
Type 2 diabetes	Fatty liver disease (not alcohol related)
Metabolic syndrome	Erectile dysfunction in men (impotence)
Polycystic ovary syndrome	Low-grade inflammation
Infertility	Gastroesophageal reflux disorder (GERD)
Elevated blood lipid levels	Psychological depression
Gallstones	Certain cancers
Sleep apnea	Skin ulcers
Osteoarthritis	Premature death

Sources: Jackson Y and others: Summary of the 2000 Surgeon General's listening session: Toward a national action plan on overweight and obesity. *Obesity Research* 10(12):1299, 2002; Virji A, Murr MM: Caring for patients after bariatric surgery. *American Family Physician*, 73(8):1403, 2006.

central-body obesity condition characterized by excessive visceral fat

Figure 10.14 Measuring waist circumference. A quick and easy method to determine a person's risk of obesity-related disorders is to measure the individual's waist circumference.

A quick and easy method to determine your risk of obesity–related disorders is to measure your *waist circumference*. Figure 10.14 shows a recommended placement of the tape measure. Note the positioning of the tape at the top of the hip bones and not necessarily at the narrowest point. It is also important to use a measuring tape that does not stretch and to hold the tape around the waist, parallel to the floor. Central–body obesity is defined by a waist circumference of greater than 40 inches in men and greater than 35 inches in women.[25]

Concept **Checkpoint 10.5**

22. A young woman's BMI is 26.2. According to this information, is this woman likely to be healthy, overweight, obese, or extremely obese?
23. List at least six different serious health problems that are associated with having too much body fat and being obese in particular.
24. What is the "stigma" of obesity?
25. Which of the two major types of body fat distribution is more likely to pose serious health risks? Which chronic diseases are more likely to develop in people who have this pattern of excess fat deposition?
26. What is a quick and easy way to determine whether a person's body fat distribution is likely to result in serious health problems, such as type 2 diabetes?

10.6 What Causes Overweight and Obesity?

Learning Outcomes

1. Identify factors that can influence the development of excess body fat
2. Discuss factors that influence hunger and satiety.
3. Discuss the roles of hormones and peptides in regulating hunger.
4. Explain what is meant by having "thrifty genes."
5. Discuss how the set-point theory can explain why people often regain the weight they lose.

Although an excess intake of calories in relation to calorie output causes weight gain, there is no simple *cause* of obesity. To lose weight, a person needs to cre–ate a negative energy state by eating fewer calories, expending more calories than the amount consumed, or taking both actions. For many people, however, it is not easy to alter calorie input and output. Numerous factors, including physiological, environmental, behavioral, and psychological forces influence a person's calorie intake and expenditure.

Physiological Factors

From a physiological standpoint, eating behavior is complex and largely involves interactions among the nervous, endocrine, and digestive systems as well as fat tis–sue. *Hunger* and *satiety* are key sensations that regulate eating behavior. **Hunger** is an uncomfortable feeling that drives a person to consume food. Thus, hunger is the need to eat. **Satiety** is the sense that enough food or beverages have been consumed to satisfy hunger.

Physical sensations influence eating behavior. As time between meals increases, the stomach signals "it's time to eat" by contracting, causing hunger

hunger uncomfortable feeling that drives a person to consume food

satiety sense that enough food or beverages have been consumed to satisfy hunger pangs. As the contractions become stronger, the person usually eats or drinks something to relieve the discomfort. The size of the stomach influences satiety. During meals, the stomach stretches as it fills. The sensation that the stomach has reached its capacity can make a person stop eating. Nevertheless, many overfat persons do not recognize the sensation of stomach fullness, and as a result, they may eat even when they should not be hungry.

An area of the *hypothalamus*, a structure in the brain, controls hunger and satiety. Scientists think this region functions as a "hunger/satiety center." The stomach, intestines, and fat tissue produce certain proteins, such as hormones and *peptide YY*, that stimulate nerve cells involved in the regulation of hunger and satiety. **Ghrelin** (*grel'−in*), a hormone secreted mainly by the stomach, stimulates eating behavior. Some scientists think that reducing ghrelin production or activity is the key to helping people lose or maintain their weight. The small and large intestines release peptide YY, a protein that signals the stomach to reduce ghrelin secretion. The small intestine also releases *cholecystokinin* (*CCK*), the hormone that stimulates the gallbladder to contract and the pancreas to release digestive enzymes (see Chapter 6). Additionally, CCK stimulates the brain and other nervous tissue, suppressing appetite as a result.

Fat cells secrete **leptin,** a hormone that reduces hunger and inhibits fat storage in the body. A person's blood leptin level is directly proportional to his or her amount of body fat.[12] The brain obtains information about the status of body fat stores by monitoring the level of leptin in blood. When researchers administer leptin to genetically engineered mice that cannot synthesize the hormone, the rodents lose weight. Studies involving humans, however, generally find that obese people produce high amounts of leptin, but their bodies resist the hormone's hunger−suppressing action.[26] Figure 10.15 illustrates the complex effects of ghrelin, leptin, CCK, and peptide YY on hunger and satiety.

ghrelin hormone that stimulates eating behavior

leptin hormone that reduces hunger and inhibits fat storage in the body

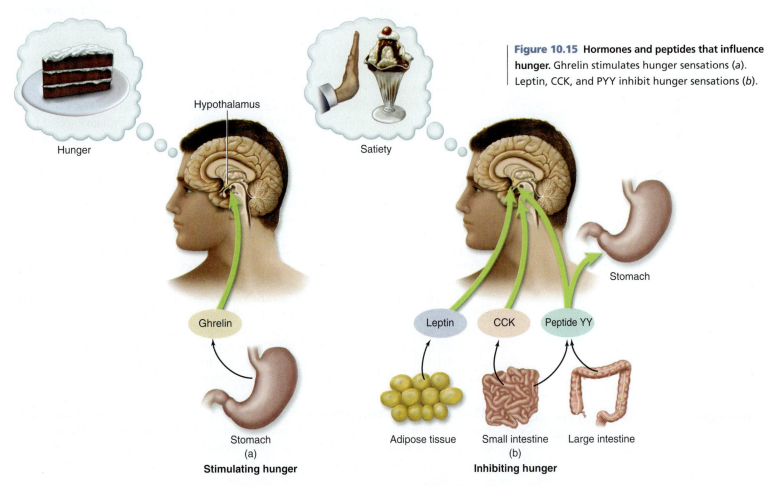

Figure 10.15 Hormones and peptides that influence hunger. Ghrelin stimulates hunger sensations (*a*). Leptin, CCK, and PYY inhibit hunger sensations (*b*).

Food Composition Factors

Dietary factors, particularly amounts of fat and certain carbohydrates in diets, can influence body fat production and appetite. Fatty foods are more energy dense than foods that contain more carbohydrate, protein, and water than fat. Thus, high–fat diets are associated with excess calorie intakes and rising obesity rates.[27] Fatty foods often contain a lot of sugar. Some medical researchers think the consumption of the simple sugar fructose is associated with the current obe–sity epidemic. High fructose intakes may result in weight gain because the sugar stimulates fat synthesis in the body.[28] For a more extensive review of the role that carbohydrates may play in weight gain, see the "Are Carbohydrates Fattening?" section of Chapter 5.

Genetic Factors

Genetics play a major role in the development of obesity. Most physical char–acteristics are inherited, including metabolic rate, hormone production, body frame size, and pattern of fat distribution. All of these characteristics affect body weight.

Some rats and mice are genetically predisposed to become obese because they have inherited genes for "thrifty metabolisms." Rodents with thrifty metabolisms have bodies that are more efficient at storing excess energy as fat than rodents who do not have such metabolisms. It is possible that humans who gain weight easily have genes that code for thrifty metabolisms as well. In ancient times, food was often scarce, and people had to eat as much as they could when food was available. During times when food was plentiful, individuals who had thrifty metabolisms stored more of the excess energy from food as body fat than per–sons who did not have such efficient metabolisms. The people who lacked thrifty metabolisms wasted the excess food energy as body heat. As a result, the energy–"thrifty" people were more likely to survive periods of starvation than the other persons. In many modern societies, however, high–calorie food is available 24 hours a day and starvation is unlikely. As a result, having thrifty metabolisms is no longer beneficial because depositing excess body fat often results in serious health problems.

If you gain weight easily, you may have inherited a thrifty metabolism. To prevent becoming overfat, you need to be physically active and make careful food choices. On the other hand, you probably do not have a thrifty metabolism if you can eat a lot of food and have difficulty gaining weight.

Medical researchers have identified several genes that contribute to human fatness. Genes also control hormones that regulate growth and metabolism, as well as ghrelin and leptin production. Certain mice, for example, become obese because they lack genes for synthesizing leptin (Fig. 10.16). Researchers are interested in developing medications that regulate the influence of certain genes over metabolism and hormone production. If research indicates that such medi–cations are safe and effective, they could help people manage their weight over the long term.

Prader–Willi syndrome is a rare genetic condition that results from the lack of genes in a particular section of a chromosome. People with this condi–tion have skeletal deformities, delayed motor development, decreased intellectual functioning, food cravings, and insatiable appetites. If their access to food is not restricted, children with Prader–Willi syndrome eat constantly and become obese. There is no cure for Prader–Willi syndrome.

set-point theory scientific notion that body fat content is genetically predetermined

What's the Set-Point Theory?   The majority of people who intentionally lose weight regain the weight over time. According to the **set–point theory,** the body's fat content (and therefore, body weight) is genetically predetermined.

The set point acts like a home thermostat, except that it regulates body weight instead of temperature. For example, a person infected with an intestinal virus tends to lose weight because he or she has no interest in eating for a few days. During and after recovery, the person generally regains the lost weight. This observation provides support for the set–point theory. Results of studies involving mice support the set–point theory.[29]

When calorie intakes are reduced, blood thyroid hormone levels decline, depressing the normal basal metabolic rate. Additionally, the caloric cost of performing weight–bearing activities decreases when a person loses weight. As a result, an activity that required 100 kcal before weight loss may burn only 80 kcal after weight loss. Furthermore, weight loss appears to make the body become more efficient at storing calories from macronutrients as fat. When a person gains weight and stays at that weight for a while, his or her body tends to establish a new and higher set point. According to the theory, all these changes protect the body from losing weight and explain why weight loss is so difficult to achieve and maintain.

Opponents of the set–point theory argue that weight does not remain constant throughout adulthood: The average person gains weight slowly, at least until old age. Thus, body weight may result more from lifestyle practices and environmental influences than predetermined biological controls such as a set point.

Figure 10.16 **Genetic obesity in mice.** Certain genetically engineered mice (the mouse on the right) become obese because they lack genes for synthesizing leptin.

appetite desire to eat appealing food

Environmental Influences

Consider your eating behavior during a typical holiday meal that includes a variety of attractive, tasty foods. After eating the meal, your hunger should be satisfied, but as soon as pie or cake is placed on the table, do you "find some room" in your stomach for some dessert? If you often eat when you are not hungry or when you see a favorite food, then you are probably aware of the effect your environment can have on your appetite. **Appetite** is the desire to eat appealing food.

Food advertising is an aspect of the environment that has a powerful influence on your food choices. To entice you to buy their products, food manufacturers usually appeal to your senses, emphasizing the appearance and taste of food, in particular. Recently, a television ad for a fast–food chain promoted a hamburger that has three beef patties, three slices of cheese, and six bacon slices topped with mayonnaise. According to information at the fast–food company's website, this burger provides 800 kcal. The site, however, does not tell you that 800 kcal is more than one–third of a day's calorie needs for an average person! How do you respond when you see food advertisements on television? Do the ads make you hungry or eager to try a new food product?

Over the past 30 years, portion sizes of many popular foods, especially restaurant items, have become larger. People may choose to purchase "supersized" portions of foods because they like the idea of getting more for their money. In many instances, however, "more" means *more* fat and calories per serving. According to some nutrition experts, consumption of oversized portions of foods and beverages contributes to increased calorie intake in the United States.[30]

How does the presence of such appealing food affect your appetite?

Our environment also affects whether we choose to be sedentary or physically active. In our homes, we rely on a variety of "energy-saving" devices such as dishwashing machines, TV remote controls, and garage door openers to work for us. Outside our homes, we use cars, elevators, escalators, and other motorized devices, instead of our feet, to move us from place to place. With the help of machines, our lives are considerably easier; however, we are consuming more calories than in the past.

In 2009–2010, the energy intake in one day of American men and women who were 20 to 29 years of age was 2626 kcal and 1949 kcal, respectively.[31] Overall, Americans are consuming more food energy than they consumed in the early 1970s. The increase in energy intake may help explain why the prevalence of overweight and obesity has increased among Americans over the past 40 years. According to the principles of energy balance, excess energy intake in relation to energy output results in weight gain.

By becoming more physically active, people can increase their energy output. Many Americans, however, have "desk jobs" that require little muscular movement. When we have some leisure time, we often spend it performing tasks that involve sitting—watching television, playing computer games, or chatting with people on the Internet. Less than 48% of American adults meet recommendations for physical activity.[32] According to experts with the Centers for Disease Control and Prevention, healthy adults should perform at least 150 minutes of moderate-intensity physical activity (brisk walking, for example) per week.[33] Adults who include exercise in their weight-loss plan may need to engage in at least 60 minutes of moderate-intensity activity each day to achieve long-term maintenance of lower body weight. ChooseMyPlate.gov has information about physical activity, including examples of activities that are moderate or vigorous.

If you live on or near a university or college campus, your environment probably provides ample opportunities for engaging in exercise and sports, such as tennis courts, swimming pools, and weight-training rooms. It is relatively easy to be physically active while you are in college, *if you choose to be*. After you graduate, consider what you will do to maintain a healthy level of physical activity each day, especially if you have a sedentary job. How likely are you to use the staircase in a building when you see the elevator? Will you keep a pair of comfortable shoes at work, so you can walk for at least 20 minutes during lunch?

Genes and Environment: Interactions

It is difficult to determine the extent to which an obese person's genetic makeup or environment contributes to his or her excess body weight. Children are more likely to become overweight or obese if their biological parents were overfat prior to becoming pregnant.[34] This finding appears to support the hypothesis that obesity is an inherited trait. Nevertheless, genes do not control everything about our health, including our weight. Environmental and other factors can modify the expression of genes. For example, children whose mothers are obese may have inherited genes that increase risk for obesity. However, these children may avoid becoming obese if they adopt a physically active lifestyle and do not overeat. On the other hand, these children may become obese if their parents have poor eating habits and sedentary lifestyles and the youngsters follow their parents' practices.

Other Factors That Influence Weight

Psychological factors such as mood and self–esteem influence eating behaviors and body weight. Many people eat not because they are hungry but because they are bored, anxious, angry, or depressed. Obesity may increase the likelihood of depression, especially in American non–Hispanic white women.[36] Researchers, however, cannot easily determine whether being obese causes depression or being depressed causes obesity.

Among some segments of American society, the ideal female figure is slim but curvy, and the ideal male physique is trim and muscular. As a result, societal pressures inspire many young women to idealize underweight. Consider the body shapes of many fashion models, professional ballerinas, and successful young actresses. These young women have so little subcutaneous fat that some of their bones protrude under their skin. In their relentless efforts to pursue such unre–alistic body shapes, many young women adopt unhealthy and potentially life–threatening eating practices. The "Nutrition Matters" section of this chapter focuses on eating disorders, including *anorexia nervosa*.

Societal pressures inspire many young women to idealize underweight people, especially thin female models and celebrities.

Concept **Checkpoint 10.6**

27. What is hunger? What is satiety?
28. Discuss the roles of leptin and ghrelin in regulating hunger.
29. Under what conditions would having "thrifty genes" benefit a person?
30. What is the set-point theory?
31. What is the difference between hunger and appetite?
32. Describe how the environment influences a person's food intake and physical activity level.
33. Provide at least three examples of ways that physiological, psychological, and societal factors can influence eating behavior.

10.7 Weight Loss and Its Maintenance

Learning Outcomes

1 Identify four key elements that are necessary for weight loss and maintenance.

2 Describe features of reliable weight-loss plans or programs.

3 Discuss practical steps that overfat people can take to reduce their body fat.

4 Explain what members of the National Weight Control Registry do to maintain their reduced body weights.

Before you embark on an effort to lose (or gain) weight, an important first step is determining whether it is even necessary to change your weight. The need for changing your weight should be based on your overall health and family history of weight–related diseases. If you are dissatisfied with your body weight and shape, consider the following questions. Are you physically healthy at your present weight? If your BMI is within the healthy range, why do you think you need to lose or gain weight?

Using a BMI calculator (http://www.nhlbi.nih.gov/health/educational/lose_wt/BMI/bmicalc.htm) or consulting a BMI table such as the one in Figure 10.17 that indicates the range of healthy weights for a particular height (BMIs of 18.5 up to 24.9) can be helpful. According to this chart, an adult who is 5–feet, 5–inches tall has a healthy weight range of about 111 to 149 pounds.

To determine your BMI range using the table in Figure 10.17, locate your height in the left–most column with your left index finger, then locate your weight along the bottom line of the graph with your right index finger. Read across the row with your left finger and up from the bottom with your right finger, until your fingers meet. Note the color of the BMI range where the two fingers meet and compare it to the color key in the upper left–hand corner of the figure. According to this graph, is your BMI in the healthy range?

The next step, if necessary, is setting a reasonable and realistic goal weight. It is important to note that an overweight or obese person does not have to shed a lot of weight to reduce risk factors associated with CVD, stroke, and type 2 diabetes. Just losing 5 to 10% of excess body fat can increase beneficial high–density lipoprotein levels (HDL cholesterol), reduce elevated blood pressure and triglyceride levels, and improve glucose tolerance.[20]

Figure 10.17 Adult BMI chart. Are you at a healthy weight?

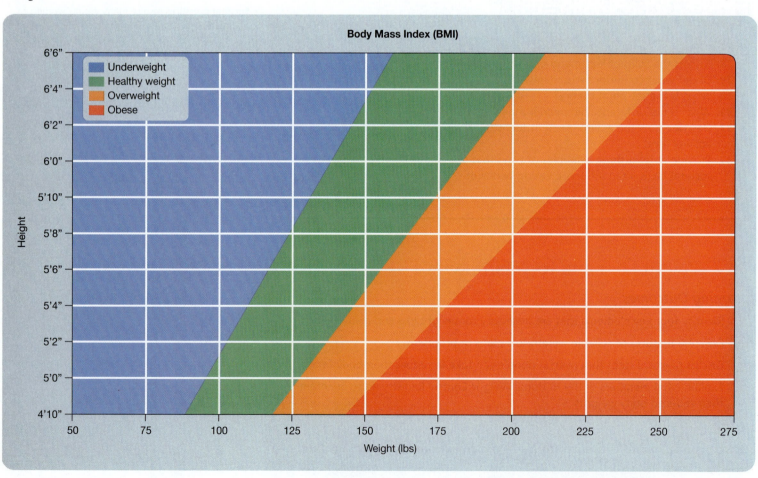

Features of Medically Sound Weight-Loss Plans

Table 10.7 presents some key features of reliable weight–loss plans. Such plans should be safe and effective, as well as flexible enough to meet the person's nutritional, psychological, and social needs. A medically sound weight–loss diet should emphasize a wide variety of low–calorie, readily available nutritious foods and be adaptable to the person's food likes and dislikes. Furthermore, reliable weight–loss plans should provide suggestions for altering environments that foster overeating and sedentary behaviors. Before beginning any weight–loss diet, overfat people need to obtain their physician's approval, especially if they have serious health conditions, such as type 2 diabetes, or they are over the age of 40 (men) or 50 (women).

Key Factors

Despite claims made in advertisements and infomercials, there are no quick cures for overweight and obesity. Successful weight loss and long–term weight maintenance involve four key elements: motivation, calorie reduction, regular physical activity, and behavior modification.

Motivation

The motivation to lose weight and keep it off requires an overfat person to recognize that there is a need to change his or her behavior and become committed to making those changes permanent. For some people, this recognition occurs when they are diagnosed with a health disorder that is associated with excess body fat. Nevertheless, many overfat people choose not to lose weight. The commitment to lose weight and enjoy better health must become far more important than the desire to overeat.

Weight–loss "triggers" often serve as motivators. For some people, seeing themselves in an unflattering photograph, being advised by their physicians to lose weight, or being unable to enjoy activities because being obese restricts their movement triggers the decision to lose weight. According to results of a large survey, adult Americans most frequently cited "medical advice" as the reason for their weight–loss efforts.[37]

Calorie Intake Reduction

According to guidelines issued by the National Institutes of Health, reasonable calorie intakes for adults who want to lose weight range from 1200 to 1500 kcal/day for women and 1500 to 1800 kcal/day for men.[25] At these calorie intake levels, careful food choices are necessary to obtain nutritionally adequate diets. Certain diets severely limit food intake and provide fewer than 800 kcal/day. Such *very–low–calorie diets* are not recommended without close medical supervision.[25] People who follow very–low–calorie diets may lose a lot of weight rapidly, but they tend to regain the weight quickly after they "go off" the diet and return to their former eating habits.

The healthy way to lower intake of total calories is to reduce consumption of added sugars, solid fats, and alcohol. People can also achieve negative energy states by reducing calorie intake *and* increasing physical activity. Nevertheless, a survey of adults who were trying to lose weight indicated that only one–third reported combining the two weight–loss strategies.[38]

Reliable weight–loss diets should follow a healthy food pattern that is lower in calories than one's usual food pattern (see http://www.choosemyplate.gov/weight–management).[39] Increasing consumption of watery, high–fiber foods that are not energy dense, such as fruits and vegetables, may be helpful for people who are trying to lose weight. Such foods are more likely to provide satiety sooner than energy–dense foods and, as a result, reduce the person's calorie intake.[27]

TABLE 10.7 Some Key Features of Reliable Weight-Loss Plans

A sound weight-loss plan:

- Is safe and effective.
- Meets nutritional, psychological, and social needs.
- Incorporates a variety of common foods from all food groups.
- Fosters slow but steady weight loss.
- Does not require costly devices or diet books.
- Accommodates family and restaurant meals, parties and special occasions, ethnic foods, and food likes.
- Does not make the person feel deprived.
- Emphasizes readily available nutritious foods.
- Promotes changing habits that lead to overeating.
- Encourages regular physical activity.
- Provides suggestions for obtaining social support.
- Can be followed for a lifetime.

No particular food has a "metabolic advantage" by promoting greater calorie burning by the body. A dieter's goal should be reducing total calorie intake while obtaining all essential nutrients.

Preparing nutritionally adequate but calorie–reduced meals and snacks can be easier when dietary experts have already done the calculations for consumers. For example, MyPlate provides patterns of food choices for 12 different calorie levels (1000 to 3200 kcal/day) that incorporate all food groups (http://www.choosemyplate.gov/MyPlate–Daily–Checklist). Chapter 3 provides more information about MyPlate. For more general information about weight control, obesity, and nutrition, visit the Weight–control Information Network (WIN) at http://www.niddk.nih.gov/health–information/health–communication–programs/win/Pages/default.aspx. Other reliable sites for weight control information include www.eatright.org.

Eventually, a person who intentionally loses weight by reducing calorie intake and increasing physical activity reaches a weight *plateau*. When this occurs, the individual is in energy balance. To continue losing weight, the person must reduce his or her calorie intake or increase physical activity beyond the present levels. For someone who is consuming only 1000 to 1200 kcal/day, cutting calories even further can lower the metabolic rate, hindering weight loss.

A pound of body fat contains about 3500 kcal. This fact is often used to estimate how changes in caloric intake relate to weight changes: You should lose or gain approximately one pound of weight in a year for every 10 kcal/day reduction or increase your caloric intake (10 kcal/day × 365 days = 3650 kcal). Scientists, however, have challenged the reliability of using the 3500 kcal rule–of–thumb for predicting weight change over the long term. According to their new formula, cutting your caloric intake by 10 kcal/day would enable you to lose only about half a pound in one year, and it would take over 3 years for you to lose a pound of weight, after which no further weight would be lost.[41] This formula helps explain why many people who reduce their usual calorie intakes do not lose as much weight as they expect over time and eventually their weight plateaus. To estimate your caloric intake to achieve weight change by using this formula, visit http://www.niddk.nih.gov/health–information/health–topics/weight–control/body–weight–planner/Pages/bwp.aspx .

Regular Physical Activity

It is difficult to burn much energy without being physically active. By increasing their physical activity level and burning more calories, people do not need to limit their food intake as excessively as they would by relying on calorie reduction alone to lose weight. You do not need to jog for 10 miles to reap the benefits of engaging in regular physical activity. Moderate–intensity activities are recommended for people who want to lose or manage their weight. Chapter 11 discusses the healthful benefits of a physically active lifestyle.

Behavior Modification

Controlling calorie intake and increasing physical activity are easier to accomplish if over–fat persons analyze their faulty behaviors, identify eating *cues* and "problem" habits, and develop ways to change the behaviors. Eating cues are usually environmental factors that stimulate eating behavior, such as seeing an ad for a fast–food restaurant or smelling freshly baked brownies when walking past a bakery. Identifying such cues can enable people to recognize effects of the signals and avoid inappropriate ones, whenever possible. By analyzing their food–related behaviors and habits, overfat individuals can often determine in which circumstances they tend to overeat.

Cues can also help overfat people lose weight. If, for example, you are trying to lose weight, posting an unflattering photograph of yourself on the refrigerator or pantry door can serve as a reminder to stay on course with your behavior modification plan.

Although the process may seem slow, people are more likely to change ingrained habits by focusing on changing one behavior at a time. For example, many people snack on energy–dense foods and drinks while watching television. To change this habit, a person could decide to eat only at the kitchen table and avoid all food and beverage consumption while sitting in front of a TV.

For individuals who want to lose (or gain) weight, keeping records of food intake and physical activities can be helpful for estimating daily calorie input and output. However, overfat persons often underestimate their calorie intake and overestimate their energy output.[42] Therefore, people need to record information about food choices and physical activity habits accurately.

Read Nutrition Facts panels to compare calorie and fat contents of packaged foods.

Tips for Modifying Food- and Exercise-Related Behaviors   The follow–ing suggestions may help a person lose excess weight as well as maintain a lower, healthier body weight.

- **Planning Menus**

  1. Plan meals and snacks to cover three or more days, then use the plan to prepare grocery lists.
  2. When menu planning, include sources of protein, unsaturated fat, and complex carbohydrates in meals and snacks.
  3. Avoid labeling certain foods as "off limits." Depriving yourself of such items can result in bingeing on the "forbidden" food. Learning to analyze why you have difficulty controlling your intake of these foods and developing strategies to learn how to reduce your intake of them can be very helpful.

- **Grocery Shopping**

  1. To reduce the likelihood of making impulsive food choices, shop for food *after* eating.
  2. Shop from a grocery list. If a food is not on your list, ask yourself if you really need to buy it and if it will hinder or help your weight–loss efforts.
  3. Read food labels to compare calorie and fat contents per serving.

- **Food Preparation**

  1. Reduce the use of solid fat in cooking; bake, broil, or roast meats instead of frying them.
  2. Add less solid fat to foods such as cooked vegetables before serving or eating them.
  3. If you sample foods while preparing them, consider the amounts you ate and at mealtimes reduce your portion sizes accordingly.
  4. Prepare only enough food to provide one limited–size portion for yourself. Using measuring cups and a small scale for weighing food can be helpful.
  5. Take your usual–size portion and return one–third to one–half of it to the serving dish or container.
  6. Remove serving dishes from the table. Keeping foods or their containers in sight can encourage overeating.

- **Eating Behavior**

  1. Keep nutrient–dense, low–calorie snack foods, such as fresh fruits and vegetables, on hand.
  2. Eat meals and snacks at scheduled times; do not skip meals, especially breakfast.
  3. Eat all food in a "dining" area; avoid eating while engaged in other activities, such as reading a book or watching television.
  4. Leave some food on your plate.
  5. Become a "defensive eater." Practice ways to refuse food graciously or request smaller portions. Be aware of people, especially relatives and friends, who

Using a small scale for weighing food can be helpful for limiting portion sizes.

Food & Nutrition tips

- When you are hungry, drink some fat-free milk or eat a banana, an apple, a few whole dates, or a handful of raisins.

- Skipping meals can contribute to fatigue. Eating breakfast and small between-meal snacks can provide the carbohydrates needed to maintain blood glucose levels.

- Include foods that supply some protein and complex carbohydrate, including fiber, in each meal to provide a sense of fullness and satiety.

sabotage your weight–loss efforts. Examples of such sabotage include a person who repeatedly offers calorie–dense foods to you, even though you have turned down the food and this person knows you are trying to lose weight.

- **Holidays and Parties**

  1. Beforehand, think about what you will eat and drink while attending the event. Practice polite ways to decline food.
  2. Consider limiting your food intake before the special occasion to avoid consuming too many calories for the day.
  3. Eat a low–calorie snack about an hour before the occasion.
  4. Drink fewer alcoholic beverages. Replace alcoholic beverages with ice water or diet soft drinks.

- **Restaurants**

  1. Avoid fried menu items or those made with butter, gravy, or cream sauce.
  2. Choose pasta with red sauce instead of white sauce.
  3. Request salad dressing "on the side" so you can control the amount.
  4. Think "small." Order an entrée and share it with another person.
  5. Do not be a member of the "clean plate club." Ask your server for a "carryout bag" when he or she brings your order to the table. Then divide the food in half, and place one–half in the container. Be sure to refrigerate the leftovers within 2 hours after the meal, and eat them for a meal the following day.
  6. If you choose a dessert item, share it with others.
  7. Avoid eating regularly at fast–food outlets.
  8. When at fast–food outlets, make substitutions, such as a salad instead of a fried fish sandwich, a regular hamburger instead of a specialty burger, or a roasted chicken sandwich instead of a breaded and fried chicken sandwich. Order a diet soft drink or water instead of a regular soft drink. If possible, order a baked potato instead of fries.

- **Physical Activity**

  1. Choose physical activities that you enjoy and can do without the need for expensive equipment.
  2. Increase the time you spend walking each day. Keep walking shoes where you can see them.
  3. Reduce the amount of time you spend sitting. For example, do more household chores yourself.
  4. Take stairs instead of elevators or escalators whenever possible.
  5. Park your car farther from your destination and walk, if you feel it is safe to do so.
  6. Perform calisthenics or lift handheld weights while watching television.
  7. Adopt moderate–intensity activities for your leisure time. For example, join a co–ed volleyball club or take a ballroom dancing class.

- **Self–Monitoring**

  1. Keep a special notebook to use as a food and exercise diary where you can see it—near the kitchen table, refrigerator, or pantry, for example.
  2. In the diary, note the time and place of eating as well as the type and amount of food eaten. Also record who was present and your mood when you ate meals and snacks.
  3. Use the diary to identify your food–related problem areas, such as eating when bored or depressed.
  4. In the exercise section of the diary, record the form of moderate–intensity exercise you performed and the number of minutes you spent engaging in that activity each day. Try to achieve at least 150 minutes of moderate–intensity activities each week.

5. Measure your waistline weekly and keep a record of the measurements.

6. Weigh yourself at least once a week, preferably at the same time and without clothing. However, do not rely only on your weight as an indication of your progress. Regular exercise often increases muscle mass that can result in weight gain or failure to lose weight. However, adding muscle mass is healthier than maintaining too much body fat.

- **Rewards for New Behaviors**

1. Plan nonfood motivators or rewards for specific behaviors. For example, "I'll buy a pair of jeans that are one size smaller than what I currently wear and hang them where I can see them," or "I'll buy that DVD I've wanted, when I lose 5 pounds."

2. Encourage family and friends to provide praise and encouragement for your efforts to manage your weight. Let family, friends, and associates know that you are trying to lose weight and you would appreciate their help and support. Thank them when you receive their praise and support.

- **Changing Negative Thought Patterns**

1. Do not get discouraged by occasional setbacks; relapses can be expected when changing behaviors. For example, instead of thinking, "I can't lose weight. I'm a failure," say to yourself, "OK, so I lost control and had too much to eat at the wedding. That's to be expected. I just need to get back on track. I'll pull in the reins on my eating for the next day and exercise more."

2. Think positively about progress. "I didn't lose any weight this week, but I didn't gain any either. I must be losing fat and getting trimmer; those slacks fit better than they did 2 months ago."

3. Counter negative thoughts with positive statements. "Next time, I'll eat two cookies instead of four. This afternoon, I'll just have to walk a little longer and harder to burn off those extra calories."

Did You Know?

A *pedometer* is a small device that records the number of steps a person takes while engaging in physical activities. According to the Shape Up America! organization (http://shapeup.org/sud10-overview/), the goal is to take at least 5000 steps per day. If you would like to monitor your steps, you can purchase an inexpensive pedometer in sporting goods stores. The one shown in the photo clips onto socks or belts.

Community-Based Weight-Loss Programs

Many communities offer a variety of weight−loss programs. Registered dietitians often conduct weight−loss classes at hospitals or universities. Dietitians have extensive training in foods, nutrition, dietetics, and counseling methods to help people design safe and effective weight−loss plans. If a physician prescribes dietary counseling by a registered dietitian, the patient's health insurance may cover the cost of such treatment.

Some commercial weight−loss programs, such as *Weight Watchers*, have diet plans that have been developed by dietitians. Members who have lost weight while following the plan often conduct local meetings. Before joining any weight−loss program, consumers should obtain answers to the following questions:

- How much does the program cost? Do I pay when I attend meetings? Do I need to sign a contract? If so, for what length of time?

- Do I have to buy special foods or dietary supplements?

- Is nutrition counseling provided? Do the persons providing nutrition counseling and information have degrees in nutrition and dietetics from accredited colleges or universities? How much contact will I have with a counselor?

- Was the diet plan developed by dietitians? Does the plan emphasize the importance of making lifestyle changes, including ways to increase physical activity?

- Does the program's advertising include questionable weight−loss claims and deceptive testimonials?

REAL PEOPLE | REAL STORIES

Jan Haapala

Early in 2005, 24-year-old Jan Haapala did not feel well. He slept poorly at night, and during the day, extreme fatigue seemed to be his constant companion. Frequent indigestion added to his general discomfort. Concerned about her husband's health, Jan's wife, Valerie, urged him to see a doctor and have a physical exam. That trip to the doctor's office would prove to be a major turning point in Jan's life.

During the physical exam, Jan was shocked to learn he had hypertension. The physician prescribed medication to reduce his dangerously elevated blood pressure.

At the time of his doctor's appointment, Jan weighed 335 pounds and his BMI was over 45, which is in the "extremely obese" range. If Jan could not reduce his blood pressure and maintain it at a healthy level, he was very likely to die prematurely. Taking medication can reduce elevated blood pressure and keep it under control, but losing excess fat often cures hypertension, making the medication unnecessary.

Jan was aware that his lifestyle contributed to his extreme obesity. He typically ate two doughnuts and a 20-ounce serving of a sugar-sweetened soft drink for breakfast. Lunches and dinners were "big" meals, often comprised of fast foods, especially double cheeseburgers and large portions of French fries and soft drinks. Candy bars were among his favorite snacks. "I knew those foods were unhealthy, but that didn't change what I ate once I sat down to eat." In addition to his poor food choices, Jan was physically inactive.

After returning home from the doctor's office, Jan made up his mind to improve his health. He recalls, "I didn't want to take medicine to stay alive." Determined to lose weight, Jan heeded his wife's suggestion to join Weight Watchers, one of the oldest and most reliable commercial group weight-loss programs in the country.

Although some people can lose weight on their own, others benefit from participating in group weight-loss programs that offer sensible and safe nutritional guidance, including tips for controlling the size of food portions and increasing physical activity. Group membership also provides emotional support from other members, a factor that is often critical for weight-loss success and maintenance.

By joining Weight Watchers, Jan acquired the information he needed to change his lifestyle to a healthier one. He also developed the motivation to follow a personalized diet and exercise plan that was very different from his past eating and physical activity patterns. In addition to choosing less fatty and sugary foods, he started a walking regimen that eventually became a running regimen. The pounds seemed to melt away from his body, and not long after he began to lose weight, he was able to discontinue taking the medication for hypertension.

When Jan joined the weight-loss program, his waistline measured 46 inches and he wore shirts with a 21-inch neck size. By the time he reached his goal weight of 210 pounds, his waistline was a trim 35 inches and his neck size measured only 15 ½ inches. Although it took 3 years, Jan had lost 125 pounds! The gradual but steady weight loss was an indication that he was making the kinds of behavioral and lifestyle changes that would be permanent.

Today, Jan is "feeling great" and running races from 5Ks to half-marathons. He has even completed his first marathon. His advice to overfat people who are worried about what strangers will think while they exercise: "Don't be embarrassed about doing something in public that's good for you. People won't judge you negatively for trying to become healthier." Clearly, Jan is a role model and inspiration for anyone who is overweight or obese and wants to get his or her weight under control.

Successful Losers: How Do They Manage Their Weight?

The National Weight Control Registry tracks a group of over 10,000 adult Americans, mostly women, who have lost at least 30 pounds and maintained the weight loss for at least 1 year.[43] Information about members' nutrition– and exercise–related practices provides some insights into lifestyle practices that foster losing excess weight and maintaining the lower weight. The majority of registry members:[43]

- eat low–calorie, low–fat diets.
- eat breakfast every day.
- weigh themselves at least once a week.
- exercise, on average, for 60 minutes each day.
- limit television watching to less than 10 hours per week.

Concept Checkpoint 10.7

34. What are the four key elements that are necessary for weight loss and maintenance?
35. List at least six features of reliable weight-loss plans or programs.
36. What questions would it be wise for consumers to have answered before they join a weight-loss group or plan?
37. List at least three steps that members of the National Weight Control Registry often take to maintain their reduced body weights.

Individuals who lose excess weight and maintain the weight loss tend to eat regular meals, including breakfast.

10.8 Medical Treatments for Obesity

Learning Outcomes

1 Discuss medications and surgeries that are options for treating overweight and obesity.

2 Explain the pros and cons of bariatric surgical procedures.

Obese patients are often unsatisfied with the amount of weight they lose while following fad as well as conventional diets. The frustration of repeated dieting leads some obese persons to turn to physicians for prescription medication and surgical procedures for managing their weight.

Weight-Loss Medication

Some obese people are candidates for taking prescribed medication to aid their weight–loss efforts. Such candidates generally have BMIs of 30 or more, or they have waist circumferences that exceed 40 inches (men) or 35 inches (women). The U.S. Food and Drug Administration (FDA) has approved a few weight–loss medications for long–term use, including Belviq®, Qsymia®, and Xenical® (orlistat). When orlistat is taken along with a meal, the medication reduces fat digestion by about 30%. The undigested fat is eliminated in the feces and can cause an oily, unpleasant discharge. The fat carries fat–soluble vitamins along with it, and these micronutrients are eliminated in feces as well. Therefore, patients using orlistat often need to take a multiple vitamin supplement. In 2007, the FDA approved sales of the nonprescription form of orlistat (Alli®) as a weight–loss aid for adults.

The typical patient who uses orlistat in addition to a weight loss diet for up to 2 years loses only about 7 more pounds than if he or she used the diet without the medication.[44] Overfat people need to recognize that in some instances, prescription medication can aid their weight−loss efforts but does not replace the need to reduce calorie intake and increase physical activity.

Bariatric Surgical Procedures

Bariatric (*bar−ee−a′−tric*) **medicine** is the medical specialty that focuses on the treatment of obesity. Bariatric surgery can an effective method of treating people who are extremely obese (have BMIs greater than or equal to 40) or have BMIs of greater than or equal to 35 and serious health problems because of their obesity.[25] Such surgical procedures drastically reduce the size of an obese person's stomach, markedly limiting his or her food intake. Patients who have bariatric surgery may lose significant amounts of their excess weight.[45] Most patients, however, regain some weight within 10 years after the surgery.[46] Aside from helping obese people lose considerable amounts of weight and maintain the loss, bariatric surgery can produce dramatic health benefits. Patients often achieve normal blood pressure, glucose levels, and triglyceride levels after surgery. Furthermore, overall death rates are lower for extremely obese people who lose weight after undergoing bariatric surgery. Such surgeries are relatively safe: Fewer than 1% of patients die as a result of a bariatric surgical procedure.[46]

In the United States, two common surgical approaches to treating obesity are the *Roux−en−Y* (*ru−en−wi′*) *gastric bypass* and *gastric banding procedures*. Both of these operations can be performed *laparoscopically*, that is, by using several small incisions that allow surgeons to insert instruments and a video camera into the abdomen. Laparoscopic bariatric surgical procedures reduce recovery time and the risk of infections.

During the Roux−en−Y operation, the surgeon staples across the upper part of the stomach to create a small pouch. This procedure reduces the obese patient's stomach capacity to about 1.5 oz, which is approximately the volume of one egg. (Normally, the stomach's capacity is about 32 oz.) Additionally, the surgeon cuts the small intestine and attaches the lower end of it to the newly formed stomach pouch (Fig. 10.18a). The "bypassed" section of the intestine does not receive food, so digestion and absorption are reduced as a result of the surgery.

Sleeve gastrectomy is another form of bariatric surgery that reduces the stomach's size. During this procedure, the surgeon staples the stomach to form a banana−shaped pouch that holds about 2 to 5 ounces of food. The surgery does not involve bypassing a section of the small intestine, so nutrient absorption is not reduced (Fig. 10.18b). People who have undergone sleeve gastrectomy can eat only small portions of solid foods, which contributes to rapid weight loss. These patients also lose weight because they are not as hungry as they were before having the surgery. Why? The portion of the stomach that secretes ghrelin is removed during surgery, and as a result, hunger sensations are reduced. Sleeve gastrectomy surgery is irreversible, because the unused portion of the stomach is removed.

Complications often associated with gastric bypass surgery include intestinal blockage and bleeding, leaks along the staple site, blood clot formation, and wound infections. After surgery, gastric bypass patients can develop micronutrient deficiencies and some bone loss. However, patients can reduce their risk of nutrient deficiencies by taking vitamin and mineral supplements.

bariatric medicine medical specialty that focuses on the treatment of obesity

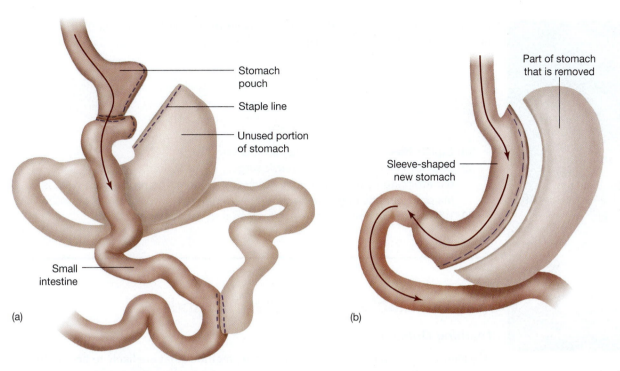

Stomach pouch

Staple line

Unused portion of stomach

Small intestine

Part of stomach that is removed

Sleeve-shaped new stomach

(a)

(b)

| **Figure 10.18 Gastric bypass surgeries.** (*a*) The Roux-en-Y gastric bypass procedure. (*b*) The sleeve gastrectomy procedure.

By performing the *adjustable gastric banding* procedure, the bariatric surgeon creates the small stomach pouch with an adjustable band instead of fixed surgical staples (Fig. 10.19). By adjusting the tightness of the band, the surgeon determines the size of the stomach. Laparoscopic gastric banding procedure is easier to perform and safer than the other types of bariatric surgery.[46] The procedure is also reversible. However, obese people who undergo the procedure lose weight more slowly and they lose less weight than those who undergo gastric bypass or sleeve gastrectomy procedures.

Bariatric surgeries result in weight loss partly because the stomach pouch fills quickly with food and patients experience satiety sooner than prior to surgery. Moreover, overeating causes discomfort or vomiting. Thus, people who undergo such surgical procedures must make major lifestyle changes, such as learning to plan and consume frequent, small meals. Engaging in regular exercise and avoiding "soft calories," energy–dense high–calorie foods such as milk shakes and ice cream, are also important for maximizing weight loss and maintaining the lower body weight over time.

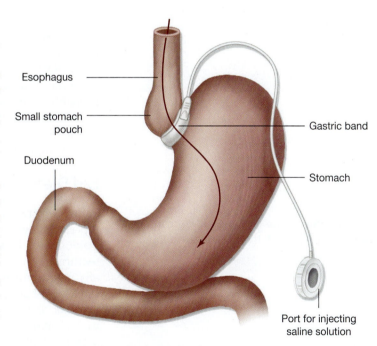

Esophagus

Small stomach pouch

Duodenum

Gastric band

Stomach

Port for injecting saline solution

| **Figure 10.19 Adjustable gastric banding.**

What Is Liposuction?

Liposuction is a surgical method of reducing the size of local subcutaneous fat deposits. Liposuction is not intended to treat obesity, but it can help a person improve the contours of his or her body. This procedure involves inserting a pencil–thin tube into an incision in the skin and suctioning the excess subcutaneous

liposuction surgical method of reducing the size of local fat deposits fat out of the body (Fig. 10.20). This procedure has risks, such as infection, and blood clots or droplets of fat that can enter the bloodstream and be deadly.

| Figure 10.20 Liposuction.

10.9 Unreliable Weight-Loss Methods

Learning Outcome

1 Identify characteristics of weight-reduction methods that are likely to be unsafe and unreliable.

There are numerous products and services available for adults who want to lose weight. Some overweight or obese people join commercial weight—loss programs that have good track records for encouraging successful weight loss and mainte—nance. Other overfat persons obtain individual dietary counseling from a regis—tered dietitian to help them lose weight. By recognizing that it took months and probably years to gain the excess fat, individuals may be more likely to accept advice and diets that result in slow but steady weight loss. However, many over—weight and obese people seek quick fixes to lose weight, such as *fad* diets and dietary supplements promoted to "burn" or "melt" fat fast.

Fad Diets

fad trendy practice that has widespread appeal for a period, then becomes no longer fashionable

A **fad** is a trendy practice that has widespread appeal among a population. After a period, however, people lose interest in the practice, and it becomes no longer fashionable. Table 10.8 presents some popular fad weight—loss diets and their features. People often lose weight while following fad diets; however, they usu—ally regain much of the weight that was lost while on the diet when they resume their prior eating and other lifestyle habits. Too often, people think of a weight—loss diet as a temporary change in their eating habits. Achieving a healthy body weight and maintaining that weight requires making lifestyle changes that a person adopts for the rest of his or her life.

Fad diets often rely on *gimmicks*. A gimmick is a novel feature that makes the diet seem to be unique and more likely to work than other diets. Some fad diets use the gimmick of emphasizing one food or food group while excluding almost all others. The cabbage soup and grapefruit diets are examples of fad diets that promote eating single foods. Overfat people may lose some weight while fol—lowing eating plans that restrict food variety, but the weight loss occurs because the diet is low in calories, not because cabbage, grapefruit, or other "special food" contains compounds that cause rapid weight loss. Following such diets for a few days often results in boredom and monotony. Eventually, people who are trying to lose weight abandon such restrictive menu plans because they just cannot face

TABLE 10.8 Examples of Popular Fad Weight-Loss Diets

Approach	Examples	Features	Outcomes
Restricted carbohydrates	Paleo Diet; Dr. Atkins' New Diet Revolution; Sugar Busters!	Generally less than 100 g of carbohydrate daily	Ketosis due to excess burning of fat; may cause fatigue, constipation, headaches, and bad breath May improve blood lipid levels and reduce the risk of CVD for up to 1 year After 1 year, amount of weight loss is comparable to that achieved by following low-fat diets.
Low fat	The Macrobiotic Diet (some versions); Pritikin Diet; Ornish Diet; TLC Diet	Generally less than 20% of calories from fat Limited or no sources of animal protein Limited nuts and seeds	Excess fiber may result in increased intestinal gas; difficult to follow for long periods because food choices are so limited Limited food choices may lead to feelings of food deprivation.
Diets with gimmicks	Wheat Belly Diet; hCG Diet; The Beverly Hills Diet; Cabbage Soup Diet; Cookie Diet; Grapefruit Diet; Eat Right for Your Type	Promotes or excludes certain substances, nutrients, foods, or combinations of foods	Undernutrition if followed for a long period Such diets generally do not encourage changing exercise and food-related habits.
Nutritionally balanced	Biggest Loser Diet; Flat Belly Diet; Flexitarian Diet; Glycemic Index Diet; Zone Diet; Spark Solution Diet; Gluten-free Diet; Anti-Inflammatory Diet; Mayo Clinic Diet	Generally include a variety of foods that supply recommended amounts of carbohydrate, protein, and fat.	Such diets may reduce risks of diabetes and heart disease, but long-term studies are needed to provide evidence that supports these benefits. Some of the diets (e.g., the Anti-Inflammatory Diet) are easier to follow than others.

another cup of cabbage soup or bowl of grapefruit. Weight regain occurs when the people return to their former eating habits—the habits that contributed to their original over–weight or obese conditions.

Fad diets will come and go. However, if you examine any diet plan carefully, you can determine whether it is probably a fad. A typical fad diet:

- offers a quick fix; that is, the diet promotes rapid weight loss without calorie restriction and increased physical activity.

- limits food selections from a few food groups and dictates specific rituals, such as eating only fruit for breakfast or eating only certain food combinations.

- requires buying a book or various gimmicks, such as expensive dietary supplements, weight–loss patches, or cellulite–reducing creams.

- uses outlandish and unscientific claims to support its usefulness. For example, *The Beverly Hills Diet* book promoted the notion that people become fat because food "gets stuck" in their bodies, rots, and produces toxins. Another author of a fad diet book claimed people can lose weight by following diet plans based on their blood types. These notions and recommendations are not supported by scientific evidence.

- relies on testimonials from famous people or connects the diet to trendy places such as Beverly Hills, California, and South Beach, Florida.

- does not emphasize the need to change eating habits and physical activity patterns.

Low-Carbohydrate Approaches

Fad weight–loss diets that limit carbohydrate intakes and are high in protein and saturated fat include the Dr. Atkins' New Diet Revolution and the early phases of the South Beach Diet. A weight−reduction diet is low carbohydrate if it eliminates or severely restricts the intake of carbohydrate−rich foods such as breads, cereals, fruits, vegetables, and sweets. The lack of variety often leads to boredom with the selection of foods, and as a result, people lose weight because they tend to eat less. On the other hand, people who follow low−carbohydrate/high−protein diets tend to like the diet plan more and have less difficulty adhering to the diets than people who are on low−fat diets.[47]

Low−carbohydrate diets usually produce rapid weight loss initially, primarily because the body loses water. Why? The body produces less glycogen when carbohydrate intake is low and uses much of its stored glycogen to supply glucose for energy. Tissues maintain about 3 grams of water with each gram of glycogen, so a reduction in body glycogen content results in the need for less water to store with it. The kidneys eliminate the excess water in urine. Furthermore, a very−low−carbohydrate intake causes the liver to produce glucose, mostly from certain amino acids supplied by the body's tissue proteins. Protein tissue also contains a lot of water. When protein−rich tissues are dismantled and their amino acids used for energy, the water that was stored with the proteins also ends up in urine.

An analysis of 13 studies indicated that after 6 months, people on low−carbohydrate/high−protein diet plans lost an average of about 9 pounds more than people on low−fat/high−carbohydrate diets.[47] After 12 months, however, people on the carbohydrate−restricted diets weighed only about 2 pounds less than people following the low−fat diets. Low−carbohydrate diets resulted in more favorable high−density lipoprotein ("good cholesterol") and serum triglyceride levels. According to the authors of this review, low−carbohydrate diets may be as effective as or even more effective than low−fat diets for reducing weight and risk of cardiovascular disease for up to 1 year. More studies, however, are needed to determine whether low−carbohydrate diets are safe and reduce the risk of CVD for longer periods.

Very-Low-Fat Approaches

Very−low−fat diets are actually very−high−carbohydrate diets. These diets supply approximately 5 to 10% of calories from fat and generally result in rapid weight loss when followed consistently. The most notable are the Pritikin Diet and Dr. Dean Ornish's "Eat More, Weigh Less" diet plans. Very−low−fat diets are not harmful for healthy adults, but they are difficult to follow for the long term. Fat contributes to the flavor and texture of foods. Extremely low−fat diets are not tasty, and they eliminate many foods that are usually high on peoples' favorite foods lists, such as ice cream and meat. Although grains, fruits, and vegetables are nutrient−dense foods, eating them repeatedly and without fat can cause "diet boredom."

Dietary Supplements for Weight Loss

Many overweight and obese people are attracted to dietary supplements for weight loss because they believe promoters' claims that their products are "magic bullets" for shedding unwanted weight quickly and effortlessly.[48] Although several different types of weight−loss supplements are available, these products generally have not been scientifically tested in humans for safety and effectiveness.

In 2004, the FDA banned the sale of most dietary supplements that contained the natural stimulant ephedra (*eh−feh'−dra*) or ephedra−related compounds, after the agency received reports of serious side effects and even deaths resulting from use of these products. The death in 2003 of Steve Bechler, Baltimore Orioles baseball player, was linked to ephedra (Fig. 10.21). Table 10.9 presents science−based findings about some popular weight−loss supplements, including their potential usefulness and safety concerns. At this point, medical experts do not recommend any dietary supplement for weight loss.[48]

Figure 10.21 Toxic herbal supplement. In 2003, Baltimore Orioles pitcher Steve Bechler's death was linked to ephedra. Bechler had taken a large dose of an ephedra-containing supplement a few hours before he died.

TABLE 10.9   Summary of Selected Weight-Loss Supplements

Supplement	Usefulness	Side Effects/Safety Concerns (Usual Doses)
Açai berry	Not effective	Potentially dangerous; may be contaminated with an FDA-unapproved drug
Beta-hydroxy-beta-methylbutyrate	May decrease adipose tissue and increase lean body mass, but more research is needed	None reported
Chia seed	No scientific support	None reported
Chinese diet pills	Not determined	Linked to illness and deaths in Japan. May contain the active drug fenfluramine
Chitosan	A few studies show some usefulness, but more research is needed.	May cause gastrointestinal discomfort including nausea, constipation, and intestinal gas
Chromium picolinate	May enhance weight loss to a small extent	None reported, but may damage DNA
Conjugated linoleic acid	Has minimal effect on reducing body weight	Appears to be safe, but can cause gastrointestinal upset
Green tea or extracts	May enhance weight loss to a small extent	Concentrated extracts linked to severe liver damage
Ephedrine (ma huang, ephedra, ephedra sinica, sida cordifolia, pinellia, and ephedrine with caffeine)	Ephedrine-containing products promote short-term weight loss but also increase risk of serious side effects. Ephedra-containing dietary supplements are banned in the United States.	May cause rapid heart rate, elevated blood pressure, dizziness, sweating, headache, and sleep disturbances. Linked to heart attacks, strokes, and deaths
Garcinia cambogia (hydroxycitric acid, HCA)	Overall evidence does not suggest usefulness.	May cause headache and gastrointestinal discomfort
Glucomannan	May be effective, but more research is needed	None reported
Guar gum	Not effective	May cause diarrhea and intestinal gas
Hoodia	Not effective	Vomiting, increased blood pressure and heart rate, signs of liver damage
Human chorionic gonadotropin (hCG)	Not effective	Unknown
Pyruvate	May be beneficial; more research is needed	None reported, but long-term safety is unknown
Raspberry ketone	Lack of scientific support for effectiveness	Unknown
Spirulina (blue-green algae)	Not effective	Unknown

Sources: Food and Drug Administration: Public notification: "Acai Berry Soft Gel ABC" contains undeclared drug ingredient. October 18, 2011; Egras AM and others: An evidence-based review of fat modifying supplemental weight loss products. *Journal of Obesity 2011,* Article ID 297315, doi: 10.1155/2011/297315; Nieman DC and others: Chia seed supplementation and disease risk factors in overweight women: A metabolomics investigation. *Journal of Alternative and Complementary Medicine 18*(7): 700, 2012. Pittler MH, Ernst E: Dietary supplements for body-weight reduction: A systematic review. *American Journal of Clinical Nutrition 79*: 529, 2004; Saper RB and others: Common dietary supplements for weight loss. *American Family Physician 70:*1731, 2004; Hursel R and others: The effects of green tea on weight loss and weight management: A meta-analysis. *International Journal of Obesity* advance online publication, 14 July 2009; doi:10.1038/ijo.2009.135; Sarma DN and others: Safety of green tea extracts: A systematic review by the US Pharmacopeia. *Drug Safety 31*(6): 469, 2008; Peregrin T: Frequently asked questions of the Academy's Knowledge Center. *Journal of the Academy of Nutrition and Dietetics* 113 (7): 887, 2013.

Analyzing Advertising Hype for Weight-Loss Supplements

Maybe you have heard or read remarkable claims for weight—loss products such as "Lose weight while you sleep," "Lose 30 pounds in just 30 days," and "Eat anything you want and still lose weight." In general, advertising claims that a product promises quick and easy weight loss are too good to be true.

A Federal Trade Commission (FTC) study identified several features, includ—ing typical claims, for popular weight—loss products and services. The agency's report also provided reasons why you should be skeptical of such features when they are used in magazine ads, in television infomercials, or on Internet websites. According to the FTC, you should be wary of claims that the product or service:

- *causes rapid and extreme weight loss.* Ads commonly use outrageous claims such as "Lose up to 18 pounds in one week!" to attract consumers. The use of the modifier "up to" means that the person using the product could lose considerably less than 18 pounds a week.

- *requires no need to change dietary patterns or physical activity.* Principles of energy balance do not support claims such as "Lose weight without dieting or strenuous exercise" and "Eat as much as you want—the more you eat, the more you'll lose." Regular exercise and moderate energy intake are necessary for weight loss and long–term maintenance.

- *results in permanent weight loss.* Claims such as "Discover the secret to permanent weight loss" and "Lose weight and keep it off" often appear in ads. These claims target consumers who have lost weight but gained it back and are wary of weight–loss products. Long–term weight loss is difficult to achieve without calorie reduction and regular exercise, and claims that permanent weight loss can result simply from using a product are questionable.[48]

- *is scientifically proven or doctor endorsed.* Some ads claim their product or service has been "clinically tested," "scientifically proven," or "physician recommended." Scientific testing of the product or service supposedly occurred at "respected" or "leading" medical centers or universities. However, most ads do not provide information about testing sites or journals where the results were published. Such information is critical for assessing the reliability of claims. Endorsements by "doctors" or medical professionals can be misleading. A doctor could be someone with a bogus doctorate degree (PhD) or a PhD in a nonscientific field. Moreover, consumers need to be aware that the "professionals" pictured or featured in the ads may be models or fictional characters.

- *includes a money–back guarantee.* Consumers should recognize that a product does not necessarily work just because it is guaranteed. The FTC frequently sues companies that fail to return money to dissatisfied consumers, as their ads guaranteed.

- *is safe or natural.* Ads may include safety–related claims, such as "proven 100% safe" or "safe, immediate weight loss." Additionally, the term *natural* often accompanies safety claims, implying that "natural" weight–loss products are safer than prescribed weight–loss treatments. Despite such assurances, weight–loss supplement manufacturers usually have little scientific evidence to support safety claims, particularly concerning long–term use of their products. Furthermore, "natural" does not indicate safety. Mushrooms are natural, but many species of the fungi are highly toxic and even deadly.

- *is supported by satisfied customers.* Ads for weight–loss products or services typically feature testimonials from satisfied users. The assumption is that if the product worked for the person providing the testimonial, it should work for anyone. According to the FTC, testimonials generally provide little reliable information about what consumers can expect from using the product.

- *displays before–and–after photos.* Many ads use photos of "satisfied" customers to support claims that their weight–loss products are effective. In the typical "before" photo, the subject has poor posture, no smile, unkempt hair, and unfashionable, unflattering clothing. In the "after" photo, the person stands with his or her shoulders held back and abdomen tucked in. Additionally, the subject is usually smiling and appears more attractive than in the "before" photo. If you read carefully, you may find disclaimers in small print, such as "results not typical," at the bottom of the "after" photo.

Did You Know?

The U.S. Federal Trade Commission (FTC) can prosecute promoters making fraudulent claims about the effectiveness of their weight-loss products. Enforma Natural Products, Inc., had to pay $10 million in fines after the company used false claims in ads for its "Fat Trapper," "Fat Trapper Plus," and "Exercise in A Bottle" products.

Concept **Checkpoint 10.9**

41. What is a "fad" diet? List at least four typical features of fad diets.
42. Why do fad diets and dietary supplements promoted for weight loss appeal to overfat people?
43. Identify at least four popular weight-loss supplements, and indicate whether each supplement is safe and effective.
44. Discuss at least three features or claims that are commonly used in ads for weight-loss products or services.

Many underweight individuals are interested in gaining weight, especially muscle mass.

10.10 Gaining Weight

Learning Outcomes

1 Explain why some people are underweight.

2 Discuss ways to gain weight safely and sensibly.

In 2007–2010 about 2% of Americans who were 20 to 39 years of age were under—weight.[49] An **underweight** individual has a BMI that is less than 18.5. Factors that contribute to underweight include genetics, lifestyle practices, chronic diseases, and psychological disturbances.

It is often difficult to pinpoint a cause of underweight; multiple factors contribute to having a lower—than—average body weight. Individuals who inherit higher resting metabolic rates, tall body frames, or both may find it difficult to gain weight. Excessive physical activity can result in low body weight. Compared to sedentary adults, the bodies of rapidly growing, physically active children and adolescents have higher energy needs. If these children do not consume enough energy, they can lose weight. Chronic diseases such as cancer, tuberculosis, AIDS, and *inflammatory bowel disease* often result in severe weight loss that is dif—ficult to treat. Some people who suffer from depression fail to eat enough food to support their energy needs, and they lose weight as a result.

If a person's BMI was within the healthy range before excessive weight loss occurred, an evaluation by a physician may be necessary to determine the cause or causes of the loss, especially when the underweight person has not tried to shed pounds. A thorough medical examination can rule out possible reasons for unintentional weight loss, such as hormonal imbalances, depression, cancer, and infectious or digestive tract diseases.

Many underweight individuals want to gain weight, especially muscle mass. For an underweight person, gaining weight can be just as challenging as losing weight is for an overfat person. To gain weight, underweight adults can gradually increase their consumption of calorie—dense foods, especially those high in healthy fats. Fatty fish, such as salmon; olives; avocados; seeds; low—fat cheeses; nuts and nut butters; bananas; and granola made with dried fruit, seeds, and nuts are high—calorie nutritious food choices with low saturated—fat content. Additionally, underweight people can replace beverages such as soft drinks with more nutritious calorie sources, such as 100% fruit juices, smoothies, and milk shakes made with peanut butter and fat—reduced ice cream. Follow—ing a regular meal and snack schedule also aids in weight gain and maintenance.

Sometimes people who are underweight are too busy to eat, and as a result, their caloric intakes are too low to support weight gain. If physical activity habits contribute to their inability to increase their weight, underweight people can find

underweight describes person with a BMI of less than 18.5

ways to be less active. If their weight remains low, underweight persons can add muscle mass through a *resistance–training* (weight–lifting) program, but they must increase their calorie intake to support the additional exercise. Otherwise, gaining muscle tissue is not likely to occur.

In many instances, healthy underweight people may have to accept their body builds. Furthermore, they can realize the health benefits of being lean and the sheer enjoyment of being able to eat a variety of foods without gaining weight. For the typical slim person, the passage of time is usually all that is necessary for weight gain to occur, as the aging process is often accompanied by increasing body fat.

Concept **Checkpoint 10.10**

45. List at least three health conditions that are often associated with being underweight.

46. Discuss at least three measures an underweight person can take to gain lean mass safely.

10.11 Nutrition Matters: Eating Disorders and Disordered Eating

Learning Outcomes

1 Explain the difference between having an eating disorder and practicing disordered eating.

2 List the major types of eating disorders and their signs.

3 Identify risk factors for eating disorders, disordered eating practices, and the female athlete triad.

4 Describe the health consequences of eating disorders and professional forms of treatment for eating disorders.

Many American adolescents and young adults are dissatisfied with their body shape and weight. Among some segments of society, the ideal female figure is slim but curvy, and the ideal male physique is lean and muscular. The media constantly bombard consumers with images of the "ideal" body. Television shows and movies often portray thin women or muscular men as happy and successful. As a result, societal pressures inspire many young people to idealize underweight. In their efforts to pursue such unrealistic slender body shapes, young people may adopt unhealthy and potentially life–threatening eating practices. This "Nutrition Matters" focuses on eating disorders and disordered eating behaviors.

Eating disorders are psychological disturbances that lead to abnormal physiological changes and dangerous health complications. An eating disorder is not the same as disordered eating. **Disordered eating** is chaotic and abnormal food–related practices, such as skipping meals, limiting food choices, following fad diets, and bingeing on food. Disordered eating behaviors are temporary, and they often occur when a person is under a lot of stress or wants to lose weight quickly. When a person adopts disordered eating behaviors as a lifestyle, the practices can become harmful and lead to serious eating disorders.

Major Types of Eating Disorders

According to guidelines published in the fifth edition of the American Psychiatric Association's (APA's) *Diagnostic and Statistical Manual of Mental Disorders* (*DSM–5*), physicians can diagnose three main types of eating disorders:[50]

- Anorexia nervosa (AN);
- Bulimia nervosa (BN); and
- Binge–eating disorder (BED).

Eating Disorders: Risk Factors There are several known risk factors for eating disorders. These factors include being female, having a poor self–image, having low self–esteem

eating disorders psychological disturbances that lead to certain physiological changes and serious health complications

disordered eating chaotic and abnormal food-related practices

TABLE 10.10

Risk Factors for Eating Disorders

Being female
Being an adolescent (AN and BN)
Having a history of frequent dieting
Having a first-degree relative with an eating disorder
Placing a high degree of importance on having an "ideal" body shape
Being dissatisfied with one's body shape
Having a poor self-image and low self-esteem
Having a perfectionist personality
Being from a dysfunctional family
Being teased about one's weight
Being in an occupation or sport that emphasizes a lean body build

and a perfectionist personality, being in a dysfunctional family environment, and being teased about weight. Table 10.10 lists these and several other risk factors.[51]

A person's age is a major factor in predicting his or her risk of a particular eating disorder. Binge—eating disorder is more likely to occur in adults, while AN and BN tend to begin during adolescence.[51] Results of studies of adolescent girls conducted over a long period of time indicated that 13% developed an eating disorder.[52] Factors that contribute to an adolescent's vulnerability to develop AN or BN generally include:

- drastic changes in body weight and shape that normally occur during this life stage;
- increased reliance on peers for support and approval; and
- greater independence from parental control over food choices.

Causes of Eating Disorders

The causes of eating disorders include genetic, biological, social, psychological, and environmental factors. The following sections discuss several of these factors.

Genetic and Biological Factors People who have a first—degree relative (a sister or mother, for example) with AN are 10 times more likely to have an eating disorder than people who do not have any relatives with AN.[53] Specific genes that modify the brain's ability to regulate eating behaviors and satiety may have a role in development of AN.[53] More research, however, is needed to clarify how genes affect eating behavior.

Psychological and Personality Factors Mood and anxiety disorders, as well as substance abuse, often accompany eating disorders. It is not clear whether eating disorders cause psychological problems or are the result of emotional disturbances. Furthermore, people with eating disorders typically have a distorted view of their body weight or

Figure 10.22 Risky occupation. People in occupations that encourage thinness, such as ballet, have an increased risk of developing an eating disorder.

shape, and they often place a great deal of importance on "ideal" body weight, shape, or specific body parts. Having a poor self—image and being dissatisfied with one's body shape are risk factors for developing an eating disorder.

Other Factors National origin, income level, occupation, and lifestyle choices contribute to the development of eating disorders in people who are vulnerable to developing them. Eating disorders are most prevalent in industrialized, high—income countries such as the United States, Australia, Canada, Japan, and many European nations.[50] Individuals who participate in activities or occupations that encourage thinness such as ballet, acting, and fashion modeling have an increased risk for developing an eating disorder, especially AN and BN (Fig. 10.22). Athletes, especially those participating in endurance running, swimming, and gymnastics, are at risk.[51] Additionally, athletes who have to "make weight," such as wrestlers and jockeys, have a higher incidence of eating disorders than athletes in other sports.

Adolescents who are at risk of an eating disorder, such as AN, may develop the condition in response to a stressful life event (a "trigger"). Moving away from home to attend college is an example of a trigger. Additionally, the manner in which a family interacts and functions can increase the risk of developing an eating disorder, especially among adolescents. Teenagers with eating disorders tend to think their parents are more controlling and less affectionate than the parents of healthy youths.[54] In general, individuals with eating disorders describe having a poor emotional connection to their family.

Parents can influence whether their children develop an eating disorder, because they play a role in establishing healthy attitudes about body weight and shape, as well as healthy eating practices. Adolescents may model unhealthy behaviors of their parents, especially when the teens' mothers are overly focused on their own weight.[55] Furthermore, parents who tease their children about their body weight may foster the development of disordered eating behaviors.[55,56] On a positive note, parents and other caregivers can play an important role in preventing eating disorders among their children by modeling healthy eating behaviors and expressing a positive attitude toward their own bodies.

The following sections provide more specific information about anorexia nervosa, bulimia nervosa, and binge—eating disorder. We also discuss other conditions that are characterized by unhealthy eating and exercise patterns, and we describe measures to prevent and treat these conditions.

Anorexia Nervosa

It is not unusual for *anorexia*, loss of appetite, to occur when a person is ill. The anorexia generally resolves as the individual recovers. **Anorexia nervosa (AN)** is a severe psychological disturbance characterized by self–imposed starvation that results in malnutrition and very low body weight (*emaciation*). A BMI of 18.5 is the lowest limit of what is generally considered a normal or healthy body weight for adults.[57]

According to estimates, about 0.5% of adolescent American females have AN.[58] Although males also develop AN, females comprise three times more cases than males.[59]

Signs and Symptoms People with AN have distorted body images and severely restrict their food intake, which leads to rapid weight loss and maintenance of an unhealthy low body weight. Even when they are emaciated, the patients deny they are too thin, and they are overly concerned about becoming fat. An intense fear of weight gain or "becoming fat" compels people with AN to act in ways that hinder weight gain. These behaviors can include frequent food restriction (dieting), fasting, or exercising excessively.

Some forms of AN involve bingeing and purging behaviors. **Purging** includes activities that limit calorie intake (self–induced vomiting after eating, for example) or increase calorie output by performing more physical activity than is necessary for optimal health. Although AN does not typically involve purging behaviors, when fasting or food restriction becomes difficult to maintain, someone with AN may try to compensate for eating by self–induced vomiting, misuse of laxatives or diuretics, or excessive exercise.[50]

Because people with AN are so thin, they lack adequate amounts of subcutaneous fat to insulate their bodies and have trouble maintaining their body heat as a result. Therefore, individuals with the disorder often wear layers of clothing to keep warm and hide their emaciated appearance. People with AN also have lanugo (*la–new'–go*), which is dense, fine white hair that grows on the face and other parts of the body. Lanugo may help retain body heat. Table 10.11 lists lanugo and some other common signs of AN.

AN has the highest mortality rate of any psychological disorder.[60] Almost 6% of people with AN eventually die as a result of the disorder.[61] Primary causes of death include starvation, electrolyte imbalances, and suicide.[60]

Bulimia Nervosa

Bulimia nervosa (BN) is a severe psychological condition characterized by repeated episodes of binge eating followed by purging, such as self–induced vomiting, to prevent

TABLE 10.11
Common Health Consequences of Anorexia Nervosa[50]

Weakened immune system
Slow heart rate
Hypotension (low blood pressure)
Loss of normal menstrual cycles (women)
Low bone mineral density
Lanugo (delicate, dense, white hair on the skin)
Low thyroid hormone and decreased metabolic rate
Muscle wasting and weakness

weight gain. **Binge eating** involves consuming an amount of food that is much larger than what a normal person would eat in a brief period of time, such as 2 hours. People with BN feel they have no control over their eating behavior during binge episodes. After a binge, people with BN attempt to prevent weight gain with inappropriate purging methods, such as self–induced vomiting, abuse of laxatives and/or diuretics, fasting, or excessive exercise. As with AN, a major underlying personal characteristic of BN is having a distorted body image.

BN usually begins in adolescence or young adulthood. An estimated 1.0 to 2.9% of Americans have bulimia nervosa.[52] Females are 10 times more likely to have BN than males.[50]

Signs and Symptoms Unlike people who have anorexia nervosa, individuals with bulimia nervosa are often difficult to identify by their appearance, because they tend to have BMIs in the normal or overweight range (18.5 to less than 30). However, people with BN are often ashamed of their food–related behaviors and attempt to conceal their binge–purge practices from others.

People with BN frequently induce vomiting by thrusting fingers deep into their mouths and, as a result, scrape their knuckles. Thus, characteristic signs of bulimia nervosa are bite marks and scars on the knuckles. Dentists often identify people who practice bulimic behaviors because the acid in vomit erodes the enamel on the surfaces of teeth, especially

anorexia nervosa (AN) severe psychological disturbance characterized by self-imposed starvation

purging activities that limit calorie intake or increase calorie output

bulimia nervosa (BN) severe psychological condition characterized by repeated episodes of binge eating followed by unhealthy behaviors to prevent weight gain

binge eating consuming a much larger amount of food than is normally eaten in a brief period the backs of teeth. Eroded teeth develop many dental caries (cavities) and may become chipped and ragged in appearance.

Persons with bulimia nervosa often have low self−esteem and feel guilty or depressed after a binge. Bingeing usually involves eating "forbidden" foods such as cakes, cookies, ice cream, and other high−fat, high−carbohydrate foods during binges. In cases of BN, different triggers may bring on a binge, including stressful situations, extensive dieting, and negative feelings about body weight, body shape, or food.

The bingeing activities can help the person with BN feel better in the short term; but guilt, emotional distress, and depression persist in the long term and worsen the disorder. The compelling need to binge and purge eventually becomes a preoccupation for people with BN, and as a result, they become less involved in social activities and more isolated.

Some people show behavioral characteristics of both anorexia nervosa and bulimia nervosa, because the illnesses can overlap. About half of the women diagnosed as having anorexia nervosa eventually develop signs or symptoms of bulimia.

Health Risks Self−induced vomiting and diuretic abuse can cause fluid and electrolyte imbalances that can be life threatening. Frequent vomiting also causes tears, ruptures, or bleeding of the esophagus and stomach. Someone who abuses laxatives may become dependent on their use in order to stimulate bowel movements. Almost 4% of people with BN die as a result of the disorder.[62] One in four of these deaths is due to suicide.[60]

Several psychological disorders are associated with BN. Compared to people who do not have an eating disorder, people with BN are more likely to have low self−esteem, bipolar, depressive, and personality disorders. Some people with BN also abuse alcohol or drugs. Even after recovery, up to 30% of former BN patients continue to struggle with alcohol or drug use.[50]

Binge-Eating Disorder

Binge−eating disorder (BED) is an eating disorder that features recurrent episodes of overeating that are not followed by purging behaviors.[50] As mentioned earlier, binge eating involves consuming a much larger amount of food than most people would eat under similar circumstances in a brief period of time, such as within 2 hours.

The prevalence of BED is difficult to estimate, but it may be more common than AN and BN.[51] According to one report, 3.5% of adult American women and 2% of adult American men have been diagnosed with binge−eating disorder.[59]

People with BED can be normal weight, overweight, and obese. Table 10.12 lists typical signs and symptoms of binge−eating disorder.

People with BED often have other psychological illnesses, such as bipolar, depressive, anxiety, and substance use disorders. Furthermore, stressful events and feelings of loneliness, anxiety, depression, anger, isolation, and

TABLE 10.12
Common Signs and Symptoms of Binge-Eating Disorder[51]

A person with BED:
• Is extremely distressed over the binge-eating behavior.
• Eats large amounts of food when not hungry.
• Eats more rapidly than normal and eats until uncomfortably full.
• Eats alone because of feeling embarrassed by how much is consumed.
• Feels depressed, guilty, or disgusted with him- or herself after the binge.
• Binge eats, on average, at least once a week for 3 months.

frustration can trigger a food binge. During binges, a person with BED typically isolates him− or herself and consumes large quantities of calorie−dense foods, such as ice cream, cookies, sweets, and potato chips. While bingeing, the person may feel better, but after the episode of overeating, the individual usually feels depressed, ashamed, guilty, and disgusted with his or her abnormal eating behavior.

As with the other eating disorders, BED usually begins during adolescence and young adulthood. However, people seeking treatment for BED are usually older than those seeking treatment for AN and BN.[50]

Other Disordered Eating Behaviors

The *DSM−5* also describes "other specified" feeding and eating disorders, which include less severe versions of the three main eating disorders, as well as a condition called *night eating syndrome*. Physicians use the specific criteria reported in the *DSM−5* to diagnose someone with one of the eating disorders. Some disordered eating behaviors, such as "diabulimia," are publicized in the media, but these unusual food−related practices are not recognized as eating disorders by the APA. The following sections describe night eating syndrome and some popularized unhealthy eating practices.

Night Eating Syndrome People with **night eating syndrome (NES)** experience episodic food binges that are not followed by purging. These binges take place after the

binge-eating disorder (BED) eating disorder featuring recurrent episodes of binge eating that are not followed by purging behaviors

night eating syndrome (NES) episodic food binges that are not followed by purging; binges take place after the evening meal and when the person wakens from sleep during the night evening meal and when the person wakens from sleep during the night. People with NES are aware of their actions and can recall their overnight eating practices the next day. Approximately 1 to 2% of the general population may have NES.[63,64]

Diabulimia Insulin treatment often causes weight gain in people who are recently diagnosed with type 1 diabetes. Accepting the weight can be difficult for a person who has a poor body image. However, some people with the chronic disease discover they can manipulate their body weight by skipping insulin injections or using less insulin than prescribed. This abusive practice, which affects an estimated 11 to 42% of young women with type 1 diabetes, is often referred to as **"diabulimia."**[65] The signs and symptoms of diabulimia include those that are associated with poorly controlled type 1 diabetes (see Table 5.9). Complications of long–term diabulimia are very serious and can include blindness, kidney failure, hypertension, heart attack, permanent heart damage, stroke, and nerve damage.[66]

Muscle Dysmorphia

Muscle dysmorphia is an unhealthy preoccupation with the body being too small or not muscular enough.[50] This condition occurs almost exclusively in men, and it is common among body builders. More than 50% of men with muscle dysmorphia have used anabolic steroids to help gain weight and increase muscle size.[67] People with muscle dysmorphia exercise obsessively and may lift weights for hours every day. They can become so obsessed with exercise that they continue to train despite injury and they allow exercise to take priority over work, school, and friends. Individuals who have muscle dysmorphia are more likely to drop out of school, and they have a high risk of suicide.[50]

Female Athlete Triad

Women and girls participating in competitive sports or sports and activities that benefit from a low body weight, such as gymnastics, dance, and distance running, are at risk of developing one or more components of the **female athlete triad** (Fig. 10.23). This condition is characterized by three interrelated components:

- **Low energy availability** (negative energy balance);
- Menstrual disturbances that often include loss of menstrual cycles; and
- Reduced bone mineral density that may lead to osteoporosis.

As many as 16% of female athletes have all three components of the triad.[68]

Female athletes may restrict their calorie intake to improve athletic performance, lose weight, or maintain a

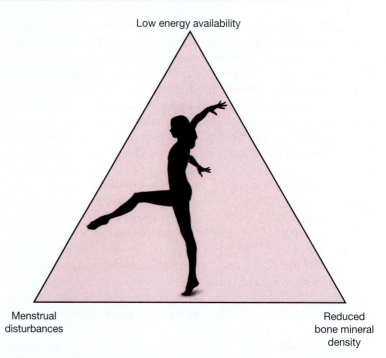

Low energy availability

Menstrual disturbances

Reduced bone mineral density

Figure 10.23 Female athlete triad. Women and girls participating in competitive sports or sports and activities that benefit from a low body weight are at risk of developing one or more components of the female athlete triad.

lean physique. Other female athletes may lack the appetite, nutrition knowledge, or time to consume enough energy to meet their high needs and maintain a healthy BMI, especially during periods of intense physical training.

Females of childbearing age need adequate amounts of energy to maintain normal menstrual cycles. Low energy availability is associated with a deficiency of the "female hormone" estrogen.[69] The lack of estrogen causes menstrual disturbances, such as longer–than–normal intervals between menstrual periods and absence of menstrual periods. Estrogen is needed to build and maintain bone mineral mass. Female athletes who have low energy availability and no menstrual periods can have low bone mineral density and an increased risk for bone fractures.

diabulimia popular term used to describe people with type I diabetes who skip insulin injections or use less insulin than prescribed to control their body weight

muscle dysmorphia unhealthy preoccupation with the body being too small or not muscular enough

female athlete triad condition that is characterized by low energy availability, menstrual problems, and reduced bone mineral density in female athletes

low energy availability state of negative energy balance

When the lack of estrogen occurs during adolescence, a critical time for bone growth, the female athlete's bone mineral density may not improve even after she recovers from the triad.[70] Premature osteoporosis is a serious and long–term consequence of the triad.

Preventing Eating Disorders

Early identification of people with risk factors for eating disorders, such as disordered eating patterns and distorted body images, can help prevent the development of eating disorders. Prevention efforts generally focus on fostering the individual's body acceptance, improving his or her self–confidence, and encouraging the person to challenge the idea that being thin is ideal.

Treating Eating Disorders If someone you know has an eating disorder, it is important to encourage the person to seek help as soon as possible to avoid serious health con–sequences. In academic environments, professional help is commonly available at student health centers and student guidance or counseling facilities on campus.

It may be difficult to talk with someone whom you suspect has an eating disorder. When approaching the

REAL PEOPLE | REAL STORIES

Sarah Marie

Twenty-year-old Sarah Marie loves animals. She loves them so much, she would like a career that involves animals. Underneath her seemingly happy and relaxed surface, Sarah suffers from a serious health condition that has no easy cure. Sarah has bulimia nervosa.

"When I was 12, I weighed 164 pounds and I was 5-feet, 1-inch tall," says Sarah." I went on a diet to lose weight. I just remember the first 10 days of the diet; all you ate was fruit. I don't recall much about the diet after that, but I followed it for 5 months and lost 45 pounds. Losing the weight made me so happy! After that, I got my first boyfriend, but the relationship didn't last and I didn't stay on the diet. I regained about 25 pounds.

"When I was 16, I tried to do 'negative' calories. I'd walk for 2 hours every single day, and I still didn't think it was enough exercise. I also really limited my food. I would eat all my calories within 2 hours early in the day, then I wouldn't eat anything for the rest of the day. I felt a lot of anxiety . . . ," Sarah says. "I worried about breaking the fast and eating, but I started losing weight again, and that made me feel good. When I looked at the scale, I thought when I reached a certain point, I would be happy. I kept losing weight, but I never felt happy. Soon my weight was 103 pounds. My dad told me that I looked like I walked out of a prison camp, and I took it as a compliment. If I hadn't started bingeing, I would've lost more weight.

"I feel relieved when I binge, but when I feel sick to my stomach, I realize what I've done and I feel disgusting. I'm fearful that I'm going to gain weight, so I exercise after the binge.

"I've been to a few therapists, but I still have the disorder. I want fast results, but of course, that's not going to happen. I remember a time when I could eat and not worry about it. I wish I could go back to then. If you have bulimia, you need to seek help: Don't keep it a secret. There's a lot of help out there."

individual to discuss your concerns, you can follow these recommendations:[71]

- Meet with the person privately and without distractions.
- Share your feelings and concerns in a caring and supportive manner.
- Describe occasions when you observed behaviors that were signs of an eating disorder.
- Avoid using harsh, judgmental language and instead explain how you feel. For example, instead of stating "You've lost too much weight: You look like you're starving!" say "I feel very worried about how much weight you've lost."
- Do not suggest simple solutions, such as: "If you'd just have meals with the family again, you'll eat and feel better."
- Suggest that he or she discuss your concerns with an expert who treats eating disorders, such as a psychotherapist, dietitian, physician, or nurse. Offer to help find such an expert, make an appointment, or accompany him or her on the first visit.
- Avoid conflict. If the person denies that he or she has an eating disorder, repeat your concerns and indicate that you will be available if the person decides to get help in the future.
- End the conversation by expressing your desire to be supportive. For example, remind the person that you want him or her to be happy and healthy.

A multidisciplinary group of experts in nutrition, mental health, and medicine is necessary for optimal treatment of eating disorders.[51] Treatment should include psychotherapy while also addressing critical nutritional needs and other medical conditions. Dietitians play a critical role in assessing and treating eating disorders, including providing nutritional counseling. Dietitians can help stabilize healthy eating patterns and improve patients' nutrient status by providing appropriate medical nutrition therapy. Furthermore, experts in nutrition can play an important role in helping patients avoid relapse once recovery is underway.[51]

Treatment for eating disorders can occur in several settings. Inpatient hospitalization or residential care in a facility that specializes in the treatment of the disorders may be required when the patient's medical complications become life threatening. However, eating disorder treatment most often occurs in outpatient care settings. Outpatient care may involve individual, group, or family counseling. Treatment of eating disorders may also include prescription medications. Participation in eating disorder support groups may help prevent relapse.

Cognitive behavioral therapy (CBT) is a major treatment approach for BN and BED.[51] CBT is a general term used to describe psychological therapy approaches that address unhealthy emotions and behaviors. The therapy teaches people healthy coping strategies to use when under stress instead of fasting, bingeing, purging, or excessive exercise.

cognitive behavioral therapy (CBT) psychological therapy approaches that address unhealthy emotions and behaviors

Concept **Checkpoint 10.11**

47. Keira usually skips breakfast. Explain whether her behavior is a sign of an eating disorder.
48. List the major types of eating disorders and their signs.
49. List at least four risk factors for eating disorders.
50. What are three serious health consequences of anorexia nervosa?

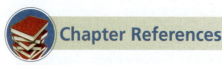

Chapter References

See Appendix H.

Summary

10.1 The Obesity Epidemic

- The prevalence of overweight and obesity has reached epidemic proportions in the United States and throughout the world. Over two-thirds of American adults were either overweight or obese in 2010; about one-third of the adults were obese. The prevalence of obese American infants, children, and adolescents has risen sharply over the past 25 years.

10.2 Body Composition

- The body is composed of two major compartments: total body fat and fat-free mass. Overfat people have excessive adipose tissue. Percentage of body fat is associated with risks of obesity-related diseases. Medical researchers use several methods to estimate body composition.

10.3 Energy for Living

- Biological fuels are foods and beverages that contain macronutrients and the nonnutrient alcohol. Under normal conditions, human cells metabolize primarily glucose and fatty acids, but small amounts of amino acids are also used for energy. Cells release the energy stored in biological fuels by breaking bonds within the molecules. Cells obtain only about 40% of the energy that was in macronutrients by forming ATP. Cells release the remaining energy as heat.

- Basal or resting metabolism, physical activity, TEF, and NEAT account for total energy use by the body. Metabolism accounts for the largest share of an average person's daily energy needs. Various factors including thyroid hormone, body composition, gender, and age influence the metabolic rate. Physical activity is energy use by skeletal muscle movement. TEF is the increase in energy needs that occurs during digestion, absorption, and processing of nutrients in food. NEAT is energy use for involuntary skeletal muscle activities, such as shivering.

10.4 Energy Balance

- Energy balance is a state in which a person's calorie intake from food and beverages equals his or her calorie output for metabolism, physical activity, TEF, and NEAT. Negative energy balance occurs when calorie output is greater than calorie intake, resulting in weight loss. Positive energy balance occurs when calorie intake is greater than calorie output, resulting in weight gain.

10.5 Classifying Overweight and Obesity

- In addition to percentage of body fat, medical experts use BMI to determine whether one's weight is healthy. BMIs of 18.5 to 24.9 are healthy; BMIs of 25.0 to 29.9 are in the overweight range. Persons with BMIs of 30.0 or more are obese.

- People with BMIs greater than 25 have increased risks of CVD, hypertension, type 2 diabetes, and certain cancers. Compared to people with healthy BMIs, obese people are more likely to die prematurely from all causes. Body fat distribution is associated with obesity-related diseases. Excessive central-body fat (apple shape) is associated with increased risks of CVD, type 2 diabetes, and hypertension. Waist circumferences that exceed 40 inches (men) or 35 inches (women) are linked to obesity-related diseases.

10.6 What Causes Overweight and Obesity?

- There is no simple cause for obesity. From a physiological standpoint, eating behavior is complex and largely involves interactions among the nervous, endocrine, and digestive systems, as well as fat tissue. Dietary and inherited factors also influence body weight. Additionally, overfat people may have inherited genes for "thrifty metabolisms." According to the set-point theory, the body's fat content is genetically predetermined. The set point may protect the body from losing weight and explain why weight loss is so difficult to achieve and maintain.

- Environmental factors can have a powerful influence on food choices and appetite. The environment also influences people's patterns of physical activity. Healthy adults under 65 years of age should perform at least 150 minutes of moderate-intensity physical activity each week.

10.7 Weight Loss and Its Maintenance

- A reliable weight-loss plan is safe and effective, and the plan should meet the person's nutritional, psychological, and social needs. Successful weight loss and long-term weight maintenance involve four key elements: motivation, calorie reduction, regular physical activity, and behavior modification.

- A pound of body fat contains about 3500 kcal. If energy output exceeds calorie intake a person can expect to lose weight. A healthy way to lower total calorie intake is to reduce consumption of added sugars, added fats, and alcohol. A goal of a person who wants to lose weight should be reducing total calorie intake while obtaining all essential nutrients.

10.8 Medical Treatments for Obesity

- At present, the FDA has approved a few medications for weight loss. Orlistat can improve weight loss to a small degree, when it is combined with a plan that includes calorie restriction and regular exercise. Bariatric surgeries reduce the stomach volume of people with extreme obesity.

10.9 Unreliable Weight-Loss Methods

- People can lose weight while following fad diets, but they usually regain much of the weight that was lost when they resume their prior eating and other lifestyle habits. Achieving a healthy body weight and maintaining that weight requires making lifestyle changes that a person adopts for the rest of his or her life. No dietary supplement is recommended for weight loss.

10.10 Gaining Weight

- Underweight can be caused by various factors, such as genetics, excessive physical activity, and certain diseases. To gain weight, an underweight person generally needs to increase portion sizes, eat more calorie-dense foods, and reduce physical activity, if excessive.

10.11 Nutrition Matters: Eating Disorders and Disordered Eating

- Disordered eating, involving temporary chaotic and abnormal food-related practices, often occurs when a person is under a lot of stress or wants to lose weight. When a person adopts disordered eating behaviors as a lifestyle, the practices can become harmful and difficult-to-treat eating disorders. Eating disorders are psychological disturbances that lead to behavioral changes and serious health complications. Anorexia nervosa, bulimia nervosa, and binge-eating disorder are the major types of eating disorders. Treatment of eating disorders is complex, involving more than just dietary counseling.

Recipe for Healthy Living

Did You Make That Dip?!

When it's time to entertain your friends, you can make a fiesta dip that will disappear quickly and provide plenty of compliments, too. Fresh cilantro and dried cumin give recipes a distinctive "Mexican" flavor. Bean dip recipes often include canned refried beans and cheeses that are high in fat. This lower-fat version uses canned red beans and reduced-fat cheese. You can save time by using canned fat-free "refried" beans (yes, there is such a product). You can also substitute commercially prepared salsa for the homemade version, but you may find that making salsa with fresh ingredients is worth the extra effort. If you like a hotter salsa, use jalapeño peppers instead of mild green chili peppers. When preparing hot peppers, be careful to avoid touching your eyes or the inside of your nose until after you have thoroughly washed your hands with soap and water. The peppers contain *capsaicin,* the highly irritating chemical used in pepper spray that causes intense burning when in contact with mucous membranes.

This recipe makes approximately eight ¼-cup servings. Each serving (without tortilla) supplies approximately 157 kcal, 10 g protein, 5 g fat, 110 mcg folate, 439 mg potassium, 1.6 mg iron, and 5 g fiber.

SALSA LAYER INGREDIENTS:

1 large, fresh ripe tomato
¼ medium onion
1 clove garlic finely minced
1 4-oz can of mild green chilies (peeled and diced)
3 Tbsp fresh cilantro leaves

GUACAMOLE LAYER INGREDIENTS:

1 ripe, black-skinned avocado (slightly soft)
juice of 1 lime
¼ tsp dried cumin (a spice)
⅛ tsp ground black pepper

OTHER LAYERS:

1 14-oz to 16-oz can red beans (no added salt)
1 cup shredded fat-reduced cheddar cheese
⅓ cup fat-free plain yogurt (optional)

PREPARATION STEPS:

1. Cover an 8" dinner plate with a sheet of heavy-duty aluminum foil.

2. Wash cilantro in cool water and shake off excess water. Wash tomato, avocado, and lime in cool water. Set cilantro and fruits aside on paper towels.

3. Use a sharp knife to *mince* (finely chop) onion, garlic, and cilantro on a cutting board. Place in small bowl.

4. Add chilies to the onion, garlic, and cilantro mixture. Stir gently until well mixed.

5. *Dice* (cut into small pieces) tomato and add to minced ingredients. You've made *salsa*.

6. To make guacamole, remove skin and seed from avocado. In a small bowl, dice avocado into small pieces and sprinkle with lime juice. Mash avocado and lime mixture. Add cumin and black pepper to avocado mixture, stir, and set aside.

7. Drain juice from beans and rinse them with cool water. Mash beans with the back of a large spoon; bean mixture will be lumpy.

8. Spread mashed beans evenly on the plate, leaving about ¾" from the edge of the plate free of beans.

9. Cover beans with individual layers of salsa and guacamole, and top with shredded cheese. If desired, place yogurt in the center as a low-fat substitute for sour cream and top with the cheese.

10. Loosely cover layered dip with clear plastic wrap and refrigerate.

11. To serve, spoon dip on pieces of soft tortillas.

Further analyze this and other recipes through activities on Connect at www.mcgrawhillconnect.com.

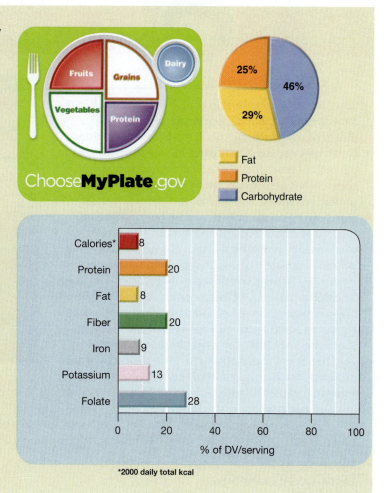

ChooseMyPlate.gov

- Fat
- Protein
- Carbohydrate

46%
25%
29%

Calories* 8
Protein 20
Fat 8
Fiber 20
Iron 9
Potassium 13
Folate 28

% of DV/serving

*2000 daily total kcal

Personal Dietary Analysis

1. Consider your eating behaviors.

   a. Explain how your emotional state influences your eating behaviors. For example, do you eat certain foods when you feel happy, "stressed out," or depressed? Which foods do you eat under these circumstances? Describe a situation in which you ate in response to an emotional state instead of being hungry.

   b. Discuss the influence that food advertising has on your eating practices.

   c. Besides emotional state and food advertising, what other factors influence your eating habits?

2. Estimate your energy requirement by using one of the following formulas; choose the appropriate formula for your sex group.

Men 19 Years and Older:

Estimated Energy Requirement (EER) = 662 – (9.53 × AGE) + PA × (15.91 × WT + 539.6 × HT)

Women 19 Years and Older:

Estimated Energy Requirement (EER) = 354 – (6.91 × AGE) + PA × (9.36 × WT + 726 × HT)

The variables in the formulas are as follows:

AGE = age in years

PA = physical activity estimate (see Table 10.4)

WT = weight in kg (lb ÷ 2.2)

HT = height in meters (inches ÷ 39.4)

 |NUTRITION

Complete this Personal Dietary Analysis activity online at www.mcgrawhillconnect.com.

Critical Thinking

1. Kim and Kevin weigh the same and have similar swimming skills. While in a swimming pool, Kim floats easily when she extends her arms and legs in the water. When Kevin extends his arms and legs and tries to float in the pool, he sinks. Why is Kim able to float more easily than Kevin?

2. An advertisement for a weight—loss supplement claims that the mixture of herbs in the product increases the metabolic rate by 150%. Explain why you would or would not recommend this product to someone who wants to lose weight.

3. Explain why it is usually difficult to pinpoint a *cause* of obesity.

4. Why are most people who lose weight unable to maintain the lower body weight over time?

5. If your BMI is within the overweight or obese range, discuss your reasons for being interested or not interested in losing weight. If you want to lose weight, what lifestyle changes will you make?

6. If your BMI is within the underweight range, discuss your reasons for being interested or not interested in gaining weight. If you want to gain weight, what life—style changes will you make?

7. If your BMI is in the healthy range, discuss steps you can take to maintain a healthy body weight as you grow older.

Practice Test

Select the best answer.

1. Body mass index (BMI) is

   a. a standard used to calculate a person's body fat percentage.
   b. based on a relationship between weight and risk of chronic disease.
   c. gradually being replaced by more reliable height/weight tables.
   d. a chart used to predict one's caloric intake.

2. _____ cells are specialized to store fat.

   a. Carcinoma
   b. Megaloblastic
   c. Neural
   d. Adipose

3. _____ fat deposits are under the abdominal muscles.

   a. Subcutaneous
   b. Visceral
   c. Cellulite
   d. Bulimic

4. _____ relies on the principle that lean tissue is denser than water.

   a. Bioelectrical impedance
   b. Underwater weighing
   c. Dual—energy x—ray absorptiometry
   d. Air displacement

5. A healthy body fat percentage for women is

   a. 3–10%.
   b. 23–31%.
   c. 32–37%.
   d. 40–50%.

6. For the typical active person, basal metabolism accounts for _____ of the body's total energy use.

   a. 10–20%
   b. 21–49%
   c. 60–75%
   d. over 75%

7. Basal metabolism includes energy needs for

   a. breathing and circulating blood.
   b. performing physical activity.
   c. digesting food.
   d. absorbing nutrients.

8. Which of the following statements is true?

   a. Women generally have higher metabolic rates than men.
   b. Thyroid hormone levels influence BMR.
   c. A person who has more muscle mass will have a lower BMR than someone with less muscle tissue.
   d. When a person has a fever, his or her BMR drops below normal.

9. Negative energy balance occurs when

   a. the body needs more calories than the diet supplies.
   b. fat storage in the body increases.
   c. energy intake is higher than energy output.
   d. the thermic effect of food equals NEAT.

10. _____ is a hormone that reduces hunger and inhibits fat storage in the body.

   a. Coumadin
   b. Leptin
   c. Ghrelin
   d. Dexadrin

11. Members of the National Weight Control Registry tend to

   a. skip breakfast regularly.
   b. follow low−carbohydrate/high−protein diets.
   c. exercise two to three times per week.
   d. eat meals regularly, including breakfast.

12. Joseph's BMI is 23. When he is under a lot of stress, he eats a large amount of empty−calorie foods. Soon after eating these foods, he goes to a bathroom and makes himself vomit. Based on this information, Joseph probably has

   a. diarexia psychosis.
   b. anorexia nervosa.
   c. cystic fibrosis.
   d. bulimia nervosa.

LEARNSMART®
ADVANTAGE

Get the most out of your study of nutrition with McGraw-Hill's innovative suite of adaptive learning products including McGraw-Hill LearnSmart®, SmartBook®, LearnSmart Achieve®, and LearnSmart Prep®. Visit www.learnsmartadvantage.com.

Answers to **Quiz Yourself**

1. You can determine whether you have an unhealthy amount of body fat simply by measuring your waistline. **True.** (p. 388)

2. The safest way to lose a lot of weight and keep it off is to follow a low-carbohydrate, high-fat diet, such as the Atkins diet. **False.** (p. 406)

3. As people age, their muscle cells turn into fat cells. **False.** (p. 380)

4. When a person consumes more protein than needed, the excess can be converted to fat and stored in fat cells. **True.** (p. 384)

5. Cellulite is a unique type of fat that can be eliminated by taking certain dietary supplements. **False.** (p. 373)

CHAPTER 11

Nutrition for Physically Active Lifestyles

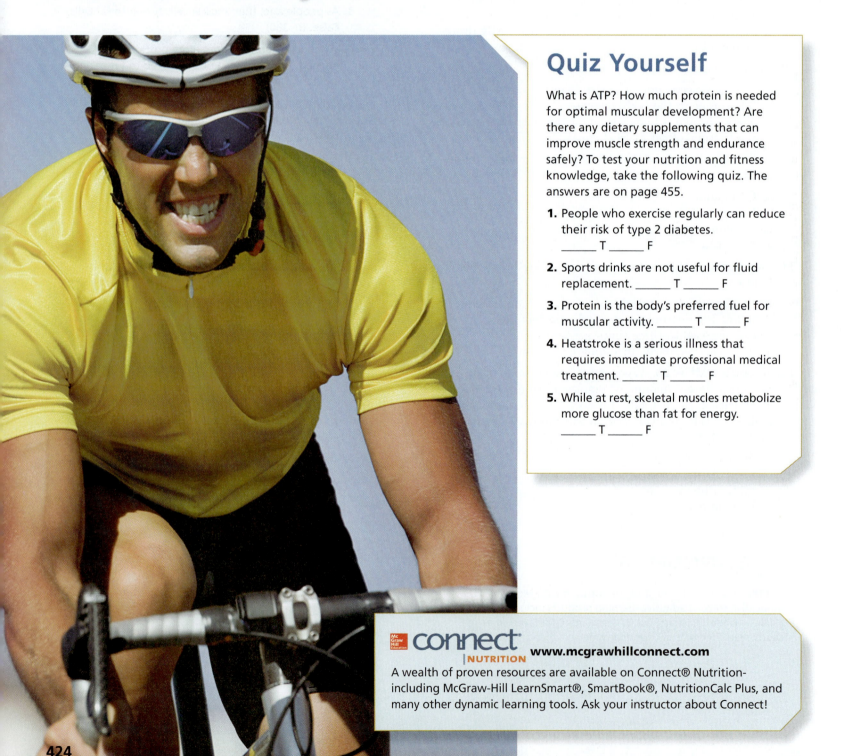

Quiz Yourself

What is ATP? How much protein is needed for optimal muscular development? Are there any dietary supplements that can improve muscle strength and endurance safely? To test your nutrition and fitness knowledge, take the following quiz. The answers are on page 455.

1. People who exercise regularly can reduce their risk of type 2 diabetes. _____ T _____ F

2. Sports drinks are not useful for fluid replacement. _____ T _____ F

3. Protein is the body's preferred fuel for muscular activity. _____ T _____ F

4. Heatstroke is a serious illness that requires immediate professional medical treatment. _____ T _____ F

5. While at rest, skeletal muscles metabolize more glucose than fat for energy. _____ T _____ F

11.1 Introduction to Nutrition for Fitness and Sport

Learning Outcomes

1 Explain the difference between physical activity and exercise.

2 Define *physical fitness.*

3 Discuss recommendations concerning the duration and intensity of physical activity to achieve good health.

Bicycling for weeks through quaint villages and over steep mountains in France; swimming for miles in the chilly English Channel while being buffeted by waves; lifting metal disks that weigh more than the weight lifter—the extent to which some people push their bodies is truly amazing. Superior athletes seem to thrive on performing grueling physical feats that require extraordinary stamina, strength, and energy. Millions of Americans admire competitive athletes for their physical accomplishments and enjoy watching them perform. Many Americans, however, lead *sedentary* lives; that is, their daily activities do not require much muscular exertion. In 2012, about 50% of adults in the United States did not obtain recommended amounts of moderate or vigorous physical activity.[1] Even when Americans have the time, many chose not to be physically active.

The human body is designed for **physical activity,** movement that results from skeletal muscle contraction. Most of the physical activities you perform each day are *unstructured*, for example, shopping for groceries or doing household tasks. **Exercise** refers to physical activities that are usually planned and structured for a particular purpose, such as having fun or increasing muscle mass. Both forms of physical activity can benefit your health.

Physical fitness is the ability to perform moderate— to vigorous—intensity activities without becoming excessively fatigued. A *physically fit* person has the strength, endurance, flexibility, and balance to meet the physical demands of daily living, exercise, and sports. Proper nutrition is essential for optimal physical fitness and sports performance.

Regardless of whether you aspire to be a world—class athlete or simply want to be healthier, regular exercise should be a part of your daily routine. Physically inactive people do not have to perform high—intensity structured workouts daily to improve their health. According to recommendations of the U.S. Department of Health and Human Services, healthy adults under 65 years of age should perform:

- moderate—intensity physical activity for 150 minutes a week,

or

- vigorous—intensity physical activity for 75 minutes a week,

and

- eight to 10 strengthening exercises (eight to 12 repetitions of each exercise) that focus on major muscle groups twice a week.[2]

By reading this chapter, you will learn about the benefits of a physically active lifestyle, different cellular energy systems, and dietary practices that are appropriate for athletes and other physically active people. This chapter also provides practical tips for planning an exercise routine that you can follow for a lifetime.

physical activity movement resulting from contraction of skeletal muscles

exercise physical activities that are usually planned and structured for a purpose

physical fitness ability to perform moderate- to vigorous-intensity activities without becoming excessively fatigued

11.2 Benefits of Regular Exercise

Learning Outcomes

1 Describe the health benefits of performing exercise on a regular basis.

2 Describe the physical activity pyramid and explain how it can be used as a guide for developing a personal exercise plan.

3 Calculate a person's target heart rate range.

People who exercise regularly can help reduce their risks of serious chronic conditions, including cardiovascular disease, type 2 diabetes, hypertension, obesity, osteoporosis, and certain cancers.[3] Maintaining a physically active lifestyle is one of the most important steps that people can take to improve their health. In 2008, the U.S. Department of Health and Human Services issued the *2008 Physical Activity Guidelines for Americans* (http://www.health.gov/paguidelines/). These guidelines provide evidence–based physical activity recommendations to help Americans reduce the risk of chronic diseases that contribute to millions of premature deaths each year.[4] The *2015–2020 Dietary Guidelines for Americans* support the Physical Activity Guidelines.

Determining the Intensity of Physical Activity

As Figure 11.1 illustrates, you can gain physical as well as psychological benefits by performing moderate–intensity physical activity regularly. Furthermore, you may achieve even greater health benefits by increasing the duration, frequency, and intensity (physical effort) of your exercise routine.

Intensity refers to the level of exertion used to perform an activity. Duration and type of physical activity, as well as body weight, influence the intensity of skeletal muscle movement. Thus, activities such as walking and bicycling can be classified as either moderate–or vigorous–intensity physical activity, depending on the rate at which the activities are performed as well as the weight of the person performing them. See http://www.cdc.gov/physicalactivity/basics/measuring/index.html for examples of physical activities that are generally classified as moderate or vigorous intensity.

There are a few ways to determine the intensity of exercise. One way is to judge your level of exertion based on physical signs, such as breathing rate and sweat production. While exercising at the moderate–intensity level, you should be aware of your muscular effort, but you should also be able to chat with an exercise partner comfortably.

A popular method of estimating the intensity of exercise is to use a percent–age of your *age–related maximum heart rate*. To calculate your age–related maximum heart rate, subtract your age from 220, the age–related maximum heart rate. (Some experts suggest using a slightly lower age–related maximum heart rate for women.) Your **target heart rate zone** is the range of heart

target heart rate zone heart rate range that reflects intensity of physical exertion

Reduces stress and improves self-image

Promotes psychological well-being

May protect the brain from changes associated with the aging process

Increases muscle mass and strength

Reduces risk of colon cancer (cancer of the large intestine)

Increases flexibility and balance

Strengthens bones and improves the function of joints

Reduces feelings of depression and anxiety

Reduces the likelihood of sleep disorders

Increases cardiovascular function and improves blood lipid profile

Reduces blood pressure

Reduces risk of breast cancer

Aids in weight loss/ weight control

Improves blood glucose regulation; reduces risk of type 2 diabetes

Entire body:

Improves immune function

Reduces the risk of dying prematurely

Figure 11.1 Benefits of being physically active. Regular physical activity improves health in several ways.

rate that reflects the intensity of your exertion during physical activity. For moderate–intensity physical activity, your target heart rate zone should be 50 to 70% of your age–related maximum heart rate.[5] To determine your moderate–intensity "zone," take your age–related maximum heart rate and multiply this figure by 0.50 and 0.70. For example, the age–related maximum heart rate of a 20–year–old person is 200 beats per minute (220 minus 20). Multiply 200 beats per minute (bpm) by 0.50 to calculate the 50% value and multiply 200 bpm by 0.70 to obtain the 70% level. This person's target heart rate zone for moderate–intensity activities is 100 to 140 bpm.

Moderate–intensity physical activities expend 3.5 to 7.0 kcal/min.[6] To "burn" (*oxidize* or *metabolize*) more energy and give your heart a more vigorous workout, you can engage in physical activities that expend more than 7 kcal/min. Such physical activities usually require considerable muscular effort and result in significant increases in breathing rate and perspiration. Examples of vigorous physical activities include jogging, running, aerobic dancing, swimming laps, and bicycling uphill.

To exercise vigorously, your target heart rate should be 70 to 85% of your age–related maximum heart rate.[5] To calculate this range, follow the same formula that you used to determine the range for moderate–intensity activity, except that you need to change "0.50 and 0.70" to "0.70 and 0.85." A 20—year—old person, for example, would have an estimated maximum age—related heart rate of 200 bpm, and the 70 to 85% levels would range from 140 to 170 bpm. If you have any serious health problems, ask your physician to help you determine your target zone.

You can measure your heart rate (pulse) easily by finding the *radial artery* in your wrist. Locate the radial artery by gently placing your index and middle fingers on the underside of your wrist by the thumb, as shown in Figure 11.2. Count your pulse for 10 seconds, and then multiply that number by 6 to determine your heart rate for 1 minute. Your heart rate begins to decline as soon as you stop exercising, so you need to practice taking your pulse while still working out.

Physical Activity Pyramid

The physical activity pyramid shown in Figure 11.3 provides practical suggestions for increasing the intensity of various routine activities. For example, you will exert more physical effort and expend more energy if you use stairs instead of ele— vators or "jog" instead of "walk" the dog.

Figure 11.2 Finding the radial artery. To locate the radial artery, gently place your index and middle fingers on the underside of your wrist by the thumb, as shown.

Sedentary Activity (occasionally)
Sitting, driving, watching TV, using a computer, taking an elevator or escalator

| Figure 11.3 Physical activity pyramid.

Light Recreational Activity (2–3 days/week)
Bowling, walking (fast pace), line dancing, and doing yoga

Aerobic Exercise (3–5 days/week, for a total of 150 minutes)
Running, cycling, in-line skating, stair stepping

Flexibility Exercise (2–3 days/week)
Static stretching of major muscle groups. Holding each stretch for 10–30 seconds.

Strength Exercise (2–3 days/week, 8–10 exercises 1 set of 8–12 reps)
Bicep curls, tricep presses, squats, lunges, push-ups

Activities of Daily Living (Most days of the week, accumulate 30+ minutes)
Gardening, raking leaves, mowing the lawn, walking the dog, cleaning the house, playing with your children

Low—intensity, unstructured physical activities that involve usual daily liv—ing activities, such as routine household chores, form the foundation of the phys—ical activity pyramid. The next level of the activity pyramid recommends adding *aerobic* exercise to foundation activities at least three times a week. **Aerobic exercise** involves sustained, rhythmic contractions of large muscle groups in the legs and arms. Such activities raise your heart rate, giving your heart a more effective workout. Running, jogging, rapid walking, and swimming are aerobic activities. Additionally, the second level of the pyramid recommends performing resistance and stretching exercises at least two times a week to increase muscle mass, strength, and flexibility. Resistance exercises, such as weight lifting, can also increase bone mass. The third level of the pyramid encourages regularly performing recreational activities that are physical, such as yoga and line danc—ing. The top of the pyramid depicts activities that expend little energy, such as watching television or using a personal computer. The pyramid recommends spending little time being sedentary. The "Nutrition Matters" section in this chapter provides information concerning how to design a more formal physical fitness plan.

| Swimming is an aerobic exercise.

Concept **Checkpoint 11.2**

4. List at least five health benefits of performing moderate-intensity exercise regularly.

5. What are at least two benefits of performing resistance exercise regularly?

6. Calculate the target heart rate range for a 24-year-old person performing moderate-intensity physical activity.

aerobic exercise physical activities that involve sustained, rhythmic contractions of large muscle groups

11.3 Energy for Muscular Work

Learning Outcomes

1 Explain how cells make and use ATP.

2 Discuss how each energy system supplies ATP for muscles and under what conditions a particular energy system functions.

3 Explain how a person can improve his or her aerobic capacity.

4 Discuss the body's use of macronutrients as energy sources.

To move, muscles must contract, and to contract, muscles must have a source of energy. Under normal conditions, most cells, including muscle cells, metabolize a mixture of biological fuels, especially glucose and fatty acids. Muscle cells also metabolize a small amount of amino acids from proteins to obtain energy.

Energy Metabolism

Cells obtain energy by means of a complex series of chemical reactions that progressively break down (*catabolize*) macronutrients and alcohol to release the energy that is stored within them. Cells lose much of this energy as heat, but

Figure 11.4 **ATP.** Cells capture and store energy by forming ATP from ADP and inorganic phosphate (P_i).

adenosine diphosphate (ADP) high-energy compound; by-product of ATP use

anaerobic conditions that lack free oxygen

aerobic conditions that require free oxygen

glycolysis first stage of glucose oxidation

pyruvate compound that results from anaerobic breakdown of glucose

mitochondria cellular structures that release energy from macronutrients; singular, mitochondrion

Figure 11.5 **Obtaining energy.**
(a) During glycolysis, the first stage of glucose oxidation, cells degrade glucose into pyruvate under anaerobic conditions.
(b) If oxygen is available, pyruvate undergoes further degradation in mitochondria, forming CO_2, H_2O, and ATP, at certain points.

they capture some of the energy in *high–energy compounds* such as adenosine triphosphate (ATP). ATP forms when an *inorganic phosphate* group (Pi) bonds with **adenosine diphosphate (ADP)** and traps energy in the process (Fig. 11.4). Note in Figure 11.4 that ADP has two inorganic phosphate groups and ATP has three inorganic phosphate groups.

Glucose is the most useful biological fuel, because the simple sugar can be catabolized when free oxygen (O_2) is unavailable **(anaerobic)** or available **(aerobic).** Catabolic processes involve *oxidation*, the removal of electrons from compounds to create new compounds. During **glycolysis** (*glyco* = carbohydrate [particularly sugar]; *lysis* = breakdown), the first stage of glucose oxidation, glucose is degraded to form **pyruvate** under anaerobic conditions (Fig. 11.5a). Glycolysis produces a small amount of ATP.

If oxygen is available, pyruvate undergoes further oxidation in a stepwise series of chemical pathways called *aerobic respiration*. Pyruvate moves from the fluid within cells (cytoplasm) into **mitochondria** (Fig. 11.5b). Mitochondria are often referred to as "powerhouses," because much of the energy stored in glucose or other biological fuels is released within these cellular structures. In mitochondria, pyruvate undergoes complete degradation, and as a result, cells generate more ATP than during glycolysis. Oxygen is a key player in this phase of the process, because the element bonds to hydrogen atoms that were released from pyruvate, forming water (H_2O) (see Fig. 11.5b). When cells completely oxidize glucose to release energy, the end products are ATP, carbon dioxide (CO_2) and H_2O. Most of the CO_2 is exhaled, and the H_2O produced metabolically can help maintain proper body water volume. Besides glucose, triglycerides (fat), amino acids, and alcohol are also sources of ATP. Figure 11.6 summarizes the pathways that dietary protein, carbohydrate, and fat follow during energy metabolism. For more detailed illustrations of the metabolic pathways that biological fuels undergo, see Appendix C.

Did You Know?

Human cells can convert certain amino acids into glucose, but the cells are unable to make glucose from fatty acids.

Figure 11.6 Summary of ATP formation. Protein, carbohydrate, and fat can be metabolized for ATP production. Amino acids from proteins may be channeled into aerobic energy pathways to generate ATP. Glucose (carbohydrate) can be broken down anaerobically, but the biological fuel generates relatively little ATP as a result. However, aerobic breakdown of pyruvate (a by-product of anaerobic glucose metabolism) in mitochondia generates more ATP. Products of fat breakdown can enter aerobic metabolic pathways as well.

Figure 11.7 Energy from ATP. When a cell needs energy to drive a chemical reaction, it uses an enzyme to break the bond between the last two phosphate groups of ATP, releasing energy and reforming ADP and P$_i$.

How Do Cells Use ATP?

ATP is the primary source of direct energy for all cells. ATP is often referred to as "energy currency," because it functions like money. Just as you save money until it is needed to make a purchase, your cells save energy in ATP until it is needed to power cellular work.

When a cell needs some energy to drive a chemical reaction, it uses an enzyme to break the bond between the last two phosphate groups of ATP (Fig. 11.7). This process releases energy ($ATP-energy$) and reforms ADP and P$_i$. Thus, cells can recycle their supplies of ADP and P$_i$. Cells do not store much ATP, so they must constantly replace their supply of the high−energy compound by recycling ADP and P_i.

Energy Systems for Exercising Muscles

Gram for gram, fat supplies more energy than carbohydrate. Fatty acids, however, are not a very useful fuel for intense, brief exercise, such as a 100−meter sprint. Why? A fatty acid molecule has fewer oxygen atoms in relation to carbon atoms than a glucose molecule. Thus, cells need more oxygen to metabolize a fatty acid molecule than to burn a glucose molecule. During a brief bout of intense exercise, the heart and lungs do not have enough time to deliver much oxygen to muscles. Under these conditions, glucose is a major source of energy. For physical activities that last longer and are less intense, muscles can use more fat for energy, because the lungs are able to supply them with enough oxygen.

Muscle cells rely on three major systems to obtain energy: the $PCr-ATP$, *lactic acid*, and *oxygen systems*. The PCr−ATP and lactic acid systems do not need oxygen to produce ATP. Thus, these systems metabolize glucose under anaerobic conditions, such as when a person holds his or her breath while sprinting or lifting a heavy load. As the duration of the activity increases, muscle cells need to form considerably more ATP. To meet this demand, muscle cells depend heavily on the oxygen system to metabolize glucose and fat.

The three energy−releasing systems do not function independently of each other during intense physical exertion; each contributes ATP−energy to power intense muscular activity. The following sections provide more information about these major energy systems.

PCr-ATP Energy System

A resting muscle cell contains only a small amount of ATP that can be used immediately. Muscle cells have another type of high−energy compound—**phosphocreatine (PCr)**—that enables the cells to produce more ATP quickly under anaerobic

During a brief bout of intense anaerobic exercise, glucose is a major source of energy for working muscles.

Figure 11.8 **PCr.** Muscle cells break down PCr into creatine and inorganic phosphate, releasing energy to form ATP from ADP and P_i (*a*). When the intense activity stops and there is no need to maintain high levels of ATP, an inorganic phosphate group bonds with creatine to recycle PCr (*b*).

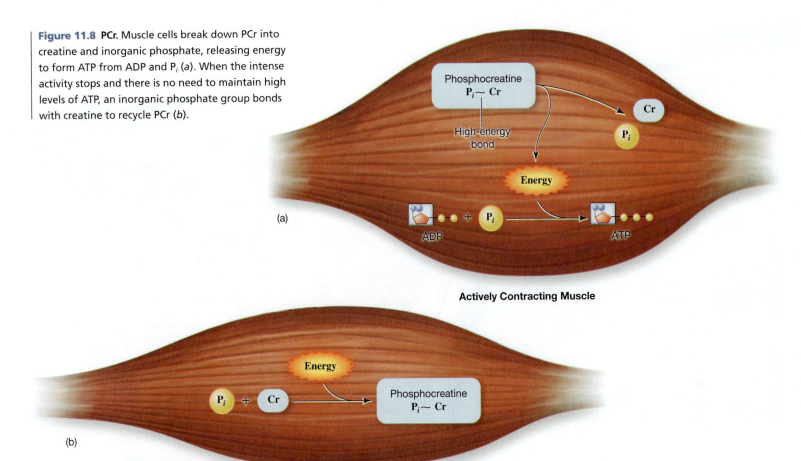

conditions. To make the ATP, cells break down PCr into *creatine* and P_i, releasing energy to form ATP from ADP and P_i (Fig. 11.8a). Cells do not use PCr directly to power their activities; the compound provides the energy to resupply ATP.

By breaking down PCr to form ATP, muscle cells can obtain enough energy to function during intense events lasting only a few seconds.[6] However, the PCr–ATP system can be activated instantly, replenishing ATP fast enough to meet the energy demands of the swiftest and most powerful muscle movements, such as jumping, lifting, throwing, and sprinting. When the intense activity stops and there is no need to maintain high levels of ATP, an inorganic phosphate group bonds with creatine to recycle PCr (see Fig. 11.8b). Muscle cells, however, do not make or store much PCr.

Lactic Acid Energy System

When physical activity lasts longer than a few seconds, the PCr–ATP energy system cannot keep up with the demand for energy, and muscle cells must metabolize glucose to generate more ATP. The immediate source of glucose for working muscles is glycogen that is stored in muscles. The liver also helps supply glucose for muscles by degrading glycogen and releasing glucose molecules into the bloodstream.

In anaerobic conditions, muscle cells metabolize glucose to pyruvate and then convert pyruvate to **lactic acid** (Fig. 11.9.1). The degradation of glucose to lactic acid produces a small amount of ATP—only enough to sustain maximum physical exertion for 30 to 40 seconds.[7] Lactic acid accumulates in muscles and converts

phosphocreatine (PCr) high-energy compound used to reform ATP under anaerobic conditions

lactic acid compound formed from pyruvate during anaerobic metabolism

Figure 11.9 Lactic acid conversion to glucose. This illustration summarizes basic steps in which lactic acid can be converted into glucose.

to a related substance, *lactate*. Although certain muscle cells can use lactate as a fuel, some of the compound enters the bloodstream (Fig. 11.9.2). The liver removes lactate from blood and can convert the compound into glucose (Fig. 11.9.3). The liver may then release the glucose into the bloodstream to help meet muscles' demand for fuel or use the simple sugar to make glycogen (Fig. 11.9.4).

Hydrogen ions (H^+) form as a result of the conversion of lactic acid to lactate. The accumulation of H^+ in muscle tissue contributes to muscle acidity, a condition that can lead to muscle fatigue and declining physical performance.

Oxygen Energy System

You would not be able to enjoy activities such as walking at a fast pace, swimming laps, playing a game of soccer or basketball, or other continuous types of physical activity, if your muscles depended only on the anaerobic energy systems. When muscle cells have plenty of oxygen, such as during low— to moderate— intensity exercise, they can metabolize glucose completely to CO_2 and H_2O. In fact, the availability of oxygen enables cells to produce about 18 times more ATP—energy than the amount produced by anaerobic systems. The ability to

Even well-trained athletes experience muscle fatigue as the time they spend performing intense muscular exertion increases. This marathon runner collapsed as she crossed the finish line of the 28th Annual U.S. Marine Corps Marathon. *Photo: LCPL Richard A. Burkdall, USMC.*

obtain this amount of energy is useful for endurance athletes, because it allows their muscle cells to contract repeatedly for hours. Table 11.1 presents various energy sources for resting and contracting muscles.

Aerobic Capacity   The ability of your heart and lungs (sometimes referred to as the *cardiorespiratory system*) to deliver oxygen to muscles determines your capacity for intense aerobic physical activity. Scientists can use special equip— ment to estimate maximal oxygen intake (*aerobic capacity* or *VO₂max*) during vigorous physical exertion. A simple way to determine if you are nearing your aerobic capacity is to engage in vigorous exercise and note when your breathing rate increases to the point that you cannot carry on a conversation.

You can increase your aerobic exercise capacity by engaging in an endurance training program that gradually increases the intensity level of activities. Such training improves your muscle cells' ability to generate ATP rapidly. However,

Did You Know?

As people grow older, their aerobic capacities decline with each passing decade. By being physically active, however, even elderly persons can maintain a higher degree of aerobic capacity than their sedentary counterparts. It is never too late to begin a training program to improve physical fitness. If you have existing health problems, you should have a complete medical checkup and obtain your physician's OK before beginning a moderate-intensity fitness program. Men older than 40 years and women older than 50 years who plan a vigorous-intensity program should also consult their physician for help designing a safe, effective program.

TABLE 11.1   Energy Sources for Muscles*

Source/System	When in Use	Examples of Activities
ATP	At all times	All types
Phosphocreatine (PCr)	All exercise initially; short bursts of exercise thereafter	Shot put, high jump, bench press
Carbohydrate		
Anaerobic	High-intensity exercise, especially lasting 30 seconds to 2 minutes	200-yard sprint
Aerobic	Exercise lasting 2 minutes to 3 hours or more; the higher the intensity of exercise, the greater the use	Basketball, swimming, jogging
Fat	At rest	Sitting
	Exercise lasting more than a few minutes; low- to moderate-intensity physical activities	30-minute brisk walk
Protein	Low amounts during all exercise, slightly more during endurance exercise, especially when carbohydrate fuel is lacking	Long-distance running

* Note that at any given time, more than one energy system is operating. Adapted from Wardlaw GM, Smith AM: *Contemporary Nutrition.* 7th ed. New York: McGraw-Hill, 2009.

even highly trained athletes experience muscle fatigue after increasing the time they usually spend performing intense muscular exertion.

Fat or Carbohydrate for Fueling Exercise?

The intensity of a physical activity largely influences the relative amounts of fatty acids and glucose that muscles metabolize for energy. Glucose supplies only about 40% of the energy needed to sustain a person who is resting or engaged in very light to light activities, such as watching TV, typing, and walking. Fat is the primary fuel muscles use while resting or engaged in low– to moderate–intensity physical activities.[8] During high–intensity exercise, the rate of fat oxidation decreases while that of glucose oxidation increases. The chart in Figure 11.10 illustrates rough estimates of carbohydrate and fat metabolism during six forms of exercise.

An individual's level of training influences the ratio of glucose to fatty acids that his or her muscles use during exercise. Trained endurance athletes tend to oxidize more fat when exercising at the same intensity than untrained persons.[9] As a result, muscle cells of trained athletes "spare" glycogen; that is, they con– serve their supply of glucose. By sparing their glycogen supplies, athletes can enhance their capacity to exercise longer.

Figure 11.10 Rough estimates of energy use during exercise. The intensity of an exercise largely influences the relative amounts of macronutrients that muscles metabolize for energy.

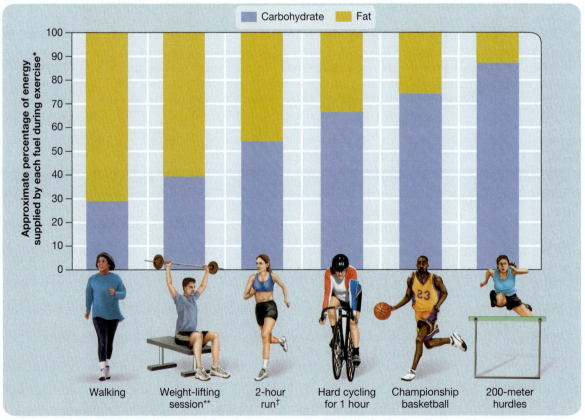

*Protein supplies a minor percentage of energy.
**Fat use generally is higher because much of the time spent weight lifting is for rest periods.
†The values shown are for a runner consuming carbohydrate during the run; more fat and less carbohydrate would be used if carbohydrates were not consumed.

Concept **Checkpoint 11.3**

7. How is glycogen used during exercise?
8. How is ATP formed? How do cells use ATP?
9. Explain how each energy system supplies ATP for muscles. Which energy systems operate under anaerobic conditions?
10. How can you improve your aerobic capacity?
11. When is fat a major source of energy for muscles?

11.4 General Dietary Advice for Athletes

genetic endowment inherited physical characteristics that can affect physical performance

Learning Outcomes

1 Estimate an athlete's energy, protein, and other nutrient needs.

2 Explain the importance of optimal nutrition for athletes.

3 Identify high-carbohydrate/low-fat foods.

4 Discuss heat-related illnesses, including prevention and treatment of these conditions.

Athletes often manipulate their diets to lose or gain weight, increase their muscular strength, and prevent or delay fatigue during exercise. Although an athlete's diet plays a major role in determining if he or she finishes first or last in a competitive event, *genetic endowment* and *physical training* are the most crucial factors that influence athletic performance.[6] **Genetic endowment** refers to inherited physical characteristics that can affect an athlete's physical performance, such as body size, shape, and composition. Regardless of how well an athlete eats, if this person lacks the physical traits that are necessary for success in his or her chosen sport, the athlete will find it difficult to compete effectively. Athletes must also be highly motivated to compete and engage in a well-designed intensive training program to maximize their physical capabilities. Nevertheless, optimizing an athlete's diet may provide a competitive advantage, especially for sporting events in which hundredths of a second can mean the difference between finishing first and finishing second.

Athletes and coaches often believe misinformation concerning the value of dietary supplements, certain foods, and fad diets for optimizing physical health and performance. Such beliefs can lead to diet-related practices that are useless and a waste of money. In some cases, these practices are harmful or even deadly.

Sports nutrition focuses on applying nutrition principles and research findings to improving athletic performance. This section provides specific dietary recommendations that are appropriate for athletes and other physically active people. If you would like additional information on sports nutrition, contact a registered dietitian. Other reliable sources of sports nutrition include websites of the American College of Sports Medicine (www.acsm.org) and *The American Journal of Sports Medicine*. If you are interested in studying sports nutrition, check with your academic advisor to determine whether your college or university offers sports nutrition courses.

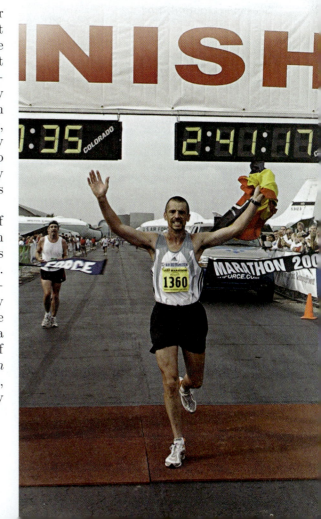

Optimizing an athlete's diet may provide a competitive advantage.

TABLE 11.2 Sample Daily 5000 kcal Menu

5000 kcal
66% carbohydrate
21% fat
13% protein

Breakfast

Fat-free milk, 1 cup

Cheerios, 2 cups

Bran muffins, 2

Orange, 1

Snack

Low-fat plain yogurt, 1 cup

Chopped dates, 1 cup

Lunch

Chicken enchilada, 1

Romaine lettuce, 1 cup

Garbanzo beans, 1 cup

Shredded carrots, ¾ cup

Chopped celery, ½ cup

Seasoned croutons, 1 oz

French dressing, 2 Tbsp

Whole-wheat bread, 2 slices

Soft margarine, 1 Tbsp

Snack

Banana, 1

Bagel, 1

Cream cheese, 1 Tbsp

Dinner

Lean broiled beef, sirloin, 5 oz

Mashed potatoes, 2 cups

Soft margarine, 2 tsp

Spinach egg noodles, 1 ½ cups cooked

Grated parmesan cheese, 2 Tbsp

Green beans, 1 cup

Oatmeal-raisin cookies, 3

Snack

Air-popped popcorn, 2 cups

Raisins, ½ cup

Cranberry juice, 2 cups

Energy for Athletic Performance

Compared to nonathletes, athletes generally need more energy to support their physically active lifestyles. Athletes who do not consume enough food energy can lose muscle mass and bone density, experience fatigue and menstrual problems (females), and be at risk of injury.[10] Thus, low energy intakes can hinder an athlete's chances of performing well.

Male athletes who train or compete aerobically for more than 90 minutes daily need at least 50 kcal/kg/day; their female counterparts need 45 to 50 kcal/kg/day.[11] Thus, athletes may require 3000 kcal/day or more to support their energy needs and maintain their weight. Table 11.2 presents a sample daily menu that is nutritionally adequate, supplies approximately 5000 kcal/day, and provides ample amounts of carbohydrate.

How can athletes tell if they are consuming enough energy? One way is to have them keep accurate food records and use the information to estimate their daily calorie intakes. Athletes can also monitor their body weights and have their skinfold thicknesses measured regularly. If their weights were within the healthy BMI range before training and they start to lose weight during training, the individuals should consume more food until they regain their pretraining weights. Consuming an additional 500 to 700 kcal/day, especially by eating calorie– and nutrient–dense foods such as nuts and dried fruit, is a healthy way for anyone to boost his or her calorie intake. Athletes who gain too much body fat can increase their energy output by spending more time in training. Overfat athletes can also reduce their food intake by about 200 to 500 kcal/day until they are in the healthy body mass index (BMI) range. In general, a good way to reduce energy intake is to limit portions of fatty foods. Chapter 3 provides general information to help you plan nutritious menus.

For most physically active people, fat should supply 20 to 35% of energy, which is within the range recommended for the general population.[12] Trained endurance athletes may adapt to long–term, very–high–fat diets (65% or more of total energy) without harming their performance.[13] Nevertheless, high–fat diets are not recommended for athletes.[6] Furthermore, very–low–fat diets (< 20% of total energy from fat) are not beneficial for athletic performance.[10]

Focusing on Carbohydrate Intake

Recommended diets for athletes should supply adequate amounts of energy from carbohydrates. To maintain adequate muscle glycogen, athletes should consume 6 to 10 g of carbohydrate per kilogram of body weight daily.[10] Glycogen depletion is a major cause of fatigue during endurance exercise. By consuming several servings of grains, starchy vegetables, and fruits daily, an athlete can obtain enough carbohydrate to maintain adequate liver and muscle glycogen stores.

To calculate your recommended range of carbohydrate intake, multiply your weight in kilograms by 6 and then by 10. For example, a 145–pound (66 kg) female athlete should consume between 396 and 660 g of carbohydrate each day. If she requires 3000 kcal/day to maintain her weight and physical activity level and she consumes 60% of her energy from carbohydrates, she will obtain about 450 g of carbohydrate, which is within the recommended range.

It is important to keep in mind that there is no "one size fits all" diet plan that specifies amounts of carbohydrate–rich foods for pre–event, event, or post–event meals and snacks. Diets for athletes should be individualized and based on factors such as the athlete's sex, body size and weight, sport and training level, and exposure to environmental conditions, as well as personal experiences and food preferences. Furthermore, athletes should test any dietary strategies during practices or trials several days or weeks before a competitive event.

TABLE 11.3   High-Carbohydrate, Low-Fat Pre-Event Meals

Meal A	Meal B	Meal C
Instant oatmeal, cinnamon-flavored, 2 packets Fat-free milk, 8 oz	Pasta salad, 1 ½ cups French bread, 4 ounces Soft margarine, 1 Tbsp	Cornflakes, ready-to-eat cereal, 1 ½ cup Fat-free milk, 8 oz Banana, medium
Canned peaches, light syrup, sliced, 1 cup	Apple juice, 8 oz	Orange juice, 8 oz
Orange juice, 8 oz Raisin bread, toasted 2 slices Soft margarine Jelly, 2 Tbsp	Frozen yogurt, 1 cup	English muffin, toasted Soft margarine, 1 Tbsp Jelly, 2 Tbsp Nutty energy bar*

*See this chapter's "Recipe for Healthy Living."

Pre-Event Meals and Snacks

About 3 to 4 hours before competing, athletes should consider eating a meal that supplies 200 to 300 g of carbohydrate, because such meals can improve perfor-mance.[10] Table 11.3 provides some menu ideas for high–carbohydrate, low–fat pre–event meals that supply approximately 200 g of carbohydrate. Eating fatty foods such as sausage, bacon, sauces, and gravies is not recommended because they take longer to empty from the stomach than low–fat foods.[6] Although some nutritionists advise athletes to exclude high–fiber foods from pre–event meals, there is a lack of scientific evidence to support this recommendation. Neverthe-less, athletes can have different responses to eating high–fiber diets prior to events; individuals who react negatively may find it necessary to avoid eating high–fiber foods until after competing.

High–carbohydrate, low–fat food choices for pre–event meals or snacks include cereal with fat–free milk, bagels, dried fruit, pretzels and a sports drink, cooked oatmeal with fruit, pasta, baked potato topped with yogurt, and toasted bread with jelly. Table 11.4 presents commonly eaten foods that are high in

TABLE 11.4   Energy and Macronutrient Contents of Selected Foods

Food and Amount	kcal	Carbohydrate (g)	Protein (g)	Fat (g)
Macaroni, plain, cooked, 1 cup	221	43.20	8.12	1.30
Spaghetti, cooked, 1 cup	220	42.83	8.12	1.30
Rice, instant, white, cooked, 1 cup	194	41.16	4.60	0.58
Egg noodles, cooked, 1 cup	221	40.26	7.26	3.31
Baked potato, ½ large	139	31.62	3.74	0.19
Corn, canned, drained, 1 cup	133	30.49	4.30	1.64
Bagel, ½, 4" diam.	144	28.04	5.51	0.84
Banana, 1 med. (approx. 7" long)	105	26.95	1.29	0.39
Crackers, 6 rectangular saltines	154	25.53	3.32	4.09
Orange juice, unsweetened, 1 cup	110	25.05	1.99	0.69
Cornflakes, 1 cup	101	24.28	1.88	0.03
Pretzels, 1 oz	108	22.61	2.93	0.75

Source: U.S. Department of Agriculture: *USDA national nutrient database for standard Reference, Release 19.* 2006. www.nal.usda.gov/fnic/foodcomp/search/

carbohydrate and relatively low in fat. Food eaten about an hour before compet—ing should be blended or liquid to promote rapid stomach emptying. Examples of such foods are low—fat smoothies or liquid meal—replacement formulas, such as "instant breakfast" products.

What Is Carbohydrate (Glycogen) Loading?

A healthy person stores about 6 g of glycogen per kilogram of body weight. Therefore, an individual who weighs 165 pounds (75 kg) stores about 450 g of glycogen. This amount of glycogen sup—plies 1800 kcal, which is enough energy to enable the person to bicycle at 13 mph for about 4 hours and 15 minutes. Endurance athletes who have more muscle glycogen at the start of an event may be able to exercise longer than those who do not have as much muscle glycogen. **Carbohydrate** or **(glycogen) loading** involves manipulating dietary and physical activity patterns 3 to 7 days before an event to increase muscle glycogen stores well above the normal range. The practice helps delay fatigue in athletes participating in events lasting more than 90 minutes.[14]

About 3 g of water are incorporated into muscle tissue along with each gram of glycogen. Thus, carbohydrate loading adds water to muscles. Although this fluid aids in maintaining proper hydration status, some individuals expe—rience muscle stiffness and unwanted weight gain as a result of carbohydrate loading. Table 11.5 presents the classic 7—day method of carbohydrate load—ing and two modified versions. Athletes who would like to determine whether a carbohydrate—loading regimen helps their performance should try one of the regimens during training to experience its effects. Rather than promote

TABLE 11.5 Carbohydrate Loading: Comparing 7-Day Methods

Day	Classic Method	Modified Method 1	Modified Method 2
1	**Exercise:** Depletion **Diet:** Low carbohydrate	**Exercise:** Depletion **Diet:** High carbohydrate	**Exercise:** Tapering (reduced physical activity) **Diet:** Moderate carbohydrate
2	**Exercise:** Tapering **Diet:** Low carbohydrate	**Exercise:** Tapering followed by supplemental carbohydrate feeding **Diet:** High carbohydrate	**Exercise:** Tapering **Diet:** Moderate carbohydrate
3	**Exercise:** Tapering **Diet:** Low carbohydrate	**Exercise:** Tapering followed by supplemental carbohydrate feeding **Diet:** High carbohydrate	**Exercise:** Tapering **Diet:** Moderate carbohydrate
4	**Exercise:** Tapering **Diet:** Low carbohydrate	**Exercise:** Tapering followed by supplemental carbohydrate feeding **Diet:** Moderate carbohydrate	**Exercise:** Tapering **Diet:** Moderate carbohydrate
5	**Exercise:** Tapering **Diet:** High carbohydrate	**Exercise:** Tapering followed by supplemental carbohydrate feeding **Diet:** Moderate carbohydrate	**Exercise:** Tapering **Diet:** High carbohydrate
6	**Exercise:** Tapering or none (rest) **Diet:** High carbohydrate	**Exercise:** Tapering followed by supplemental carbohydrate feeding **Diet:** Moderate carbohydrate	**Exercise:** Tapering or rest **Diet:** High carbohydrate
7	**Exercise:** Tapering or rest **Diet:** High carbohydrate	**Exercise:** Tapering followed by supplemental carbohydrate feeding **Diet:** Moderate carbohydrate	**Exercise:** Tapering or rest **Diet:** High carbohydrate
8	Competitive event	Competitive event	Competitive event

Sources of data: Goforth HW Jr: Effects of depletion exercise and light training on muscle glycogen supercompensation in men. *American Journal of Physiology, Endocrinology, & Metabolism* 285(6): E1304, 2003; Kreider RB and others: ISSN exercise & sport review: Research & recommendations. *Journal of International Society of Sports Nutrition* 7: 7, 2010. Published online February 2, 2010. doi: 10.1186/1550-2783-7-7; Williams MH and others: *Nutrition for Health, Fitness, & Sport.* 10th ed. New York: McGraw-Hill, 2013.

carbohydrate loading, many nutrition and human performance experts simply recommend that athletes routinely follow a high—carbohydrate diet and consume certain forms of carbohydrate during prolonged exercise.

Consuming Carbohydrate During Events

When athletes exercise vigorously for longer than 60 minutes, their glycogen supplies become depleted. At this point, athletes report they have "hit the wall"; that is, they feel unable to maintain a competitive pace. While performing pro—longed physical activity, athletes can delay reaching "the wall" by consuming 30 to 60 g of carbohydrate per hour of activity.[10]

Sports drinks are a convenient way to obtain a source of glucose during lengthy and vigorous physical activities. Commercially available sports drinks are usually sweetened with nutritive sweeteners such as sucrose, glucose, fructose, or maltodextrin. Such beverages typically provide 15 to 27 g of carbohydrate per 12—ounce serving. Foods or drinks that are concentrated sources of fructose are not recommended, because large amounts of this particular simple sugar may cause gastrointestinal upset. In addition to supplying carbohydrate, sports drinks contain water and electrolytes, such as sodium, that can benefit athletes during prolonged physical effort. Sports gels are also good sources of simple carbohy—drate, but they generally supply very little fluid. Therefore, it is important for athletes who consume these products to drink enough water to maintain proper hydration during endurance events.

Consuming Carbohydrates During Exercise Recovery

After completing exhaustive physical activity, trained athletes can replenish nearly all of their glycogen stores within a few days, provided they rest and eat a high—carbohydrate diet. During a post—event meal, starchy foods such as whole—grain bread, mashed potatoes, rice, and pasta can be served to boost ath—letes' carbohydrate consumption.

Athletes who train intensely each day need to consume 8 to 10 g of carbohydrate/kg of body weight to replenish their muscle glycogen stores.[6] To restore their supply of muscle glycogen quickly after an event, athletes can con—sume sports drinks, candy, sugar—sweetened soft drinks, and fruit or fruit juices.

What About Protein?

One of the most controversial topics in nutrition is the amount of protein needed to support athletic performance. Many athletes are convinced that consum—ing ample amounts of protein from animal foods and taking protein or amino acid supplements are necessary to improve their physical performance and body build. The adult RDA for protein is 0.8 g/kg of body weight.[12] A review of the nutritional practices of elite athletes indicated that individuals training for aerobic sports consumed 1.1 to 3.0 g of protein/kg of body weight per day (g/kg/day), whereas those training for anaerobic sports, such as weight lifting, consumed 1.1 to 3.2 g/kg/day.[11] Are such high—protein intakes recommended or even necessary?

Under normal conditions, carbohydrate and fat are the primary fuels for cellular activity, and protein only a minor percentage of the body's energy needs. Thus, protein is not a major biological fuel. During prolonged physical activ—ity, muscles lose some protein because they metabolize certain amino acids for energy. To spare protein so the nutrient can be used for muscle tissue growth and repair instead of for energy, it is very important for physically active people to consume adequate amounts of carbohydrate and fat.

carbohydrate (glycogen) loading practice of manipulating physical activity and dietary patterns to increase muscle glycogen stores

During a post-event meal, starchy foods, such as pasta, can be served to boost an athlete's carbohydrate consumption.

After strenuous exercise, muscle cells repair damaged muscle tissue by using available amino acids to synthesize new proteins. Thus, having adequate amounts of amino acids in muscle tissue promotes positive nitrogen balance after exercise.[17] After engaging in intense physical activity, athletes may be able to enhance protein synthesis in their muscles by eating protein—rich foods.[6] Compared to nonathletes, however, the typical athlete consumes more food to meet his or her increased energy needs and, as a result, obtains plenty of dietary protein.[10] Therefore, healthy active Americans who eat varied diets that supply adequate energy do not need to take protein or amino acid supplements. If people consume excess protein from foods or supplements and they do not need the energy, the amino acids in these proteins will not be used for building or repairing muscles. Instead, the body converts the extra amino acids into fat for storage in adipose tissue.

Protein: Recommendations for Athletes

Despite conventional wisdom that athletes have higher protein requirements than nonathletes, there are no specific protein RDAs for endurance or resistance athletes. According to the Institute of Medicine, "no additional dietary protein is suggested for healthy adults who undertake resistance or endurance exercise."[12] Nevertheless, the RDA for protein may not apply to athletes involved in training or competition. According to joint recommendations issued by the Academy of Nutrition and Dietetics, Dietitians of Canada, and the American College of Sports Medicine, endurance and resistance athletes should consume 1.2 to 1.4 g of protein/kg of body weight/day and 1.2 to 1.7 g of protein/kg of body weight/day, respectively (Table 11.6).[10] Although these amounts of protein are considerably higher than the RDAs for nonathletes, they do not appear to be harmful for *healthy* physically active people.

Raising the Bar?

"Lasting energy," "fast fuel," "optimal energy"—such claims are used to promote so—called "energy" bars, gels, and drinks. Energy or sports bars are essentially cookies made from soy and milk proteins that are fortified with vitamins, minerals, and fiber. Sugary syrups hold these ingredients together. *High—protein* energy bars may appeal to athletes who think proteins are a source of energy and enhance muscular development. However, proteins are not a major biological fuel, and they are not "quick energy" sources, because the liver must process amino acids before they can be used for energy. Moreover, eating more protein than the body needs does not build muscle tissue. People need to follow a resistance training program to enlarge their skeletal muscles safely.

Granola bars, fruit—filled cookies, and fresh or dried fruits are less expensive and more natural sources of energy and nutrients than energy or sports bars. You can make your own "energy" bars by following the recipe in the "Recipe for Healthy Living" feature. If you prefer to eat commercial energy bars, check the products' Nutrition Facts panels to determine amounts of carbohydrates and other nutrients that are in a serving. By eating several energy bars daily, you may ingest high amounts of iron, vitamin A, and other micronutrients. Therefore, consider energy bars as occasional snacks and not as meal replacements. Table 11.7 presents approximate energy and macronutrient contents per 100 g of various popular energy bars and gels.

Energy drinks usually contain sugars and a lot of **caffeine,** a stimulant drug that is naturally in coffee and tea. When consumed in moderate amounts, caffeine can increase alertness and decrease fatigue. Some energy drinks also contain the amino acid *taurine* and herbal substances such as ginseng. Although the body uses taurine, the compound is not required by humans. Ginseng may enhance the stimulating effects of caffeine.[18] The "Ergogenic Aids: Separating

---

TABLE 11.6 Daily Protein Recommendations

Physical Activity Classification	g Protein/kg of Body Weight/Day
Adult RDA (nonathletes)	0.8
Endurance athlete	1.2 – 1.4
Resistance athlete	
Muscle-building phase	1.6 – 1.7
Maintenance phase	1.2 – 1.4

Adapted from Williams MH and others: *Nutrition for health, fitness, and sport.* 10th ed. New York: McGraw-Hill, 2013.

caffeine naturally occurring stimulant drug

TABLE 11.7 Popular Energy Bars and Gels: Energy and Macronutrient Contents/100 g

Product	Energy kcal/100 g	Carbohydrates g/100 g	Protein g/100 g	Fat g/100 g
PowerBar Performance (cookies & cream)	370	66.2	12.3	4.6
PowerBar ProteinPlus (cookies & cream)	385	48.7	29.5	7.7
PowerBar PowerGel (vanilla)	268	65.9	0	0
Luna Bar (peanut butter cookies)	375	47.9	28.8	12.5
Clif Bar (chocolate chip)	368	66.2	28.8	7.4
Clif Shot (vanilla gel)	312	78.1	0	0
Balance Bar (chocolate)	400	44.0	28.0	12.0
Balance CarbWell (chocolate peanut butter)	400	44.0	28.0	16.0

Sources: Clif Bar & Company, www.clifbar.com/; Luna Bar, www.lunabar.com/index_main.cfm; Balance Bar Food Company, www.balance.com/; Power Bar, www.powerbar.com/

Fact from Fiction" section of this chapter provides more information about caffeine, ginseng, and some other substances that are promoted for enhancing physical performance.

Focusing on Fluids

The Adequate Intake (AI) for total water intake is approximately 11 cups (2.7 L) and 15.5 cups (3.7 L) for young women and men, respectively. Athletes generally require more water than nonathletes to keep their bodies cool during muscular activity. Many factors, however, influence a person's hydration status. Among athletes in particular, differences in sports, fitness levels, and environmental conditions affect fluid needs. For example, sweating can cause runners to lose 3 to 8 cups (750 to 2000 ml) of water per hour.[19] Even a small degree of dehydration can lead to declines in an athlete's endurance, strength, and overall performance. Moreover, body temperature rises when dehydration occurs, increasing the risk of heat–related illness.

Heat-Related Illness

As the environmental temperature and humidity increase, the evaporation of sweat from skin slows, and the body has difficulty cooling itself by perspiring. Ineffective sweating contributes to fatigue, makes the heart work harder, and raises the risk of *heat–related illness*. Table 11.8 presents three major types of heat–related illness and their common signs and symptoms.

Many athletes are familiar with **heat cramps.** These painful muscle *spasms* (involuntary contractions) can affect any muscle, but they usually occur in the back, abdominal, or calf muscles. The cause of heat cramps is unclear, but the spasms may partially result from the loss of electrolytes in sweat.[6] Treatment of heat cramps includes resting, drinking juice or a sports drink, and gently stretching and massaging the affected muscles.[20]

Heat exhaustion can occur after heavy exercise in warm conditions, especially when fluid and salt intakes have been inadequate. A person suffering from heat exhaustion experiences heat cramps, sweats excessively, and feels faint or dizzy.[21] Other signs of the illness include cool, moist, gray–colored skin and rapid, weak pulse. To treat heat exhaustion, move the victim to a cool or shady place and have the person lie on his or her back with legs slightly elevated. Furthermore, cool the person by fanning, spraying with cool water, or giving a cool sponge bath. It is also very important to have the victim drink cool water or a sports drink. People with heat exhaustion should be monitored closely, because the condition can rapidly develop into *heatstroke*.

heat cramps heat-related illness characterized by painful muscle contractions

heat exhaustion heat-related illness that can occur after intense exercise

TABLE 11.8 Heat-Related Illnesses: Signs and Symptoms

Heat cramps

- Painful muscle spasms

Heat exhaustion

- Muscle ("heat") cramps
- Low-grade fever
- Heavy sweating
- Weakness
- Light-headedness or dizziness
- Headache
- Nausea

Heatstroke

- Severe weakness
- High fever (over 104°F)
- Lack of sweating
- Rapid, shallow breathing
- Irritability and confusion
- Coma

heatstroke most dangerous form of heat-related illness

Sports drinks provide some nutritional benefits beyond those of plain water.

Heatstroke is the most dangerous form of heat−related illness. Signs of heatstroke include elevated body temperature (often more than 104°F); lack of sweating; rapid, shallow breathing; irritable and confused behavior; and loss of consciousness (coma).[22] Heatstroke is a medical emergency that needs to be treated by trained medical staff. If you suspect that a person has heatstroke, summon emergency medical assistance immediately (dial 911) and move the victim to a cool environment. While waiting for professional medical care to arrive, you can give the patient cool water to drink (if he or she is conscious) and spray the person with cool water.

Replenishing Fluids

To reduce the risk of heat illnesses, athletes and other physically active people should avoid exercising under extremely hot, humid conditions and should replace fluid losses that occur during prolonged exertion. According to recommendations recently established by the International Marathon Medical Directors Association (IMMDA), thirst protects athletes from consuming too little or too much fluid.[23] Experts with this organization no longer recommend drinking fluids even if you are not thirsty, because this practice can lead to water intoxication (*hyponatremia*). However, athletes should avoid losing more than 2% of their body weight during exercise.[19]

To estimate the amount of fluids needed to replace water loss during exercise (*rehydration*), athletes can weigh themselves prior to exercising and then calculate 2% of their body weight (0.02 × weight). After working out, athletes should weigh themselves again. If the difference between preexercise and postexercise body weights is more than 2%, fluid replacement is necessary during such activities. For example, if you weigh 150 pounds, 2% of that weight is 3 pounds (0.02 × 150). Therefore, you should drink enough watery fluids to avoid losing 3 or more pounds when you train or compete. In general, you can replace each pound that you lose during exercise by drinking 1 ¼ to 1 ½ pints (2 ½ to 3 cups) of water.[6] For example, if your usual weight is 150 pounds and you weigh 149 pounds immediately after exercising, you have lost 1 pound of body water during the activity. The next time you exercise under similar conditions, you can consume 3 cups of water during the activity to maintain your body's water balance. Why do you need to drink more fluids than you have lost in sweat? After exercise, rehydration may stimulate the kidneys to produce more urine than normal; thus, you need to drink the extra watery fluids to achieve proper hydration. As noted in Chapter 9, alcoholic beverages have a diuretic effect on the body and are not recommended for rehydration.

Do I Need a Sports Drink? Sports drinks provide some nutritional benefits beyond those of plain water. These beverages usually contain simple carbohydrates, a source of energy that can enhance performance during endurance activities. Recommended products contain about 21 g of carbohydrate per 12−ounce serving, or about 6% carbohydrate by weight. Drinks with sugar contents above 10%, such as soft drinks or fruit juices, are not recommended because they may cause intestinal discomfort. Sodium and other electrolytes in sports beverages help maintain blood volume, enhance the absorption of water and carbohydrate from the intestinal tract, and stimulate thirst.

Should you drink water or a sports drink during competition? According to the Association of International Marathons and Road Races (IMMDA), sports drinks are necessary when workouts or events last longer than 30 minutes.[23] Although electrolytes are lost in sweat, the quantities lost in shorter periods can be easily replaced by consuming foods and beverages, such as water or fruit juice, after the event.

It is possible to drink too much water and develop water intoxication (see Chapter 9). Endurance athletes, especially poorly trained individuals, may compete at relatively low exercise intensities for prolonged periods. Under these conditions, the athletes do not sweat as much; therefore, they do not need to replace as much water as better–trained athletes who exercise at higher intensities. Regardless of training level, athletes who drink too much water can dilute the level of sodium in their blood and develop serious and even deadly side effects. Although sports drinks generally contain sodium, these beverages are mostly water; therefore, consuming excessive amounts of sports drinks can contribute to fluid overload. To avoid water intoxication, athletes should drink water according to their thirst. If an athlete gains weight while exercising, he or she may be retaining too much fluid.

Antioxidant Vitamins

During aerobic physical activities, skeletal muscles use more oxygen and generate more free radicals than resting muscle tissue.[24] Exercise can produce a temporary imbalance between free radical generation and the ability of antioxidants to counteract them. Scientific evidence suggests that such *oxidative stress* may contribute to muscle fatigue and damage. Nevertheless, results of studies that examined whether antioxidant vitamin supplements enhanced athletic performance generally concluded that performance was not improved, unless there was a preexisting deficiency of those particular vitamins.

Findings of some scientific studies indicate that free radicals generated during intense exercise may stimulate the body's natural antioxidant defense system. Thus, the oxidative stress produced during exercise might have benefits, and blocking this process by taking antioxidant vitamin supplements may not be desirable.[24,25]

Antioxidant vitamin supplements are not recommended for athletes.[24] Athletes should be cautious about taking such supplements based on anecdotes or advertising claims, because there is not enough scientific evidence concerning the long–term effects of using these products. Rather than experiment on themselves with antioxidant supplements, athletes should follow diets that contain foods naturally rich in antioxidants, such as fruits, vegetables, whole–grain breads and cereals, and vegetable oils.

Iron

The body needs iron to produce red blood cells, transport oxygen, and obtain energy. Thus, iron deficiency can negatively affect athletic performance. Young female athletes are likely to develop iron deficiency because of their menstrual blood losses: Bleeding is a cause of iron deficiency. Athletes who follow low-calorie or vegetarian (especially vegan) diets are also at risk of iron deficiency, because their food choices may be low in iron. Additionally, distance runners may develop low iron status, because intense prolonged workouts can lead to gastrointestinal bleeding.

In the early phase of their training, endurance athletes often develop *sports anemia*, a temporary condition that results from an increase in the liquid portion of blood (*plasma*), rather than iron deficiency.[6] The effects of sports anemia on physical performance are unknown. Nevertheless, it can be difficult to differentiate between sports anemia and true iron deficiency anemia. It is a good idea for athletes, especially females, to have their iron status checked at the beginning of a training season and at least once during midseason. If an athlete is iron deficient, a physician needs to determine the cause and prescribe treatment.

Intense exercise may stimulate the body's natural antioxidant defense system.

Calcium

Athletes, especially those who are total vegetarians or restrict their consumption of dairy products to lose weight, can have marginal or low calcium intakes. This practice may result in weak bones that fracture easily, as well as in osteoporosis later in life. Additionally, female athletes who have irregular or no menstrual cycles may be deficient in the hormone estrogen. Although weight—bearing exercise, such as jogging, improves bone density, estrogen is also necessary for maintaining healthy bones. Female athletes who develop menstrual cycle abnormalities should consult a physician to determine the cause. Decreasing the amount of training or gaining weight may restore a regular menstrual pattern. For information about the *female athlete triad*, see the Chapter 10 "Nutrition Matters"; Chapter 9 provides information about osteoporosis.

Concept **Checkpoint 11.4**

12. What are some practical ways to assess whether an athlete's energy intake is adequate?
13. Why should athletes be concerned about their carbohydrate intakes before, during, and after prolonged intense physical activity?
14. Identify at least five high-carbohydrate/low-fat foods.
15. Explain why athletes do not need to take protein or amino acid supplements.
16. Why should athletes be concerned about their bodies' fluid status?
17. What are major signs and symptoms of heat cramps, heat exhaustion, and heatstroke?
18. When is consuming a sports drink a better choice than plain water for rehydration?
19. Explain why you would or would not recommend that an athlete take antioxidant supplements.
20. Explain why iron deficiency can impair an athlete's physical performance.
21. For young female athletes, what is the significance of having irregular or no menstrual cycles for bone health?

11.5 Ergogenic Aids: Separating Fact from Fiction

Learning Outcomes

1 Discuss the pros and cons of using amino acid supplements and other ergogenic aids for athletic performance.

2 Identify three ergogenic aids that have been banned by at least one athletic association.

3 Identify rich sources of caffeine, and discuss the effects that the substance can have on the body.

ergogenic aids foods, devices, dietary supplements, or drugs used to improve physical performance

Athletes often use **ergogenic aids**—foods, devices, dietary supplements, and even drugs ("doping")—to improve their physical performance. Bee pollen, dried adrenal glands from cattle, seaweed, freeze—dried liver flakes, and ginseng are among the dietary supplements that athletes consume as they hope to gain the competitive edge over their rivals. However, no reliable scientific evidence sup-ports the effectiveness of most dietary supplements purported to have ergo-genic effects. Nevertheless, many athletes firmly believe in the value of the performance–enhancing aids that they use. In many instances, the perceived benefits are more likely to result from the placebo effect than from actual physi-ological changes (see Chapter 2).

A few dietary substances and practices can enhance physical performance. These ergogenic aids include sufficient water and electrolytes, carbohydrates, and a balanced and varied diet consistent with MyPlate recommendations. For ath-letes, meeting carbohydrate and fluid needs—along with overall nutrient needs—is the most important ergogenic aid.

Athletes should be skeptical of claims made for any substance until its ergogenic effects and long–term safety have been determined by researchers who are not associated with the supplement industry. Rather than searching for a "magic bullet" to enhance their performance, athletes should concentrate their efforts on improving their dietary habits, training routines, and sports tech-niques. Nutrient supplements should be used for specific dietary deficiencies, such as preventing iron deficiency or boosting calcium intakes.

Table 11.9 summarizes science–based findings regarding caffeine, creatine, and some other dietary supplements and ergogenic aids that are popular among athletes. It is important to note that certain dietary supplements are known to be unsafe, and the use of others is restricted or banned by major athletic orga-nizations. For example, in 2004, the U.S. Food and Drug Administration (FDA) banned the use of ephedrine–containing supplements. Ephedrine (ephedra, ma huang) increases central nervous system activity, but the drug can cause serious, even deadly side effects. The following section discusses the ergogenic properties of caffeine.

Caffeine

Worldwide, caffeine is the most widely used ergogenic aid. Caffeine raises the level of fatty acids in blood, and as a result, exercising muscles can use more fat for energy. Caffeine also enhances the ability of skeletal and heart muscles to contract and increases mental alertness. Although consuming even small amounts of caffeine may help endurance athletes, the National Collegiate Athletic Asso-ciation limits the amount of caffeine that athletes can have in their bodies during competition. Athletes who have more than 15 micrograms of caffeine per mil-liliter (mcg/ml) of their urine can be banned.[26] Nevertheless, the World Anti-Doping Agency does not prohibit the use of caffeine.[27]

People who are not regular caffeine consumers may experience shaki-ness, rapid heart rate, sleep disturbances, diarrhea, and frequent urination after ingesting relatively high amounts of the stimulant drug. Caffeine is addictive; discontinuing its use results in *withdrawal*, temporary unpleasant side effects, especially headache.

It is important to understand that the quick "energy" boost provided by "energy drinks" is a result of caffeine or other stimulants contained in the prod-ucts. Nevertheless, energy drinks also provide calories if they are sweetened with added sugars. Table 11.10 compares the caffeine and calorie contents of popular beverages, including an energy drink (e.g., "Red Bull®"). "Stay awake" pills and chewing gums are concentrated sources of caffeine that can be purchased without a prescription. In July 2014, the FDA warned consumers to avoid "powdered" caffeine. At that time, the agency was aware of one death that was attributed to use of the product.[28]

Caffeine raises the level of fatty acids in blood, and as a result, exercising muscles can use more fat for energy.

TABLE 11.9 Evaluation of Some Popular Ergogenic Supplements/Aids

Substance	Claim	Current Evidence-Based Findings Concerning Claims	Side Effects
Anabolic steroids	Increase muscle mass and strength	Increase protein synthesis In the United States, legal use requires a physician's prescription.	Side effects include blood liver cysts; increased risk of cardiovascular disease, hypertension, and reproductive problems; mood swings and aggressive behavior ("roid rage"); sleep disturbances. Banned by many sports organizations
Bee pollen	Shortens muscle recovery time Increases muscular strength and endurance	No benefit	May cause allergic reactions in sensitive persons
Beta-hydroxy-beta-methylbutyrate (HMB)	Decreases protein metabolism, increasing muscle mass	May increase muscle mass, but evidence is weak	None reported, but results of long-term use are unknown
Branched-chain amino acids	Provide energy for muscles	May enhance muscle recovery after intense physical activity	None reported
Caffeine	Enhances fat metabolism Delays depletion of muscle glycogen Increases alertness	Consuming 3 to 6 mg of caffeine/kg of body weight about 1 hour before exercise can benefit certain athletes.	High doses can cause nervousness, shakiness, and sleep disturbances Intakes of more than 600 mg (6 to 8 cups of coffee) can produce levels of caffeine in urine that are banned by the National Collegiate Athletic Association.
Chromium picolinate	Increases lean mass	No benefit	Toxic reactions reported
Creatine	Enhances muscular endurance and strength Increases lean muscle mass	May enhance performance of sprinters and weight lifters	High doses may cause kidney damage, especially in persons with kidney disease
DHEA and androstenedione ("andro")	Increases the body's steroid production	No benefit	May be dangerous Banned by the International Olympic Committee In 2004, the FDA warned companies to stop manufacturing products that contain "andro".
Energy drinks	Increase alertness and focus Enhance anaerobic and endurance performance Increase fat metabolism	Results vary based on the composition of the energy drink Some energy drinks may enhance the performance of athletes and promote a small amount of fat loss	See "Caffeine." Elevated heart rate and blood pressure Increased likelihood of engaging in risky behaviors
Gamma hydroxybutyric acid (GHB)	Increases muscle mass by acting like an anabolic steroid	Illegal: FDA has not approved GHB for production or sale in the United States	Vomiting, dizziness, shakiness, and seizures May cause death
Ginseng	Combats fatigue and improves stamina	May have mild stimulant effects	Adverse effects on the immune system Headache, nausea, and sleep disturbances
Glucosamine	Aids in repairing damaged joints	Mixed results, but generally no beneficial results	None reported
Human growth hormone	Increases muscle mass and fat metabolism	Most studies indicate no benefit	May increase height as well as the size of the heart and other internal organs Very dangerous, can be deadly International Olympic Committee bans the use of growth hormone
Sodium bicarbonate (baking soda)	Reduces lactic accumulation	May enhance performance, particularly in exercises that rely primarily on the lactic energy system (e.g., 400-meter sprint)	May cause nausea, vomiting, and diarrhea

Sources: American Dietetic Association: Position of the American Dietetic Association, Dietitians of Canada, and the American College of Sports Medicine—Nutrition and athletic performance. *Journal of the American Dietetic Association* 109:509, 2009; Campbell B and others: International Society of Sports Nutrition position stand: Energy drinks. *Journal of the International Society of Sports Nutrition* 10:1, 2013; Higgins JP and others: Energy beverages: Content and safety. *Mayo Clinic Proceedings* 85:1033, 2010; Williams MH and others: *Nutrition for health, fitness, and sport.* 10th ed. New York: McGraw-Hill, 2013.

TABLE 11.10 Caffeine Content of Selected Beverages

Beverage and Amount	Energy (kcal)	Caffeine (mg)
Chocolate drink, 8 oz	120	2
Coffee, Starbucks Dark Roast, 16 oz*	5	330
Coffee, brewed from grounds, unsweetened, 8 oz	2	95
Coffee, instant plain, prepared, 8 oz	5	62
Cola with caffeine, 12-oz can	136–151	29–99
5-Hour energy shot®, original, 2-oz bottle**	4	215
Monster® energy drink, 8-oz can**	100	92
Mountain Dew®, 20-oz bottle***	290	91
Red Bull®, 8.3-oz can	115	76
Rockstar energy shot, 2.5-oz bottle**	10	229
Tea, brewed, unsweetened, 8 oz	2	47
Tea, ready-to-drink, 12-oz can	89	11

Sources

*Starbucks Beverages: *Nutrition information.* www.starbucks.com Accessed July 24, 2014;

**Consumer Reports:* The buzz on energy drink caffeine. December 2012. http://www.consumerreports.org/cro/magazine/2012/12/the-buzz-on-energy-drink-caffeine/index.htm Accessed July 24, 2014;

***Pepsico: *Brands: Pepsi-Cola.* www.pepsicobeveragefacts.com Accessed July 24, 2014; U.S. Department of Agriculture: *USDA national nutrient database for standard reference, Release 26.* 2013.

Concept **Checkpoint 11.5**

22. Why do many athletes use ergogenic aids?

23. Identify three ergogenic aids that have been banned by at least one athletic association.

24. Identify at least three beverages that are rich sources of caffeine.

25. Discuss the ergogenic effects that caffeine can have on the body.

11.6 Nutrition Matters: Developing a Personal Fitness Plan

Learning Outcomes

1 Identify the key components of an aerobic workout regimen.

2 Design a personal fitness program that suits your interests and lifestyle.

When developing your personal physical fitness plan, first consider your fitness goals. For example, if you want to lose weight, how much do you want to lose and how many weeks will it take to lose that amount? Do you want to focus more on strengthening your muscles or on improving your aerobic capacity? Then determine when you can work out and whether you'll need to join a fitness facility such as a gym or purchase special equipment, such as hand-held weights. For a comprehensive fitness program, make sure to include aerobic, resistance, and stretching activities in your weekly exercise regimen. The following fitness plan has three stages: initial, improvement, and maintenance phases.

Initiation

The first 3 to 6 weeks of your new exercise program is the *initiation* stage. Start by incorporating short periods of physical activity into your daily routine. For example, you can walk more often, take the stairs instead of the elevator, and do more housework, gardening, or other activities that cause you to "huff and puff" a bit. Furthermore, you can strive to reduce the time that you spend in sedentary activities.

The goal is to accumulate a total of 150 minutes of moderate−intensity types of activity each week. If necessary, the time that you spend engaging in the activity each day can occur in three short intervals lasting at least 10 minutes. If you do not have 150 minutes to spend on exercising, try increasing the intensity of the activities during shorter bouts of exercise to obtain some health benefits.

Improvement and Maintenance

The next 5 or 6 months of the program is the *improvement* stage, in which you increase the intensity and duration of exercises. When you begin the improvement phase, exercise at an intensity that is near the lower end of your target heart rate zone. As you progress and become more physically fit, you can increase the intensity by exercising at a higher heart rate.

By the end of the improvement stage, you may notice that you have reached your goals, and you do not seem to be making further gains in your fitness. This plateau marks the beginning of your *maintenance* stage. At this point, you can evaluate your personal fitness plan, and if you would like to make new goals, this is the time to develop them. If you are satisfied with your fitness level, continue with your present program. Discontinuing exercise gradually results in *detraining*, declining physical fitness.

Components of an Aerobic Workout Regimen

Ideally, you should establish a regular time for exercising that fits into your daily routine. To be effective, your aerobic workout program needs to include the following components:

1. **Warm−up** Warming up muscles can increase your joints' range of motion (flexibility) and may decrease your risk of injury. Stretching for 5 to 10 minutes is a good way to warm up. Start with smaller muscle groups such as the arms and progressively work toward stretching larger muscle groups in the legs and abdomen. Hold your position in the stretch for 15 seconds and do not bounce. If stretching causes pain, stop immediately. "No pain, no gain" is not true: Pain is an indication of injury. Another way to warm up is to perform 5 to 10 minutes of the anticipated activity but at a low intensity. For example, if you walk for fitness, warm up by walking at a slower pace.

2. **Aerobic workout** To obtain substantial health benefits, you should engage in some form of aerobic activity regularly. A comprehensive aerobic workout emphasizes the *type*, *duration*, *frequency*, *intensity*, and *progression* of exercise.

   - **Type:** The kinds of exercise you choose should increase your heart and breathing rates and involve rhythmic movements of large muscle groups in the legs. Examples include brisk walking, running, swimming, and cycling. If you swim, add some *weight−bearing activities*, such as walking, to your comprehensive fitness plan. Weight−bearing exercises place stress on your bones, increasing their strength.

   - **Duration:** Duration is the amount of time spent in an exercise session. A session should generally last at least 20 to 30 minutes, depending on intensity, not including time spent warming up and cooling down. Ideally, the exercise session should be continuous (without stopping), but multiple 10−minute bouts of moderate to intense activity with rest periods in between are also acceptable.

   - **Frequency:** The frequency of exercise describes the number of times that the activity is performed, generally on a weekly basis. To derive significant health benefits, the frequency of aerobic exercise should be at least five times per week. By exercising daily, you can enjoy even greater benefits.

   - **Intensity:** Health benefits can occur when you achieve at least a moderate level of intensity during exercise.

   - **Progression:** Progression, the final component of a comprehensive fitness plan, refers to the gradual increase in the frequency, intensity, and duration of exercise that occurs over a period.

3. **Cool—down** To cool down, you can repeat the same stretches you performed during warming up. Stretch for 5 to 10 minutes. Cooling down may prevent injury and reduce muscle soreness.

What About Strength (Resistance) Training?

Strength training, such as weight lifting, is an important part of a comprehensive physical fitness plan. Strength training should be done at least 2 days per week. To start, warm up by stretching for 5 to 10 minutes. Then perform a group of 8 to 10 exercises that strengthen major muscle groups of the upper body and lower body. Cool down for 5 to 10 minutes at the end of each session.

Fitness centers have machines that provide resistance for various muscle groups. For resistance training outside of gymnasiums or fitness clubs, you can purchase simple elastic exercise cords designed to increase muscular strength (Fig. 11.11). For increasing upper arm strength, a set of inexpensive handheld weights can be kept in a convenient location for performing resistance exercise regularly, such as near the TV. The weights should allow you to perform at least one set of 8 to 15 repetitions. When you can do more than 15 repetitions with relative ease, consider increasing the weight slightly.

Mixing It Up

To make your exercise routine more enjoyable, include several types of physical activity in your weekly regimen. For example, jogging one day might be followed by

Figure 11.11 **Increasing muscle strength.** This individual is using a simple rubber exercise cord to increase muscular strength.

swimming the next day. Adding variety to a program not only keeps you from becoming bored with your workouts but also strengthens different muscle groups in your body and reduces your risk of injury. Additionally, invite a friend or relative to be your exercise partner. Having an exercise partner may provide additional motivation and encouragement to exercise regularly.

Some overfat people do not experience significant weight loss while following an exercise regimen. However, they still benefit from regular physical activity. Initially, exercise programs for obese people should emphasize non—weight—bearing activities, such as swimming, water aerobics, and bicycling. As obese people lose weight and become more fit, they can add weight—bearing activities to their plans.

Whatever physical activities you choose to include in your fitness program, they should be enjoyable and easy to incorporate into your routine. You can apply the dietary principles of variety, balance, and moderation to your exercise routine:

- **Variety:** Perform several different activities to exercise different muscle groups.
- **Balance:** For overall fitness, balance your exercise regimen by including activities that build cardiovascular endurance, muscular strength, and flexibility.
- **Moderation:** Focus on exercising to keep fit without overdoing it and injuring yourself. You do not need to work out vigorously every day to become healthier.

To learn more about the health benefits of physical fitness, determine your level of fitness, or develop a personal fitness program, access the following websites:

www.shapeup.org
www.fitness.gov
www.presidentschallenge.org

Concept **Checkpoint 11.6**

26. List three key components of an aerobic workout regimen.
27. Develop a personal fitness regimen that you can follow for the rest of your life.

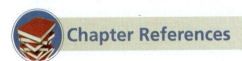 **Chapter References**

See Appendix H.

Summary

11.1 Introduction to Nutrition for Fitness and Sport

- Many Americans lead sedentary lives. People can manage their weight more effectively and reduce their risk of developing the major causes of death and disability by engaging in at least 30 minutes of moderate-intensity physical activity on five days of the week. Furthermore, most people can achieve even greater health benefits by increasing the duration, frequency, and intensity of their physical activities.

11.2 Benefits of Regular Exercise

- Regular physical activity reduces the risk of dying prematurely and developing heart disease, diabetes, and high blood pressure. Additionally, regular exercise builds and maintains healthy bones, muscles, and joints; helps reduce blood pressure in people who have high blood pressure; reduces the risk of developing certain cancers; aids weight-control efforts; helps older adults become stronger and reduces their risk of falls; reduces risk of sleep disorders, depression, and anxiety; and promotes psychological well-being. Millions of Americans suffer from chronic illnesses that can be prevented or improved by exercising more often.

11.3 Energy for Muscular Work

- ATP is the major form of energy used by cells. Phosphocreatine (PCr) can rapidly reform ATP from its breakdown product ADP, but PCr supplies are limited. To generate ATP, muscle cells can metabolize carbohydrate, fat, and protein. In muscle cells, glucose molecules are broken down through a series of steps to yield lactic acid (in anaerobic conditions) or CO_2 plus H_2O (in aerobic conditions).

- The proportions of macronutrients used for energy largely depend on the intensity of the physical activity. Fat is a key aerobic fuel for muscle cells, especially at low-intensity exercise. At rest and during light activity, muscles burn primarily fat for energy needs. In comparison, little protein generally is used to fuel muscles. During brief bouts of intense physical effort, the cardiorespiratory system is unable to deliver adequate oxygen to muscles. Under such anaerobic conditions, muscle cells metabolize glucose rather than fat for energy, but their ability to sustain the release of energy for intense activity is limited. Muscle cells can obtain far more energy when in aerobic conditions.

11.4 General Dietary Advice for Athletes

- Sports nutrition focuses on applying nutrition principles and research findings to improving athletic performance. Athletes often manipulate their diets to enhance their body contours, increase their muscular strength, and prevent or delay fatigue during exercise. Although diet is important, genetic endowment and physical training are the most crucial factors that influence athletic performance.

- A high-carbohydrate diet can be beneficial for athletes, and carbohydrate-rich foods should form the foundation of pre-event meals. Many athletes consume more protein than they require. Despite marketing claims, protein supplements are unnecessary. By eating their usual food choices, most athletes can meet their protein needs.

- Physically active people need to be concerned about their fluid intakes. Fluid replacement should be based on thirst and loss of body weight while exercising. Consuming a source of electrolytes, such as a sports drink, can be helpful, especially when the duration of intense exercise exceeds 30 minutes. It is important to avoid overconsumption of water because of the risk of water intoxication.

11.5 Ergogenic Aids: Separating Fact from Fiction

- Athletes often ingest certain substances, including herbal products, because they believe these substances have ergogenic effects. Scientific evidence, however, does not suggest that most of these substances are effective. Furthermore, long-term safety of many ergogenic aids has not been determined, and use of some substances is restricted or banned by various athletic organizations.

11.6 Nutrition Matters: Developing a Personal Fitness Plan

- The three components of an aerobic workout are warming up, performing the moderate or vigorous intensity activity, and cooling down.

Recipe for Healthy Living

Nutty Energy Bars

You can use the following recipe to make your own "energy bars." This recipe makes eight 4-by-2-inch bars. Each bar supplies approximately 253 kcal, 8 g protein, 13 g fat, 26 g carbohydrate, 3 g fiber, and 4.9 mg iron.

INGREDIENTS:

Oil cooking spray
1 egg, large
1 ½ cups instant oats, dry
¼ cup almonds, slivered
¼ cup enriched wheat flour
½ cup smooth peanut butter
1 Tbsp vegetable oil
½ cup honey
½ tsp ground cinnamon
1 tsp vanilla

ChooseMyPlate.gov

Fat
Protein
Carbohydrate

PREPARATION STEPS:

1. Preheat oven to 350°. Spray "nonstick" oil on the inside bottom and sides of an 8" × 8" pan.

2. Crack open the egg, drop the egg's contents into a medium-size bowl, and discard the shell. Using a fork, beat the egg until its yolk is completely mixed with the egg white.

3. Add remaining ingredients to the egg and stir until well blended. Mixture will be thick, like cookie dough. Using a large spoon, press dough into the bottom of the pan, covering the inside of the pan evenly.

4. Bake for 12 to 14 minutes. Cool completely before cutting into eight 4-by-2-inch bars.

*2000 daily total kcal

Further analyze this and other recipes through activities on Connect at www.mcgrawhillconnect.com.

Critical Thinking

1. Analyze your weekly physical activity habits. Does your participation in various physical activities meet the minimum recommendations? If not, which physical activities are you willing to include in your weekly routine to improve your fitness level?

2. Calculate your target heart rate zone for moderate–intensity as well as vigorous–intensity activities.

3. Why do human cells rely far more on glucose and fat for energy than on protein?

4. What advice would you give a runner concerning fluid intake before and during a marathon?

5. One of your friends is a student athlete who uses gin–seng, bee pollen, and glucosamine to enhance his physical performance. What would you tell your friend concerning the pros and cons of taking these substances?

Practice Test

Select the best answer.

1. Miranda is physically fit. She has
   a. an increased risk of osteoporosis.
   b. the strength, endurance, and flexibility to meet the demands of daily living.
   c. a greater need for vitamins and minerals than other women.
   d. no need to exercise regularly.

2. During glycolysis, the body
   a. converts two fatty acid molecules into one glucose molecule.
   b. synthesizes one amino acid molecule from one carbon dioxide molecule and two oxygen molecules.
   c. breaks down one glucose molecule to form two pyruvate molecules.
   d. metabolizes fatty acids into carbon monoxide and peroxide.

3. A _____ physical activity generally requires a high degree of exertion.
   a. vigorous   c. moderate
   b. basic   d. precise

4. Aerobic activities
   a. enable muscles to use less oxygen than normal.
   b. do not require voluntary muscular contractions.
   c. force muscle cells to use more vitamins and minerals for energy.
   d. involve sustained, rhythmic contractions of certain large skeletal muscles.

5. Which of the following statements is true?
   a. Resistance exercises do not help build bone mass.
   b. Sedentary activities do not require much energy to perform.
   c. Anaerobic energy systems need large quantities of oxygen to produce ATP.
   d. All of the above are correct.

6. Amy is studying quietly. Under these conditions, her muscles are using primarily _____ for energy.
   a. fat   c. amino acids
   b. glucose   d. ketone bodies

7. Carbohydrate loading
   a. provides a competitive edge for award–winning sprinters, bodybuilders, and weight lifters.
   b. involves manipulating dietary patterns and physical activities prior to an endurance event.
   c. often results in short–term weight loss and positive energy balance.
   d. is generally recommended for long–term weight control for athletes.

8. Which of the following foods is high carbohydrate and low fat?
   a. roast chicken
   b. Swiss cheese
   c. peanut butter
   d. toast spread with strawberry jam

9. Caffeine

   a. is the most widely used ergogenic aid in the world.
   b. reduces the level of fatty acids in blood.
   c. is nonaddictive.
   d. decreases mental alertness.

10. Human cells release much of the energy stored in car—bohydrates, fats, and amino acids as

   a. electricity.   c. ATP.
   b. phosphocreatine. d. heat.

11. To obtain energy under aerobic conditions, cells need

   a. ribose.   c. methionine.
   b. oxygen.   d. alanine.

12. _____ is an immediate and direct source of energy for cells.

   a. LDP   c. ATP
   b. Glycogen d. Phospholipid

Answers to Quiz Yourself

1. People who exercise regularly can reduce their risk of type 2 diabetes. **True.** (p. 426)

2. Sports drinks are not useful for fluid replacement. **False.** (p. 444)

3. Protein is the body's preferred fuel for muscular activity. **False.** (p. 441)

4. Heatstroke is a serious illness that requires immediate professional medical treatment. **True.** (p. 444)

5. While at rest, skeletal muscles metabolize more glucose than fat for energy. **False.** (p. 436)

LEARNSMART®
ADVANTAGE

Get the most out of your study of nutrition with McGraw-Hill's innovative suite of adaptive learning products including McGraw-Hill LearnSmart®, SmartBook®, LearnSmart Achieve®, and LearnSmart Prep®. Visit www.learnsmartadvantage.com.

CHAPTER 12

Food Safety Concerns

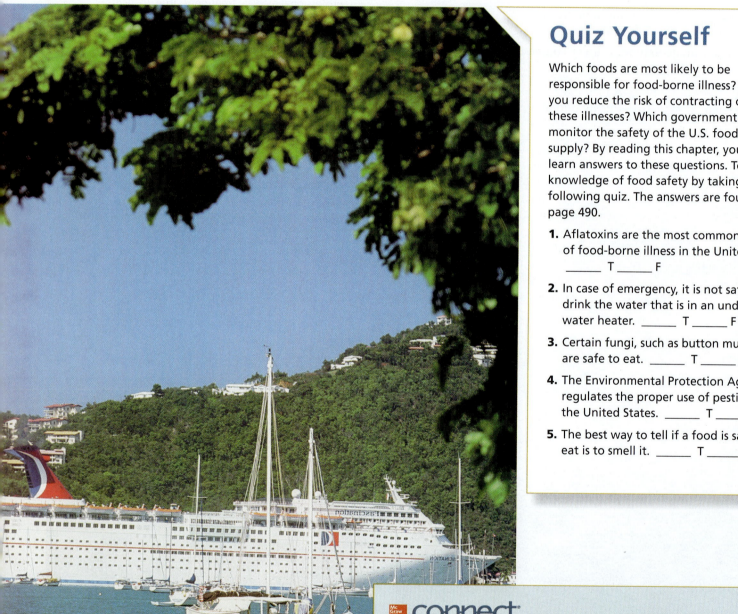

Quiz Yourself

Which foods are most likely to be responsible for food-borne illness? How can you reduce the risk of contracting one of these illnesses? Which government agencies monitor the safety of the U.S. food supply? By reading this chapter, you will learn answers to these questions. Test your knowledge of food safety by taking the following quiz. The answers are found on page 490.

1. Aflatoxins are the most common sources of food-borne illness in the United States. _____ T _____ F

2. In case of emergency, it is not safe to drink the water that is in an undamaged water heater. _____ T _____ F

3. Certain fungi, such as button mushrooms, are safe to eat. _____ T _____ F

4. The Environmental Protection Agency regulates the proper use of pesticides in the United States. _____ T _____ F

5. The best way to tell if a food is safe to eat is to smell it. _____ T _____ F

12.1 Introduction to Food Safety

Learning Outcomes

1 Identify the most common cause of food-borne disease outbreaks in the United States.

2 Explain the difference between a food-borne infection and a food-borne intoxication.

Most Americans look forward to taking vacations, and for many people, this involves boarding a cruise ship to visit tropical, Caribbean island destinations such as Montego Bay, the Bahamas, or Grand Cayman. The attractions of a cruise vacation include enjoyable activities for people of all ages, as well as dining opportunities that showcase plenty of delicious food. Every year, however, some people's dream vacation becomes a cruising nightmare, as hundreds of guests and crew members become miserably ill with stomach pain, diarrhea, and vomiting as a result of *norovirus* infection. In the United States, norovirus is the most common cause of **food—borne illness** outbreaks.[1]

People who are infected with norovirus will have the virus in their vomit and feces. If people with the infection do not wash their hands thoroughly after vomiting or having bowel movements, they can spread the infection to others by handling food or ice cubes, shaking hands, or touching objects that other people touch. The infection spreads rapidly among people who are living in close quarters, such as persons on a cruise ship. To control the spread of the infection, sick passengers should be isolated from healthy people, and bathrooms, guest rooms, and any surface that may have been touched by ill persons should be disinfected with a strong bleach solution.[2]

Pathogens

Disease—causing microbes, such as norovirus, are referred to as **pathogens.** When pathogens are in food, they can make the item unsafe to eat. Many kinds of food—borne pathogens infect the digestive tract, inflaming the tissues and causing an "upset stomach" within a few hours after being ingested. A few types of food—borne pathogens multiply in the human intestinal tract, enter the bloodstream, and cause general illness when they invade other tissues. Such illnesses are called **food—borne infections.** Other pathogens do not sicken humans directly, but these microbes contaminate food and secrete poisons (toxins). When the contaminated food is eaten, the toxins irritate the intestinal tract and cause a type of food—borne illness called **food intoxication** (or food poisoning).

Food—borne illnesses spread through the ingestion of food or beverages are common, debilitating, and sometimes life—threatening diseases for millions of people around the world. Each year, an estimated 48 million Americans become sick from various food—borne illnesses.[3] Of those persons who contract such ailments, 128,000 require hospitalization and 3000 die. There are more than 250 food—borne illnesses; preventing these diseases is a major U.S. public health objective.

food-borne illness disorder that is caused by consuming disease-causing agents in food or water

pathogens disease-causing microbes

food-borne infection illness that results when a pathogen in food inflames the intestinal tract or other body tissues

food intoxication illness that results when poisons produced by certain microbes contaminate food and irritate the intestinal tract

In the United States, water–borne disease–causing microbes are not major health threats, because of basic waste water and potable (drinkable) water treat–ment systems. Therefore, this chapter focuses primarily on food–borne illness, including common sources of these infections in the United States. Additionally, this chapter presents safe food handling practices.

Concept **Checkpoint 12.1**

1. Which microbe is responsible for most cases of food-borne illness in the United States?
2. Is the illness caused by norovirus the result of a food-borne infection or food intoxication?

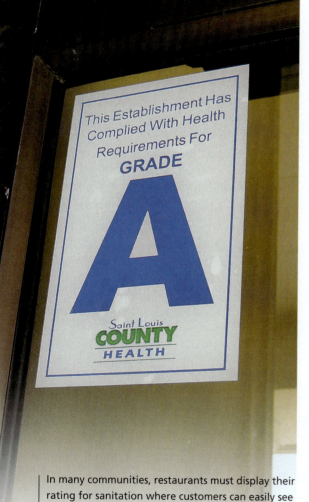

In many communities, restaurants must display their rating for sanitation where customers can easily see it. Local health departments can close restaurants that do not receive high enough ratings and not allow them to reopen until food safety hazards have been corrected.

12.2 Protecting Our Food

Learning Outcomes

1 Identify government agencies that are responsible for ensuring the safety of the food supply in the United States.

2 Discuss the roles of the FDA, FSIS, and EPA.

The United States has one of the safest food supplies in the world, primarily the result of a team effort conducted by cooperating federal, state, and local agencies that regulate and monitor the production and dis–tribution of food. The Food and Drug Administration (FDA) of the U.S. Department of Health and Human Services and the U.S. Department of Agriculture (USDA) are the key federal agencies that protect consumers by regulating the country's food indus–try. Other team members include the Environmental Protection Agency (EPA), the CDC, the Federal Trade Commission (FTC), and state and local governments.

To help protect our food supply, the FDA performs many important tasks, such as regulating nearly all domestic and imported food sold in inter–state commerce and enforcing federal food safety laws. Additionally, the FDA establishes standards for safe food manufacturing practices, such as Hazard Analysis and Critical Control Point (HACCP) programs. HACCP is a science–based, systematic approach to preventing food–borne illness by predicting which hazards are most likely to occur in a food production facility. When a hazard is identified, food manufacturers can then take appropriate measures to prevent the illness. If necessary, FDA officials can take certain enforcement actions, such as requesting that a food manufacturer recall an unsafe item, so that it is removed from store shelves. Another important function of the FDA is educating the general public about safe food handling practices.

Although the FDA oversees the safety of most foods, the USDA's Food Safety and Inspection Service (FSIS) enforces food safety laws for domestic and imported meat and poultry products. FSIS staff inspect beef, poultry, and other food animals for diseases before and after slaughter, and the agency also ensures that meat and poultry processing plants meet federal standards. Additionally, FSIS staff collect and analyze food samples to check for the presence of microbial and other unwanted and potentially harmful material in foods. If a food hazard is identified, FSIS officials can ask meat and poultry processors to recall their unsafe products. Additionally, food safety experts with FSIS conduct programs to educate people about proper food handling practices. For more information, visit the FSIS website at http://www.fsis.usda.gov/wps/portal/fsis/home.

The EPA oversees the quality of our drinking water. EPA staff establish safe drinking water standards and assist state officials in their efforts to moni-tor water quality. Furthermore, EPA staff regulate toxic substances and wastes to prevent their entry into foods and the environment.

State and local officials work with the FDA and other federal agency staff to implement national food safety standards for foods produced and sold within their state's borders. Local health departments, for example, are responsible for inspecting restaurants, grocery stores, dairy farms, and local food processing companies. In many communities, restaurants are required to post their sani-tation rating where customers can easily see it. Local health departments can close restaurants that do not receive high enough ratings and prevent them from reopening until food safety hazards have been corrected.

After you obtain foods and bring them into your home, it becomes your responsibility to reduce the risk of food–borne illness by handling the items properly. However, if you suspect that something you consumed made you or a family member very sick, you should contact your physician for treatment. The physician may decide to report the case of food–borne illness to local public health officials, so they can investigate and determine the source of your infection.

Concept Checkpoint 12.2

3. Discuss the roles of the FDA, FSIS, and EPA in protecting the U.S. food supply.
4. How do local health departments protect consumers from food-borne illness?

12.3 Microbes in Food

Learning Outcomes

1 Discuss ways that pathogens can contaminate human foods.

2 Explain how cross-contamination of food occurs.

3 Discuss the purpose of pasteurization.

4 Discuss conditions that favor the survival and multiplication of food-borne pathogens.

5 Identify foods that are high risk for supporting pathogens.

For thousands of years, people have used certain microbes to produce a variety of foods, including hard cheeses, raised breads, and alcoholic beverages. When microorganisms metabolize nutrients in food, they often secrete substances that

Wine production relies on the use of certain kinds of microbes.

parasite organism that lives in or on another organism, often deriving nourishment from its host

contaminated food item that is impure or unsafe for human consumption

cross-contamination unintentional transfer of pathogenic microbes from one food to another

pasteurization process that kills the pathogens in foods and beverages as well as many microbes responsible for spoilage

alter the color, texture, taste, and other characteristics of the food in beneficial and desirable ways. Other kinds of microbes grow and multiply in food, but their metabolic byproducts spoil the food, making it unfit for human consumption.

Some microorganisms are parasites. A **parasite** needs to live on or within a "host" organism to survive. Parasites often obtain their nourishment from the host's tissues, so the host's health suffers as a result of a parasitic infection.

A **contaminated food** (or beverage) is no longer wholesome—pure or safe for human consumption. Contamination generally occurs when something that may or may not be harmful enters food or beverages unintentionally. Such contaminants include pathogens, insect parts, residues of compounds used to kill insects that destroy food crops, and metal fragments from food processing equipment. The following section discusses how pathogens can contaminate our food.

Sources of Pathogens

The microbes that cause food−borne illness can live practically anywhere—in air, water, soil, sewage, and on various surfaces. Our skin, nasal passages, and large intestines have vast colonies of various kinds of microbes, some of which can be pathogenic. Animals, including cats, dogs, reptiles, cattle, and poultry, can also harbor harmful microbes on and in their bodies, especially in their intestinal tracts. Because pathogens are found throughout your environment, there are numerous ways that the microbes can contaminate your food. To reduce your risk of food−borne illness, you need to be aware of how pathogens can enter foods. The "Preventing Food−Borne Illness" section of this chapter discusses specific steps you can take to reduce the chances of contracting or spreading food−borne illness.

Common Routes for Transmitting Pathogens

One common route for transmitting harmful microbes involves *vermin*, animals that often live around sewage or garbage, such as flies, cockroaches, mice, and rats. When vermin land on or crawl across filth, they pick up pathogens on their feet. When the vermin come in contact with food, they can transfer the pathogens to humans. To reduce your risk of food−borne illness, keep flies, cockroaches, and other vermin away from your food.

Poor personal hygiene practices frequently transfer microbes to food. People can contaminate their hands with pathogens when they come in contact with feces, such as while using the toilet or changing a baby's soiled diaper. Furthermore, animals harbor pathogens in their feces as well as on their skin and fur. If children prepare or eat foods after stroking animals at petting zoos or playing with pets, they can transmit these microbes to themselves or others. Thus, it is important for people to wash their hands before preparing or eating foods. Children (and many adults) often need to be reminded to wash their hands.

Improper food handling frequently results in food−borne illness. A common practice is failing to wash cutting boards and food preparation utensils after they come in contact with raw meat or poultry. The contaminated boards and utensils are then used to prepare other foods. As a result of this practice, **cross−contamination** is likely to occur, because the pathogens in one food are trans−ferred to another food, contaminating it. If that food is eaten raw, such as carrots in a salad, it carries a high risk of food−borne illness. Failing to cook foods properly can also increase the likelihood of food−borne illness. **Pasteurization** is a special heating process used by many commercial food producers to kill

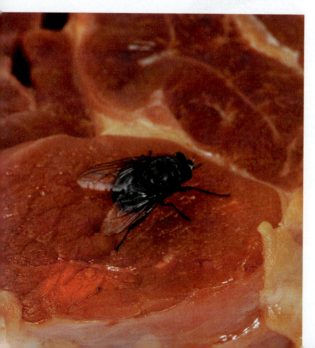

To reduce your risk of food-borne illness, keep flies, cockroaches, and other vermin away from your food.

pathogens. In the United States, for example, most juices and milk have been pasteurized before they are marketed. The "Food Preservation" section of this chapter discusses other ways of preserving foods.

High-Risk Foods

Not all foods are likely to harbor pathogens. To survive and multiply, most microbes need warmth, moisture, and a source of nutrients, and some also require oxygen. In general, high—risk foods are warm, moist, and protein—rich, and they have a neutral or slightly acidic pH. Many of the foods we eat every day, such as meats, eggs, milk, and products made from milk, fit this description. Table 12.1 presents some high—risk foods and the primary food—borne pathogens they may contain.

People who touch turtles or other potential *Salmonella* carriers should wash their hands thoroughly after handling the animals.

TABLE 12.1 Some High-Risk Foods and Their Primary Pathogens

Raw or Undercooked Animal Food	Typical Menu Item	Common Pathogens
Beef	Rare hamburger	*Salmonella* species *E. coli* O157:H7
Pork	Undercooked pork (rarely in the United States)	*Trichinella*
Poultry	Chicken, turkey, duck	*Salmonella* species *Campylobacter jejuni*
Eggs	Salad dressings or sauces made with raw eggs, cream-filled desserts or toppings made with raw eggs	*Salmonella enteritidis*
Fresh produce	Tomatoes, peppers, cantaloupes, lettuce, spinach, sprouts	*Salmonella* species *E. coli* O157:H7
Raw fish/finfish	Sushi; lightly cooked fish	*Anisakis*
Shellfish	Oysters	*Vibrio vulnificus*
	Clams	*Vibrio* species Hepatitis A virus *Norovirus*
Milk and milk products	Raw or unpasteurized milk, some soft cheeses such as Camembert and Brie	*Listeria monocytogenes* *Salmonella* species *Campylobacter jejuni*, *E. coli* O157:H7 *Brucella* species

Source of data: Food and Drug Administration: *Bad bug book,* 2nd ed. 2012. http://www.fda.gov/Food/FoodborneIllnessContaminants/CausesOfIllnessBadBugBook/default.htm Accessed February 5, 2014

Concept **Checkpoint 12.3**

5. Discuss at least three ways pathogens can contaminate human foods.
6. With regard to food preparation, what is cross-contamination?
7. What is pasteurization?
8. List at least three conditions that favor the survival and multiplication of food-borne pathogens.
9. Identify at least four foods that are high risk for supporting pathogens.

12.4 Food-Borne Illness

Learning Outcomes

1 Describe typical signs and symptoms of food-borne illness.

2 Explain when a person who has a food-borne illness should seek professional medical help.

3 Explain why it is incorrect to call a food-borne illness the "flu" or "stomach flu."

Did You Know?

Honey, even commercially processed brands of the sweetener, should not be fed to infants because it may contain *Clostridium botulinum* spores. The spores can grow in an infant's intestinal tract, produce toxin, and cause botulism (see Chapter 5). Older children and adults can consume honey safely, because their digestive systems prevent the spores from growing.

Signs and symptoms of food–borne (and water–borne) illnesses generally involve the digestive tract and include nausea, vomiting, diarrhea, and intestinal cramps. However, most pathogens have an *incubation period*, a length of time in which they grow and multiply in food or the digestive tract before they can cause illness. Thus, if you develop signs and symptoms of a food–borne illness, you might have difficulty identifying the source of the infection or intoxication. Was the vomiting and diarrhea that you experienced at 3 A.M. the result of eating soft–cooked eggs for breakfast 18 hours earlier or the sliced deli chicken you ate for lunch 2 days ago?

Various factors influence whether an individual becomes ill after consuming a food or beverage that has been contaminated with a pathogen or toxin. The number of pathogenic microbes in a food or the amount of toxin it contains can contribute to the risk and severity of a food–borne illness. Furthermore, individuals vary in their vulnerability to many food–borne pathogens. In general, high–risk groups are pregnant women, very young children, older adults and persons who suffer from serious chronic illnesses or weakened immune systems.

In most cases, otherwise healthy individuals who suffer from common types of food–borne illness recover completely and without professional medical care within a few days. However, vomiting, diarrhea, and other signs of illness can be so severe, the patient requires hospitalization. You should consult a physician when an intestinal disorder is accompanied by one or more of the following signs: fever (oral temperature above 101.5°F), bloody bowel movements, prolonged vomiting that reduces fluid intake, diarrhea that lasts more than 3 days, or dehydration.[4]

Many people mistakenly report that they have the "stomach *flu*," when they actually are suffering from a food– or water–borne illness. "Flu," or *influenza*, is an infectious disease caused by specific viruses that invade the respiratory tract. Influenza is characterized by coughing, fever, weakness, and body aches. On the other hand, food–borne illness primarily affects the digestive system and not the respiratory system. Intestinal cramps, diarrhea, and vomiting are *not* typical signs and symptoms of influenza, and coughing is not a usual sign of a food–borne illness. Thus, it is inaccurate to call a bout of diarrhea and intestinal cramps the "flu" or the "stomach flu."

Concept **Checkpoint 12.4**

10. Identify at least three typical signs and symptoms of food-borne illness.
11. When should a person suffering from a food-borne illness seek professional medical help?
12. Discuss the differences between a food-borne illness and the "flu."

12.5 Common Food-Borne Pathogens

Learning Outcomes

1 Identify common pathogens that are sources of food-borne illness in the United States.

2 Discuss typical signs, symptoms, and incubation periods of food-borne illnesses that are caused by each major pathogen.

3 Identify high-risk foods that are often sources of pathogens or their toxins.

Improperly cooked or handled beef, poultry, eggs, and foods made with eggs are common sources of *Staphylococcus aureus*.

The major kinds of pathogens are bacteria, viruses, protozoans, and fungi. In the United States, *bacteria* and *viruses* are responsible for most cases of food−borne illness. The following sections take a closer look at some of the major pathogens that can cause food−borne illness.

Bacteria

Bacteria are single−cell microorganisms that do not have the complex array of organelles that plant and animal cells contain. Some bacteria can live without oxygen, such as in canned or vacuum−packed foods. Other types of bacteria transform into inactive resistant forms called *spores* when living conditions are less than ideal. If the environment becomes more hospitable, the spores revert to the active bacterial state.

Many kinds of bacteria are pathogens that cause food−borne illness, includ−ing forms of *Campylobacter, Clostridium, Escherichia, Listeria, Salmonella* and *Staphylococcus* (*kam′−pih−low−bak′−ter, kloss−trid′−ee−um, esh′−er−ee′−she−ah, liss−tear′−ee−ah, sal′−mo−nell−ah, staff′−il−lo−cawk′−kiss*). Some types of pathogenic bacteria do not cause infections when they are con−sumed in food, but these microbes produce toxins that cause food intoxication. Table 12.2 summarizes some general information about common bacterial sources of food−borne illness in the United States.

bacteria simple single-celled microorganisms

virus microbe consisting of a piece of genetic material coated with protein

Viruses

Viruses are another common source of food−borne infection (Table 12.3). A **virus** is simply a piece of genetic material coated with protein (Fig. 12.1). Viruses must invade a living cell to produce more viruses. Unlike certain bacteria, viruses do not secrete toxins, and therefore, they do not cause food intoxication. Con−taminated food or water, however, can transmit viruses to humans and cause food infection.

Vaccines that protect against hepatitis A virus and rotaviral infections are available. A vaccine to prevent norovirus infections is in development.

| **Figure 12.1** Norovirus.

TABLE 12.2 Common Sources of Food-Borne Illness: Bacteria

Bacterium	High-Risk Foods	Approx. Time of Onset	Typical Signs and Symptoms
Bacillus cereus (toxin)	Starchy foods (rice, potatoes, puddings, some soups)	6–15 hours	Abdominal cramps, watery diarrhea, nausea
Campylobacter jejuni	Raw, undercooked poultry; raw milk; contaminated water	2–5 days	Diarrhea (sometimes bloody), abdominal cramping, vomiting, fever
Clostridium botulinum (toxin)	Vacuum-packed foods, improperly canned foods, low-acid foods. Honey may contain spores.	18–36 hours	Vomiting, diarrhea, blurry or double vision, difficulty swallowing, muscular weakness. Can be fatal
Clostridium perfringens (toxin)	Cooked meat, poultry, casseroles, gravies	8–16 hours	Watery diarrhea (may be bloody), mild abdominal cramps
Escherichia coli O157:H7 (toxin)	Raw ground beef, raw seed sprouts, raw leafy greens, fresh fruit, raw milk, unpasteurized juices, foods contaminated with feces	3–4 days	Intestinal cramps, bloody diarrhea, kidney failure. Can be fatal
Listeria monocytogenes	Raw meat and poultry, raw milk, fresh soft cheese made from raw milk, liver paté, smoked seafood, deli meats, hot dogs, raw vegetables	Few hours to 3 days; 3 months for invasive disease	Fever, muscular aches, vomiting, diarrhea. In pregnant women, the infection can lead to stillbirth (birth of a dead fetus) or premature birth. Can be fatal
Salmonella species	Meat poultry, seafood, and eggs; raw seed sprouts; raw vegetables; unpasteurized juice	6 hours to 3 days	Nausea, vomiting, fever, headache, abdominal cramps, diarrhea. Infection can be fatal in infants, older adults, and people with a weak immune system.
Shigella species	Unclean water; raw vegetables, herbs, and other foods that were contaminated with feces as a result of poor food handling and personal hygiene practices	8–50 hours	Abdominal cramps, fever, diarrhea that may contain blood and mucus. Can be fatal in infants, older adults, and people with a weak immune system
Staphylococcus aureus (toxin)	Meat and meat products, poultry, and eggs; foods made with eggs, such as potato, egg, macaroni, and tuna salads; custards, and cream-filled pastries. Cooked foods are often contaminated as a result of improper food handling practices.	1–7 hours	Diarrhea, nausea, vomiting, abdominal cramps
Vibrio vulnificus	Raw oysters, clams, crabs and other raw or under-cooked seafood; unclean water	12 hours to 3 weeks	Fever, vomiting, diarrhea, abdominal cramps. Can be fatal
Yersinia enterocolitica	Raw vegetables, undercooked pork, contaminated water, unpasteurized milk, oysters	1 day to 2 weeks	Diarrhea, high fever, abdominal pain, vomiting (in some cases)

Source of data: Food and Drug Administration: *Bad bug book,* 2nd ed. 2012. http://www.fda.gov/Food/FoodborneIllnessContaminants/CausesOfIllnessBadBugBook/default.htm Accessed February 5, 2014

TABLE 12.3 Common Sources of Food-Borne Illness: Viruses

Virus	High-Risk Foods	Approx. Time of Onset	Typical Signs and Symptoms
Norovirus	Food or water that has been contaminated with infected feces Virus can be spread person to person	12 hours to 2 days	"Explosive" vomiting; watery, nonbloody diarrhea; abdominal cramps; nausea; low-grade fever (occasionally)
Rotavirus	Food, water, or objects that have been contaminated with infected feces	2 days	Fever, abdominal pain, vomiting, watery diarrhea
Hepatitis A (HAV)	Food or water that has been contaminated with HAV from feces	2 to 4 weeks	Fever, loss of appetite, nausea, vomiting, diarrhea, muscle aches, general weakness May have signs of liver inflammation, such as jaundice, liver enlargement, and dark-colored urine Most people recover after a few weeks, but in rare cases, the illness is deadly.

Source of data: Food and Drug Administration: *Bad bug book,* 2nd ed. 2012. http://www.fda.gov/Food/FoodborneIllnessContaminants/CausesOfIllnessBadBugBook/default.htm Accessed February 5, 2014

Protozoans and Parasitic Worms

Giardia (*jee—ar'—de—ah*) and *Cryptosporidium* (*krip'—toe—spo—rid'—ee—um*) are **protozoans** (*pro—toe—zoe'—ans*), single—celled microorganisms that have a more complex cell structure than bacteria. Table 12.4 lists some protozoans that often cause food—borne and water—borne illnesses in the United States. The "Nutrition Matters" section discusses traveler's diarrhea, which frequently results from a protozoan infection.

Certain types of worms such as *Trichinella* (*trick'—ah—nell'—ah*) and *Anisakis* (*ah'—ni—sa'—kis*) are food—borne pathogens. (Fig. 12.2). Most Americans who become infected with parasitic worms that are found in the United States recover when they receive proper treatment. Nevertheless, some infected persons suffer long—term health problems and even die as a result of the illnesses. Table 12.4 provides information about the kinds of parasitic worms that can infect people.

Fungi

Fungi such as molds, yeast, and mushrooms are simple life forms that live on dead or decaying organic matter. Certain fungi, such as button mushrooms and the mold in blue cheese, are beneficial and edible. Other fungi are responsible for spoiling foods, such as bread molds, or causing respiratory problems or allergic reactions in sensitive people.[5] A serious concern is the toxicity of several varieties of wild mushrooms. Cases of severe illness and death have been reported as a result of people picking and eating toxic wild mushrooms after mistaking them for edible varieties (Fig. 12.3). Nevertheless, fungi are not a major source of food—borne illness in the United States.

Certain molds produce *aflatoxins*, substances that can cause severe illness, particularly liver damage, and even death when consumed. Tree nuts, peanuts, and corn that are stored under warm, humid conditions can become sources of aflatoxins. In some regions of the world, especially Africa and Southeast Asia, people often eat foods that are contaminated with aflatoxin—producing molds. Rates of liver cancer are high in these places. Thus, medical researchers think there is an association between exposure to aflatoxins and development of liver cancer. No outbreaks of food—borne intoxication caused by aflatoxins have been reported among the U.S. population.[6]

| Figure 12.2 *Anisakis.*

protozoans single-celled microorganisms that have complex cell structures

fungi simple organisms that live on dead or decaying organic matter

Figure 12.3 Deadly mushrooms. Severe illness and even death can occur if people pick and eat toxic mushrooms, such as this *Amanita* mushroom.

| Giardia

TABLE 12.4 Common Sources of Food-Borne Illness: Protozoans and Parasitic Worms

Pathogen	High-Risk Foods	Approx. Time of Onset	Typical Signs and Symptoms
Protozoans			
Cryptosporidium	Foods prepared by people whose hands were contaminated with infected feces; fresh juices, produce, and milk	7–10 days	Profuse, watery diarrhea; abdominal pain; fever; nausea; vomiting
Giardia	Consumption of contaminated water, including water from lakes, streams, swimming pools High-risk groups include travelers to certain countries Hikers, and people who swim in or camp by lakes and streams.	1–2 weeks	Diarrhea, abdominal pain, weight loss
Toxoplasma	Raw or partially cooked wild game (especially bear and wild pig), clams, oysters Accidentally ingesting infected cat feces	5–23 days	Fever, headache, muscle aches, rash Pregnant women should avoid contact with cat feces, because the parasite can infect their unborn offspring, causing eye or brain damage and even fetal death.
Parasitic Worms			
Trichinella	Raw or undercooked infected meat, especially pork, bear, seal, and walrus meat	1 to 4 weeks	Nausea; vomiting; diarrhea; fatigue; fever; abdominal discomfort; facial swelling, especially around the eyes; muscle pain Death can occur in severe cases.
Anisakis	Raw or undercooked infected seafood	1 day to 2 weeks	Abdominal pain, nausea, vomiting, diarrhea

Source of data: Food and Drug Administration: *Bad bug book,* 2nd ed. 2012. http://www.fda.gov/Food/FoodborneIllnessContaminants/CausesOfIllnessBadBugBook/default.htm Accessed February 5, 2014

| Certain fungi, such as button mushrooms and the mold in blue cheese, are beneficial and edible.

12.6 Preventing Food-Borne Illness

Learning Outcomes

1 Explain how to reduce the risk of food-borne illness when purchasing, preparing, cooking, and storing foods and beverages.

2 Explain why ground meat and poultry often are sources of food-borne illness.

3 Identify the temperature range that encourages rapid multiplication of pathogens.

4 Discuss the federal government's simple actions for reducing the risk of food-borne illness.

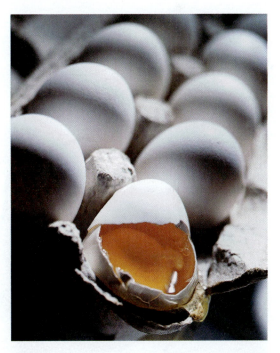

Before purchasing eggs, open the carton and check the eggs. Do not buy cartons that have any cracked eggs.

In many instances, you cannot control the safety of foods that are prepared in restaurants or other places outside your home. However, you can greatly reduce your risk of food—borne illness by following some important rules, most of which require changing risky food selection, preparation, and storage practices.

Purchasing Food

The following tips can help reduce your risk of food—borne illness:

- When shopping in a supermarket, select frozen foods and highly perishable foods, such as meat, poultry, or fish, last.

- Check "best by" dates on packaged perishable foods. Choose meats and other animal products with the latest dates.

- Do not buy food in damaged containers; for example, avoid containers that leak, bulge, or are severely dented, or jars that are cracked or have loose or bulging lids.

- Open egg cartons and examine eggs; do not buy cartons that have cracked eggs.

- Purchase only pasteurized milk, cheese, and fruit and vegetable juices (check the label).

- Pack meat, fish, and poultry in separate plastic bags, so their drippings do not contaminate each other and your other groceries.

- After shopping for food, take groceries home immediately. Refrigerate or freeze meat, fish, egg, and dairy products promptly.

- Store whole eggs in their cartons, even if your refrigerator has a place for storing eggs. Egg cartons are designed to keep eggs fresh longer than a refrigerator's egg compartment.

Setting the Stage for Food Preparation

Contaminated hands and food preparation surfaces spread pathogens. The following tips can help reduce the risk of food–borne illness:

- Wash hands thoroughly with very warm, soapy water for at least 20 seconds before and after touching food. If clean water for handwashing is not available, use sanitizing hand wipes.

- Before preparing food, clean food preparation surfaces, including kitchen counters, cutting boards, dishes, knives, and other food preparation equipment with hot, soapy water. You can kill most pathogens when you clean and *sanitize* food preparation surfaces with a solution made by adding a tablespoon of bleach to 1 gallon of water.

- The FDA recommends cutting boards with unmarred surfaces made of easy–to–clean, nonporous materials, such as plastic, marble, or glass. If you prefer to use wooden cutting boards, make sure they are made of a nonabsorbent hardwood, such as oak or maple, and have no obvious seams or cracks.

- Replace cutting boards when they become streaked with cuts, because these grooves can be difficult to clean thoroughly and may harbor bacteria.

- If possible, have a cutting board reserved for meats, fish, and poultry; have another cutting board for fruits and vegetables; and have a third board for breads. Clean all cutting boards in the dishwasher or with hot, soapy water. You can also sanitize cutting boards with a dilute bleach solution.

Wash hands thoroughly with hot, soapy water for at least 20 seconds before and after touching food.

- Sanitize food preparation surfaces and equipment that have come in contact with raw meat, fish, poultry, and eggs as soon as possible to destroy pathogens that may be present. In addition, sanitize damp kitchen sponges by heating them in a microwave oven for 60 seconds and machine—wash and —dry kitchen towels frequently.

Preparing Food

The following tips can help reduce your risk of food—borne illness:

- Do not use foods from containers that leak, bulge, or are severely dented or from jars that are cracked or have loose or bulging lids.

- Do not use foods from containers that have damaged safety seals, because the food they contain may have been contaminated.

- Do not taste or use food that spurts liquid or has a bad odor when the can is opened.

- Read product labels to determine whether foods need to be refrigerated after their packages are opened.

- Before preparing fresh produce, carefully wash the foods under running water to remove dirt and bacteria clinging to the surface. Bacteria can be sticky, so scrub the peel with a vegetable brush if it is to be eaten. Even if you plan to remove the skin or peel, wash the produce before you cut it.

- Avoid eating moldy foods. Mold does not grow well on low—moisture foods. Thus, small amounts of mold on hard cheeses and on firm fruits and vegetables can be removed by cutting away the mold along with at least 1 inch of food that surrounds the moldy area.[5]

- **When in doubt, throw the food out.**

Wash produce in water before eating or preparing it.

Maintaining the Proper Temperature of Foods

Most microbes grow well when the temperature of a high—risk food is between 40°F and 140°F—the "danger zone" (Fig. 12.4).[7] Cooking foods to the proper tem—perature destroys food—borne viruses and bacteria, such as *Norovirus* and *E. coli* O157:H7. To be safe, a product must be cooked to an internal temperature that is high enough to destroy harmful pathogens and bacterial toxins. Using a meat thermometer is a reliable way to ensure that meat, poultry, thick pieces of fish, and egg—containing dishes have reached the proper internal temperature without overcooking. Table 12.5 indicates recommended minimum internal temperatures for cooking these foods.

Meat thermometers must be used properly. In general, the thermometer should be placed in the thickest part of the muscle tissue, away from bone, fat, or gristle (Fig. 12.5). If the thermometer is inserted incorrectly or placed in the wrong area, the reading may not accurately reflect the internal temperature of the product.

Microwave cooking can result in uneven heating that does not destroy microbes in the cool spots. While cooking a food in a microwave oven, keep the dish covered, and stop the oven occasionally to stir the food. Stirring the food reduces uneven heating. Cook the food until it reaches 165°F. Microwave cooking is not recommended for stuffed foods, because during cooking, the temperature of the stuffing may not be high enough to kill pathogens.[8]

Chilling food slows the growth of microbes in the items, but some bacte—ria can grow even at proper refrigeration temperatures. Freezing does not kill

Figure 12.4 Temperature guide for food safety. Most pathogenic microbes grow well when the temperature of risky food is between 40°F and 140°F—the "danger zone."

| Figure 12.5 **Use of a meat thermometer.**

TABLE 12.5 USDA Recommended Safe Minimum Internal Temperatures

Food	Safe Minimum Internal Temperature (°F)
Beef steaks and roasts	145
Fish	145
Pork	145
Ground beef, pork, lamb, and veal	160
Egg dishes	160
Poultry products	165

Source: U.S. Department of Agriculture, Safe minimum cooking temperature. http://www.foodsafety.gov/keep/charts/mintemp.html

bacteria or inactive viruses in food; the process just halts the microbes' ability to multiply. As frozen food thaws, the bacteria and viruses resume their activities and can cause illness.

A major challenge for food handlers involves keeping large amounts of high–risk foods at safe temperatures when they are served from a single container. Food that is near the sides of the container may stay hotter or colder than food that is near or in the center of the container. As shown in Figure 12.6, chilled foods should be kept covered and served from a shallow container filled with ice. Hot foods should be kept covered and be served from shallow, heated pans. The best simple advice to follow: "Keep hot foods hot and cold foods cold."

The following tips can help reduce your risk of food–borne illness:

- Always thaw high–risk foods in the refrigerator, under cold running water, or in a microwave oven.

- Cook foods immediately after thawing.

- Marinate food in the refrigerator, and if marinating meat, fish, or poultry, discard the marinade.

- Do not remove cold foods from the refrigerator or hot foods from the stove until it is time to serve them.

Raw Fish

Eating raw fish, such as sushi, can be safe for most healthy people if the fish is very fresh before being commercially frozen and then thawed. While frozen, the fish must maintain an internal temperature of 10°F for 7 days. The freezing step is important because very cold temperatures can kill parasites that are often in fish tissues. If you choose to eat uncooked fish, purchase it from reputable establishments that have high standards for quality and sanitation. Nevertheless, it is prudent to not eat any raw animal products, including fish.

Ground Meats, Poultry, and Fish

Ground meats, poultry, and fish are highly perishable and must be thoroughly cooked to avoid being a source of food–borne illness. The interior portion of an intact piece of raw animal flesh is free of bacteria, because the tissues are not exposed to air. However, ground meats, fish, and poultry products are often contaminated with microbes. Prior to being ground up, the surface of a chunk of

Did You Know?

Have you heard about the "5-second rule"? Supposedly, food that drops on the floor will not pick up microbes if it is picked up within 5 seconds. A study determined that this is a food-related myth. As soon as food touches a contaminated surface such as a floor, microbes adhere to it.[9]

Figure 12.6 Keep cold foods cold. Chilled foods, especially picnic items, should be kept covered, in a shallow container, and placed in another container that is filled with ice.

Eating raw fish, such as some forms of sushi, can be safe for most healthy people if the fish is very fresh before being commercially frozen and then thawed.

meat, fish, or poultry may contain relatively harmless concentrations of pathogens. The grinding process, however, mixes the pathogens throughout the meat. At the same time, grinding the meat greatly increases its surface area, exposing more of the protein–rich tissues to microbes in air. Furthermore, the meat grinder can be a source of pathogens and spread them to the food product, especially if the machine was not properly cleaned after its last use. The particles of food that remained in the grinder can provide food for pathogenic microorganisms. Therefore, surfaces that touch ground meats should be cleaned carefully.

The following tips can help reduce your risk of food–borne illness:

- Cook beef, poultry, pork, thick pieces of fish, and egg–containing dishes thoroughly, using a meat thermometer to check for doneness.

- Cook eggs until the yolk and white have solidified and no "runniness" remains.

- Bake stuffing separately from poultry or wash the poultry cavity thoroughly and stuff the bird immediately before cooking. Make sure the temperature of the stuffing reaches 165°F. After cooking, transfer the stuffing to a clean bowl for serving or storage.

- Serve meat, poultry, and fish on a clean plate. Never use the same plate that held the raw product. For example, when grilling hamburgers, do not put cooked items on the plate that was used to carry the raw meat to the grill.

The grinding process mixes pathogens throughout the raw meat.

Storing and Reheating Food

After food is cooked, careless food handling continues to set the stage for the growth of pathogens. Food–borne pathogens thrive at "room temperature," temperatures that are between 60°F and 110°F. A common practice is to let hot or cold foods remain on the table at room temperature for a few hours. Although you may not feel like clearing the table after eating, it is a good idea to cover leftovers and refrigerate or freeze them as soon as you have finished eating, or within 2 hours. If environmental temperatures are above 90°F, refrigerate the leftovers within 1 hour.[10] There is no need to let hot foods cool before chilling or freezing them.

To reduce your risk of food—borne illness, follow these food storage tips:

- Check your refrigerator's temperature regularly to make sure it stays below 41°F. Keep the refrigerator as cold as possible without freezing milk and lettuce.

- Cook ground meats and poultry soon after purchasing. If this is not possible, freeze the ground items.

- Note that raw fish, shellfish, and poultry are highly perishable. It is best to cook these foods or freeze them the day they are purchased.

- Use refrigerated ground meat and patties within 1 to 2 days, and use frozen meat and patties within 3 to 4 months after purchasing them. Table 12.6 presents recommended time limits for refrigeration and freezer storage of foods. Foods that are stored in the freezer for longer than recommended periods often develop unappealing flavors. Note that ground meats are more perishable than intact cuts of meat.

- Use refrigerated leftovers within 4 days.

Cross—contamination is a threat not only during food preparation; it can also become a problem during food storage. Therefore, keep all foods, including left—overs, covered while they are in the refrigerator. This practice can prevent drippings

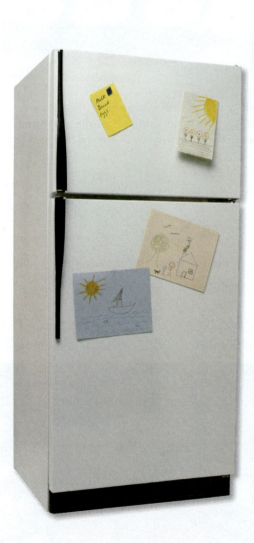

TABLE 12.6   Cold Storage Time Limits for Perishable Foods

Product	Storage Period in Refrigerator (40°F)	Storage Period in Freezer (0°F)
Fresh meat		
Ground meat	1–2 days	3–4 months
Steaks and roasts	3–5 days	4–12 months
Fresh pork		
Chops	3–5 days	4–12 months
Ground	1–2 days	3–4 months
Cured meats		
Luncheon meat, open package	3–5 days	—
Unopened package	2 weeks	—
Fresh fish	1–2 days	—
Fresh chicken or turkey (whole)	1–2 days	12 months
Parts	1–2 days	9 months
Dairy products		
Cheese (Swiss, brick, processed cheese)	3–4 weeks	(Not recommended)
Milk	5 days	—
Eggs		
Fresh, in shell	3–5 weeks	—
Hard-cooked	1 week	—

Source: USDA, FSIS: Kitchen companion. 2008. http://www.fsis.usda.gov/PDF/Kitchen_Companion.pdf; *Freezing and food safety.* 2013. http://www.fsis.usda.gov/wps/portal/fsis/topics/food-safety-education/get-answers/food-safety-fact-sheets/safe-food-handling/freezing-and-food-safety/ct_index Accessed February 9, 2014 from foods that are often contaminated, such as raw chicken, from tainting other foods. Furthermore, store raw meats, fish, poultry, and shellfish on lower shelves of the refrigerator, so they are separated from foods that are to be eaten raw. Examine Figure 12.7. Can you find two examples of improperly stored refrigerated foods?

Food safety educators with the federal government condensed these rules into four simple actions as a part of their Check Your Steps program:

1. **CLEAN.** Wash hands and surfaces often.

2. **SEPARATE.** Do not cross—contaminate.

3. **COOK.** Cook to proper temperatures.

4. **CHILL.** Refrigerate promptly.

You can find reliable information about food—borne illness at www.foodsafety.gov. For general food safety questions, you can call the FDA's food safety hotline at 1−888−723−3366.

Figure 12.7 Storing risky foods in the refrigerator. In this photograph, can you identify two risky foods that are improperly stored? What can be done to store the foods safely?

17. List at least four rules for reducing the risk of food-borne illness when you purchase foods and beverages.

18. List at least five rules for reducing the risk of food-borne illness when you prepare and cook foods.

19. List at least three rules for reducing the risk of food-borne illness when you store cooked foods.

20. Explain why ground meat and poultry often are sources of food-borne illness.

21. What preparation step can be taken to make fish safer to eat raw?

22. What temperature range encourages rapid multiplication of pathogens?

23. What are the federal government's four simplified actions for reducing the risk of food-borne illness?

12.7 Food Preservation

Learning Outcomes

1 Discuss food preservation methods, including how each method extends the shelf life of foods.

2 Explain how to prepare home-canned, low-acid foods that are safe to eat.

shelf life period of time that a food can be stored before it spoils

fermentation process used to preserve or produce a variety of foods, including pickles and wine

sterilization process that kills or destroys all microorganisms and viruses

If nothing is done to preserve a fresh food, the item soon undergoes various chemical changes that eventually result in spoilage. Preserving food extends its shelf life. **Shelf life** refers to the period of time that a food can be stored before it spoils. Heating is one of the oldest ways to preserve foods. Heat can kill or deactivate pathogens, and the process also destroys naturally occurring enzymes in foods that can contribute to food spoilage.

Fermentation is an ancient method of food preservation that is still used to produce a variety of foods, including yogurt, wine, pickles, and sauerkraut. The fermentation process involves adding certain bacteria or yeast to food. These microbes use sugars in the food to make acids and alcohol, chemicals that hinder the growth of other types of bacteria and yeast that can spoil food.

For centuries, people preserved meats, fruits, and other foods that had high water contents by adding salt or sugar to them. To grow, bacteria need plenty of water; yeasts and molds can grow when less water is available. Adding sugar or salt to foods draws water out of cells, including bacteria, fungi, protozoans, and worms. As a result, these pathogens are less likely to survive in sugary or salty foods. Drying reduces a food's water content. Dried fruits such as raisins, for example, have a longer shelf life than grapes, their natural counterparts.

Today, we can add pasteurization, refrigeration, freezing, canning, irra—diation, additives, and *aseptic* processing to the list of food preservation techniques (Table 12.7). Aseptic processing involves sterilizing a food and its package separately, before the food enters the package. The **sterilization** pro—cess destroys all microorganisms and viruses. After undergoing aseptic packag—ing, boxes of sterile foods and beverages, such as milk or juices, can remain free of microbial growth for several years while sitting on supermarket or pantry shelves. However, once the containers of these products are opened, the foods or beverages have the same shelf life as their counterparts that have not under—gone aseptic processing.

TABLE 12.7 Summary of Food Preservation Methods

Method	Means of Effectiveness	Examples of Foods
Heating (cooking, pasteurization, aseptic processing)	Kills or deactivates spoilage and pathogenic microbes, destroys enzymes that result in food spoilage	Most foods
Adding salt/sugar	Binds water, decreasing the amount available for microbes	Ham, bacon, fish, pickled foods
Smoking	Kills spoilage microbes, destroys enzymes that result in food spoilage Smoking is a method of heating. The process involves salting food before smoking and refrigerating or freezing the food after smoking.	Meats, fish
Curing	Retards the growth of *C. botulinum* and stabilizes the flavor of the food Additives such as sodium nitrate and nitrite are used to cure meat, fish, or poultry.	Luncheon meats, smoked fish
Chilling/freezing	Slows molecular movement, retarding microbial and enzymatic activity	Most foods
Drying (dehydration)	Removes much of the moisture in food that microbes need to survive	Fruit, herbs, meat jerkies, seeds
Fermenting	Produces acids and alcohol that interfere with the survival of unwanted microbes	Alcoholic beverages, yogurt, cheeses, soy sauce
Canning	Kills spoilage microbes, destroys enzymes in food that result in spoilage, removes oxygen that certain microbes need to survive	Meat, fish, poultry, fruits, vegetables, milk
Irradiating	Destroys most pathogens, delays sprouting (potatoes)	Spices, raw meat and poultry, fresh fruits and vegetables

Source: National Center for Home Food Preservation: *USDA complete guide to home canning, 2009 revision.* http://nchfp.uga.edu/publications/publications_usda.html

Home-Canned Foods

When food is canned, commercial food production methods require heating the food to certain temperatures for specified times. Thus, unless the can or jar has been damaged, properly processed canned foods should be free of pathogens. Certain home–canned foods, however, may contain the microorganism *Clostridium botulinum* (*C. botulinum*) that causes *botulism* or its toxin. The home–canning process may kill *C. botulinum* bacteria in the food, but their spores or toxin may remain. That is why home–canned, *low–acid* foods such as beans and corn should be boiled for 10 minutes before eating. Foods made with vinegar, tomatoes, or citrus juices are usually high–acid foods, and as a result, such items are not likely to be sources of *C. botulinum*. The botulinum toxin is highly poisonous; never taste a home–canned, low–acid food before boiling it. For more information about proper home canning of foods, obtain a copy of the U.S. Department of Agriculture's *Complete Guide to Home Canning* (http://www.uga.edu/nchfp/publications/publications_usda.html) or contact a food and nutrition specialist at your community's university extension office.

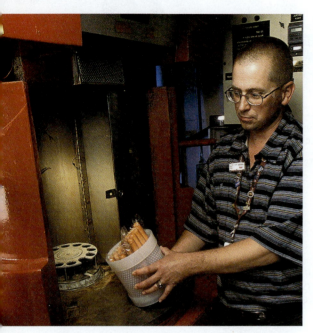

Figure 12.8 Irradiating food. U.S. Department of Agriculture microbiologist Glenn Boyd places a batch of hot dogs into the gamma radiation source to rid them of food-borne pathogens.

Figure 12.9 Radura symbol. The Radura symbol indicates the food in this package has been irradiated.

Irradiation

The process of food irradiation preserves food by using a high amount of energy to kill pathogens such as *Salmonella* and *E. coli* O157:H7 (Fig. 12.8). The processes used to irradiate foods do not make the items radioactive. The energy passes through the food, as in microwave cooking, and no radioactive material is left behind. The energy is strong enough to destroy the genetic material as well as cell membranes or cell walls of insects and microbes. As a result, irradiation is a highly effective way of killing insects and microorganisms that may be in foods. However, irradiation is not always an effective way to destroy viruses.[12] It is important to recognize that even when foods, especially meats, have been irradiated, once their packaging has been opened, the foods can still become contaminated.

Irradiation extends the shelf life of spices, dry vegetable seasonings, meats, seeds, shell eggs, and fresh fruits and vegetables. Except for dried seasonings, packages that contain irradiated foods must be labeled with the international food irradiation symbol, the Radura, and include a statement indicating the product has been treated by irradiation (Fig. 12.9).

According to medical experts with the World Health Organization, FDA, and CDC, irradiated foods are safe to eat.[12] Furthermore, irradiation causes few or no nutritive losses. Despite such assurances, many Americans are skeptical about the safety of irradiated foods, and they avoid purchasing such products.

Concept **Checkpoint 12.7**

24. Define *shelf life.*
25. Identify four methods of food preservation and explain how each method extends the shelf life of foods.
26. What preparation step can be taken to make home-canned, low-acid foods safe to eat?
27. List three foods that may undergo irradiation to extend their shelf life.

12.8 Preparing for Disasters

Learning Outcomes

1. Explain actions people in households can take to have safe food and water available after a disaster.

2. Discuss ways to safely prepare food when a power outage occurs.

On October 29, 2012, Hurricane Sandy moved onto land in New Jersey and proceeded to batter much of the East Coast of the United States with high winds and severe flooding. The hurricane took the lives of 117 Americans and caused billions of dollars in property damage.[13] Immediately after the storm struck, more than 8.5 million utility customers in the affected region lost power.[14] What steps can you take to have enough water and food available to survive hurricanes, earthquakes, or other serious emergency situations?

A supply of clean water and wholesome food is necessary for surviving disasters such as hurricanes and earthquakes. This chapter's "Nutrition Matters" provides instructions for sanitizing water. The following recommendations may help sustain you and your loved ones for several days:

- Store at least 1 gallon of water per person per day. Ideally, you should have at least a 3– to 5–day supply of drinking water, or at least 5 gallons of water for each person in a household. Children and breastfeeding women may need more than 1 gallon of water per day. Also, more water may be necessary for people living in warm climates. Furthermore, store extra water for food preparation, personal hygiene, dishwashing, and pets.

- Water should be maintained in a cool place and in sturdy plastic bottles with tight–fitting lids.

- Change stored water every 6 months.

- Drink only bottled, boiled, or treated water until you are certain the public water supply is safe.

- If you have time to prepare, fill a bathtub with water to use if it becomes necessary. The water, however, will need to be sanitized before being consumed.

- If you drink bottled water, make sure the seal has not been broken.

    If your emergency water supply is inadequate, you can consume melted ice cubes from the freezer, canned fruit juices, and water drained from an undamaged water heater. Water stored in the tank of the toilet (not the bowl) is also fit to drink. Water in swimming pools and spas can be used for personal hygiene needs but not for drinking. Never drink water from car radiators, home heating systems, or water beds. Alcoholic beverages contribute to dehydration and therefore should be avoided.

| Aftermath of Super Storm Sandy (2012)

Emergency Food Supply

A disaster can easily disrupt your access to safe food; therefore, you should store at least a 3–day supply of food for emergency use. Choose foods that have a long storage life, require no refrigeration, and can be eaten without cooking, such as canned meats, fruits, and vegetables. Table 12.8 lists foods that can be included in your emergency food supply. Also store a manual can opener, paper plates, and eating utensils.

    If stored under proper conditions, unopened canned or boxed foods will remain fresh for about 2 years. Before storing food, use a permanent marking pen to write the date on the package. You should use and replace foods before they lose their freshness or reach their expiration dates. An ideal food storage location is a cool, dry, dark place. Do not store foods near gasoline, oil, paints, or petroleum–based solvents, because some food products absorb their odors. You can protect foods from rodents and insects by storing them in airtight containers or plastic storage bins.

    If you have no electricity, consume perishable food in your refrigerator or freezer before using your emergency food supply. However, discard cooked foods after they have been at room temperature for 2 hours. Do not eat food that appears spoiled or is from cans that are leaking or bulging.

    To prepare meals safely after a disaster, you will need to store:

- a camp stove or charcoal grill.

- fuel for cooking, such as charcoal. **Never** cook food on a camp stove or charcoal grill indoors. The fumes contain *carbon monoxide*, an odorless deadly gas.

TABLE 12.8 Foods to Store for Emergency Situations

- Canned meats, fish, fruits, and vegetables
- Canned fruit juices
- Unopened boxes of cereal, low-salt crackers, and trail mix
- Prewrapped fruit-filled granola bars
- Peanut or other nut butters
- Raisins and other dried fruit
- Dry milk powder
- Baby foods

- matches.
- cooking and eating utensils.
- paper plates, cups, and towels.

For more information about emergency preparedness, visit http://www.cdc.gov/ healthywater/emergency/preparedness/index.html and http://www.fda.gov/Food/ RecallsOutbreaksEmergencies/Emergencies/ucm2006925.htm .

Concept **Checkpoint 12.8**

28. Develop an emergency food and water supply plan for your home. Identify at least five foods that are appropriate for an emergency food supply.

29. In case public water supplies are disrupted, identify at least three sources of drinking water in homes that are safe for humans. Identify at least two sources of water that are unsafe to drink.

12.9 Food Additives

Learning Outcomes

1 Explain the difference between direct and indirect food additives, and provide examples of each type of additive.

2 Discuss the impact of the GRAS list and the Delaney Clause on the use of food additives.

3 Identify unintentional food additives.

4 Discuss pesticides, including the pros and cons of their use.

5 Explain the usefulness of integrated pest management.

food additive any substance that becomes incorporated into food during production, packaging, transport, or storage

color additives dyes, pigments, or other substances that provide color to food

Food Additives Amendment U.S. legislation that requires evidence that a new food additive is safe before it can be marketed for use

Generally Recognized as Safe (GRAS) ingredients considered to be safe

A **food additive** is any substance that becomes incorporated into food during production, packaging, transport, or storage. Food manufacturers incorporate *direct* or *intentional additives* into their products for various reasons. Such additives may make food easier to process, more nutritious, able to stay fresh longer, or better tasting. Most additives are added to influence a food's sensory characteristics, including taste or color.

Many direct food additives help maintain the safety of foods by limiting the growth of bacteria that cause food–borne illness. Other additives protect against the action of enzymes that can lead to undesirable changes in the food's color and taste. Such unwanted chemical changes occur when enzymes that are natu–rally in certain foods are exposed to the oxygen in air. *Antioxidant additives*, including vitamins E and C and a variety of *sulfites*, can prevent oxygen from reacting with these enzymes. **Color additives** are dyes, pigments, or other sub–stances that provide color to foods, drugs, or cosmetics, such as beta–carotene in margarine and FD&C (Food, Drug, & Cosmetic) Red No. 40 in cherry–flavored cough syrup. Table 12.9 lists common types of direct food additives (including color additives), their uses, examples of products that contain the additives, and names of specific additives.

TABLE 12.9   Common Types of Direct Food Additives

Type of Additive	Functions	Typical Products	Examples of Specific Ingredients
Preservatives	Prevent food spoilage	Jellies, beverages, baked goods, cured meats, cereals, snack foods	Ascorbic acid, citric acid, sodium benzoate, calcium propionate, sodium erythorbate, BHA, BHT, EDTA, sodium nitrite
Sweeteners	Add sweetness	Processed foods, beverages, baked goods, sugar substitutes	Sucrose, glucose, mannitol, corn syrup, aspartame, sucralose
Flavors and spices	Add specific flavors	Puddings, pie fillings, gelatins, cake mixes, candies, soft drinks	Natural flavorings, artificial flavorings, spices
Flavor enhancers	Enhance flavors already present	Many processed foods	Monosodium glutamate (MSG), hydrolyzed soy protein
Nutrients	Replace nutrients lost during processing, boost levels of nutrients naturally in food	Flour, cereals, margarine, fruit beverages, energy bars	Thiamin hydrochloride, riboflavin, niacin, niacinamide, folic acid, beta-carotene, ascorbic acid
Emulsifiers	Keep oily and watery ingredients from separating	Salad dressings, peanut butter, chocolate, frozen desserts	Soy lecithin, mono- and diglycerides, polysorbates
Leavening agents	Promote rising of certain baked goods	Baked goods	Baking soda, monocalcium phosphate, calcium carbonate
Stabilizers, thickeners, binders	Provide uniform texture and improve "mouth feel"	Frozen desserts, puddings, sauces	Gelatin, pectin, guar gum, carrageenan, whey
Color additives	Enhance natural colors, provide color to colorless and "fun" foods as well as medications and cosmetics	Processed foods, including candies, snack foods, margarine, cheese, soft drinks, gelatin	FD&C Blue No. 1, FD&C Red No. 40, beta-carotene, caramel color

Modified from: International Food Information Council and U.S. Food and Drug Administration: *Food: Overview of food ingredients, additives & colors.* Last updated March 2013. http://www.fda.gov/food/ingredientspackaginglabeling/foodadditivesingredients/ucm094211.htm Accessed February 10, 2014

Indirect additives, such as compounds from a food's wrapper or container, can enter food as it is packaged, transported, or stored. Indirect additives, how—ever, have no purpose. The FDA and certain international organizations regulate all food additives to ensure that processed foods and their packaging are safe.[15]

Food Safety Legislation: Food Additives

By the 1950s, hundreds of ingredients were being added to foods during processing. Many of these substances had long histories of being safe; others were deemed safe after undergoing scientific testing. In 1958, the U.S. Congress enacted the **Food Additives Amendment.** According to this amendment, an ingredient that had been in use prior to 1958 was **Generally Recognized as Safe (GRAS)** when qualified experts generally agreed that the substance was safe for its intended use. The Food Additives Amendment excluded GRAS substances from being defined as food additives.[15] Thus, mod—ern food manufacturers can include substances on the GRAS list as ingredients without testing them for safety or getting prior approval from the FDA.

As a result of the 1958 Food Additives Amendment, the manufacturer of a *new* food additive (one developed after 1958) must provide evidence of the

Color additives are dyes, pigments, or other substances that provide color to foods, drugs, or cosmetics.

Delaney Clause component of the 1958 Food Additives Amendment that prevents manufacturers from adding carcinogenic compounds to food

unintentional food additives substances that are accidentally in foods

substance's safety to the FDA before the additive can be used.[15] When evaluating the safety of a newly developed food additive, FDA experts consider the chemical composition and characteristics of the substance, the amount of the substance that Americans would typically ingest, and the additive's effects on the body. If the additive is safe in amounts that people are likely to consume, FDA experts establish a level of the substance that can be added to foods.

According to the **Delaney Clause** of the Food Additives Amendment, food manufacturers cannot add a new compound that causes cancer at *any* level of intake. Thus, if an additive causes cancer, even though very high doses may be necessary to cause the disease, no amount of the additive is considered to be safe, and none is allowed in food. Evidence for cancer risk could come from either laboratory animal or human studies. The FDA allows very few exceptions to this clause.

The FDA cannot ban **unintentional food additives**—various industrial chemicals, pesticide residues, and mold toxins—from foods, even though some of these contaminants may be carcinogenic. The Food Quality Protection Act of 1996 established the safety standard of "a reasonable certainty of no harm" for pesticide residues in foods. As a result of this act, the "no risk" provision of the Delaney Clause does not apply to pesticide residues. However, the Delaney Clause remains in effect for food additives.[16] The following section discusses chemical contaminants and other unintentional food additives.

Other Substances in Foods

Various substances can accidentally enter food during processing. Although such contaminants can blend into a food, they are not food additives. Common biological and physical food contaminants are insect parts, rodent feces or urine, dust and dirt, and bits of metal or glass from machinery used to process food. Although some of these substances may not be harmful to health, most people find it unappealing to have filth and other unintentional ingredients in their foods.

According to the Federal Food, Drug, and Cosmetic Act, adulterated food contains objectionable and unsanitary material, and it cannot be distributed. However, the FDA permits very small amounts of unavoidable, naturally occurring substances such as dirt and insect parts in foods, because they are not harmful when consumed in minute amounts. The FDA established guidelines concerning amounts (*action levels*) of certain materials that are permitted in specific foods, such as mold and rodent hairs in paprika or insect eggs in canned orange juice. According to the FDA, ". . . it is economically impractical to grow, harvest, or process raw products that are totally free of non–hazardous, naturally occurring, unavoidable defects. Products harmful to consumers are subject to regulatory action whether or not they exceed the action levels."[17]

Chemical contaminants also enter foods unintentionally. Toxic metals, such as lead, cadmium, and mercury, are naturally in our environment, and these elements may also be in our food. Poisonous human–made compounds such as *benzene* and *polychlorinated biphenols* (*PCBs*) are in the environment as well. Toxic metals or poisonous compounds resulting from human manufacturing practices can pollute sources of water used by consumers (well water, for example). Americans who drink water from municipal supplies can be assured that the water is analyzed regularly to determine its concentrations of toxic substances. However, people who rely on privately owned wells should have the water tested routinely.

Common biological and physical food contaminants include rodent feces or urine.

What Are Pesticides?

A **pesticide** is any substance that people use to control or kill unwanted insects, weeds, rodents, fungi, or other organisms. There are several different kinds of pesticides. **Insecticides** control or kill insects; **rodenticides** kill mice and rats; **herbicides** destroy weeds; and **fungicides** limit the spread of fungi, such as mold and mildew. Herbicides are the most widely used type of pesticide in agriculture.[18]

Pesticide Residue Tolerances The use of pesticides in modern farming practices has helped increase crop yields, reduce food costs, and protect the quality of many agricultural products. However, many pesticides leave small amounts (*pesticide residues*) in or on treated crops, including fruits, vegetables, and grains, even when they are applied correctly. Concentrations of pesticide residues often decrease as food crops are washed, stored, processed, and prepared. Nevertheless, some of these substances may remain in fresh produce, such as apples or peaches, as well as in processed foods, such as canned applesauce or peaches.

The EPA regulates the proper use of pesticides. The agency can limit the amount of a pesticide that is applied on crops, restrict the frequency or location of the pesticide's application, or require the substance be used only by specially trained, certified persons. The EPA also sets pesticide **tolerances,** maximum amounts of pesticide residues that can be in or on each treated food crop. A pesticide tolerance includes a margin of safety, so the maximum pesticide residue that is allowed to be in or on a food is much lower than amounts that can cause negative health effects.[18]

Nonchemical Methods of Pest Management Although the EPA focuses on chemical methods of managing pests, the agency also promotes nonchemical pest management techniques that may be safer for humans and the environment. Integrated pest management (IPM) involves using a variety of methods for controlling pests while limiting damage to the environment. IPM methods include growing pest–resistant crops, using predatory wasps to control crop–destroying insects, and trapping adult insect pests before they can reproduce. Biologically based pesticides, such as sex hormones (*pheromones*) that attract pesky insects to predators or traps and viruses that infect insects and weeds, are becoming increasingly popular among farmers (Figure 12.10). Such methods are often safer for humans than traditional chemical pesticides.

It is important to note that IPM permits the use of chemical pesticides but only as needed to enhance the effects of nonchemical methods. Studies suggest that IPM techniques generally increase crop yields and economic profits, while reducing the use of chemical pesticides.[18] As IPM programs become more widely adopted, conventional farmers will depend less on the use of chemical pesticides.

Fruits and vegetables grown without use of pesticides are available and may bear an "organic" label (see Chapter 3 for information about organic foods). These products generally are more expensive than those grown using pesticides, and they are not necessarily safer or more nutritious than conventionally produced foods.

How Safe Are Pesticides? Pesticides used in agriculture have both beneficial and unwanted effects. Pesticides help protect the food supply and make food crops available at reasonable cost. Nevertheless, pesticides have the potential to harm humans, animals, or the environment because they are designed to kill

pesticide substance that people use to kill or control unwanted insects, weeds, or other organisms

insecticides substances used to control or kill insects

rodenticides substances used to kill mice and rats

herbicides substances used to destroy weeds

fungicides substances used to limit the spread of fungi

tolerances maximum amounts of pesticide residues that can be in or on each treated food crop

Did You Know?

Lead is a highly toxic mineral that may be in candies imported from Mexico and traditional ethnic folk remedies, especially *greta, azarcon, ghasard,* and *ba-baw-san.* Therefore, it is prudent to avoid ingesting these candies or folk remedies.

Figure 12.10 Helpful insect. The spined soldier bug (*left*) makes a meal of a Mexican bean beetle larva. Bean beetle larvae are devastating pests of snap beans and soybeans. The spined soldier bug's pheromone may help farmers control many insects that eat crops.

or otherwise negatively affect organisms. If a pesticide is applied improperly to cropland, it may remain in the soil, be taken up by plant roots, decompose to other compounds, or enter groundwater and waterways. Winds may carry pesticides in air and dust to distant locations. Each path can be a route to the human food chain (Fig. 12.11).

The potential harmful effects of a pesticide in food depend on the particular chemical and how effectively the body can eliminate it, its concentration in the food, how much and how often it is eaten, and the consumer's vulnerability to the substance. Tolerable amounts of pesticide residues on or in foods are extremely small. However, it is possible that regular exposure to small amounts of these chemicals may enable the substances to accumulate in the body and produce toxicity or initiate cancer.[19] Health experts have studied rates of cancers among people who have close contact with pesticides, such as farmers and pesticide applicators. People who are exposed to certain pesticides have a greater risk of developing specific cancers, particularly bladder and colon cancer, than people who have not been exposed to the chemicals.[20] More research is needed to confirm these findings and explain how exposure to pesticides influence cancer risk. Thus, environmental health experts continue to monitor the effects of pesticides on humans.

Figure 12.11 Pesticide pathways. If a pesticide is applied improperly to cropland, it may remain in the soil, be taken up by plant roots, decompose to other compounds, or enter groundwater and waterways. Winds may carry pesticides in air and dust to distant locations. Each path can be a route to the human food chain.

Concept **Checkpoint 12.9**

30. What is a food additive? What is the difference between direct and indirect food additives?
31. What is a color additive?
32. What is the GRAS list?
33. Explain the role of the Delaney Clause in protecting the U.S. food supply.
34. What is an unintentional food additive? Provide at least three examples of such additives.
35. What is a pesticide? Provide at least three examples of types of pesticides.
36. Define *integrated pest management,* and provide an example of this method.
37. Which U.S. agency regulates the use of pesticides?
38. What is a pesticide tolerance?
39. Explain how pesticides can enter the human food chain.

12.10 Nutrition Matters: Avoiding "The Revenge"

Learning Outcomes

1 Discuss ways to prevent traveler's diarrhea.

2 Identify nations where visitors are most likely to develop traveler's diarrhea.

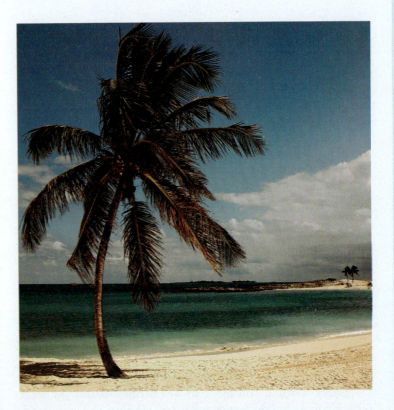

If you like traveling to foreign countries and enjoy sampling exotic cuisines in these places, one thing you do not need to encounter is *travelers' diarrhea* (*TD*). Also referred to as "Montezuma's Revenge" and "Tut's Tummy," TD can ruin your vacation. By taking some precautions, however, your digestive system can stay healthy while you travel abroad.

TD results from consuming food or water contaminated with pathogens. The illness is characterized by the abrupt onset of abdominal cramps and loose or watery bowel move—ments. Additional symptoms may include nausea, vomiting, intestinal bloating, and fever. TD generally lasts 3 to 5 days without treatment, but signs and symptoms may persist in a small percentage of infected travelers.

Unless precautions are taken, TD is likely to occur during or shortly after traveling in regions where sanitary water supplies are not always available, people who prepare food have less than ideal personal hygiene practices, and untreated human feces are used for fertilizer. Health experts estimate that bacterial pathogens are responsible for 80 to 90% of cases of TD.[21] Protozoans such as *Giardia* account for about 10% of TD cases. When travelers suffer from per—sistent symptoms, the illness is likely to be the result of a protozoal rather than a bacterial infection.

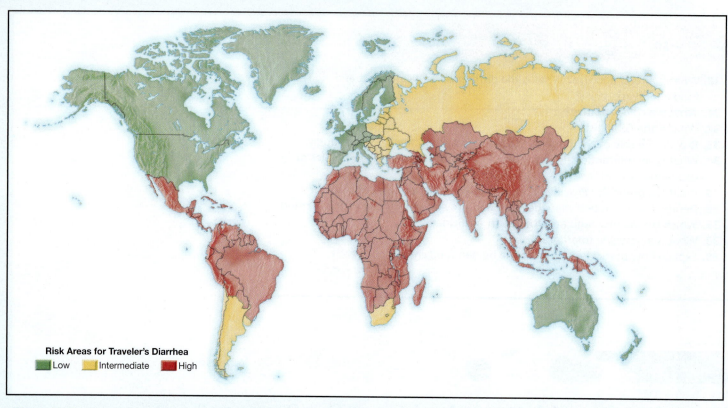

Risk Areas for Traveler's Diarrhea
☐ Low ☐ Intermediate ☐ High

| **Figure 12.12 Areas of risk for travelers' diarrhea.** This map presents regions of the world where the risks are low, intermediate, and high.

Thirty to 70 percent of travelers to international places will develop TD, depending on their destinations.[21] However, it is important to note that a trip to every foreign destination is likely to include the risk of TD. Figure 12.12 presents regions of the world where the risks are low, intermediate, and high. Low–risk countries include the United States, Canada, Australia, New Zealand, Japan, and countries in Northern and Western Europe. Intermediate–risk countries include those in Eastern Europe, South Africa, and some of the Caribbean islands. High–risk areas generally have high–density populations, widespread pollution, and inadequate water treatment systems.[22] These regions include Mexico and other Central American countries, and most of Asia, the Middle East, Africa, and South America.

Reducing Your Risk of TD

Experts at the CDC recommend several approaches for reducing your risk of TD. These include following instructions regarding food and beverage selection, avoiding contact with contaminated waterways, sanitizing drinking water, and using medications that may prevent TD.

Carry a small container of an alcohol–based (at least 60% alcohol) hand cleaner with you. Before you eat, wash your hands with the hand cleaner. When you visit places where risk of contracting TD is moderate to high, avoid consuming food or beverages purchased from street vendors.

Before you eat meat or other high–risk foods, make sure they are fully cooked and served hot. Avoid raw foods that have been washed in water, such as fresh fruits, raw vegetables, and salads. Do not eat fresh fruit without peeling it first. Avoid water, ice, and beverages diluted with water or ice, such as reconstituted fruit juices and iced drinks. Do not drink fresh fluid milk or milk products that have not been pasteurized. Safe beverages include those that are bottled and sealed; bottled beer and wine may also be safe to drink. If boiled water is used to make tea and coffee, these beverages may be safe to consume. Use bottled water to wash hands, brush teeth, and take medication.

TD can be spread when pathogens from human or animal feces are in sources of water, including swimming pools, lakes, rivers, and other bodies of water. Accidentally swallowing even small amounts of contaminated water can cause illness. Swimming pools that contain chlorinated water may be safe places to swim, if the disinfectant and pH levels are properly maintained. However, some pathogens are resistant to levels of chlorine commonly used to disinfect swimming pools. Thus, you should also avoid swallowing chlorinated swimming pool water.

How Can I Sanitize Drinking Water?

Boiling is the most reliable method to make impure water safe to drink.[23] Water should be boiled for 1 minute, covered, and allowed to cool to room temperature without adding ice. To inactivate microbes at altitudes greater than 6562 feet, water should be boiled for 3 minutes.

Chemical Disinfection Disinfection methods kill large numbers of microorganisms, reducing the likelihood of infection. Chemical disinfection with chlorine (in household bleach) or iodine is an alternative method of sanitizing water when boiling water is not practical. Iodine and chlorine are available in tablets and drops. To reduce the risk of TD, follow the manufacturer's instructions for sanitizing water with these chemicals.

Filtering Water Microstrainer filters can remove bacteria and protozoans from drinking water, but they may not remove viruses (Fig. 12.13). To destroy viruses, you should disinfect the water with iodine or chlorine after using microstrainer filters. Filters collect organisms from water, so wash your hands with sanitized water after handling used filters. For more information about water filters and other water disinfection methods, visit http://wwwnc.cdc.gov/travel/page/water−disinfection .

Preventive Medications Before you leave the United States to enter a high−risk region, see your physician for his or her recommendations for preventing TD. You can also take medications that contain bismuth subsalicylate (BSS), the active ingredient in Pepto−Bismol, to reduce the risk of TD. Side effects of BSS commonly include nausea, constipation, and blackening of the tongue and bowel movements. BSS is not recommended for children under 12 years of age, and the medication should be avoided by people who are allergic to aspirin or have certain chronic conditions. Therefore, check with your physician before taking BBS along when you travel to other countries.

Treating TD

Because pathogenic bacteria are often the cause of TD, antibiotics are the primary method of treating the condition. In the United States, physicians often prescribe antibiotics for their patients to bring with them when they travel out of the country. When used in combination with antibiotics, *antimotility* agents can be helpful. These medications, such as loperamide, the active

Figure 12.13 Microstrainer filters. Microstrainer filters can remove bacteria and protozoans from drinking water.

ingredient in Imodium, slow the muscular activity of the digestive tract and can provide relief from the diarrhea associated with TD.

Dehydration can be a serious complication of TD. To prevent dehydration, it is important for people suffering from TD to replace fluids and electrolytes lost by vomiting and diarrhea. However, travelers should remember to use only beverages that are in sealed containers, including carbonated soft drinks. If fluid loss is severe, it is best to obtain professional medical treatment.

Concept **Checkpoint 12.10**

40. List three ways to reduce the risk of traveler's diarrhea.
41. List three countries where visitors have a high likelihood of developing traveler's diarrhea.

Chapter References

See Appendix H.

Summary

12.1 Introduction to Food Safety

- In the United States, millions of people become ill from various food-borne illnesses each year. Food-borne illness occurs when microscopic pathogens or their toxic by-products enter food (or beverages) and are consumed. Many kinds of pathogens infect the digestive tract; other types of food-borne pathogens do not sicken humans directly, but these microbes secrete toxins into food. When the food is eaten, the toxins irritate the intestinal tract and cause food intoxication.

12.2 Protecting Our Food

- The United States has one of the safest food supplies in the world, primarily the result of a team effort conducted by cooperating federal, state, and local agencies that regulate and monitor the production and distribution of food. The FDA and the USDA are the key federal agencies that protect consumers by regulating the country's food industry.

12.3 Microbes in Food

- When certain microorganisms metabolize nutrients in food, they often secrete substances that alter the color, texture, taste, and other characteristics of the food in beneficial and desirable ways. When pathogens are in food, they can make the item unsafe to eat. Food contaminants include pathogens, insect parts, residues of compounds used to kill insects that destroy food crops, and metal fragments from food processing equipment.

- The microbes that cause food-borne illness can live practically anywhere. Common routes for transmitting harmful microbes to food involve vermin, poor personal hygiene practices, and improper food preparation and storage practices.

- To grow, most microbes need warmth, moisture, and a source of nutrients, and some microorganisms also need oxygen. In general, high-risk foods are warm, moist, and protein-rich, and they have a neutral or slightly acidic pH. Such foods include meat, poultry, milk and milk products, and eggs.

12.4 Food-borne Illness

- Many factors influence whether an individual becomes ill after eating food or drinking a beverage that has been contaminated with a pathogen. The number of pathogens in a food or the amount of toxin it contains can contribute to the risk and severity of a food-borne illness. In general, high-risk groups are pregnant women, very young children, older adults and persons who suffer from serious chronic illnesses or weakened immune systems.

- Signs and symptoms of food- or water-borne illnesses primarily involve the digestive tract and include nausea, vomiting, diarrhea, and intestinal cramps. Medical treatment should be obtained when an intestinal disorder is accompanied by fever, bloody bowel movements, prolonged vomiting and diarrhea, and/or dehydration.

12.5 Common Food-Borne Pathogens

- The major kinds of pathogens are bacteria, viruses, protozoans, and fungi. In the United States, bacteria and viruses are responsible for most cases of food-borne illness.

12.6 Preventing Food-Borne Illness

- People can reduce their risk of food-borne illness by following some important rules, most of which require changing risky food selection, preparation, and storage practices. Cooking foods is an effective way to destroy pathogens. After food is cooked, however, careless food handling sets the stage for the growth of pathogens. A simple rule to follow is this: "Keep hot foods hot and cold foods cold." Other simple rules include these: Wash hands and surfaces often, do not cross-contaminate, heat foods to proper temperatures, and chill foods promptly.

12.7 Food Preservation

- Modern methods of food preservation include pasteurization, refrigeration, freezing, canning, aseptic processing, using preservative additives, and irradiation.

12.8 Preparing for Disasters

- It is important to have a supply of clean water and wholesome food on hand to survive disasters.

12.9 Food Additives

- Direct food additives can make food easier to process, more nutritious, able to stay fresh longer, better tasting, or more attractive in appearance. An indirect food additive is a substance that becomes incorporated into food during production, packaging, transport, or storage. The 1958 Food Additives Amendment established the GRAS list and requires the manufacturer of a new food additive to provide evidence of the substance's safety to the FDA before the additive can be marketed for use. According to the Delaney Clause of the Food Additives Amendment, food manufacturers cannot add a new compound that causes cancer at *any* level of exposure.

- Unintentional food additives are substances that accidentally are in foods. A pesticide is any substance that people use to kill or control unwanted insects, weeds, rodents, or other organisms. The EPA regulates the proper use of pesticides and sets pesticide tolerances. IPM methods control agricultural pests while limiting damage to the environment.

  Agricultural pesticides have both beneficial and unwanted effects. Pesticides help protect the food supply and make food crops available at reasonable cost. Nevertheless, these substances may harm humans, animals, or the environment. Environmental health experts continually monitor the effects of pesticides on humans.

12.10 Nutrition Matters: Avoiding "The Revenge"

- Traveler's diarrhea (TD) results from consuming food or water contaminated with pathogens. TD is likely to occur during or shortly after travel in regions where sanitary water supplies are lacking, people who prepare food have less than ideal personal hygiene practices, and untreated human feces are used for fertilizer. To reduce the risk of TD, follow instructions regarding safe food and beverage selection, avoid contact with contaminated waterways, sanitize drinking water, and use medications that may prevent the condition.

Recipe for Healthy Living

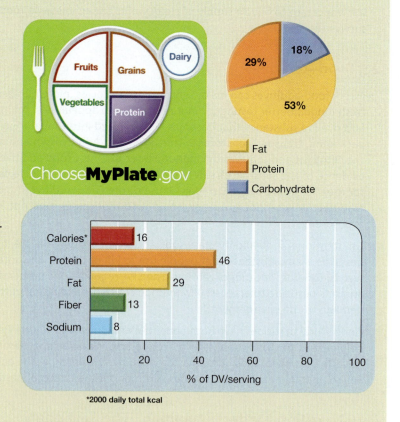

Very Easy Chicken Salad

Chicken that is properly prepared, cooked, and stored is a safe, nutritious, economical food. A good way to use up day-old cooked chicken is to make chicken salad. This recipe is unusual, because it includes seedless grapes and sunflower seeds. (You can substitute day-old cooked turkey for the chicken and chopped apple or dried apricots for the grapes.)

The chicken salad recipe makes approximately three 1-cup servings. A serving of this salad supplies approximately 320 kcal, 23 g protein, 19 g fat, 3.3 g fiber, and 190 mg sodium.

INGREDIENTS:

1 ¼ cups cooked and chilled, skinless, boneless chicken meat
   (approximately 1 whole chicken breast)
1 medium stalk celery, washed and chopped
½ cup raw onion, skinned and finely chopped
½ cup washed seedless red or green grapes, halved
½ cup unsalted roasted sunflower seeds
⅛ tsp curry powder
⅛ tsp ground black pepper
¼ cup low-fat mayonnaise-type salad dressing

PREPARATION STEPS:

1. Cut chicken into small pieces and place in a large bowl.

2. Add the rest of the ingredients to the chicken and gently mix until well blended.

3. Serve on a bed of washed leaf lettuce or as a sandwich filling.

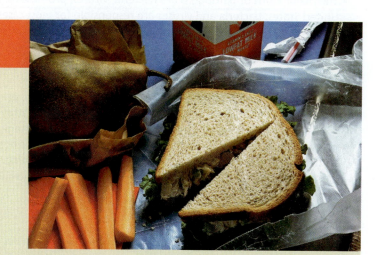

ChooseMyPlate.gov

Fat 53%
Protein 29%
Carbohydrate 18%

Nutrient	% of DV/serving
Calories*	16
Protein	46
Fat	29
Fiber	13
Sodium	8

% of DV/serving

*2000 daily total kcal

Further analyze this and other recipes through activities on Connect at www.mcgrawhillconnect.com.

Critical Thinking

1. Consider your usual food preparation practices. After having read this chapter, list any food preparation practices you have that are unsafe.

2. Consider your usual food storage practices. After having read this chapter, list any of your food storage practices that are unsafe.

3. For lunch on Monday, you visited a restaurant and ordered a hamburger, French fries, baked beans, and a container of orange juice. Two days later, you developed nausea, vomiting, fever, chills, headache, abdominal cramps, and diarrhea. You suspect Monday's lunch made you sick. Considering the foods that you ate for lunch on Monday, which one was the most likely source of your infection? Why? Which food–borne pathogen was the most likely suspect for causing the intestinal disorder? In the future, what steps can you take to reduce the likelihood that the food will make you sick again?

4. Develop a pamphlet to educate consumers about food–borne illness.

Practice Test

Select the best answer.

1. _____ are disease–causing microbes.

   a. Pathogens
   b. Toxins
   c. Teratogens
   d. Oxidants

2. The _____ is the primary government agency that oversees the safety of most foods in the United States.

   a. Food and Drug Administration (FDA)
   b. Agricultural Research Service (ARS)
   c. Centers for Disease Control and Prevention (CDC)
   d. Environmental Protection Agency (EPA)

3. Which of the following foods is most likely to support the growth of pathogens?

   a. overripe bananas
   b. pasteurized milk
   c. raw ground meat
   d. commercially canned tomato soup

4. Food–borne illnesses are usually characterized by

   a. flulike signs and symptoms.
   b. coughing, sneezing, and respiratory inflammation.
   c. megaloblastic anemia and nervous system defects.
   d. abdominal cramps, diarrhea, and vomiting.

5. In the United States, common sources of food–borne illness include all of the following, except

   a. *Norovirus*.
   b. *Staphylococcus aureus*.
   c. fungi.
   d. *Salmonella*.

6. Aflatoxins are

   a. responsible for 30% of food–borne illnesses in the United States.
   b. harmful compounds produced by certain molds.
   c. a type of parasitic worm.
   d. medications that are effective against viral toxins.

7. Which of the following practices can help reduce the growth of food—borne pathogens?

    a. washing hands before preparing food
    b. keeping cold foods cold and hot foods hot
    c. cooking foods to proper internal temperatures
    d. All of the above are correct.

8. Which of the following substances are *not* direct food additives?

    a. sulfites
    b. enrichment nutrients
    c. pesticide residues
    d. emulsifiers

9. Irradiation of food is

    a. an untested technology.
    b. not recommended, because the process increases nutrient losses.
    c. considered to be a safe process by the FDA.
    d. a widely accepted method of food preservation in the United States.

10. Which of the following food preservation processes effectively destroys microbes?

    a. freezing
    b. sterilization
    c. smoking
    d. chilling

11. _____ is the commercial heating process that destroys harmful bacteria in milk and fruit juices.

    a. Sporulation
    b. Sedimentation
    c. Detoxification
    d. Pasteurization

12. When you travel to countries outside the United States, you can reduce your risk of "traveler's diarrhea" by

    a. eating whole fresh fruits and vegetables.
    b. avoiding water that has not been bottled and sealed.
    c. purchasing foods from street vendors.
    d. consuming ice with beverages.

Answers to Quiz Yourself

1. Aflatoxins are the most common sources of food-borne illness in the United States. **False.** (p. 465)

2. In case of emergency, it is not safe to drink the water that is in an undamaged water heater. **False.** (p. 477)

3. Certain fungi, such as button mushrooms, are safe to eat. **True.** (p. 465)

4. The Environmental Protection Agency (EPA) regulates the proper use of pesticides in the United States. **True.** (p. 481)

5. The best way to tell if a food is safe to eat is to smell it. **False.** (p. 459)

CHAPTER 13

Nutrition for a Lifetime

Quiz Yourself

What steps can young women take to prepare for pregnancy? Compared to breast milk, do infant formulas provide the same health benefits for infants? When is the best time to begin feeding solid foods to infants? Which nutrients are most likely to be deficient in diets of older adults? While reading this chapter, you will learn answers to these questions. Test your knowledge of nutrition during various life stages by taking the following quiz. The answers are found on page 535.

1. During pregnancy, a mother-to-be should double her food intake because she's "eating for two." _____ T _____ F

2. The natural size of a woman's breasts is not a factor in determining her ability to breastfeed her baby. _____ T _____ F

3. Caregivers should add solid foods to an infant's diet within the first month after the baby is born. _____ T _____ F

4. Over the past few decades, the prevalence of obesity has increased among American children. _____ T _____ F

5. Compared to younger persons, older adults have lower risks of nutritional deficiencies. _____ T _____ F

13.1 Introduction to Nutrition for a Lifetime

Learning Outcomes:

1 Identify the life stages.

2 Explain why it is important to learn about nutrition concerns for pregnancy, lactation, childhood, and the older adult years.

The chapter opening portrait features a young woman during her eighth month of pregnancy, looking forward to a bright future. Thanks to technological and medical advances that occurred during the twentieth century, her baby has an excellent chance of enjoying a long, healthy life.

If you are a woman, are you pregnant? Do you already have children? If you have children, were they breastfed or formula—fed? Do you live with and help care for an elderly parent or grandparent? These may seem to be personal questions, but many undergraduate college students do not fit the stereotype of being 18 to 22 years of age, having no children, and residing away from home.

Most of the nutrition recommendations presented in this textbook apply to people who are "adults"—loosely defined as the period when a person is 19 to 70 years of age.[1] This chapter focuses on the differing nutrition needs and health concerns of people who are in specific *life stages*. These particular life stages are the **prenatal period** or pregnancy, the time between conception and birth; **lactation** (milk production for breastfeeding); infancy; childhood; adolescence; and the older adult period that generally spans from 70 years of age until death.

prenatal period time between conception and birth; pregnancy

lactation milk production

Why is it necessary to learn some basic information about nutrition—related concerns during various life stages? If you do not have children, you may become a parent in the future. If your parents and grandparents are relatively young and vigorous now, you can expect them to experience declining physical functioning as they grow older. Finally, you need to recognize that most of these changes are normal and will affect you as well.

Today in the United States, many of the leading causes of death are chronic diseases, such as heart disease and cancer. Long—term health—related practices, including dietary and physical activity habits, often contribute to the development of these diseases. Whether you enjoy overall good health or suffer from one or more disabling physical ailments as you grow older depends not only on your lifestyle choices but also on several other factors, including your heredity, relationships, environment, income, education level, and access to health care. Achieving and maintaining a healthy body weight is critical to enjoying good health throughout life. This chapter also includes information about obesity during childhood and adolescence.

Concept **Checkpoint 13.1**

1. John is 79 years of age. According to the general definition of *adult,* is he an adult or an "older adult"?

2. For women, which life stage involves milk production for breastfeeding?

conception moment when a sperm enters an egg (fertilization)

uterus female reproductive organ that protects the developing organism during pregnancy

embryo human organism from 14 days to 8 weeks after conception

fetus human organism from 8 weeks after conception until birth

13.2 Pregnancy

Learning Outcomes

1 Discuss the roles of the placenta and uterus during pregnancy.

2 Explain why an infant's birth weight is an important aspect of the baby's health during its first year of life.

3 List major physiological changes that occur during pregnancy, and identify typical nutrition-related discomforts associated with this stage of life.

4 Discuss the importance of appropriate weight gain during pregnancy, and identify recommended ranges of weight that pregnant women should gain.

5 Explain why prenatal care and a nutritious diet are important for the health of the pregnant woman and her unborn offspring.

"It's positive!" Each day, the results of pregnancy testing are a source of excitement, relief, or concern for thousands of women. About 50% of pregnancies are unplanned in the United States.[2] Therefore, all sexually active women of child-bearing age should be aware of their likelihood of becoming pregnant. Regardless of whether a pregnancy is planned or not, dietary practices before and during pregnancy play a major role in the course of the pregnancy and the primary outcome—a healthy infant.

The prenatal period (*gestation*) encompasses the time from **conception,** the moment a male sperm cell enters a female egg cell, until the birth of a *full-term* infant, about 38 to 42 weeks later. During the first 2 weeks after conception, the fertilized egg (*ovum*) divides repeatedly, forming a mass of cells that enters the woman's **uterus,** the female reproductive organ that protects the developing organism. The mass of cells buries itself into the nutrient-rich lining of the uterus (implantation) and continues to develop. For the next 6 weeks, the rapidly dividing mass of cells, called an **embryo,** increases in size and forms organs. Eight weeks after conception, the developing human being is referred to as a **fetus** (Fig. 13.1).

Figure 13.1 Prenatal development: Conception to fetus. During the first 2 weeks after conception, the fertilized egg divides repeatedly, forming a mass of cells that eventually enters the uterus and buries itself into the organ's nutrient-rich lining. From 14 days through 8 weeks after conception, the rapidly dividing mass of cells is called an embryo. Eight weeks after conception and until its birth, the developing human being is referred to as a fetus.

The prenatal period is often divided into three stages or *trimesters*. During the first trimester, the embryo/fetus develops most of its organs, and by the end of this period, the fetus can move. The first trimester is a critical stage in human development because nutrient deficiencies or excesses and exposure to toxic compounds, such as alcohol, are most likely to have devastating effects on the embryo/fetus. However, many women who are in their first trimester do not realize they are pregnant.

As the second trimester begins, the fetus is still very tiny, about 2½ to 3 inches in length, and weighs only about an ounce. However, the fetus is beginning to look more like a human infant: It has fully formed arms, hands, fingers, legs, feet, and toes. The fetus's organs continue to grow and mature in their ability to function. As the fetus moves around, its mother becomes increasingly aware of its presence within her body.

By the beginning of the third trimester, the fetus is approximately 10 inches long (from crown to rump) and weighs about 2 pounds. During this trimester, the fetus will nearly double in length and multiply its weight by three to four times. Thus, a healthy fetus usually weighs about 6 to 8 pounds and is 19 to 21 inches long by the time it is full-term and ready to be born.

Throughout the prenatal period, the embryo/fetus depends entirely on its mother for survival. During most of the pregnancy, the expectant mother nourishes her embryo/fetus through the **placenta,** the organ of pregnancy that connects the uterus to the embryo/fetus via the *umbilical cord* (see Fig. 13.1). The role of the placenta is to transfer nutrients and oxygen from the mother's bloodstream to the embryo/fetus. Additionally, the placenta transfers wastes from the embryo/fetus to the mother's bloodstream, so her body can eliminate them. Unfortunately, the placenta does not filter many microbes and toxic substances, such as alcohol and nicotine, from the mother's blood. Thus, agents of infection and harmful chemicals can pass through the placenta, enter the embryo/fetus, and cause disease, birth defects, or embryonic/fetal death.

A fetus generally needs to spend at least 37 weeks developing within the uterus to be physiologically mature enough to survive after birth without the need for special care. A fetus's weight depends on the supply of nutrients that it receives through the placenta.[3] If the placenta fails to grow properly, the developing fetus is likely to be born too soon and be lighter than average at birth.

Low-Birth-Weight and Preterm Newborns

Birth weight is a major factor that determines whether a baby is healthy and survives his or her first year of life. A **high-birth-weight (HBW)** baby weighs more than approximately 8.8 pounds at birth. A large baby is difficult to deliver vaginally and in many cases requires birth by *caesarian section* (C-section). A C-section involves surgical removal of the fetus from the mother's uterus.

Low-birth-weight (LBW) infants generally weigh less than 5½ pounds at birth. LBW is the leading cause of death among American infants who are less than 28 days of age.[4] In 2012, 8% of infants born in the United States were low birth weight.[5] Pregnant females who are under 15 years of age or 45 to 54 years of age are more likely to give birth to LBW infants than women in other age groups.[4] Additionally, women who smoke during pregnancy are at risk to have LBW babies.[6] Low birth weight is often associated with premature or preterm births. In 2012, 11.5% of births in the United States were preterm; that is, they occurred before the thirty-seventh week of pregnancy.[5]

Early preterm infants are born before 34 weeks of gestation.[7] In 2010, 3.5% of babies born in the United States were early preterm infants. Such infants are more likely to have serious health problems or die soon after birth than babies delivered after 34 weeks of pregnancy.[8] An early preterm infant who is born after about 26 weeks of pregnancy may survive if cared for in a hospital nursery for high–risk newborns (Fig. 13.2). However, the tiny infant's body will not have stores of fat and certain minerals that normally accumulate during the last month of pregnancy. Additionally, early preterm babies are likely to have conditions that complicate their medical care and food intake, such as breathing difficulties and weak sucking and swallowing abilities.

Nutrition-Related Signs of Pregnancy

During pregnancy, a woman's body undergoes major physiological changes, such as increased blood volume, breast size, and levels of several hormones. These adaptations enable her body to nourish and maintain the developing embryo/fetus, as well as produce milk for her infant after its birth. However, some of the physical changes cause discomfort for the pregnant woman.

In the first trimester, most women experience physical signs that they are pregnant, such as enlarged breasts and "morning sickness." Other common nutrition–related signs as well as complaints of pregnancy include extreme tiredness, swollen feet, constipation, and heartburn. In most cases, such discomforts do not create serious complications, and they resolve within a few months.

Breast Changes

During pregnancy, hormones signal the breasts to increase in size in preparation for lactation. The mother's pituitary gland in the brain produces **prolactin,** a hormone that stimulates the development of milk–producing tissue in the breasts. However, a pregnant woman's breasts do not form milk, because high levels of progesterone, a hormone that helps maintain pregnancy, inhibit milk production.[9] After birth, the level of progesterone drops rapidly, essentially removing the "brakes" from the breasts' ability to produce milk.

Morning Sickness

A common sign of pregnancy is **morning sickness,** nausea that is sometimes accompanied by vomiting. The name "morning sickness" is misleading because the queasy feeling can occur at any time of the day. The cause of this unpleasant condition is unclear, but it may be the result of the pregnant woman's body adapting to higher levels of female hormones. Additionally, emotional stress and certain foods can contribute to nausea. The condition generally begins early in the first trimester, and most women are no longer affected by the sixteenth week of pregnancy.[10] However, some women experience nausea and vomiting occasionally throughout their pregnancies.

To help control mild morning sickness, pregnant women can avoid odors and foods, such as fried or greasy foods, that trigger nausea. Some women find that eating crackers and drinking some water helps reduce the likelihood of feeling nauseated, especially before they get out of bed in the morning. Furthermore, eating smaller but more frequent meals and nutritious snacks can be helpful.

If the nausea and vomiting contribute to weight loss of more than 2 pounds, the pregnant woman should contact her physician for treatment. Morning sickness that persists beyond the fourth month of pregnancy should also be brought to the attention of a physician. During pregnancy, excessive vomiting is harmful because it can lead to dehydration and nutritional deficiencies.

Fatigue in Pregnancy

Early in pregnancy, the mother's blood volume expands to approximately 150% of normal. The number of red blood cells, however, increases by only 20 to 30%, and

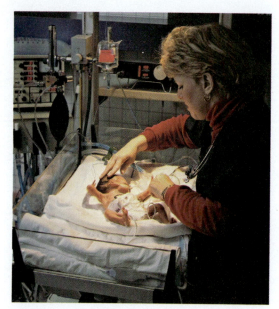

| Figure 13.2 **Early preterm infant.**

prolactin hormone that stimulates milk production after delivery

morning sickness nausea and vomiting associated with pregnancy

Did You Know?

In 2012, Kate Middleton, wife of Great Britian's Prince William, was hospitalized for 3 days because of excessive vomiting during early pregnancy. She recovered and gave birth to a healthy baby boy on July 22, 2013. In 2014, she experienced severe morning sickness with her second pregnancy.

this change occurs more gradually. As a result, the pregnant woman develops *physiological anemia*, a condition characterized by a lower concentration of red blood cells in the bloodstream. This form of anemia is a normal response to pregnancy, rather than the result of inadequate nutrient intake. Nevertheless, physiological anemia may be responsible for the extreme tiredness experienced by pregnant women during their first trimester. As their red blood cell numbers increase, expectant mothers report having more energy, especially during the second trimester. By the third trimester, however, most pregnant women are easily fatigued again, possibly because carrying a rapidly growing fetus is physically demanding.

What Is Edema?

High levels of certain hormones can cause various tissues to retain fluid during pregnancy. Although the extra fluid causes some minor swelling (edema), especially in the hands and feet, the condition is normal. In most cases, mild edema does not require treatment such as restricting salt intake or taking diuretics. Edema, however, can be a sign of trouble if hypertension and the appearance of extra protein in the urine accompany the swelling. The "Importance of Prenatal Care" section of this chapter discusses hypertension during pregnancy.

Digestive Tract Discomforts

During pregnancy, certain hormones produced by the placenta relax muscles of the digestive tract. As a result, intestinal movements slow down and digested material takes longer to pass through the tract, increasing the likelihood of constipation (see the "Fiber and Health" section of Chapter 5). To help prevent constipation, pregnant women should consume adequate amounts of fiber and fluids. During pregnancy, the Adequate Intake (AI) for fiber is 28 g/day, and the AI for total water is 3 L/day.[1] If constipation still persists after making these dietary changes, the pregnant woman should discuss this concern with her physician.

Heartburn is another common complaint of pregnant women. As the fetus grows, the uterus pushes upward in the mother's abdominal cavity and applies pressure on her stomach. When this occurs, stomach acid can enter the esophagus, causing heartburn (see the Chapter 4 "Nutrition Matters"). To help avoid heartburn, the pregnant woman can consume smaller meals, avoid lying down after eating, eat less fatty foods, and learn to identify and avoid foods that seem to contribute to heartburn. If heartburn continues to be bothersome, the woman should consult her physician and discuss other ways to treat the condition.

Pregnancy: General Dietary Recommendations

Ideally, women of childbearing age should take steps to ensure good health before becoming pregnant. For example, women can analyze the nutritional adequacy of their diets and choose to eat foods that correct any marginal or deficient intakes. Prior to pregnancy, sedentary women can begin an exercise regimen; overweight or obese women can lose some excess weight; and women who smoke can join smoking cessation programs. The time to remedy faulty lifestyle practices and increase chances of having a healthy pregnancy and baby is long before pregnancy occurs.

During pregnancy, the mother-to-be should follow a diet that meets her own nutritional needs as well as those of her developing offspring. Depending on the trimester, an expectant woman's requirements for energy (calories), protein, and many other nutrients are greater than her needs prior to pregnancy. Nevertheless, a pregnant woman does not need to double her usual food intake just because she is "eating for two." Table 13.1 compares Recommended Dietary Allowances (RDAs) for energy and selected nutrients that apply to healthy 25-year-old nonpregnant and pregnant women.

TABLE 13.1 Comparing Selected DRIs: 25-Year-Old Nonpregnant and Pregnant Women

Energy/Nutrient*	Nonpregnant	Pregnant
Kilocalories	Estimated Energy Requirement (EER)	First Trimester = EER + 0
		Second Trimester = EER + 340
		Third Trimester = EER + 452
Protein	46 g/day	71 g/day
Vitamin C	75 mg/day	85 mg/day
Thiamin	1.1 mg/day	1.4 mg/day
Niacin	14 mg/day	18 mg/day
Folate	400 mcg/day	600 mcg/day
Vitamin D	15 mcg/day	15 mcg/day
Calcium	1000 mg/day	1000 mg/day
Iron	18 mg/day	27 mg/day
Iodine	150 mcg/day	220 mcg/day

* RDA

Source: Data from Institute of Medicine: *Dietary Reference Intakes.*

TABLE 13.2 Sample Menu for a 25-Year-Old Pregnant Woman (Second Trimester)

Breakfast
¾ cup cooked oatmeal, made with ½ cup fat-free milk and sprinkled with ¼ cup raisins
½ cup calcium-fortified orange juice
Mid-morning snack
½ cup calcium-fortified orange juice
1 rectangular graham cracker
2 Tbsp peanut butter
Lunch
Cheese sandwich
2 slices whole-grain bread
1 slice American cheese
2 slices tomato
¼ cup leaf lettuce
2 tsp mayonnaise-type low-calorie salad dressing
1 cup apple slices
1 cup fat-free milk
½ cup orange sherbet
Mid-afternoon snack
1 whole-grain English muffin, toasted
1 Tbsp soft margarine
2 tsp jelly
½ cup fat-free milk
Dinner
Broiled salmon filet, 5 oz
1¼ cups mixed salad greens
1 Tbsp low-calorie Italian dressing
½ cup enriched white rice
1 cup steamed broccoli
2 small dinner rolls
1 Tbsp soft margarine
Evening snack
1 cup frozen yogurt

Energy Needs

In the first trimester, a pregnant woman's daily energy requirement (*Estimated Energy Requirement* or *EER*) is essentially the same as a nonpregnant woman's, because the embryo/fetus is quite small (see Table 13.1). However, the fetus grows rapidly during the second and third trimesters, and the pregnant woman requires more energy and nutrients to support its growth as well as her own body's needs. During the second trimester, the expectant mother should consume approximately 340 more kilocalories per day than her prepregnancy EER. Throughout the third trimester, she should add about 450 kcal per day to her prepregnancy EER (see Table 13.1). If a woman is physically active during her pregnancy, she may need to increase her kilocalorie intake by even more than these levels. Why? As the pregnant woman gains weight, her muscles require more energy to move her body. The average expectant mother, however, reduces her physical activity level during the third trimester, conserving energy.

Folate and Iron Needs

A pregnant woman's requirements for folate and iron are 50% higher than those of a nonpregnant woman. It is important for women to enter pregnancy with adequate folate status, because embryos need the vitamin to support rapid cell division. As discussed in Chapter 8, pregnant women who are folate deficient have high risk of giving birth to infants with neural tube defects, such as spina bifida (see Fig. 8.25). To obtain adequate folate, women of childbearing age as well as pregnant women should include rich food sources of folate in their diets, such as green leafy vegetables, and take a vitamin/mineral supplement that supplies at least 400 mcg of *folic acid*, a form of folate.

As the pregnant woman's blood volume expands, her need for iron increases because her body must make more hemoglobin for the extra red blood cells. Additionally, the woman's body transfers iron to the fetus to build its stores of the mineral. If women fail to meet their iron needs during pregnancy, their iron stores can be severely depleted, and they can develop iron deficiency anemia. Pregnant women who are iron deficient have high risk of giving birth prematurely and having low-birth-weight infants.[11]

Even when their diets include good sources of iron such as red meats and enriched cereals, pregnant women often need a supplemental source of iron. Thus, most physicians recommend special prenatal multiple vitamin/mineral supplements that contain iron for their pregnant patients.

Menu Planning for Pregnant Women

Rather than view pregnancy as a time to splurge by eating energy-dense empty-calorie foods, the mother-to-be should obtain the extra calories from nutrient-dense foods. For example, drinking an additional cup of fat-free milk, eating a bowl of an enriched whole-grain cereal, and taking a prenatal supplement each day can supply extra kilocalories as well as protein, fiber, and micronutrients. Table 13.2 presents a day's meals and snacks for a sedentary 25-year-old woman who is in her second trimester of pregnancy. Her prepregnancy EER was 2000 kcal, so her sample menu is based on MyPlate recommendations for 2400 kcal, enough to cover her increased EER during this trimester.

Is Fish Safe to Eat During Pregnancy? Fish and shellfish (e.g., clams, shrimp, and crabs) are excellent sources of many minerals, omega-3 fatty acids, and high-quality protein. However, most fish and shellfish contain very small amounts of methylmercury, a compound that contains the toxic mineral mercury.[12] Certain kinds of fish and shellfish, however, contain higher levels of methylmercury than others. When a pregnant woman eats these foods, the methylmercury in them can eventually reach the developing fetus and damage its nervous system. Chapter 3 provides recommendations for safe levels of fish consumption by pregnant women.

What About Cravings?

The stereotype of a pregnant woman who craves pickles and ice cream is not simply a myth. Cravings are common during this stage of life. However, ask pregnant women to identify the foods they crave, and you are likely to get a variety of responses. The causes of cravings are unknown, but they may be responses to the hormonal changes associated with pregnancy or to the emotional state of the mother-to-be. In other instances, specific food cravings may simply reflect the pregnant woman's family traditions. Unless food cravings contribute to excess weight gain, they are generally harmless.

Some women develop **pica,** the practice of eating nonfood items such as laundry starch, chalk, cigarette ashes, and soil. Some studies have linked pica with iron and zinc deficiency, but it is not clear if pica is the result or the cause of such deficiencies. Pregnant women should refrain from practicing pica, especially eating clay or soil. Soil may contain substances that interfere with the absorption of minerals in the intestinal tract. Furthermore, eating soil can be harmful because the dirt may be contaminated with toxic substances, such as lead and pesticides, and pathogenic microbes.

pica practice of eating nonfood items

Weight Gain During Pregnancy

Nearly all pregnant women experience weight gain. In fact, gaining an appropriate amount of weight is crucial during pregnancy. How much weight a woman should gain depends on her prepregnancy weight. Women who were underweight prior to pregnancy should gain 28 to 40 pounds; women whose prepregnancy weights were within the healthy range can expect to gain 25 to 35 pounds.[13] Women who were overweight before they became pregnant should gain 15 to 25 pounds, and obese women should gain 11 to 20 pounds during pregnancy. The recommendations are higher for women who are pregnant with more than one fetus. For example, a healthy woman who is carrying twins may gain as much as 54 pounds during pregnancy.[14]

In 2011, 48% of women in the United States gained more than the recommended amount of weight during pregnancy.[13] Women who gain excess weight during pregnancy are likely to retain the extra pounds long after their babies are born. Furthermore, expectant mothers who gain excessive amounts of weight are more likely to give birth to high-birth-weight (HBW) babies. When compared to newborns with healthy weights, HBW infants have higher risk of being injured during the birth process and of having birth defects. Furthermore, HBW infants are more likely to develop obesity, diabetes, and hypertension at some point in their lives.[15] In 2011, about 7% of babies born in the United States were HBW.[13]

Underweight women who do not gain enough weight during pregnancy are at risk of having preterm or low-birth-weight (LBW) infants. Underweight pregnant women should try to reach healthy weights by the end of the first trimester and then meet the recommended weight-gain goals. Obese women have a greater risk of developing hypertension as well as type 2 diabetes during pregnancy. Obese pregnant women are also at risk of giving birth to HBW babies.[15] However, women should not try to lose weight while they are pregnant because calorie restriction may harm the fetus.

TABLE 13.3 Distribution of Weight Gain During Pregnancy

Tissue	Approximate Pounds
Maternal	
Blood	3
Breasts	2
Uterus	2
Fat, protein, and retained fluid	11
Fetus	7.5
Placenta	1.5
*Amniotic fluid**	2.0

* Protective fluid that surrounds fetus.

Source: March of Dimes, *Your pregnant body.* 2009. http://www.marchofdimes.org/pregnancy/your-pregnant-body.aspx Accessed September 12, 2014

Figure 13.3 Rate of weight gain: Healthy pregnancy. This chart illustrates the rate of maternal weight gain that typically occurs during a healthy pregnancy.

Accounting for the Weight Gain

It is important to understand that much of the weight a woman gains during a healthy pregnancy is not body fat. By the end of a full–term pregnancy, the average fetus weighs about 7½ pounds, and the placenta and *amniotic fluid* that surrounds the fetus account for about 3½ pounds. The remaining weight is comprised of tissues and fluids the mother's body gains during pregnancy (*maternal weight* gain). Table 13.3 indicates the typical distribution of weight that is gained during this life stage.

Rate of Weight Gain

For an expectant mother, the rate of weight gain is important, as well as the amount of weight gained. Most pregnant women add up to 4 pounds of weight during the first trimester. Throughout the rest of their pregnancies, healthy women typically gain at a faster rate, 3 to 4 pounds *each* month. Figure 13.3 charts the course of weight gain in a healthy pregnancy. Note how the rate reaches a steady pace of about 1 pound/week during the second and third tri—mesters. During the second and third trimesters, recommended weight gains are higher for underweight women and lower for overweight or obese women.

The Importance of Prenatal Care

Ideally, women of childbearing age should plan for pregnancy and receive dietary advice before becoming pregnant. If this is not possible, *prenatal care* should begin early in pregnancy, because many medical problems that may occur during this life stage can be diagnosed and treated before the health of the mother or her fetus are threatened. **Prenatal care** is specialized to meet the health care needs of pregnant women. Routine prenatal health care includes measuring and monitoring the pregnant woman's weight, blood pressure, blood glucose level, and uterine growth. The prenatal health care provider may also discuss various con—cerns with the expectant mother, such as morning sickness, safe types of physical activity, what to expect during the birth process, and basic infant care skills. Additionally, the health care pro—vider can advise the pregnant woman to make appropriate lifestyle choices, such as avoiding the use of tobacco, alcohol, and illegal substances. Women who receive adequate prenatal care are more likely to have good pregnancy outcomes, including babies who have healthy birth weights, than women who do not receive such care.[16]

During pregnancy, it is important for a woman to decide whether she will breastfeed her baby. Pregnant women who decide to breastfeed their babies should inform their physicians and learn as much as they can about breastfeeding early in their pregnancy.

Gestational Diabetes

According to estimates, 2 to 10% of pregnant women in the United States develop type 2 diabetes during pregnancy (*gestational diabetes*).[17] When a woman has gestational diabetes, her fetus receives too much glucose and converts the excess into fat. Thus, women with this form of diabetes often give birth to HBW babies. After birth, these infants often have difficulty controlling their own blood glu—cose levels and are at risk of becoming overweight as children.

Gestational diabetes can be detected during routine prenatal care. For more information about diabetes during pregnancy, see Chapter 5.

prenatal care specialized health care for pregnant women

190.0

High blood pressure

Sudden weight gain

Protein in urine

Edema

Major signs of preeclampsia include sudden weight gain, elevated blood pressure, edema, and protein in urine.

Gestational Hypertension

Hypertension is a common complication of pregnancy. In the United States, 3 to 5% of pregnant women develop high blood pressure.[18] Rapid weight gain, especially after the fifth month of pregnancy, could be a sign **gestational hypertension** (formerly called "pregnancy–induced" hypertension). Approximately 15 to 25% of women with gestational hypertension develop a more severe form of the con–dition, called *preeclampsia* (*pre–e–klamp'–see–a*).[18] Preeclampsia is charac–terized by sudden, dramatic increase in weight that is due to edema, particularly of the hands, calves, and face; hypertension; and protein in urine.

Pregnant women who have high risk of preeclampsia are those who are under 20 or over 35 years of age, are obese, have a history of diabetes or hypertension, are African American, and are carrying more than one fetus.[18] If a woman suffering from preeclampsia develops convulsions, her condition is called *eclampsia* (*e–klamp'–see–a*). In the United States, eclampsia is the second leading cause of death among pregnant women.[19]

At present, the only effective treatment for preeclampsia and eclampsia is delivering the fetus, but infants born before the twenty–fourth week of preg–nancy are unlikely to survive. If the fetus is older than 24 weeks, its mother may be hospitalized for treatment. This practice helps physicians monitor the mother's condition and enables the fetus to mature until it has a better chance of surviving after a premature birth.

gestational hypertension type of hypertension that can develop during pregnancy

Drug Use

Exposure to alcohol and tobacco is harmful to the embryo/fetus. Women who drink alcohol during pregnancy are at risk of having a child with a fetal alcohol spectrum disorder such as FAS (see Fig. 6.27). Scientists do not know if there is a "safe" amount of alcohol that pregnant women can consume; therefore, women of childbearing age who are sexually active or pregnant should avoid alcoholic beverages. The Chapter 6 "Nutrition Matters" provides more information about fetal alcohol spectrum disorder.

Compared to pregnant women who do not smoke cigarettes, expectant mothers who smoke have higher risk of giving birth too early and having LBW babies. Furthermore, expectant mothers who smoke cigarettes may increase the risk of having babies with birth defects or that die of *sudden infant death syndrome* (*SIDS*). SIDS is the sudden, unexplained death of an infant younger than 1 year of age and the leading cause of death for babies between 1 month and 1 year of age.[20]

The use of illegal drugs, herbal supplements, and medications during pregnancy can also harm the embryo/fetus. Ideally, the time to quit abusing illegal drugs is before pregnancy. Pregnant women should consult their physicians before using herbal supplements or taking any drugs, even over-the-counter medications.

What About Physical Activity?

Women can derive many benefits from being physically active during pregnancy, including enhanced muscle tone and strength, reduced edema, and improved mood and sleep. Most pregnant women can continue their prepregnancy exercise regimens, especially those that included low- or moderate-intensity activities. However, the exercise routine should not result in weight loss. Recommended activities generally include walking, cycling, swimming, or light aerobics. Pregnancy is not the time to begin an intense fitness regimen or perform high-risk physical activities. Activities that are risky and should be avoided include downhill skiing; contact sports such as volleyball, soccer, and basketball; and horseback riding.[21] Pregnant women should discuss their physical activity practices and needs with their physicians. Some expectant women, such as those experiencing hypertension or premature labor contractions, may need to restrict their physical activity.

Most pregnant women can continue their prepregnancy exercise regimens, especially those that included low- or moderate-intensity activities.

Concept **Checkpoint 13.2**

3. When is an embryo referred to as a fetus?
4. What is the role of the placenta?
5. What is a major factor that determines whether a newborn baby is healthy and survives its first year of life?
6. Why is gestational hypertension dangerous?
7. Identify at least three different nutrition-related signs of pregnancy.
8. How much weight should a woman at a healthy weight gain during pregnancy; how much weight should she gain if she was underweight before becoming pregnant? How much weight should she gain if she was overweight or obese before pregnancy?
9. Why is having adequate folate and iron status important for pregnant women?
10. Discuss the harmful effects that a pregnant woman's alcohol consumption and cigarette smoking can have on her embryo/fetus.

13.3 Infant Nutrition

Learning Outcomes

1 Discuss the physiological processes of lactation and breastfeeding.

2 Discuss the nutrient and energy needs of a lactating woman.

3 Describe benefits that women derive from breastfeeding and infants derive from consuming their mother's milk.

4 Compare the energy and nutrient contents of human milk, cow's milk, and infant formulas.

5 Describe signs that an infant is ready to eat solid foods, and identify appropriate foods for infants.

6 Discuss a healthy infant's rate of growth.

(a)

Rapid physical growth characterizes infancy, the life stage that extends from birth to about 2 years of age. During the first 4 to 6 months of life, a healthy baby doubles its birth weight, and by 1 year of age, an infant's birth weight has tripled. Additionally, an infant's length increases by 50% during its first year of life. Thus, if a baby girl weighs 7 pounds and is 20 inches long at birth, you would expect her to weigh 21 pounds and be 30 inches long by her first birthday (Fig. 13.4).

Compared to older children, an infant needs more energy and nutrients per pound of body weight to support its rapid growth.[1] If an infant's diet lacks adequate energy and nutrients, the baby's growth may slow or even stop. The following sections take a closer look at infant nutrition, including breastfeeding and other infant feeding practices.

Breast Milk Is Best Milk

Two hundred years ago, if a new mother was unable to breastfeed her baby, the child faced certain death—unless a woman who was producing breast milk could be located to suckle (*nurse*) the infant. Today, a new mother can choose to nurse her baby or feed the child an **infant formula,** a synthetic food that simulates human milk. Although both foods provide adequate nutrition for young babies, breast—feeding provides benefits beyond nutrition for the new mother as well as her infant.

Human milk is uniquely formulated to meet the nutrient needs of a newborn baby. During the first couple of days after giving birth, the new mother's breasts produce **colostrum** (*co−loss'−trum*), a yellowish fluid that does not look like milk. (Some women report that colostrum leaked from their breasts late in the pregnancy.)[22] By the end of the first week of lactation, colostrum has undergone a transition to *mature milk*. If you compare the appearance of mature human milk to cow's milk, you will notice that breast milk is more watery than cow's milk and may have a slightly bluish color.

If they are unaware that colostrum is secreted by breasts soon after birth, women may think something is wrong with their ability to produce milk. How—ever, colostrum is a very important first food for babies, because the fluid contains antibodies and immune system cells that can be absorbed by the infant's immature digestive tract. Colostrum also contains a substance that encourages the growth of a type of bacteria, *Lactobacillus bifidus* (*L. bifidus*), in the infant's GI tract. Such biologically active substances help an infant's body fight infections and hasten the maturation of the baby's immune system. Thus, breastfed infants, especially those who are exclusively breastfed, have lower risks of allergies and gastrointestinal, respiratory, and ear infections than formula—fed infants.[23] Furthermore, breastfed babies are less likely to develop childhood asthma, leukemia, obesity, sudden infant death syndrome, and type 1 diabetes than infants who are not breastfed.

(b)

Figure 13.4 Growth rates during infancy. A healthy newborn baby (*a*) grows rapidly during its first year. During the first 4 to 6 months of life, a baby doubles its birth weight, and by 1 year of age, an infant's birth weight has tripled (*b*). Additionally, an infant's length increases by 50% during its first year of life.

infant formula synthetic food that simulates human milk

colostrum initial form of breast milk that contains anti-infective properties

American infants who are breastfed have a lower infant mortality rate than American babies who are not.

Human milk is a rich source of lipids, including cholesterol, and fatty acids such as linoleic acid, *arachidonic acid (AA)*, and *docosahexaenoic acid (DHA)*. An infant's nervous system, especially the brain and eyes, depends on AA and DHA for proper development. Furthermore, the fat in breast milk helps supply the energy needed to maintain the infant's overall growth.

The practice of breastfeeding also provides some important advantages for parents, particularly the new mother. Breastfeeding is more convenient and economical than using infant formula. Human milk is readily available; there is no need to purchase cans of infant formula and have them on hand. As milk leaves the breast, it is always fresh, free of bacteria, and ready to feed without mixing, bottling, or warming. Because human milk production requires a considerable amount of energy, lactating women can lose the extra body fat gained during pregnancy faster than mothers who use infant formula. Additionally, women who breastfeed their babies have lower risks of breast cancer (before menopause) and ovarian cancer than women who do not breastfeed. Some of these benefits depend on whether a woman breastfeeds exclusively, that is, provides no other foods, and the number of months the mother nurses her infant. Table 13.4 lists these and several other advantages of breastfeeding.

The Milk Production Process: Lactation

When an infant suckles, nerves in the mother's nipple signal her brain to release prolactin and **oxytocin** (*ox—e—tose'—in*) into her bloodstream. Prolactin stimulates specialized cells in breasts to form milk. These cells carry out the lactation process by synthesizing some nutrients and removing others from the mother's bloodstream and adding them to her milk. Oxytocin plays a different role in establishing successful lactation. This hormone signals breast tissue to "let down" milk. The *let—down reflex* enables milk to travel in several tubes (ducts) to the nipple area. A reflex is a physical response that is automatic and not under conscious control. When let—down occurs, the infant removes the milk by continued sucking (Fig. 13.5). Shortly before the flow of milk begins, the lactating woman often feels a tingling sensation in her nipples, a signal that let—down is occurring.

oxytocin hormone that elicits the "let-down" response and causes the uterus to contract

TABLE 13.4 Advantages of Breastfeeding

Advantages for Infants
Human milk
• Is free of bacteria as it leaves the breast.
• Supplies antibodies and immune cells.
• Is easily digested.
• Reduces risk of food allergies, especially to proteins in infant formulas and cow's milk.
• Changes in composition over time to meet the changing needs of a growing infant.
• Contains zinc, iron, and other minerals in highly absorbable forms.
• Decreases risks of ear, intestinal, and respiratory infections.
• May reduce the risk of asthma, obesity, and type 1 diabetes in childhood.

Advantages for New Mothers
Breastfeeding
• Reduces uterine bleeding after delivery.
• Promotes shrinkage of the uterus to its prepregnancy size.
• Decreases the risk of breast cancer (before menopause) and ovarian cancer.
• May promote maternal weight loss.
• May enhance bonding with the infant.
• Is less expensive and more convenient than feeding infant formula.

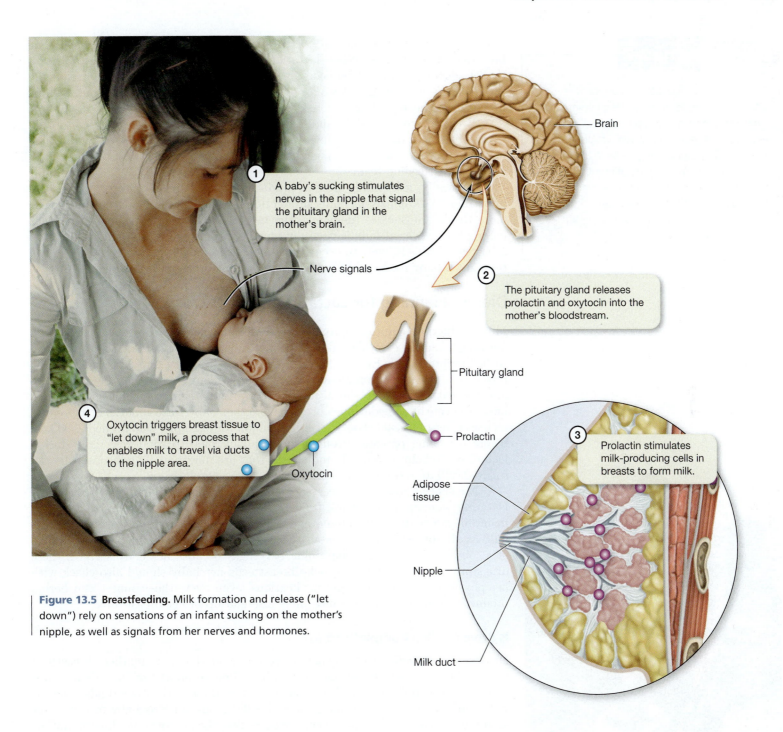

Figure 13.5 Breastfeeding. Milk formation and release ("let down") rely on sensations of an infant sucking on the mother's nipple, as well as signals from her nerves and hormones.

Embarrassment, emotional stress and tension, pain, and fatigue can easily block the let−down reflex. For example, if a lactating mother is tense or upset, let−down does not occur, and her infant will not be able to obtain milk when it suckles. When this happens, the hungry infant becomes frustrated and angry, and the mother may respond by becoming even more tense and upset, setting up a vicious cycle. At this point, new mothers often give up breastfeeding, reporting that they tried to suckle their babies but were unable to "produce" milk.

Lactating women need to be aware of the connection between their emo−tional state and failure to let down. To smooth the path to successful lactation, it helps if new mothers are in a comfortable, relaxed environment when they breastfeed their babies. When lactation and breastfeeding are well established, the let−down response often occurs without the need for suckling. For example, the mother's let−down reflex may be triggered just by thinking about nursing her infant or hearing it cry.

Breastfeeding is a skill, and like other skills, it takes some practice to fully master. Thus, it may take a few weeks for the new mother to feel comfortable with the process. By persevering, she and her baby are likely to become a suc−cessful breastfeeding team.

Typically, a lactating woman produces over 3 cups of milk per day.[9] It is important to recognize that milk production relies on "supply and demand." The more the infant suckles (demand), the more milk its mother's breasts produce (supply). However, if milk is not fully removed from the breasts, milk production soon ceases. This is likely to occur when infants are not hungry because they have been given baby food and formula to supplement breast milk feedings.

Dietary Planning for Lactating Women

Milk production requires approximately 800 kcal every day. However, the lactat−ing woman's daily energy needs can be met by adding only about 300 to 400 kcal to her prepregnancy EER. The difference between the energy needed for milk production and the recommended energy intake can enable the new mother to lose the extra body fat she accumulated during pregnancy. This loss is more likely to occur if she continues breastfeeding her baby for 6 months or more and increases her physical activity level. A woman, for example, who needed 2000 kcal before becoming pregnant would require about 2300 to 2400 kcal daily during lactation. To help plan meals and snacks that are nutritionally adequate, she can follow MyPlate recommendations at www.choosemyplate.gov.

No special foods are necessary to sustain milk production. However, a lactating woman should drink fluids every time her infant suckles to help her maintain adequate milk volume and keep her body properly hydrated. For as long as she breastfeeds her baby, the lactating mother should limit her intake of alcohol− and caffeine−containing beverages because her body secretes these drugs into her milk. A woman who breastfeeds her baby should also check with her physician before using any medications, even over−the−counter and herbal products, because such substances may also end up in her breast milk.

Is Breast Milk a Complete Food?

Dietitians and pediatricians generally recommend that new mothers breastfeed their infants exclusively during their babies' first 6 months of life.[23,25] It is not necessary to supplement healthy young infants' diets with other fluids, such as water, infant formula, and juices, or with solid foods, such as baby food.[25] After an infant reaches 6 months of age, breastfeeding should continue, but the infant can also be offered some appropriate solid foods. Breastfeeding may be combined with infant foods until the child's first birthday. However, there is no reason why children cannot be breastfed for longer periods. Throughout the world, many mothers continue to nurse their babies well past the babies' first birthdays, but in the United States, this practice is uncommon.

Although breast milk is highly nutritious, it is not a complete food for all infants. Human milk may contain inadequate amounts of vitamins D and B−12, and the minerals iron and fluoride. The American Academy of Pediatrics (AAP) recommends all breastfed infants be given a supplement that supplies 400 IU of vitamin D per day until they are consuming that amount of the vita−min from food or infant formula. Exposing the infant to some sun can also help meet part of the child's vitamin D needs (Fig. 13.6). If a lactating woman is a

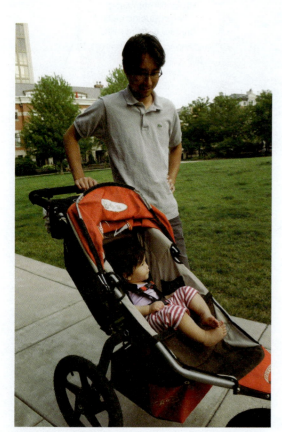

Figure 13.6 Vitamin D and infants. Exposing an infant's skin to some direct sunlight enables the baby's body to form vitamin D.

total vegetarian and she does not consume a source of vitamin B–12, she should consult her physician concerning the need for vitamin B–12 supplementation. When breastfed infants are about 6 months old, they should also be consuming some iron–containing solid foods, because the amount of iron in their mother's milk may no longer meet their needs. Furthermore, a fluoride supplement may be necessary for breastfed babies. Before giving any dietary supplements to their baby, parents or caregivers should discuss their infant's nutritional needs with the child's physician.

Quitting Too Soon

Nearly all healthy women are physically capable of breastfeeding their infants. In 2011, 79.2% of American women started breastfeeding their babies soon after birth.[26] Within 2 days of birth, 19.4% of the breastfed babies were also consuming formula. By the time the infants were 6 months old, 49.4% continued to be breastfed. By their first birthday, only about 27% of the babies were still being nourished with their mother's milk.

Women who breastfeed their newborns often stop the practice within 6 months. There are many reasons why women discontinue nursing their infants too soon. New mothers often quit because they lack information about and support for breastfeeding their babies. Some women discontinue breastfeeding because of uncertainty over how much milk their babies are consuming. Baby bottles are marked to indicate ounces, so a mother who bottle–feeds her infant can easily measure the amount of formula consumed. A lactating mother, however, has to observe her baby for cues indicating the child is full. When a breast–feeding baby is no longer interested in nursing and stops, its mother has to assume the infant is satisfied with the feeding. A well–nourished breastfed infant will gain weight normally and generally have six or more wet diapers as well as one or two soft bowel movements per day. Parents or caregivers who are concerned about their infants' food intake or nutritional status should consult their physician immediately.

Many new mothers discontinue breastfeeding before their babies are 6 months old because they need to return to work and have caregivers feed their babies. Although lactating women can learn to express milk from their breasts and preserve it for later feedings, many workplaces do not have comfortable, private facilities for women to express milk and then store it safely.

To enhance the likelihood that a nursing mother continues to breastfeed, it is helpful to enlist the support of a female relative or friend who has successfully breastfed her children. Furthermore, the woman's partner needs to understand and appreciate the function of the human breast as a source of nearly perfect nourishment for infants. New mothers are unlikely to begin and continue nursing their babies without their partners' support. La Leche League is an international organization dedicated to providing education and support for breastfeeding women (1–877–4–LALECHE or www.llli.org). Also, hospitals may employ lactation consultants or specialists. Lactation consultants are often nurses who are trained to provide information and advice about breastfeeding. For more information about breastfeeding, visit http://www.cdc.gov/breastfeeding/.

Infant Formula Feeding

Not every woman wants or is able to breastfeed her baby. Infant formulas are a safe and nutritionally adequate source of nutrients for babies who are not breastfed (Fig. 13.7). To produce artificial milk for babies, infant formula manufacturers alter cow's milk to improve its digestibility and nutrient content. Infant

This mother is using an electric device to express milk in a private room at her workplace. She will chill the milk and give it to her baby's caregiver for bottle-feeding.

Figure 13.7 Infant formulas. Infant formulas provide a safe and nutritionally adequate source of nutrients for babies who are not breastfed.

casein major protein in cow's milk

formulas generally contain heat—treated proteins from cow's milk, lactose and/or sucrose, and vegetable oil. Infant formulas generally lack cholesterol, but some of these products have the fatty acids DHA and AA added to them. Vitamins and minerals are added to the product, and in some instances, infant formula contains higher levels of micronutrients than human milk. Although infant formulas mimic the water, macronutrient, and micronutrient content of human milk, their compositions are not identical to human milk (Table 13.5). Formula manufacturers have been unable to duplicate human antibodies and other unique immune system factors that are in breast milk.

An interesting feature of human milk is that its fat content changes during each feeding, which usually lasts about 20 minutes. In the beginning of the session, the mother's milk is low in fat, but as her infant continues to suckle, the fat content of her milk gradually increases.[27] The higher fat content of the "hind milk" may make the baby feel satisfied and, as a result, discontinue feeding. Infant formulas, however, have uniform composition; that is, they do not change their fat content during a feeding session. Thus, the mother or infant caregiver is more likely to control the amount of formula the baby consumes, possibly leading to overfeeding. Nevertheless, the overall energy content of human milk is about the same as that of infant formulas (about 20 kcal per ounce).

Experts with the AAP recommend that caregivers provide an iron—fortified infant formula for babies who are not breastfed. Not all infant formulas contain iron, so it is important to read the product's label before purchasing it. Formula—fed babies may also need a source of fluoride, but caregivers should check with their infants' physicians before providing a supplement containing the mineral. For babies who are allergic to infant formulas made from cow's milk proteins, similar products made with soy or other proteins are available.

What About Cow's Milk?

Why not feed fresh fluid cow's milk to an infant? Cow's milk is too high in minerals and protein and does not contain enough carbohydrate to meet an infant's nutrient needs (see Table 13.5). In addition, infants have more difficulty digesting **casein** (*kay'—seen*), the major protein in cow's milk, than the major proteins in human

TABLE 13.5 Comparing Approximate Compositions of Human Milk, Cow's Milk, and Iron-Fortified Infant Formulas (per Ounce)

Milk or Iron-Fortified Formula	Energy (kcal/oz)	Protein (g/oz)	Carbo-hydrate (g/oz)	Fat (g/oz)	Choles-terol (mg/oz)	Iron (mg/oz)	Calcium (mg/oz)
Human milk	22.0	0.32	2.12	1.35	4.00	0.01	10.0
Cow's milk, whole	19.0	0.96	1.46	0.99	3.00	0.01	34.0
Cow's milk, fat-free	10.0	1.03	1.52	0.02	1.00	0.01	37.0
Cow's milk protein-based formulas							
Similac with iron	20.0	0.41	2.10	1.08	1.00	0.36	16.0
Enfamil with iron	19.0	0.42	2.19	1.07	0.00	0.36	16.0
Soy protein-based formulas							
ProSobee with iron	19.0	0.50	1.86	1.07	0.00	0.36	21.0
Similac Isomil with iron	20.0	0.49	2.04	1.09	0.00	0.36	21.0

Source: Data from U.S. Department of Agriculture, Agricultural Research Service. What's in the foods you eat *search tool, 5.0.* http://www.ars.usda.gov/services/docs.htm?docid=17032 Accessed February 20, 2014 milk. Cow's milk can also contribute to intestinal bleeding and iron deficiency.[28] Thus, whole cow's milk should not be fed to infants until they are 1 year of age.[29]

Whole milk is major source of saturated fat in young children's diets. According to the AAP, reduced–fat forms of milk can be given to children who are between 1 and 2 years of age, but only as part of a diet that supplies 30% of total calories from fat.[29] To reduce the risk of developing cardiovascular disease later in life, children over age 2 years should consume low–fat or fat–free dairy products.[29]

Allergies   Allergies are immune system responses to the presence of foreign proteins in the body. Allergies to proteins in foods, especially cow's milk proteins, often begin in infancy and may persist through childhood. Signs and symptoms of food allergies typically include the following:

• Vomiting, diarrhea, intestinal gas and pain, bloating, or constipation

• Itchy, swollen, or reddened skin

• Runny nose and breathing difficulties, such as asthma

Compared to breastfed infants, formula–fed babies have a greater risk of food allergies. When a woman has a personal or family history of food allergies, she may be able to prevent her children from developing such allergies if she breastfeeds her babies exclusively for 6 months. Infants rarely develop allergic reactions to food proteins that enter breast milk from the mother's bloodstream.

Introducing Solid Foods

Before 6 months of age, babies' nutritional needs can generally be met with human milk and/or infant formula. Solid ("complementary" or "baby") foods should not be introduced to infants until they are about 6 months of age.[30] At this age, many infants need the additional calories supplied by solid foods. Breastfed babies may also need a dietary source of iron, because their stores of the mineral are usually exhausted about 6 months after birth. Nevertheless, caregivers should continue to provide human milk or iron–fortified infant formula as the foundation of the baby's diet for the first year.

Many new parents are anxious to start feeding their young infants solid food. However, babies are not physically mature enough to consume solids before they are 4 to 6 months of age. For example, a baby's kidney functions are quite limited until the child is about 4 to 6 weeks of age. Additionally, an infant's digestive tract cannot readily digest starch before the child is about 3 months old.

Infants are born with the **extrusion reflex,** an involuntary response that occurs when a solid or semisolid object is placed in an infant's mouth. As a result of this reflex, a young baby thrusts its tongue forward, pushing the object out of its mouth. Thus, trying to feed the infant solid foods is a messy, frustrating process, as the child automatically pushes the food out of its mouth. Liquid foods, such as breast milk or infant formula, do not elicit the extrusion reflex, so the baby swallows fluids.

As the infant reaches 4 to 6 months of age, the extrusion reflex disappears, and the child has developed the physiological abilities to digest, metabolize, and excrete a wider range of foods. Moreover, a 6–month–old infant can usually sit up with back support and coordinate muscular control over his or her mouth and neck movements. These signs indicate the baby is ready physically to eat solid foods, is less likely to choke on such foods, and can turn his or her head away from food when full.

Weaning is the gradual process of shifting an infant from breastfeeding or bottle–feeding to drinking from a cup and eating solid foods. Pediatricians often

Food & Nutrition tip

Do not heat infant formula or human milk in a microwave oven. The heat can destroy immune factors in human milk and create hot spots that can scald an infant's tongue.

extrusion reflex involuntary response in which a young infant thrusts its tongue forward when a solid or semisolid object is placed in its mouth

weaning gradual process of shifting from breastfeeding or bottle-feeding to drinking from a cup and eating solid foods

Did You Know?

Many parents think adding solid foods to infants' diets helps babies sleep through the night. Actually, this developmental milestone generally occurs around 3 to 4 months of age, regardless of what infants are eating.

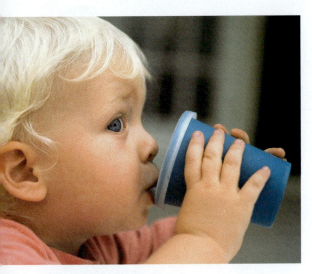

| Figure 13.8 **Learning to drink from a 'sippy' cup.**

| Babies need to practice self-feeding skills, even if it means playing with food and creating messes.

recommend introducing an iron–fortified infant cereal made from rice as the first solid food. However, pureed meat or chicken are better sources of iron for babies. After feeding the infant a solid food for the first time, caregivers should offer the food to the baby for at least 5 days and observe the infant for signs and symptoms of food allergy. If the infant appears to tolerate the food, caregivers can add a new food to the baby's diet, such as another type of meat or a cooked, strained vegetable. As each new food is introduced, caregivers should wait 3 to 5 days before adding a different food to the child's diet.[30] If the infant develops diarrhea, vomiting, or a rash during this period, he or she may be allergic to the new food.

It is a good idea to avoid giving mixed foods such as casseroles or commercially prepared baby food "dinners" to infants. If the baby has an allergic response after eating a food mixture, it will be difficult to determine which ingredient was responsible. Serving mixed foods is acceptable when the child has eaten each ingredient individually without having an allergic response.

Infants who have a high risk of food allergy have a parent or sibling who has a history of allergies, including food allergy. Foods that are associated with allergic responses in infants include egg whites, chocolate, nuts, and cow's milk. Therefore, caregivers should not offer these foods to high–risk babies under 6 months of age. Many babies outgrow food allergies during childhood, but some children remain allergic to the foods through adulthood.

Many varieties of strained baby food are available at the supermarket. Single–food items, such as carrots or peas, are more nutrient–dense choices for feeding infants than mixed dinners and desserts. Most brands have no added salt, but some fruit desserts contain a lot of added sugar. As an alternative, caregivers can prepare their own baby food by taking plain, unseasoned cooked foods and pureeing them in a blender. If a large amount of the item is blended, the pureed food can be poured into an ice cube tray, covered with a plastic bag, and frozen. When it is feeding time, an ice cube portion of the baby food can be popped out of the tray and warmed.

At about 6 to 8 months of age, the baby's first set of teeth, the "primary teeth," begin to appear. These teeth are important for proper nutrition because they help the child bite and chew food. By 8 to 12 months of age, most infants can use their fingers to pick up and chew "finger foods" such as crackers, toast, and cooked string beans. Babies can also hold a bottle and practice drinking from a special cup ("sippy cup") that has a lid with a spout (Fig. 13.8). Babies need to practice self–feeding skills, even if it means playing with food and creating messes. By about 10 months of age, many infants are mastering self–feeding and making the transition from baby foods to menu items that the rest of the family enjoys.

What Not to Feed an Infant

By the end of the first year, an infant should be consuming many different foods—grain products, meats, fruits, and vegetables—along with breast milk or infant formula. Introducing a baby to various foods helps the child learn about different tastes, odors, and textures. However, certain foods and beverages are not appropriate for infants. Avoid feeding an infant these things:

- **Honey.** This product may contain spores of *Clostridium botulinum* that can produce a potentially fatal toxin in children who are under 1 year old (see Chapter 12).

- **Excessive infant formula or human milk.** Depending on their age, most infants need less than 30 ounces of human milk or infant formula daily. A

When feeding solid foods to an infant:

• Use a baby-sized spoon—a small spoon with a broad handle.

• Hold the infant comfortably on your lap, as for breastfeeding or bottle-feeding, but in a more upright position to ease swallowing.

• Add some breast milk or infant formula to the cereal, and place a small dab of the semisolid food on the spoon's tip. Gently place the spoon on the infant's tongue and tilt it so the food slides onto the tongue. If the infant spits it out, do not continue with the feeding.

• Expect the infant to take only two or three bites during these early feeding sessions.

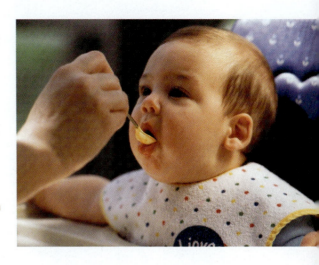

child who drinks too much milk may not eat enough solid foods that contain nutrients lacking in milk.

• **Semisolid baby cereal in a baby bottle that has the nipple opening enlarged.** This practice contributes to overfeeding and does not help the child learn self–feeding skills.

• **Candy, flavored gelatin water, or soft drinks.** These items provide few micronutrients.

• **Small pieces of hard or coarse foods.** Foods such as hot dogs (unless finely cut into sticks, not coin shapes), whole nuts, grapes, chunks of cooked meat, raw carrots, popcorn, and peanut butter can cause choking. Caregivers should supervise meals to keep young children from stuffing too much food in their mouths.

• **Excessive amounts of apple or pear juice.** The fructose and *sorbitol*, a sugar alcohol, contained in these juices can lead to diarrhea. Also, if the infant drinks fruit juice or fruit drinks rather than breast milk or infant formula, the child may not be receiving adequate amounts of calcium and other essential minerals.

• **Unpasteurized (raw) milk.** Raw milk may be contaminated with bacteria or viruses.

• **Goat's milk.** Goat's milk is low in iron, folate, and vitamins C and D.

Baby Bottle Caries

At bedtime, many caregivers place infants in their cribs with a baby bottle contain–ing formula, juice, or a sugar–sweetened drink. This practice is not recommended, because the sleepy infant sucks slowly, allowing the carbohydrate–containing fluid to bathe the child's teeth and provide a source of nutrients for bacteria that stick to teeth. These bacteria produce acids that dissolve tooth enamel, causing cavities to form in the teeth (*dental caries*). Dentists often refer to this condition as "baby bottle caries." To reduce the risk of baby bottle caries, infants should be given only water in their bedtime bottles.

Concept **Checkpoint 13.3**

11. What is the "let-down reflex"?
12. How does lactation affect a new mother's energy needs?
13. What is colostrum, and why is it a valuable first food for breastfed babies?
14. Dietitians and other health experts recommend that infants be breastfed exclusively during their first _____ months of life.
15. List at least five benefits that infants derive from breastfeeding.
16. Identify at least three benefits that women derive from breastfeeding their babies.
17. Compare the energy, macronutrient, and calcium contents of an ounce of human milk with those of an ounce of cow's milk.
18. Identify at least three physiological indications that an infant is ready to eat solid foods.
19. How much should a healthy infant's weight increase during its first year of life?

13.4 The Preschool Years

Learning Outcomes

1 Identify some major nutrition-related health concerns facing American preschool children.

2 Summarize practical suggestions for encouraging healthy eating habits among preschool children.

3 Describe steps caregivers can take to improve the nutritional status of preschool children.

Figure 13.9 Age-appropriate portion sizes. Healthy young children should not be expected to eat adult-size portions of food. Each of these children is eating half a sandwich, a reasonable amount for their age.

Childhood can be divided into the preschool period (2 to 5 years of age), the school–age period (6 to 11 years of age), and adolescence (12 to 19 years of age). In this section, we focus on some major nutrition concerns of preschool children. The rapid growth rate that characterizes the first 12 months of life tapers off quickly during the preschool years and proceeds at a slow but steady rate until the end of childhood. If an average infant's growth rate did not slow down, he or she might weigh about 190 pounds and be about 5 feet, 7 inches tall by 3 years of age! However, the average 3–year–old weighs about 32 pounds and is about 3 feet in height.

The preferred growth standard for children who are 2 to 20 years of age is the *body mass index (BMI)–for–age*. The BMI–for–age is a number calculated from the child's height and weight. BMI charts for children are both sex– and age– specific (see Appendix F). An *overweight* child has a BMI– for–age that is at or above the 85th percentile and lower than the 95th percentile for children of the same age and sex.[31] An *obese* child has a BMI–for–age that is at or above the 95th percentile for children of the same age and sex.

TABLE 13.6 Preschool Children: Daily Food Plan Based on MyPlate Recommendations

Energy/Food Group	2 Years	3 to 5 Years
*Kilocalories**	1000	1400
Grains	3 oz	5 oz
Vegetables	1 cup	1½ cups
Fruits	1 cup	1½ cups
Dairy	2 cups	2½ cups
Protein foods	2 oz	4 oz

* Kilocalorie estimates are based on age and 30 to 60 minutes of physical activity.

Source: U.S. Department of Agriculture: *MyPlate*. www.choosemyplate.gov/myplate/index.aspx. Accessed July 26, 2014

As the growth rate slows after infancy, preschoolers' appetites decrease because they do not need as much food. Parents and other caregivers must recognize that a 3–year–old child should not be expected to eat as eagerly as he or she did as an infant. Furthermore, children do not have the stomach capacity to eat adult–size portions of foods (Fig. 13.9). When planning meals and snacks for children, caregivers should emphasize nutrient–dense foods, such as lean meats, low–fat dairy products, whole–grain cereals, fruits, nuts, and vegetables. Although many ready–to–eat cereals are sweetened with sugar, it is not necessary to eliminate such foods. Caregivers, however, should read product labels and choose varieties with less added sugar. Additionally, it is important to monitor children's intake of sweets, because sugary items can crowd out more nutritious foods from their diets. Table 13.6 presents a day's food group selections, based on MyPlate recommendations, that are appropriate for children who are 2 to 5 years of age.

Snacks

Snacking is not necessarily a bad habit, especially if snacks are nutrient dense and fit into the child's overall diet. Nutritious snacks can be offered at midmorning or midafternoon, when the child is likely to become hungry between meals. A healthy 4– or 5–year–old child can safely eat raw vegetables without fear of choking. Nutritious dips, such as the yogurt dip in this chapter's "Recipe for Healthy Living," may make raw vegetables more appealing to children. Table 13.7 lists some nutritious snacks that children tend to like.

Fostering Positive Eating Behaviors

Parents often refer to their preschool children as "picky eaters" because the youngsters do not eat everything offered to them. Furthermore, it is not unusual for children to have "food jags," periods in which they refuse to eat a food that they liked in the past or want to eat only a particular food, such as peanut butter and jelly sandwiches or cereal and milk. Picky eating and food jags may be expressions of a child's growing need for independence. Caregivers should avoid nagging, forcing, and bribing children to eat. Instead, caregivers can offer the children a variety of healthy foods each day and allow the youngsters to choose which items and how much to eat.

Many children, especially preschool children, resist eating new foods. The temperature, appearance, texture, and taste of a food influence whether children will sample it. For example, young children often reject lumpy or hot–temperature

TABLE 13.7 Nutritious Snacks

- Peanut butter spread on graham crackers
- Fruit smoothies (see Chapter 9 "Recipe for Healthy Living")
- Fruit salad (or cut-up fruit)
- Mini-pizzas (half an English muffin, topped with tomato sauce and mozzarella cheese, and heated in toaster oven or microwave oven)
- Plain, low-fat yogurt topped with granola or fresh fruit
- Peanuts, cashews, or sunflower seeds
- Cheese melted on whole-wheat crackers
- Dried fruit
- Trail mix
- Ready-to-eat cereal
- Vegetable sticks dipped in hummus

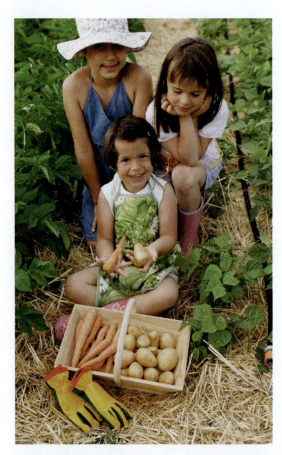

Eating vegetables may become more appealing when children help grow, select, or prepare fresh produce.

Food & Nutrition tips

• Foods with bright colors, crisp textures, and sweet or mild flavors usually appeal to children. When planning meals, consider including foods with these attractive characteristics.

• As a parent, you may want to consider having the "one bite policy." According to this policy, your child should try at least one bite of each new food provided at mealtimes.

• To stimulate your child's appetite, try serving food on a small colorful plate that is designed to appeal to young children.

• Keep in mind that you are your children's role model for food choices and physical activity habits. If you eat a variety of nutrient-dense foods and are physically active, your children are likely to eat such foods and be active as well.

foods. Sometimes children object to having foods mixed together such as in stews and casseroles, even though they like the ingredients when served separately. It is not unusual for young children to dislike vegetables that have strong flavors or odors, such as broccoli, onions, and asparagus. The idea of eating vegetables may become more appealing when children help grow, select, or prepare fresh produce. Nevertheless, it is important to recognize that everyone, including a child, is entitled to dislike certain foods.

The social atmosphere can make mealtimes enjoyable or unbearable, which in turn influences a child's desire to eat. Mealtimes should be happy, social occasions to enjoy healthful foods with parents or other caregivers. The kitchen table should not become a battleground in which adults use threats or bribes to force children to eat unfamiliar foods. For example, avoid telling a child, "You'll just sit there until you clean your plate" or "You can have a cupcake if you eat your peas." When a child refuses to eat, have the youngster remain at the table for a while. If the child continues to be disinterested in eating, remove the food and wait until the next scheduled meal or snack.

Healthy children are not in danger of starving if they skip a meal. A child who is not hungry at mealtimes may have eaten a snack before the meal at a friend's home. If a child's lack of appetite persists, caretakers should consult the child's physician to rule out illness.

Common Food-Related Concerns

Nutrition−related problems that often affect preschool children are iron deficiency, dental caries, food allergies, and obesity. Food allergies are dis−cussed in Chapter 7. Section 13.7 focuses on obesity during childhood and adolescence.

Iron Deficiency

Iron deficiency can lead to decreased physical stamina and learning ability, and resistance to infection. The best way to prevent iron deficiency in children is to provide foods that are good sources of iron, such as lean meat and enriched breads and cereals. Milk and other dairy products are poor sources of iron, so caregivers may need to limit daily servings of foods from this food group. Preschool children should consume 2 to 2.5 cups/day of fat−free or low−fat milk or equivalent dairy products.[32] Chapter 9 provides more information about iron deficiency.

Dental Caries

Many preschool children have had one or more dental caries by the time they enter school. If dental caries are not treated, jaw pain, gum infection, and tooth loss can occur. The following tips can help reduce the risk of dental caries in children:

• Brush teeth with a pea−sized amount of fluoride−containing toothpaste twice daily.

• Provide routine pediatric dental care and fluoridated drinking water.

• Any carbohydrate can contribute to dental caries, so reduce the number of snacks the child eats. Also, provide the child with more nutrient−dense snacks, such as raw fruits and vegetables or pieces of cheese.[33]

• If preschoolers want to chew gum, have them chew sugarless gum to reduce the risk of dental caries.[34]

13.5 School-Age Children

Learning Outcomes

1 Compare the typical eating patterns of school-age children with those of preschool children.

2 Identify some major nutrition-related health concerns facing American school-age children.

3 Summarize practical suggestions for encouraging healthy eating habits among school-age children.

Many school–age children adopt diets that are nutritionally inadequate.[35] Compared to preschoolers, older children often skip breakfast. Furthermore, school–age children typically consume more foods away from home and more fried items and sweetened beverages than younger children. Diets of school–age children tend to provide excessive amounts of solid fat, added sugars, and sodium.[35,36] Excessive intakes of fat and sugar contribute to the development of obesity, and high intake of sodium may contribute to hypertension among children.

School–age children often do not eat recommended amounts of fruits and vegetables, and the youngsters typically consume less than recommended amounts of dietary fiber. Low fiber intake contributes to constipation; as many as 10% of American children suffer from chronic constipation.[37]

Table 13.8 presents a day's food recommendations for healthy school–age children, based on MyPlate. The www.choosemyplate.gov website has a special

TABLE 13.8 Six- to 11-Year-Old Children: Daily Food Plan Based on MyPlate Recommendations

Energy/Food Group	Age/Sex 6 Years		Age 7–8 Years	Age/Sex 9 Years		Age 10–11 Years	
	Girls	Boys	Both	Girls	Boys	Girls	Boys
Kilocalories*	1400	1600	1600	1600	1800	1800	2000
Grains	5 oz	5 oz	5 oz	5 oz	6 oz	6 oz	6 oz
Vegetables	1.5 cups	2 cups	2 cups	2 cups	2.5 cups	2.5 cups	2.5 cups
Fruits	1.5 cups	1.5 cups	1.5 cups	1.5 cups	1.5 cups	1.5 cups	2 cups
Dairy	2.5 cups	2.5 cups	3 cups	3 cups	3 cups	3 cups	3 cups
Protein foods	4 oz	5 oz	5 oz	5 oz	5 oz	5 oz	5.5 oz

* Kilocalorie estimates are based on age, sex, and 30 to 60 minutes of physical activity.

Source: U.S. Department of Agriculture: ChooseMyPlate.gov: Supertracker & other tools: Daily food plans & worksheets. http://www.choosemyplate.gov/supertracker-tools/daily-food-plans.html Accessed February 23, 2014 series of web pages for children who are 6 to 11 years of age. Children can visit the "MyPlate Kids' Place" website and play the interactive "Blast Off Game." To test the game, visit http://www.choosemyplate.gov/kids/index.html.

Caregivers can help improve children's diets by encouraging youngsters to eat breakfast regularly. Children who routinely eat breakfast are more likely to have better diets and healthier body weights than children who skip this meal.[38] Breakfast menus do not need to feature traditional fare such as bacon, eggs, waffles, or pancakes. For example, leftovers from the previous night's dinner can be eaten for breakfast. Convenient "fast breakfasts" that school–age children can prepare quickly include ready–to–eat cereal with milk and fruit, cottage cheese and fruit, a peanut butter and jelly sandwich, or yogurt topped with trail mix or pieces of fresh fruit.

Parents and other caregivers need to be concerned about foods that are available at school and obtain answers to the following questions: What kinds of foods are offered for school breakfasts and lunches? Does the school have vend–ing machines accessible to youngsters? If so, what kinds of foods and beverages are sold from these machines? Do vending machines offer competitively priced, nutrient–dense foods? What can be done to ensure that the machines and the school's cafeteria provide nutritious foods that children will eat? Furthermore, what efforts are being made to teach children about proper nutrition while they are in school?

Food & Nutrition tips

The following tips can help you improve your child's diet:

- Guide your family's food choices instead of dictating what they eat.
- Eat meals together as a family as often as possible.
- If necessary, reduce the amount of fat, especially saturated and trans fat, in your family's diet.
- Do not place your child on a restrictive diet, unless the diet is recommended by the child's physician.
- Avoid using food as a reward or punishment.
- Encourage the child to drink water instead of sugar-sweetened beverages.
- Keep healthy snacks (such as fat-free or low-fat milk, fresh fruit, and vegetables) on hand.
- Serve at least 5 servings of fruits and vegetables each day.
- Discourage eating meals or snacks while watching TV.
- Encourage the child to eat a nutrient-dense breakfast daily.

Parents and other caregivers need to be concerned about their children's food choices.

Concept **Checkpoint 13.5**

23. Discuss how young children's eating patterns often change when they enter school.

24. List at least three tips for improving diets of school-age children.

13.6 Adolescence

adolescence life stage in which a child matures physically into an adult

Learning Outcomes

1 Discuss puberty and how it affects an adolescent's energy and nutrient needs.

2 Identify some major nutrition-related health concerns facing American adolescents.

Adolescence is the life stage in which a child matures physically into an adult. During adolescence, the reproductive organs increase in size and begin functioning properly. Furthermore, individuals typically attain their full height by the end of adolescence.[39] During this life stage, youth also develop emotionally, intellectually, and socially as they prepare for their adult roles.

Healthy adolescents learn to function independently of their adult caregivers. Thus, youths face a variety of lifestyle choices, including decisions regarding eating and physical activity habits. Such decisions often set the stage for the quality of their health in adulthood. For many teens, however, pressure to conform to fads and be influenced by other adolescents ("peer pressure") negatively affects their diets and overall health.

Puberty signals the end of childhood. Most boys begin puberty when they are between 10 and 12 years of age; most girls begin puberty between 8 and 10 years of age.[39] Puberty is a period characterized by dramatic physical changes, including increases in height and weight, known as the adolescent "growth spurt."

Most girls begin their growth spurt between 10 and 13 years of age. Boys begin their growth spurt later than girls—generally when they are between 12 and 15 years of age. Girls usually begin menstruating during their growth spurt. A girl's skeletal growth is almost complete about 2 years after her first menstrual period, whereas boys typically continue to gain stature until they are in their early twenties. The timing of puberty and growth spurts can vary widely, primarily due to genetic, environmental, and nutritional factors. Figure 13.10 shows a group of adolescents who are about the same age but are at different stages of physical maturity.

When their growth spurts begin, adolescents eat more to support their higher energy needs. If maturing boys and girls choose to eat nutritious foods and maintain a high level of physical activity, they can take advantage of their increased hunger and gain lean body mass without gaining excess body fat.

Did You Know?

Many teenagers are plagued by *acne*—pimples, blackheads, and reddening of the skin—that often occurs on the face, upper back, and chest. Many people think acne is caused by eating certain foods, especially greasy foods and chocolate. However, there is a lack of scientific evidence that links specific foods with acne. According to physicians who treat skin disorders (*dermatologists*), hormonal changes normally associated with puberty cause acne.[40]

Figure 13.10 Different rates of physical maturity. Although these adolescents are about the same age, they are in different stages of physical maturity.

Nutrition-Related Concerns of Adolescents

People generally establish their future eating habits and physical activity practices when they are teenagers. According to results of a nationwide survey, many youth are not following healthy diets. In 2013, 19% of the students had not consumed milk and 13% had skipped breakfast during the same period of time.[41] According to findings of this survey, only about 47% of the high school students met recommended levels of physical activity during the 7 days before the survey.

Adolescents whose diets rely heavily on energy–dense foods purchased at fast–food restaurants or vending machines may be setting the stage for the development of obesity, type 2 diabetes, heart disease, and other serious chronic diseases. Obesity, eating disorders, and low iron and calcium intakes are major nutrition–related concerns of adolescents. Youth, especially teenage girls, are at risk of developing disordered eating practices and eating disorders. You can learn more about eating disorders by reading the Chapter 10 "Nutrition Matters." In this chapter, Section 13.7 discusses adolescent obesity.

Iron and Calcium Intakes

Adolescent boys may become iron deficient during their growth spurt because their iron intakes do not keep up with their bodies' needs for the mineral. Adolescent girls are also at risk of iron deficiency, especially if their diets lack iron–rich foods and they have heavy menstrual blood losses. Iron deficiency leads to increased fatigue and decreased ability to concentrate and learn. Teenagers need to understand why iron is important for good health and incorporate reliable food sources of the mineral in their diets (see Chapter 9). Over the last 20 years, many adolescents have switched from drinking milk to drinking soft drinks. Dietitians and other nutrition experts are concerned that many adolescents have inadequate calcium intakes because of this practice. Inadequate calcium intake during adolescence is associated with decreased bone mass and increased likelihood of bone fractures later in life. To encourage youth to consume adequate amounts of calcium, parents or other caregivers should explain the importance of the mineral to bone health and provide calcium–rich foods and beverages during meals and snacks. Adolescents should consume 3 cups/day of fat–free or low–fat milk or equivalent dairy products. Furthermore, teenagers need to be aware that physical activity can strengthen bones, whereas smoking cigarettes is a risk factor for *osteoporosis*, a condition characterized by loss of bone density. To learn more about this condition, see the "Major Minerals" section of Chapter 9.

Vegetarianism

Some teenagers adopt vegetarian diets as a way of defining their identity and asserting independence from their caregivers. Although vegetarian diets can be healthy alternatives to the typical American diet, some youth use vegetarianism to mask disordered eating behaviors (see Chapter 10's "Nutrition Matters").[42] When planning their diets, teenage vegans need to include foods that supply adequate amounts of calcium, iron, and zinc, and vitamins D and B–12. For information to help plan well–balanced, nutritionally adequate diets, teens can use the recommendations of the MyPlate food guide that are appropriate for their age, sex, and physical activity level. Chapter 7 discusses vegetarianism in more detail.

Adolescents should consume 3 cups/day of fat-free or low-fat milk or equivalent dairy products.

Concept **Checkpoint 13.6**

25. At what age does the adolescent growth spurt usually occur in boys? At what age does the growth spurt generally occur in girls?

26. Why are intakes of iron and calcium important during adolescence?

13.7 Childhood Obesity

Learning Outcomes

1 Provide definitions for *overweight, obesity,* and *extreme obesity* in childhood and adolescence.

2 Identify health consequences of childhood obesity.

3 Discuss the prevalence of and factors that contribute to childhood obesity.

4 Discuss strategies for preventing and treating childhood obesity.

Over the past few decades, U.S. public health officials became concerned about the increasing prevalence of obesity among children and adolescents ("childhood obesity"). Approximately 17% of American children who are between the ages of 2 and 19 years are obese.[43] Between 1980 and 2008, the prevalence of obesity among American children who are between 6 and 19 has almost tripled (Fig. 13.11).[44] There is some good news: Obesity rates among low−income preschoolers are declining.[45] Nevertheless, more obese American children are classified as having extreme obesity than in the past.[46]

Defining Obesity in Children

Health care professionals use BMI−for−age charts that are available from the Centers of Disease Control and Prevention to determine children's and adolescents' weight status. The BMI for children is calculated in the same way as for adults, but BMIs for children are plotted on sex−specific growth charts (see Appendix F). Children and adolescents whose BMI−for−age is greater than or equal to (≥) the 85th percentile and less than (<) the 95th percentile are overweight, and youngsters who are at or above the 95th percentile are obese (Table 13.9). Although there is no generally accepted definition for extreme obesity that applies to children, BMI−for−age at or above the 97th percentile is typically used to identify children who have extreme obesity.[44]

Health Problems Associated with Childhood Obesity

Compared to children who have healthy body weights, obese children and adolescents are more likely to have elevated blood pressure, cholesterol, and glucose levels.[45] These chronic conditions are risk factors for cardiovascular disease (CVD). According to results of one study, 70% of obese children had at least one risk factor for CVD, and 39% of obese children had two or more risk factors.[31] Table 13.10 lists chronic health problems that obese children are more likely to have than children who have healthy body weights.

Many obese children and adolescents do not "grow out" of their excess body. Overweight or obese preschool−age children are five times as likely as preschool children who have healthy weights to be overweight or obese as adults.[45] Furthermore, overweight or obese children are more likely to be *extremely* obese when they are adults.[31]

Childhood Obesity: Contributing Factors

There is no single cause of excess body fat in children, but researchers have identified multiple factors that are associated with the development of the condition.[47] As in cases of adult obesity, the development of childhood obesity results

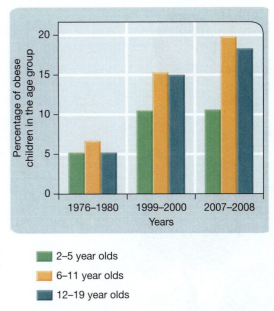

- **2–5 year olds**
- **6–11 year olds**
- **12–19 year olds**

Figure 13.11 Prevalence of obesity among American children aged 2 to 19 years, for selected years 1980 through 2008.

TABLE 13.9 Weight Status Classifications: Children and Adolescents (Ages 2 to 19)

Age	BMI-for-Age Percentile
Desirable weight	> 5th to < 85th
Overweight	≥ 85th to < 95th
Obese	≥ 95th
Extreme obesity*	≥ 97th

* No official definition

TABLE 13.10 Chronic Health Problems Associated with Childhood Obesity

- Impaired glucose tolerance, insulin resistance, and type 2 diabetes
- Breathing problems, including sleep apnea and asthma
- Musculoskeletal problems, including joint discomfort
- Fatty liver disease, gallstones, and gastroesophageal reflux (heartburn)
- Social and psychological problems, such as discrimination and poor self-esteem

Source of information: Centers for Disease Control and Prevention: Overweight and obesity: *Basics about childhood obesity.* Updated April 2012. http://www.cdc.gov/obesity/childhood/basics.html Accessed January 23, 2014

from complex interactions among multiple factors (see Chapter 10). The following sections examine the roles of genetic, biological, and environmental factors that contribute to childhood obesity.

Genetic and Other Biological Factors

Scientific evidence supports the role of inherited (genetic) and other biological factors in the development of childhood obesity, especially in cases of obesity that begin early in life.[48] Some of the biological factors that contribute to obesity include:[48]

- **Having overfat parents.** Children of overfat parents have a greater risk of obesity than children whose parents have healthy weights. If both parents are obese, the child has 10 times the risk of obesity as a child who has only one obese parent.

- **Having a mother who was overfat during pregnancy.** A mother's weight during pregnancy is a more important predictor of childhood obesity than the father's body weight. When compared to children whose mothers have a healthy body weight during pregnancy, babies born to overweight mothers are nearly three times as likely to be overweight. Furthermore, obese women are more likely than women who have healthy body weights to have large babies, and such infants have a high risk of childhood obesity.

- **Having a mother who gained too much weight and/or had diabetes during pregnancy.** Women who gain too much weight during pregnancy or have diabetes are more likely to give birth to high-birth-weight (HBW) babies. Such children are also at risk of developing excess body fat in childhood.

- **Having a mother who smoked during pregnancy.** Although the reasons are unclear, women who smoke during pregnancy set the stage for the future development of overweight and obesity in their babies.

- **Being undernourished during prenatal development.** Poor nutrition (undernutrition) during pregnancy contributes to delivery of a low-birth-weight (LBW) infant. Such infants are more likely to develop hypertension, CVD, and type 2 diabetes later in life, which are chronic diseases associated with obesity. At this point, scientists have been unable to explain why prenatal undernutrition contributes to hypertension, CVD, and type 2 in adulthood.

Biological factors, however, are not entirely responsible for the current obesity epidemic. In many cases, it is difficult to determine whether genes play a more important role than environmental factors in the development of childhood obesity. Is a child obese because the youngster inherited genes from his or her parents that "program" for obesity? Or is a child obese because his or her caregivers provide an excess of empty-calorie, energy-dense foods and do not encourage the child to be physically active?

Impact of the Child's Environment

In the United States, many children are exposed to an environment that encourages overeating and consumption of empty-calorie foods. Additionally, the environment often does not provide children with opportunities to participate in enough physical activity. Table 13.11 lists these and other environmental factors that contribute to childhood obesity. Public health measures to prevent obesity among children generally focus on modifying the environment.

Preventing Childhood Obesity

In 2010, the White House Task Force on Childhood Obesity published the report *Solving the Problem of Childhood Obesity Within a Generation.*[49] The task force report included recommendations to reduce the percentage of American children who are obese to 5% within the next 20 years. To download the entire report of the White House Task Force on Childhood Obesity, visit www.letsmove.gov/about .

Fostering Healthy Lifestyles

The Institute of Medicine developed a set of policy recommendations that may reduce the likelihood of obesity among preschool-age children.[51] Some of the institute's major recommendations focused on specific physical activity and dietary behaviors:

- New mothers should breastfeed their babies exclusively for the first 6 months of life and continue breastfeeding along with introducing appropriate foods after 6 months.

- Communities and child care providers should provide opportunities for children to be physically active throughout the day.

- Limit children's exposure to TV and forms of digital media ("screen time") to less than 2 hours per day.

    Specific steps that caregivers can take to help children achieve and maintain a body weight are listed in the "Food & Nutrition Tips" box on page 516.

Treating Childhood Obesity

The treatment goal for managing overweight and obese young children and adolescents is to slow the rate of weight gain without interfering with normal growth and physical development. This goal can be accomplished by balancing the calories children consume with the calories they use for physical activity and need for

Did You Know?

Let's Move! America's Move to Raise a Healthier Generation of Kids is a comprehensive national program that focuses on ways to prevent childhood obesity in the United States. Major components of the program include making healthier foods available in schools and increasing opportunities for children to be physically active.[50] To learn more about *Let's Move!,* visit http://www.letsmove.gov/.

TABLE 13.11 Environmental Factors That Contribute to Childhood Obesity

- Easy access to empty-calorie foods and drinks at or near schools
- Limited access to healthy and affordable foods, particularly in areas that have many convenience stores and fast-food restaurants
- Advertising of empty-calorie foods that targets youth
- Lack of set periods for daily physical activity in schools and safe places to be active in many communities
- Large portion sizes of foods sold from vending machines and in restaurants and grocery stores
- Excess exposure to television and other media
    - TV viewing and use of other digital media contribute to childhood obesity because the sedentary activities can reduce the time children spend being physically active.

Source: Centers for Disease Control and Prevention: *Overweight and obesity: A growing problem: What causes childhood obesity?* Last updated April 2013. http://www.cdc.gov/obesity/childhood/problem.html Accessed February 25, 2014 growth. Encouraging more physical activity, especially for sedentary children, is also recommended.

Caregivers should not place a child or youth on a weight reduction diet without consulting the child's physician.[52] For severely obese adolescents, treatment approaches that go beyond dietary changes and increased physical activity are often necessary. Such interventions may include prescription medication and weight loss surgery (see Chapter 10).

Bariatric Surgery for Youth

Bariatric (weight loss) surgery can improve the health of adolescents with extreme obesity.[53] According to a review of bariatric surgery outcomes in the United States, the surgeries are safe for adolescents. At this time, however, the adjustable gastric banding procedure has not been approved for use with patients who are under 18 years of age.

To qualify for bariatric surgery, an adolescent should have:

- extreme obesity (BMI>40);

- failed to lose weight after 6 months of trying to reduce his or her weight;

- attained his or her adult height (skeletal maturity), which is generally at 13 years of age for girls and 15 years of age for boys; and

- developed serious chronic conditions that are associated with obesity, such as type 2 diabetes or sleep apnea, which may improve after surgery.[53]

Regardless of one's age, bariatric surgery is a drastic measure to lose excess body weight and involves some risks. Thus, caregivers and health care providers should carefully determine whether an extremely obese adolescent is a suitable candidate for bariatric surgery. For example, is the adolescent emotionally ready to handle the surgery and make the necessary lifestyle changes to achieve good health and well-being after the procedure?

Concept **Checkpoint 13.7**

27. Define *overweight, obese,* and *extremely obese* for children as defined by the Centers for Disease Control and Prevention.
28. List at least three health consequences of childhood obesity.
29. List at least three factors that contribute to the development of childhood obesity.
30. What information is used to determine whether an obese adolescent qualifies for bariatric surgery?

13.8 Nutrition for Older Adults

Learning Outcomes

1 Explain the difference between life expectancy and life span.

2 Identify physiological changes that are associated with the normal aging process.

3 Discuss nutrient needs for older adults.

4 Identify nutrients that are often lacking in diets of older adults.

5 Discuss steps caregivers can take to improve nutrient intakes of older persons.

In 1900, the life expectancy of a baby born in the United States was only 47 years. **Life expectancy** is the length of time a person born in a specific year, such as 1900, can expect to live. One hundred years ago, the top three leading causes of death for Americans were pneumonia, influenza, and other infectious diseases. By 2011, life expectancy in the United States rose to almost 79 years.[54] Major factors that contributed to increased life expectancy during the past century include improved diets, housing conditions, and public sanitation, as well as advances in medicine.

According to the U.S. Census Bureau, 13.7% of the U.S. population were 65 years of age or older in 2012.[55] By 2060, government experts estimate that a little over 20% of Americans will be in this age group. Americans who are the "oldest old"—85 years of age or older—comprise one of the fastest-growing segments of the U.S. population. In 2000, 1.5% of Americans were in that age group. By 2010, 1.8% of the population were 85 years of age or older. By 2060, about 4.3% of Americans will be 85 years of age or older.[56]

Although more Americans are living longer than their ancestors, they are not necessarily living well. Chronic diseases are among the leading causes of death in the United States (see Figure 1.2). These diseases are associated with lifestyles that include smoking, eating a poor diet, and being physically inactive.[57]

George John Blum of St. Louis, Missouri, circa 1900. In 1900, the life expectancy of a baby born in the United States was only 47 years.

The Aging Process

The aging process begins at conception and is characterized by numerous predictable physical changes. By the time you are 65 years of age, you will have reached the final life stage, *older adulthood*. What causes people to age is unclear. Scientists who study the aging process have learned that cell structure and function inevitably decline with time, leading to many of the physiological changes shown in Table 13.12. Eventually, most cells lose the ability to regenerate their internal parts, and they die. As more and more cells in an organ die, the organ

life expectancy length of time an average person born in a specific year can expect to live

TABLE 13.12 Aging: Normal Physiological Changes

Body System	Changes
Digestive	Reduced saliva, gastric acid, and intrinsic factor secretion; increased heartburn and constipation
Skin, hair, and nails (integument)	Graying hair; drier skin and hair; skin loses elasticity and forms wrinkles; skin bruises easily
Musculoskeletal	Bone-forming cells become less active, resulting in bone loss that can lead to tooth loss and bones that fracture easily; fractures heal more slowly; joints become stiff and painful; muscle mass declines, resulting in loss of strength and stamina
Nervous	Decreased brain weight, reduced production of neurotransmitters, delayed transmission of nervous impulses, loss of short-term memory, and reduced sensory abilities (e.g., vision, hearing, smell, and taste)
Lymphatic (immune)	Reduced functioning resulting in increased vulnerability to cancer and infections
Circulatory	Hardening of the arteries, reduced cardiac output, increased risk of blood clots
Endocrine	Decreased production of reproductive, growth, and thyroid hormones
Respiratory	Reduced lung capacity, increased vulnerability to respiratory infections
Urinary	Increased loss of functional kidney cells, resulting in decreased blood filtration rate; loss of bladder control
Reproductive	Men: Decreased male hormone production and sperm count Women: Declining female hormone production, cessation of menstrual cycles, and loss of fertility

senescence declining organ functioning and increased vulnerability

life span maximum number of years an organism can live

loses its functional capacity, and as a result, other organs fail and body systems are adversely affected. When this happens, the person soon dies. **Senescence** (*se–ness'–enz*) refers to declining organ functioning and increased vulnerability to disease that occur after a person reaches physical maturity.

Extending the Human Life Span

Life span refers to the maximum number of years an organism such as a human can live. To date, a Frenchwoman, Jeanne Calment, had the longest documented human life span—122 years. Some scientists think the human life span can be lengthened considerably just by making certain dietary changes. This chapter's "Nutrition Matters" takes a closer look at the role of diet and longevity.

Growing old is a normal and natural process. Your body ages, regardless of dietary and other health–related practices you follow. Nevertheless, scientists have found a strong genetic component to human longevity. If you have ances– tors who are very old or lived to be 90 years of age or more, you may have inher– ited "longevity genes." If your ancestors were not so fortunate, to some extent, you can control the rate at which you age. How? By making responsible healthy lifestyle decisions while you are still young, such as selecting a nutritious diet, exercising regularly, and avoiding tobacco. Your focus should not be simply on living longer but on living longer *and* healthier.

Common Nutrition-Related Concerns

Compared to younger persons, older adults have greater risk of nutritional defi– ciencies because of physiological changes associated with the normal aging pro– cess. Other factors that can influence an older person's nutritional status include illnesses, medications, low income, and lack of social support.

Diets of older Americans, particularly older women, often provide inad– equate amounts of vitamins A, D, and B–12 and minerals, particularly calcium and potassium.[36] In the United States, fewer than half (41.8%) of older adults consume 2 or more servings of fruit each day, and less than a third (29.6%) of this population eats 3 or more servings of vegetables each day.[58] Furthermore, over 80% of people who are 71 years of age and older consume more empty calories than recommended.[59] Table 13.13 shows recommended amounts from

TABLE 13.13 What Americans 71 Years of Age and Older Eat Compared to USDA Recommendations

	Food Group				
	Fruit (cups)	Vegetables (cups)	Grains (oz. equivalents)	Dairy (cups)	Protein (oz. equivalents)
MyPlate Recommendations*					
Men (51 years of age and older)	2	2.5	6	3	5.5
Women (51 years of age and older)	1.5	2	5	3	5
Percentage of people who consumed recommended amount (estimated)					
Men	23	12	55	7	46
Women	34.5	13	53	3.6	40

* Amounts are for people who obtain fewer than 30 minutes/day of moderate physical activity, beyond their normal daily activities.

Adapted from Krebs-Smith SM and others: Americans do not meet federal dietary recommendations. *Journal of Nutrition* 140 (10): 1832, 2010.

U.S. Department of Agriculture (USDA) MyPlate food groups and percentages of men and women ages 71 years and older who meet the recommendations. The following sections discuss some of the major health concerns that often affect the nutritional status of older adults. Some of these conditions have been discussed in previous chapters.

Changes in Body Weight

As the human body ages, its need for energy decreases.[1] In senescence, muscle mass declines as some muscle cells shrink or die. The loss of muscle mass leads to a decrease in muscular strength and basal metabolism. The aging body typically loses lean tissue and gains fat tissue. Increased body fat results from overeating and lack of physical activity, but even athletic men and lean women usually gain some central body fat after they are 50 years of age. Being overfat may increase the bone density of older adults and result in stronger bones,[60] but having too much body fat increases the risk of type 2 diabetes, hypertension, cardiovascular disease, and osteoarthritis. For more information about overweight and obesity, see Chapter 10.

Compared to healthy younger adults, people who are over 70 years of age have a higher risk of nutrient deficiencies, because their food intake tends to decrease as their metabolic rates and physical activity levels decline. Despite having lower energy needs, however, older adults need the same or even higher amounts of vitamins and minerals. Meeting micronutrient needs while eating less food can be difficult for older persons to accomplish.

After reaching 70 years of age, it is not unusual for people to lose some weight. Several factors can contribute to weight loss among older adults (Table 13.14). Older adults may eat less because they have lost the ability to taste and smell food. Loss of teeth and difficulty swallowing can also result in decreased food consumption. Declines in normal *cognitive* functioning (thought processes) resulting from conditions such as Alzheimer's disease or reduced blood flow to the brain can contribute to poor nutritional status. People who lack normal cognitive functioning may be unable to make decisions regarding plan-ning nutritious meals, as well as to shop for and prepare food. Conditions that interfere with mobility and flexibility, such as arthritis and osteoporosis, can also interfere with food shopping and preparation activities. Social and economic fac-tors often play a role in reduced food intake. Many older people live alone and on fixed incomes, circumstances that are associated with depression and inability to afford adequate amounts of nutritious food. In many instances, very old people refuse to eat and, as a result, lose considerable amounts of weight, a situation that hastens their death.

For older adults who find that food no longer tastes "good," adding more spices may improve the taste of food and, as a result, stimulate weak appetites. Efforts to make mealtimes social events, such as inviting friends to share potluck meals together, can enhance older adults' mental outlooks and spark their inter-est in eating. Older adults can increase or maintain their weight by consuming energy-dense snacks between meals, such as cheese, milkshakes, nuts, or oatmeal cookies. If weight loss becomes significant, a physician should be consulted to determine the cause.

Physical Inactivity

Many of the undesirable physical changes we associate with growing old are the result of a lifetime of physical inactivity. Regardless of a person's age, a physically active lifestyle increases muscle strength and mobility, improves balance, slows bone loss, and boosts emotional well-being. Most older adults can benefit from performing aerobic and strength-training activities

TABLE 13.14 Reduced Food Intake Among Older Adults: Contributing Factors

- Reduced ability to taste and smell food
- Difficulty swallowing
- Loss of teeth
- Loss of normal cognitive function
- Lack of income
- Depression
- Reduced mobility and flexibility

Did You Know?

You are never too old to gain some benefits from exercise. Any form of physical activity, from swimming to performing household chores, can help extend an older person's longevity.[61]

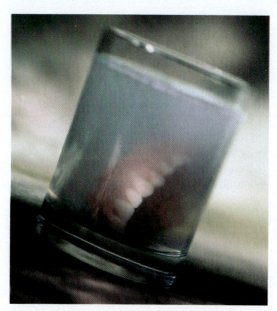

Many older adults do not like to wear dentures because they can be uncomfortable.

regularly. Before embarking on a program to increase physical fitness, however, sedentary older adults should consult their physicians concerning appropriate activities.

Tooth Loss

In the 1950s, surveys of Americans indicated that the majority of older adults had lost all their natural teeth. Since then, the percentage of older adults who retain all or most of their teeth has increased in the United States. Adults should have 28 natural teeth. In 2010–2012, about 8% of Americans who were 18 years of age or older had lost all of their teeth.[62] Moreover, approximately 23% of Americans who were 65 years or older had lost all their natural teeth. Tooth loss is related to long–term poor dental hygiene, cigarette smoking, and poor dietary practices. By following recommended dental hygiene practices, obtaining regular dental care, and avoiding tobacco use, you can greatly increase your chances of keeping most of your teeth as you age.

Excessive tooth loss can lead to faulty eating habits. People who lack teeth often avoid crisp or chewy foods, such as fresh fruits, vegetables, whole–grain cereals, and meat. According to results of a study involving over 300 older adults, subjects who had 10 or fewer teeth consumed considerably less than the recommended amounts of fruits, vegetables, meat and beans, and oils when compared to older adults who had more than 10 teeth.[63] Although dentures that replace natural teeth can enable some people to chew normally, many older adults do not like to wear them because they can be uncomfortable. When a person has difficulty chewing food, serving soft foods such as ground meats, cooked vegetables, pureed fruits, and puddings can stimulate the individual's appetite.

Intestinal Tract Problems

Constipation is a major complaint of older adults. By increasing their intakes of fiber–rich foods, such as whole–grain products and vegetables, older adults may be able to have more regular bowel movements (see the "Fiber" section of Chapter 5). Dehydration contributes to constipation, so older persons should make sure their fluid intake is adequate.

As a person ages, his or her stomach secretes less hydrochloric acid (HCl) and intrinsic factor. These changes can contribute to poor absorption of vitamin B–12 and the development of vitamin B–12 deficiency and pernicious anemia. Older adults may be able to meet their vitamin B–12 needs by eating foods fortified with the micronutrient or taking vitamin B–12 supplements. Some older adults, however, must take injections of the B vitamin to prevent pernicious anemia (see Chapter 8). Older persons are also at risk of iron deficiency because reduced stomach acid production may hinder iron absorption. Furthermore, many older adults take aspirin regularly, and this practice can cause intestinal bleeding that can lead to iron deficiency anemia. Intestinal ulcers and cancer can also cause blood loss from the digestive tract. The discovery of blood in bowel movements needs to be reported to a physician—regardless of one's age.

Many older adults take one or more prescription drugs daily. Although such medications can improve health and quality of life of older adults, some drugs interfere with the body's absorption and/or use of certain nutrients. Additionally, older adults often take one or more dietary supplements regularly. According to results of a national survey conducted in 2003–2006, 70% of adults ages 71 and older took at least 1 dietary supplement regularly.[64] Nutrient supplements, such as multivitamin/multimineral supplements, were the most widely used type of dietary supplement. Certain dietary supplements, including herbal products, can reduce or amplify the effects of prescribed medications. Therefore, older adults should notify their physicians about their use of all dietary supplements. A few foods also interfere with prescribed drugs. Grapefruit juice, for example, can alter the potency of certain medications that are used to lower blood pressure or cholesterol.

Depression in Older Adults

In 2008, 16% of women and 11% of men age 65 and over reported having symptoms of depression.[65] Situations that contribute to depression among the older adult population include coping with chronic illness or loss of mobility, and isolation and loneliness as family members and friends move away or die. If the depressed person loses interest in cooking and eating, weight loss and nutrient deficiencies are likely to occur. In many instances, depression can be managed with medication, but social support and psychological counseling may be necessary as well. Without proper treatment, depressed persons, especially males, are at risk of alcoholism and suicide. In 2009, non–Hispanic white men who were 85 years of age and older were more likely to commit suicide than other Americans.[65]

Dietary Planning in Older Adulthood

MyPlate can provide the basis for planning nutritionally adequate meals and snacks for healthy older adults. However, amounts of foods recommended in these diet plans may not provide enough vitamin D and vitamin B–12 for older adults. By regularly consuming fortified and/or enriched foods, older

Food & Nutrition tips

The following suggestions can help caregivers improve nutrient intakes of older adults:

• Emphasize nutrient-dense foods when planning daily menus.

• Try new foods, seasonings, and ways of preparing foods.

• Have easy-to-prepare, nutrient-dense foods on hand for times when the older person is too tired to cook large meals.

• Serve meals in well-lit or sunny areas, and plan appealing meals by using foods with different flavors, colors, shapes, textures, and smells.

• Plan occasions for the older adult to share cooking responsibilities and eat meals with friends or relatives.

• Encourage the older person to eat at a senior center whenever possible. Investigate community resources for helping the older adult obtain groceries, cook, or manage other daily care needs.

• Encourage the older adult to be physically active.

• If biting and chewing are difficult for an older adult, chop, grind, or blend tough or crisp foods.

• Prepare extra amounts of soup, stew, or casserole, so leftovers can be frozen for future meals.

People enjoying the social benefits of dining together at a community center for independent older adults.

Many communities in the United States offer the Meals on Wheels program in which volunteers deliver nutritious meals prepared at a senior center to qualified, homebound older adults.

adults can increase their intakes of these micronutrients. In many instances, older adults can also benefit from taking a daily multiple vitamin/mineral supplement.

Friends, relatives, and health care personnel should be alert for indications of poor nutrient intakes among older people, especially those who are at risk and live in nursing homes or other long–term care facilities. For example, family members can make sure the older adult's nutrient needs are met by visiting the person's residence during mealtimes, observing the foods that are offered, and, if necessary, helping the older adult eat. Additionally, monitoring the older person's weight can indicate whether long–term food intake has been adequate. Older adults who live at home may need help planning nutritionally adequate diets. In these instances, registered dietitians can be consulted to provide personalized dietary advice.

Community Nutrition Services for Older Adults

The Chapter 1 "Nutrition Matters" provides information about popular community–based nutrition services for American older adults. You can obtain information regarding locally available nutrition services for older people from medical clinics, private practitioners, hospitals, and health maintenance organizations in your area. To learn more about nutrition–related programs for older adults, visit the following websites: National Institute on Aging, www.nia.nih.gov/; American Geriatrics Society, www.americangeriatrics.org/; and Administration on Aging, www.aoa.gov/.

Concept **Checkpoint 13.8**

31. What is the difference between *life expectancy* and *life span*?
32. Identify at least five physiological changes that are associated with the normal aging process.
33. Explain why nutrient needs for older adults are often higher than those for younger persons.
34. List at least four nutrients that are often lacking in diets of older adults.
35. Suggest at least three ways caregivers can improve nutrient intakes of older persons.

13.9 Nutrition Matters: In Search of the Fountain

Learning Outcomes

1. Discuss at least two aging theories.
2. Explain the effects of calorie restriction on the aging process.
3. Identify steps people can take to extend their life expectancy.

In 1513, Spanish explorer Juan Ponce de León sailed to the southeastern coastal region of North America and discovered an area he named "Land of Flowers" (Florida). Ponce de León was on a mission to find gold, but he was also eager to locate a natural spring that supposedly had magical powers. According to Native Americans in the area, elderly people who drank the spring's water regained their youthful looks and vigor. Unfortunately, Ponce de León never found gold or the mythical "fountain of youth" in Florida. Nevertheless, many older adults still seek ways to combat aging, especially by taking certain hormones and dietary supplements promoted as having age–defying properties. Older Americans spend considerable amounts of money on such products, some of which may be harmful in the long run. Promoters of antiaging formulas or therapies claim their treatments can stop, and even reverse, the process of aging. Is there any reliable scientific evidence to support claims that you can take something to stay young longer?

Claims that a nutritional fountain of youth exists are simply not true. Currently, scientific evidence does not support the use of antiaging therapies that include taking antioxidants and hormones.[66] Scientists have determined that consuming a nutritious diet and obtaining adequate amounts of physical activity can promote good health as one ages.[66] Nevertheless, researchers are conducting experiments to better understand the process of aging and the keys to longevity.

Biogerontologists are scientists who study the biology of aging. Biogerontologists have proposed several theories to explain why aging occurs and why some people live longer than others. According to one of these theories, longevity results from the body's ability to maintain and repair the damage done by a lifetime of exposure to the environment and the effects of everyday "wear and tear." Some multicellular organisms are able to live longer when they can improve their abilities to repair damage to their DNA, reduce the toxicity of free radicals, and replace nonfunctioning cells. Antioxidants reduce the toxic effects of free radicals (see Chapter 8), and organisms produce a variety of antioxidants to control free radical production.

Ponce de León.

Scientific studies, however, provide little evidence that increasing one's intake of antioxidants slows the aging process.[66]

One area of biogerontological research that shows some promise is the use of *calorie restriction (CR)* to extend longevity. Although CR provides fewer calories than an organism's usual diet, the dietary pattern supplies all essential nutrients. Since the 1930s, scientists have studied the effects of CR on the health and life spans of various species of multicellular organisms. According to some research findings, CR can increase life spans of various organisms, including some kinds of rodents, fruit, flies, and yeast.[66] Results of other studies, however, were not so promising, because the animals either had the same or shorter life spans when compared to controls.

Even if scientists provide evidence that any form of CR adds some years to the human life span, would you be interested in reducing your food intake considerably to extend your life? How enjoyable would your life be if you ate only 900 kcal daily? What is important to you: how long you can live, or how *well* you live?

The science of biogerontology is still in its beginning stages; researchers have much to learn about the aging process before they can develop safe ways to enhance longevity. We already know that you can reduce your risk of dying prematurely from chronic diseases such as heart disease, hypertension, type 2 diabetes, and many forms of cancer by adopting healthy lifestyles. Rather than wait until the fountain of youth becomes a reality, you can take charge of your health now by consuming a nutritionally adequate diet, obtaining regular moderate— to vigorous—intensity physical activity, maintaining a healthy weight, avoiding tobacco products, limiting your alcohol consumption, and having regular physical checkups.

Concept **Checkpoint 13.9**

36. According to scientific evidence, which dietary modification may extend the life expectancies of organisms that include fruit flies and rodents?

37. List three steps you can take that may extend your life expectancy.

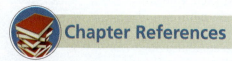

Chapter References

See Appendix H.

Summary

13.1 Introduction to Nutrition for a Lifetime

- The leading causes of death for Americans are chronic diseases: heart disease, cancer, and stroke. Lifestyles, especially dietary practices and physical activity patterns, contribute to the development of these chronic conditions. Other factors that influence a person's overall health include heredity, relationships, environment, income, education level, and access to health care.

13.2 Pregnancy

- Embryonic/fetal life is characterized by rapid rates of cell division, resulting in a dramatic increase in cell numbers. The first trimester of pregnancy is a critical stage in human development because inadequate or excessive nutrient intakes as well as exposure to toxic compounds can have devastating effects on the embryo/fetus during this period. The placenta is the organ of pregnancy that transfers nutrients and oxygen from the mother's bloodstream to her embryo/fetus. The placenta also transfers wastes from the embryo/fetus to the mother's bloodstream so her body can eliminate them.

- Women of childbearing age should take steps to ensure they are in good health prior to becoming pregnant. During pregnancy, the woman's body undergoes various physiological changes. These changes enable her body to nourish and maintain the developing fetus, as well as to produce milk for her infant after its birth. A pregnant woman should follow a diet that meets her own nutritional needs as well as those of her developing offspring. The mother-to-be can use MyPlate to develop nutritionally adequate daily menus, but she may also need to take a prenatal vitamin/mineral supplement.

- Women whose prepregnancy weights were within the healthy range can expect to gain 25 to 35 pounds during pregnancy. Women who gain excess weight during pregnancy may retain the extra weight long after delivery.

- Monitoring weight gain is an important aspect of prenatal care. Rapid weight gain, especially after the fifth month of pregnancy, could be a sign of gestational hypertension. Underweight women who do not gain enough weight during pregnancy are at risk of having preterm or low-birth-weight infants. Obese women have a greater risk of developing hypertension and type 2 diabetes during pregnancy.

13.3 Infant Nutrition

- Breast milk is the best first food for infants. Compared to babies who are not breastfed, breastfed infants have lower risks of allergies and of gastrointestinal, respiratory tract, and ear infections. Women who breastfeed their babies can also derive some important benefits from the practice, such as losing extra fat gained during pregnancy.

- When an infant suckles, nerves in the nipple signal the mother's brain to release prolactin and oxytocin into her bloodstream. Oxytocin is necessary for the let-down reflex and causes the uterus to contract. Milk production relies on "supply and demand." If the breasts are not emptied fully, milk production soon ceases. To support milk production, the lactating mother needs about 400 to 500 extra kilocalories daily.

- Growth is very rapid during infancy. Health care practitioners can assess growth in infants and children by measuring body weight, height (or length), and head circumference over time. For the first 6 months, the infant's nutrient needs can be met by human milk or iron-fortified infant formula. Breastfed babies need vitamin D and possibly iron and fluoride supplements.

- Most infants do not need solid foods before 6 months of age. The first solid food offered to babies should be an iron-containing food such as an iron-fortified infant cereal, meat, or poultry. New foods should be added one at a time, and the child should be observed for allergy signs and symptoms. Whole cow's milk should not be fed to babies until they are 1 year of age.

13.4 The Preschool Years

- It is normal for a preschooler's appetite to decline as the child's growth rate tapers off. Additionally, it is not unusual for preschool children to be "picky eaters" or embark on "food jags." Caregivers should avoid nagging, forcing, and bribing children to eat, but instead offer a variety of healthy food choices and allow the child to choose what and how much to eat. Nutrition-related problems that often affect preschool children are iron deficiency, dental caries, obesity, and food allergies.

13.5 School-Age Children

- School-age children often skip breakfast, and they tend to consume more foods away from home, larger portions of food, and more fried foods and sweetened beverages. Children who eat breakfast are more likely to have better diets and healthier body weights than children who skip this meal. Diets of many school-age children fail to supply recommended amounts of calcium and potassium while providing too much sodium.

13.6 Adolescence

- A child matures physically into an adult during adolescence. For many teens, pressure to conform to fads and be influenced by other adolescents negatively affects their diets and overall health. Obesity, eating disorders, and low iron and calcium intakes are major nutrition-related concerns of adolescents.

13.7 Childhood Obesity

- Public health experts are very concerned about the increasing prevalence of obesity among children in the United States. Overfat children have higher risks of elevated blood pressure, cholesterol, and glucose levels than children whose weights are within the healthy range. Overfat children may also have higher risk of hypertension, heart disease, and type 2 diabetes later in life. Such children are also more likely to have low self-esteem and become obese as adults.

13.8 Nutrition for Older Adults

- The aging process is characterized by numerous predictable physical changes. Senescence refers to declining organ functioning and increased vulnerability to disease that occurs after a person reaches physical maturity. Although genetics play a role in determining longevity, lifestyle practices and environmental conditions influence a person's rate of aging. People may be able to live longer and healthier by making responsible healthy lifestyle decisions while they are still young.

- Factors that can influence an older person's nutritional status include illnesses, tooth loss, medications, low income, depression, and lack of social support. Diets of older adults, particularly older women, often provide inadequate amounts of vitamins D, A, and B-12 and minerals such as calcium and potassium. Friends, relatives, and health care personnel should be alert for indications of poor nutrient intakes among older people, especially those who live in nursing homes or other long-term care facilities.

13.9 Nutrition Matters: In Search of the Fountain

- According to biogerontologists, longevity results from the body's ability to maintain and repair the damage done by a lifetime of exposure to the environment and the effects of everyday "wear and tear." Little credible scientific evidence exists to support the use of antiaging therapies that include taking hormones or megadoses of vitamins and antioxidants. Researchers are conducting experiments to better understand the process of aging and the keys to longevity.

Recipe for Healthy Living

Vegetable Dip

You can make low-fat versions of fruit or vegetable dips by replacing sour cream or mayonnaise in recipes with plain, low-fat yogurt. This vegetable dip recipe makes approximately five ¼-cup servings of dip. Each serving provides approximately 46 kcal, 3 g protein, 2 g fat, 90 mg calcium, 160 mg sodium, and 120 mg potassium

INGREDIENTS:

1 cup plain, low-fat yogurt
3 Tbsp calorie-reduced ranch dressing
¼ tsp curry powder (optional)

PREPARATION STEPS:

1. In a small bowl, combine yogurt with the dressing and stir until well blended.

2. Refrigerate until ready to serve.

3. Serve chilled in a bowl that is surrounded with fresh pieces of raw vegetables.

4. Discard any remaining dip.

 Further analyze this and other recipes through activities on Connect at www.mcgrawhillconnect.com.

ChooseMyPlate.gov

- Fat — 39%
- Protein — 26%
- Carbohydrate — 35%

Calories* 2
Protein 6
Fat 3
Calcium 9
Sodium 7
Potassium 3

% of DV/serving

*2000 daily total kcal

Critical Thinking

1. One of your friends just found out that she is pregnant. Although her BMI is within the healthy range, she is concerned about gaining too much weight during pregnancy. What advice would you provide concerning the need to gain some weight during this life stage? If your friend's prepregnancy weight was 125 pounds, how much weight would be appropriate for her to gain during pregnancy?

2. Your pregnant friend wants your advice concerning whether she should breastfeed or formula-feed her baby. After reading Chapter 13, what information would you provide to help your friend decide to breastfeed?

3. Olivia is a healthy 2-month-old baby. Olivia's mother, Kara, wants to replace Olivia's iron-fortified infant formula with the same fresh fluid 2% milk that she drinks. What advice would you give to Kara concerning the appropriateness of making such a decision?

4. Marcus is 8 years old, and his weight is in the overweight range. His caregivers are also overweight, but they seem to be concerned about Marcus's excess body weight. What advice would you provide his caregivers to help Marcus achieve a healthy body weight?

5. Are your parents, grandparents, and great-grandparents still alive? If any of your ancestors died before they were 60 years of age, can you identify their causes of death and factors that contributed to their deaths? What lifestyle changes can you make now that can help you achieve a longer, healthier lifetime?

Practice Test

Select the best answer.

1. The embryo/fetus develops most of its organs during the
   a. preconception period.
   b. first trimester.
   c. second trimester.
   d. third trimester.

2. The placenta cannot
   a. transfer nutrients from the mother's bloodstream to the embryo/fetus.
   b. eliminate waste products from the embryo/fetus.
   c. prevent all toxic substances from reaching the embryo/fetus.
   d. transfer oxygen from the mother's bloodstream to the embryo/fetus.

3. During the first trimester, a pregnant woman's daily energy requirement is _____ her daily energy needs before she became pregnant.
   a. 300 kcal lower than
   b. about the same as
   c. 300 kcal higher than
   d. 500 kcal higher than

4. Women with prepregnancy weights within the healthy range should gain _____ pounds during pregnancy.
   a. 10 – 20
   b. 20 – 25
   c. 25 – 35
   d. 35 – 50

5. Preeclampsia is a form of _____ that can develop during pregnancy.
   a. hypertension
   b. diabetes
   c. cancer
   d. anemia

6. Which of the following statements is true?
   a. A woman's energy needs are higher during the first trimester than at any other time in pregnancy.
   b. Using infant formula to bottle-feed a baby is more convenient and less expensive than breastfeeding a baby.
   c. Oxytocin is necessary for the "let-down" reflex to occur.
   d. The American Pediatric Association recommends feeding fresh whole milk to infants when they are 6 months of age.

7. A healthy infant who weighs 6.5 pounds at birth can be expected to weigh _____ pounds by her first birthday.
   a. 13.0
   b. 16.5
   c. 19.5
   d. 23.5

8. Breastfed infants are _____ than babies who are fed infant formula.
   a. more likely to have diarrhea
   b. less likely to have cystic fibrosis
   c. more likely to have respiratory infections
   d. less likely to have ear infections

9. Which of the following factors is associated with increased risk of obesity during childhood?

a. having a family history of obesity

b. eating 3 to 5 servings of fresh fruit daily

c. being a full—term infant

d. taking dietary supplements that contain zinc and vitamin C

10. Which of the following practices has been scientifi—cally shown to extend the life spans of certain flies and rodents?

a. taking antioxidant supplements

b. eating a high—protein diet

c. performing vigorous physical exercise

d. consuming a calorie—restricted diet

LEARNSMART®
ADVANTAGE

Get the most out of your study of nutrition with McGraw-Hill's innovative suite of adaptive learning products including McGraw-Hill LearnSmart®, SmartBook®, LearnSmart Achieve®, and LearnSmart Prep®. Visit www.learnsmartadvantage.com.

Answers to **Quiz Yourself**

1. During pregnancy, a mother-to-be should double her food intake because she's "eating for two." **False.** (p. 497)

2. The natural size of a woman's breasts is not a factor in determining her ability to breastfeed her baby. **True.** (p. 506)

3. Caregivers should add solid foods to an infant's diet within the first month after the baby is born. **False.** (p. 509)

4. Over the past few decades, the prevalence of obesity has increased among American children. **True.** (p. 519)

5. Compared to younger persons, older adults have lower risks of nutritional deficiencies. **False.** (p. 525)

English-Metric Conversions and Metric-to-Household Units

English-Metric Conversions

Length

English (USA)	Metric
inch (in)	= 2.54 cm, 25.4 mm
foot (ft)	= 0.30 m, 30.48 cm
yard (yd)	= 0.91 m, 91.4 cm

Metric	English (USA)
millimeter (mm)	= 0.039 in (thickness of a dime)
centimeter (cm)	= 0.39 in
meter (m)	= 3.28 ft, 39.4 in
kilometer (km)	= 0.62 mi, 1091 yd, 3273 ft

Weight

English (USA)	Metric
ounce (oz)	= 28.35 g
pound (lb)	= 453.60 g, 0.45 kg

Metric	English (USA)
milligram (mg)	= 0.000035 oz
gram (g)	= 0.04 oz ($\frac{1}{28}$ of an oz)
kilogram (kg)	= 35.27 oz, 2.20 lb

Volume

English (USA)	Metric
teaspoon (tsp)	= 5 ml
tablespoon (Tbsp)	= 15 ml
fluid ounce	= 0.03 liter (30 ml)
cup (c)	= 237 ml
pint (pt)	= 0.47 liter
quart (qt)	= 0.95 liter
gallon (gal)	= 3.79 liters

Metric	English (USA)
milliliter (ml)	= 0.03 oz
liter	= 1.06 qt
liter	= 0.27 gal

Metric and Other Common Units

Unit/Abbreviation	Other Equivalent Measure
milligram/mg	$\frac{1}{1000}$ of a gram
microgram/mcg	$\frac{1}{1,000,000}$ of a gram
deciliter/dl	$\frac{1}{10}$ of a liter (about ½ cup)
milliliter/ml	$\frac{1}{1000}$ of a liter (5 ml is about 1 tsp)

Fahrenheit-Celsius Conversion Scale

To convert temperature scales:
Fahrenheit to Celsius $°C = (°F - 32) \times 5/9$
Celsius to Fahrenheit $°F = 9/5(°C) + 32$

Household Units

3 teaspoons	= 1 tablespoon
4 tablespoons	= ¼ cup
5⅓ tablespoons	= ⅓ cup
8 tablespoons	= ½ cup
10⅔ tablespoons	= ⅔ cup
16 tablespoons	= 1 cup
1 tablespoon	= ½ fluid ounce
1 cup	= 8 fluid ounces
1 cup	= ½ pint
2 cups	= 1 pint
4 cups	= 1 quart
2 pints	= 1 quart
4 quarts	= 1 gallon

Appendix B

Daily Values Table

Dietary Constituent	Unit of Measure	RDA or Other Current Daily Dietary Standard	
		Daily Values for People Over 4 Years of Age (as of January 2016)	Proposed Daily Values*
Total fat	g	65	65
Saturated fatty acids	"	20	20
Protein	"	50	50
Cholesterol	mg	300	300
Total carbohydrate	g	300	300
Fiber	"	25	28
Vitamin A	μg (RAEs)	1500	900
Vitamin D	μg	10	20
Vitamin E	mg (ATEs)	14–20	15
Vitamin K	μg	80	120
Vitamin C	mg	60	90
Folate	μg	400	400
Thiamin	mg	1.5	1.2
Riboflavin	"	1.7	1.3
Niacin	"	20	16
Vitamin B-6	"	2	1.7
Vitamin B-12	μg	6	2.4
Biotin	mg	0.03	30
Pantothenic acid	"	10	5
Calcium	"	1000	1300
Phosphorus	"	1000	1250
Iodine	μg	150	150
Iron	mg	18	18
Magnesium	"	400	420
Copper	"	2	0.9
Zinc	"	15	11
Sodium	"	2400	2300
Potassium	"	3500	4700
Chloride	"	3400	2300
Manganese	"	2	2.3
Selenium	μg	70	55
Chromium	"	120	35
Molybdenum	"	75	45

Abbreviations: g = gram, mg = milligram, μg = microgram, RAEs = retinol activity equivalents, ATE = alpha tocopherol equivalent

*Proposed standards from: U.S. Department of Health and Human Services, Food and Drug Administration: Food labeling: revision of the Nutrition and Supplement Facts labels. 21 CFR Part 101 [Docket No. FDA–2012–N–1210] RIN 0910–AF22. *Federal Register* 79(41), March 3, 2014.

Energy Metabolism

Energy-investment steps

Glucose

① ATP → ADP

① Adding phosphate to glucose using ATP produces an activated molecule.

Glucose 6-phosphate

ATP Yield

−2 ATP

Fructose 6-phosphate

② ATP → ADP

② Rearrangement, followed by a second addition of phosphate using ATP, produces fructose 1, 6-biphosphate.

Fructose 1, 6-biphosphate

③

③ The 6-carbon molecule is split into two 3-carbon-phosphate molecules.

2X Glyceraldehyde 3–phosphate

Energy-harvesting steps   2P ← 2X NAD⁺

④ 2X NADH + H⁺

④ Oxidation, followed by the addition of phosphate produces 2 NADH + 2H⁺ molecules and two 3-carbon-phosphate-phosphate molecules.

2X 1, 3–bisphosphoglycerate

+2 ATP

⑤ 2 ADP → 2 ATP

⑤ Removal of 2 phosphate groups by 2 ADP molecules produces 2 ATP molecules and two 3-carbon-phosphate molecules.

2X 3–phosphoglycerate

⑥ H₂O ←

⑥ Removal of water produces two 3-carbon-phosphate molecules.

2X Phosphoenolpyruvate

+2 ATP
———
2 ATP

(Net Gain ATP)

2 ADP → 2 ATP   ⑦

⑦ Removal of 2 phosphate groups by 2 ADP molecules produces 2 ATP molecules.

⑧ 2X Pyruvate

⑧ Pyruvate is the end product of the glycolysis pathway. Generally pyruvate enters mitochondria for further breakdown.

Figure C.1 Glycolysis, step by step. This metabolic pathway begins with glucose and ends with pyruvate. Net gain of two ATP molecules can be calculated by subtracting those used during the energy-investment steps from those produced during the energy-harvesting steps. Text in boxes explains the reactions.

Pyruvate is first metabolized in a transition reaction to acetyl-CoA. It is acetyl-CoA that actually enters the citric acid cycle. In the process, NADH + H⁺ is produced and CO₂ is lost.

Intermediates of the citric acid cycle, such as oxaloacetate, can leave the cycle and go on to form other compounds, such as glucose.

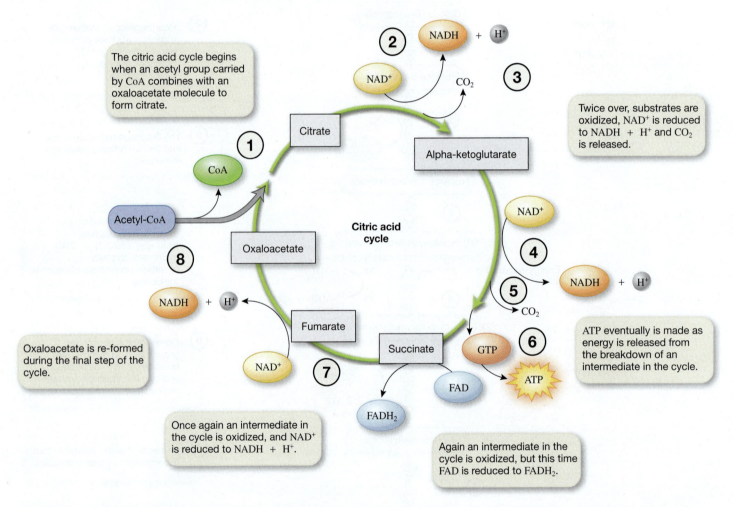

The citric acid cycle begins when an acetyl group carried by CoA combines with an oxaloacetate molecule to form citrate.

Twice over, substrates are oxidized, NAD⁺ is reduced to NADH + H⁺ and CO₂ is released.

ATP eventually is made as energy is released from the breakdown of an intermediate in the cycle.

Oxaloacetate is re-formed during the final step of the cycle.

Once again an intermediate in the cycle is oxidized, and NAD⁺ is reduced to NADH + H⁺.

Again an intermediate in the cycle is oxidized, but this time FAD is reduced to FADH₂.

Figure C.2 The transition reaction and the citric acid cycle. The net result of one turn of this cycle of reactions (steps 1–8) is the oxidation of an acetyl group to two molecules of CO_2 and the formation of three molecules of NADH + H⁺ and one molecule of $FADH_2$. One GTP molecule also results, which eventually forms ATP. The citric acid cycle turns twice per glucose molecule. Note that oxygen does not participate in any of the steps in the citric acid cycle. It instead participates in the electron transport chain.

Figure C.3 Simplified depiction of electron transfer in energy metabolism. High-energy compounds, such as glucose, give up electrons and hydrogen ions to NAD^+ and FAD. The $NADH + H^+$ and $FADH_2$ that are formed transfer these electrons and hydrogen ions, using specialized electron carriers, to oxygen to form water (H_2O). The energy yielded by the entire process is used to generate ATP from ADP and Pi.

Amino Acids

Histidine (His)
(essential)

Tryptophan (Trp)
(essential)

Glycine (Gly)

Methionine (Met)
(essential)

Leucine (Leu)
(essential)

Alanine (Ala)

Arginine (Arg)
(essential in infancy)

Lysine (Lys)
(essential)

Proline (Pro)

Glutamic Acid (Glu)

Aspartic Acid (Asp)

Serine (Ser)

Phenylalanine (Phe)
(essential)

Isoleucine (Ile)
(essential)

Tyrosine (Tyr)

Glutamine (Gln)

Asparagine (Asn)

Threonine (Thr)
(essential)

Valine (Val)
(essential)

Cysteine (Cys)

Vitamins Involved in Energy Metabolism

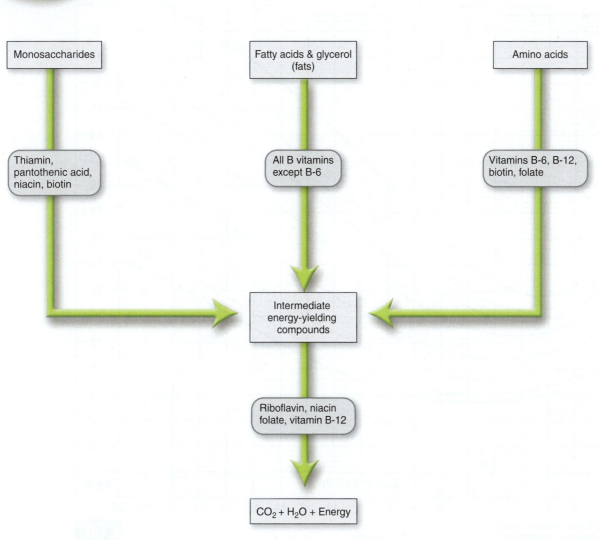

Figure E.1 The metabolism of monosaccharides, fats, and amino acids for energy requires several vitamins.

Body Mass Index-for-Age Percentiles

2 to 20 years: Boys
Body mass index-for-age percentiles

NAME _____

RECORD # _____

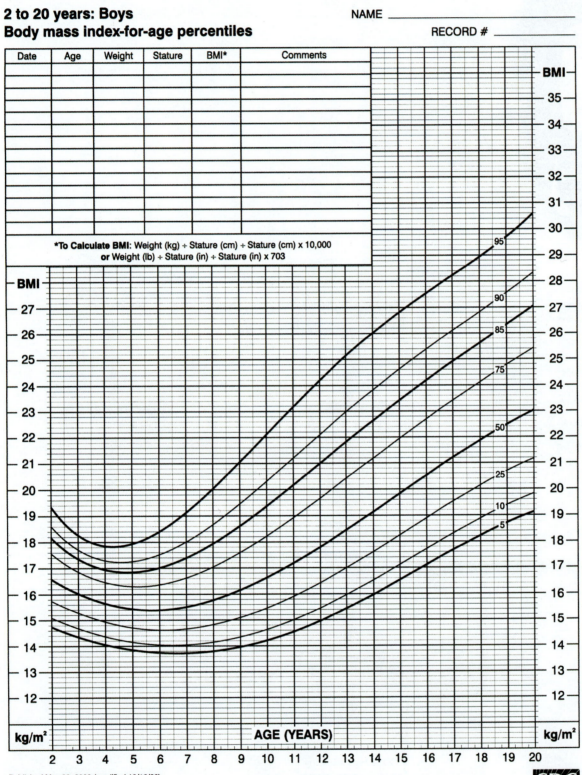

*To Calculate BMI: Weight (kg) ÷ Stature (cm) ÷ Stature (cm) x 10,000
or Weight (lb) ÷ Stature (in) ÷ Stature (in) x 703

Published May 30, 2000 (modified 10/16/00).
SOURCE: Developed by the National Center for Health Statistics in collaboration with
the National Center for Chronic Disease Prevention and Health Promotion (2000).

2 to 20 years: Girls
Body mass index-for-age percentiles

NAME _____

RECORD # _____

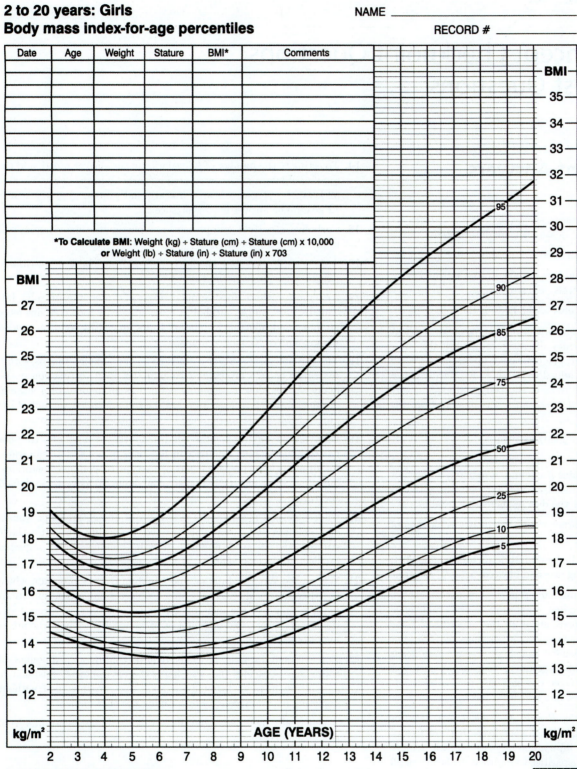

Date	Age	Weight	Stature	BMI*	Comments

*To Calculate BMI: Weight (kg) ÷ Stature (cm) ÷ Stature (cm) x 10,000
or Weight (lb) ÷ Stature (in) ÷ Stature (in) x 703

AGE (YEARS)

Published May 30, 2000 (modified 10/16/00).
SOURCE: Developed by the National Center for Health Statistics in collaboration with
the National Center for Chronic Disease Prevention and Health Promotion (2000).

Appendix G

Answers to Concept Checkpoint Questions and Practice Test Questions

Concept Checkpoint Answers

Chapter 1

1. Heart disease, some types of cancer, stroke, and type 2 diabetes are among the 10 leading causes of death that are diet related.

2. Answers will vary but should include factors shown in Figure 1.1.

3. The six major classes of nutrients are carbohydrates, fats and other lipids, proteins, vitamins, minerals, and water.

4. The smallest functional living unit in the body is the cell.

5. The key features that indicate a substance is an essential nutrient include the following: a deficiency disease results when the substance is missing from the diet; the deficiency disease is corrected when the missing substance is added to the diet; and scientists can identify the nutrient's specific roles in the body and explain why abnormalities occurred when the substance was missing from the diet.

6. A phytochemical is a substance made by plants.

7. According to the DSHEA, a dietary supplement is a product (excluding tobacco) that contains a vitamin, a mineral, an herb or other plant product, an amino acid, or a dietary substance that is taken by mouth to supplement the diet by increasing total intake.

8. A risk factor is a personal characteristic that increases chances of developing a chronic disease.

9. Answers will vary but should include lifestyle factors such as diet; alcohol, tobacco, and other drug use; and physical activity patterns.

10. Americans eat less red meat, milk, and eggs, and more fish, cheese, and poultry, than in 1970. The diet supplies more grain and cereal products, but refined grain foods make up the majority of these products. Americans are eating additional servings of fruit, but not enough to meet recommended amounts. Today, Americans eat higher amounts of fruits and vegetables than in the past, but choices tend to lack variety. Over the past 40 years, Americans' intake of calories, added sugars, and added fat has increased.

11. The main objectives of *Healthy People 2020* encourage ways for Americans to attain higher−quality, longer lives that are free of preventable disease, disability, injury, and premature death; achieve health equity by eliminating disparities to improve the health of all groups; create social and physical environments that promote good health for all; and promote quality of life, healthy development, and healthy behaviors across all life stages.

12. Scientists generally use liters, grams, and meters to report volume, weight, and length.

13. A 154−pound person weighs 70 kg. To obtain the answer, divide 154 by 2.2 (70 kg).

14. To estimate the number of kilocalories in the slice of bread, add the number of kilocalories contributed by carbohydrate (13 g × 4 kcal = 52 kcal), fat (1 g × 9 kcal = 9 kcal), and protein (3 g × 4 kcal = 12 kcal). The answer is 73 kcal/slice.

15. Carbohydrates, fats, and proteins are macronutrients; vitamins and minerals are micronutrients.

16. Answers will vary but should be taken from the key nutrition−related concepts listed in Table 1.7.

17. An empty−calorie food supplies excessive amounts of solid fat, added sugars, and/or alcohol. A nutrient−dense food contains more vitamins and minerals in relation to its unhealthy solid fat, added sugars, and/or alcohol contents.

18. The physiological dose of a nutrient is the amount that is within the range of safe intake and enables the body to function opti−mally. A megadose is generally defined as an amount of a vitamin or mineral that is at least 10 times the recommended amount of the nutrient. Megadose amounts of certain nutrients can be toxic.

19. Unfavorable environmental conditions that contribute to poor health in developing countries include lack of access to clean water for drinking and preparing foods. Disruptive political conditions, including wars and civil unrest, contribute to poverty and food shortages.

20. Undernutrition increases the risk of death among pregnant women and children. Children who survive undernutrition often have stunted and delayed physical growth, blindness, and impaired intellectual development.

21. WIC is the Women, Infants, and Children feeding program, which is federally subsidized. WIC provides access to specific nutritious foods to improve the diets of low−income infants, children under the age of 5 years, and pregnant or breastfeeding women who are at nutritional risk.

22. Conventional farming methods require considerable amounts of water and pesticides that can harm the environment. Sustainable agriculture involves farming methods that provide food without depleting natural resources or harming the environment.

23. A genetically modified organism is a living thing that results from genetic engineering.

Chapter 2

1. Epidemiology is the study of the occurrence, distribution, and causes of health problems in a population.

2. A control group is used to compare results of having a treatment against those of not having a treatment.

3. A prospective study follows a large group of healthy people over time to determine whether those with a certain characteristic

develop a disease and those without that characteristic remain disease free. A retrospective study follows a group of people who already suffer from a disease and compares them to a group of people with similar characteristics who do not have the disease.

4. A placebo is a fake treatment, such as a sham pill, injection, or medical procedure. Providing placebos to members of the control group enables scientists to compare the extent of the treatment's response with that of the placebo.

5. In a double–blind study, both the investigators and the subjects are unaware of the subjects' assignments in treatment or control groups.

6. A peer–reviewed article is one that has been critically analyzed by a group of "peers." If peers agree that a study was well conducted, its results are fairly represented, and the research is of interest to the journal's readers, these scientists are likely to recommend that the journal's editors publish the article.

7. Conflicting research findings often result from differences in the ways various studies are designed and results analyzed. For example, the numbers, ages, and physical conditions of subjects; the type and length of the study; the amount of the treatment provided; and the statistical tests used to analyze results typically vary among studies. Other factors, such as genetic and lifestyle differences among human subjects, can influence the results of nutrition research.

8. A testimonial is a personal endorsement of a product. Anecdotes are reports or personal experiences.

9. Answers will vary but should be clues that indicate a source of nutrition information is unreliable.

10. Answers will vary but should include points presented in Table 2.1.

11. Although some states regulate and license people who call themselves nutritionists, consumers cannot always rely on someone who refers to him– or herself as a "nutritionist" because there are no standard legal definitions and registered dietitian nutritionists for this descriptor. Registered dietitians and registered dietitian nutritionists are college–trained professionals who have extensive knowledge of foods, nutrition, and dietetics, the application of nutrition and food information to treat many health–related conditions. The title "registered dietitian" is legally protected.

12. Consumers may find reliable nutrition experts, including registered dietitians, among faculty members in universities or colleges. Registered dietitians may also be listed in telephone directories. Other ways to find registered dietitians include contacting the local dietetic association, calling the dietary department of a local hospital, or visiting the Academy of Nutrition and Dietetics website (www.eatright.org) or the Dietitians of Canada website (www.dietitians.ca).

13. Answers may vary but can include chiropractic manipulations, homeopathy, naturopathy, massage therapy, and use of herbal remedies and nonvitamin, nonmineral products.

14. According to the FDA, a drug is a substance, natural or human–made, that alters body functions. Although many dietary supplements act as drugs in the body, the FDA regulates dietary supplements as foods, not medications. Therefore, consumers do not need to obtain a physician's prescription to purchase a dietary supplement.

15. Answers will vary but can include the dietary supplements listed in Table 2.2.

Chapter 3

1. RDAs are standards for recommending daily intakes of several nutrients. RDAs meet the nutrient needs of nearly all healthy individuals (about 98%) in a particular life stage/sex group. In some instances, scientists set AIs for certain nutrients because they do not have enough information to establish RDAs for them. An AI represents a group's average daily intake that appears to be adequate for health.

2. To establish an RDA for a nutrient, nutrition scientists first determine its estimated average requirement. Then scientists add a "margin of safety" amount to the EAR that allows for individual variations in nutrient needs and helps maintain tissue stores.

3. The EER is more specific than RDAs or AIs because it takes into account the person's physical activity level, height, and weight, as well as sex and life stage. Furthermore, the EER does not include an additional number of kilocalories to serve as a margin of safety.

4. Dietitians refer to DRIs as standards for planning nutritious diets for groups of people and evaluating the nutritional adequacy of a population's diet. Pharmaceutical companies refer to DRIs when developing formulas that replace breast milk or regular foods. For nutrition labeling purposes, the FDA uses RDAs to develop Daily Values (DVs).

5. Answers will vary but should include grains, such as products made from wheat, rice, and oats. Pasta, noodles, and flour tortillas are grains because wheat flour is their main ingredient. Corn is a type of grain; therefore, cornmeal and popcorn are usually grouped with grains.

6. Enrichment is the addition of iron and certain B vitamins to cereal grain products such as flour and rice. Fortification is the addition of nutrients to food.

7. Foods generally classified as dairy include forms of fluid milk, yogurt, hard cheese, cottage cheese, ice cream, pudding, frozen yogurt, and ice milk.

8. Dry beans are protein–rich foods that can substitute for meats.

9. One–half cup of dried fruit is nutritionally equivalent to 1 cup of fresh fruit. Therefore, 1 cup of dried apricots is nutritionally equivalent to 2 cups of fresh apricots.

10. Eggs and nuts are protein–rich foods that can substitute for meats.

11. Solid fats are usually hard at room temperature, such as beef fat, butter, lard, and shortening. Cream and coconut oil are also considered solid fats.

12. Answers will vary but should include the guidelines listed in Table 3.3.

13. A healthy person should limit his or her sodium intake to less than 2300 mg/day.

14. Answers will vary but should include the recommendations listed in Table 3.4.

15. Replace solid fats with oils.

16. Your diet should have less than 10% of total calories from saturated fat.

17. Limit added sugars intake to less than 10% of total calories.

18. At least one–half of your grains should be whole grains.

19. Adult men who drink alcohol should limit their intake to no more than two drinks/day.

20. Women who drink alcohol and are not pregnant should limit their intake to no more than one drink/day.

21. Calcium, vitamin D, potassium, and dietary fiber are nutrients that Americans tend to consume in limited amounts.

22. Answers will vary but should include four of the following tips: Make at least half of your grains foods whole grains; vary vegetable choices; focus on fruit; consume sources of calcium; and choose lean protein sources.

23. Answers may vary but should include comparing dietary intakes against recommended amounts of foods and beverages within one's diet pattern. Furthermore, a response can involve using the inter–active tracking features at the www.choosemyplate.gov website to monitor food and nutrient intakes.

24. Answers should include cakes, cookies, pastries, and dough–nuts; sugar–sweetened soft drinks, sports drinks, and fruit drinks; cheese; pizza; and ice cream.

25. The Exchange System focuses on the energy, protein, carbohy–drate, and fat content of foods. Unlike the MyPlate food groupings, classification of foods into exchange lists is based on energy and macronutrient contribution.

26. Answers may vary but should discuss how %DVs can be confusing, because a goal is to obtain at least 100% of the DVs for fiber, vita–mins, and minerals each day. On the other hand, a goal should be to consume less than 100% of the DV for total fat, saturated fat, and sodium each day. Also, fresh or raw foods generally do not have labels indicating %DVs. Therefore, people may underestimate their intakes of nutrients if they rely on nutrition labels for the information.

27. Information provided on food labels and dietary supplements can be used to compare ingredients as well as energy and nutrient con–tributions of similar products.

28. A health claim describes the relationship between a food, food ingredient, or dietary supplement and the reduced risk of a nutrition–related condition. Examples of health claims can vary, but students can use the ones listed in Table 3.8. A structure/function claim describes the role a nutrient or dietary supplement plays in maintaining a structure, such as "calcium strengthens bone," or in promoting a normal function, such as "fiber aids bowel regularity." Examples of nutrient claims can vary, but students can use the ones listed in Table 3.9.

29. The FDA does not permit manufacturers to market a dietary supplement product as a treatment or cure for a disease, or to relieve signs or symptoms of a disease. If FDA officials question the safety of a dietary supplement or the truthfulness of claims that appear on supplement labels, manufacturers are responsible for providing the agency with evidence that their products are safe and the claims on labels are honest and not misleading. The FDA requires dietary supplement manufacturers to evaluate the purity, quality, strength, and composition of their products before mar–keting them.

30. The Nutrition Facts panels on food labels, nutrient analysis soft–ware programs, and government websites can be reliable sources of information about the energy and nutrient contents of foods and beverages.

31. Many Americans enjoy Mexican and Chinese foods, but traditional dishes are often modified to appeal to consumers who do not have Mexican or Chinese ancestry. Authentic Mexican meals are based primarily on rice, tortillas, and beans, depending on the region. To appeal to many non–Mexican Americans, "Mexican" fast–food restaurants in the United States often serve dishes that contain large portions of high–fat beef topped with sour cream and cheese. Although Chinese food is popular among Americans, many non–Asian members of the population do not like dishes that feature seafood and contain large portions of vegetables and grains. To appeal to these individuals, many North American Chinese res–taurants offer menu items that contain much larger portions of beef and chicken than authentic dishes. Furthermore, American–Chinese foods are often prepared with more fat than is used in true Chinese cooking.

32. Answers will vary but should include information from Table 3.12.

Chapter 4

1. Electrons are negatively charged particles that surround the nucleus; protons are positively charged particles in the nucleus of an atom. An element is a substance that cannot be broken down into distinctive components under usual conditions. A chemical bond is an attraction that forms when atoms interact. A molecule results from the formation of chemical bonds. A compound is a molecule that contains two or more different elements. A solution is an evenly distributed mixture of two compounds. The solvent is the primary compound of a solution, and the solute is the sub–stance dissolved in the solvent.

2. An ion is an atom or group of atoms that has an electrical charge because it has gained or lost one or more electrons.

3. Acids are substances that lose H^+ when dissolved in water; bases are substances that remove and accept H^+ when dissolved in water.

4. The pH of a watery solution refers to its hydrogen ion concentration.

5. A chemical reaction is a process that changes the arrangement of atoms in molecules.

6. Enzymes are proteins that initiate or facilitate (catalyze) chemical reactions.

7. Enzymes are sensitive to environmental conditions, including pH, temperature, and the presence of certain vitamins and minerals.

8. A cell is the smallest living functional unit in an organism. An organelle is a structure within the cell that has specific functions. DNA is a molecule that provides coded instructions for synthesiz–ing proteins. A tissue is comprised of cells usually joined together that have similar characteristics and functions.

9. Homeostasis is an internal chemical and physical environment that supports life and good health.

10. Answers will vary but should include information from Table 4.2.

11. Answers will vary but should relate to Figure 4.21 and begin with the mouth and end with the anus.

12. Examples of mechanical digestion include the biting and grind–ing actions of teeth and the muscular contractions of the GI tract. Chemical digestion includes actions of enzymes and HCl.

13. Answers may vary but should include four of the following known tastes for humans: sweet, salty, bitter, sour, and umami.

14. Choking can occur while eating if the epiglottis does not function properly and food enters the windpipe (trachea).

15. Peristalsis and segmentation, normal muscular movements of the digestive tract, keep food and chyme from becoming stuck in the tract.

16. The gastroesophageal sphincter keeps stomach contents from backing up into the esophagus.

17. The three sections of the small intestine are the duodenum, jejunum, and ileum. Most nutrient digestion and absorption takes place in the upper portion of the small intestine, primarily in the jejunum.

18. Removal of the pancreas would reduce nutrient digestion because the pancreas produces digestive enzymes.

19. Answers will vary but should include transport proteins or pumping mechanisms within the absorptive cell's plasma membrane, diffusion, or plasma membrane "swallowing" large substances.

20. Vomiting and diarrhea can cause dehydration, which develops more quickly in infants and young children as compared to adults.

21. Answers will vary but should include the information in Table 4.5.

22. Answers will vary but should include the information in Table 4.6.

23. Common signs and symptoms of irritable bowel syndrome are intestinal cramps, diarrhea, constipation, or alternating episodes of both diarrhea and constipation. Loose stools are often accompanied with mucus, and after bowel movements, the affected person feels as though elimination of stools was incomplete.

Chapter 5

1. Plants use carbon dioxide and water to make carbohydrates.

2. Plants use sunlight to obtain energy they need to live.

3. A human cell needs glucose to obtain energy.

4. The three most important dietary monosaccharides are glucose, fructose, and galactose.

5. Glucose is blood sugar; sucrose is table sugar; lactose is milk sugar; and maltose is malt sugar. Maltose is comprised of two glucose molecules; glucose and galactose comprise lactose; and glucose and fructose comprise sucrose.

6. A nutritive sweetener provides energy, whereas a nonnutritive sweetener does not provide energy in the amounts typically used to sweeten foods.

7. The parents should give their child the beverage sweetened with sucralose because the sweetener does not provide phenylalanine.

8. Starch and glycogen are both storage forms of polysaccharides, but starch is in plant foods and glycogen is primarily in liver and muscle tissue.

9. Most forms of dietary fiber are nondigestible carbohydrates. Oat bran and oatmeal, beans, apples, carrots, oranges and other citrus fruits, and psyllium seeds are rich sources of soluble fiber; whole-grain products, including brown rice, contain high amounts of insoluble fiber.

10. A minor amount of starch is digested in the mouth by the action of salivary amylase. Starch digestion stops soon after the food enters the acid environment of the stomach. In the small intestine, pancreatic amylase breaks down remaining starch molecules into maltose molecules. The enzyme maltase splits each maltose molecule into two glucose molecules. The glucose molecules are absorbed by small intestinal cells; they enter the bloodstream and travel to the liver via the portal vein. In the small intestine, sucrase splits the sucrose molecules in the grape jelly into glucose and fructose molecules. These monosaccharides are absorbed by small intestinal cells and eventually enter the hepatic portal vein and travel to the liver. The fiber in the crackers was not digested. The fiber moves through her intestinal tract and may be fermented by bacteria in her large intestine or contribute to her feces.

11. Insulin helps regulate blood glucose levels because the hormone enables glucose to enter most cells. The hormone enhances energy storage by promoting fat, glycogen, and protein production. Glucagon opposes insulin's effects by promoting the breakdown of glycogen. This process releases glucose into the bloodstream and, as a result, boosts the blood glucose level back to normal. Glucagon also stimulates liver and kidney cells to produce glucose from certain amino acids, the basic molecules that make up proteins. Furthermore, glucagon stimulates the breakdown of triglyceride into glycerol and fatty acids. As a result, glycerol and fatty acids rapidly enter into the bloodstream.

12. A ketone body is a chemical that results from the incomplete breakdown of fat. Cells form ketone bodies when they must use greater-than-normal amounts of fat for energy. Under these conditions, there is not enough glucose available for cells to metabolize the fat efficiently, and excessive ketone bodies form as a result.

13. Sugar-sweetened beverages are the main sources of added sugars in Americans' diets.

14. Fruit juice is a better choice because juice is a natural product that contains nutrients and phytochemicals in fruit. "Orange-Ade" is not a nutritionally equivalent substitute for orange juice, because it may contain only 10% fruit juice.

15. To estimate the grams of starch in the serving of the cereal, subtract the amount of starch and sugars in a serving (15 grams) from the amount of total carbohydrates (44 grams), and the remainder is the amount of starch (29 grams).

16. Answers will vary but should be the signs and symptoms listed in Table 5.9.

17. To reduce her risk of developing type 2 diabetes, Lata should avoid overweight, be physically active, and eat a healthy diet.

18. Answers may vary but should include signs presented in Table 5.11.

19. Lactose intolerance is a condition characterized by the inability to digest lactose completely.

20. Answers will vary but should include increasing one's intake of plant foods, especially whole-grain breads and cereals.

21. Eating soluble fiber can reduce the risk of cardiovascular disease by reducing blood cholesterol levels. The liver recycles the cholesterol from bile that is absorbed by the intestinal tract to make new bile. Soluble fiber interferes with the absorption of bile salts in the intestinal tract. As a result, the liver must use other sources of cholesterol, such as blood cholesterol, to produce bile. The fiber in food attracts water and swells in the digestive tract, forming a large soft mass that applies pressure to the inner muscular walls of the large intestine, stimulating the muscles to push the residue quickly through the tract. As a result, people who eat adequate amounts of fiber are less likely to strain while having bowel movements than people whose diets lack fiber.

22. Of this group of foods, raw apple has the lowest glycemic index.

Chapter 6

1. Rose's excess body fat can provide a source of energy for her, if she is ill and cannot eat. Also, the fat provides some insulation against cold temperatures and may protect her bones from break−ing if she falls.

2. The cake is likely to taste better and have a more desirable texture, because the fat in the milk contributes to flavor and "mouth feel."

3. Major lipids include fatty acids, triglycerides, phospholipids, and sterols, particularly cholesterol.

4. A saturated fatty acid has each carbon within the fatty acid chain completely filled with hydrogen atoms. An unsaturated fatty acid has two neighboring carbons within the chain that are missing two hydrogen atoms. Monounsaturated fatty acids have one double bond within the carbon chain; polyunsaturated fatty acids have two or more double bonds within the carbon chain.

5. Answers will vary but will relate to Table 6.2.

6. Alpha−linolenic acid and linoleic acid are essential fatty acids.

7. Trans fats are unsaturated fatty acids that have at least one trans double bond. The trans shape enables the hydrocarbon chain to be relatively straight. Foods that are rich sources of trans fat contain partially hydrogenated fat, such as shortening and stick margarine.

8. An omega−3 fatty acid has the first double bond in the polyunsaturated fatty acid's carbon chain appearing at the third carbon, when you start counting carbons at the omega end of the molecule. Alpha−linolenic acid, eicosapentaenoic acid (EPA), and docosahexaenoic acid (DHA) are omega−3 fatty acids.

9. Egg yolk or whole egg would keep the oil and milk emulsified.

10. Cholesterol is found only in animal foods. Egg yolk, liver, meat, poultry, whole milk, cheese, and ice cream are rich sources of cho−lesterol. Cholesterol is a component of every cell membrane; cells use cholesterol to synthesize vitamin D, bile, and steroid hormones.

11. Answers will vary but should follow the steps outlined in Figure 6.9 and the summary of lipid digestion and absorption presented in Figure 6.11.

12. Plants contain substances that interfere with enterohepatic cir−culation. This interference can reduce blood cholesterol levels, because the liver must remove cholesterol from the bloodstream to make new bile salts.

13. The body needs energy to survive. The triglycerides stored in fat cells can be used for energy. Thus, a person with excessive body fat has more energy stored in his or her body than a slim person.

14. Fat contributes 33% of the typical American diet's total energy intake.

15. The AMDR for fat is 20 to 35% of total calories.

16. According to the Dietary Guidelines, people should consume less than 10% of their total calories from saturated fatty acids.

17. The serving of chips provides 9 g of fat. Each gram of fat supplies 9 kcal. Thus, fat contributes 81 of the 150 kcal in a serving of the chips (9 g × 9 kcal/g).

18. Atherosclerosis is a long−term disease process in which plaques build up inside arterial walls. Arteriosclerosis is a condition that results from atherosclerosis and is characterized by loss of arte−rial flexibility. A thrombus is a fixed bunch of clots that remains in place. An embolus is a thrombus or part of a plaque that breaks free and travels through the bloodstream. Atherosclerosis can occur when something in the bloodstream irritates the lining of an artery. The body's immune system responds by producing inflamma−tion within the artery. Inflammation can stimulate healing, but the process can also trigger certain cells within the arterial wall to deposit cholesterol and other substances under the artery's lining. As a result, arterial plaque forms. Plaque interferes with or blocks circulation in the affected area. Plaque also roughens the normally smooth surface that lines the artery. The rough lining slows blood flow in the area and makes clots more likely to form. If a plaque ruptures, repairing the damage also involves clot formation, and such blood clots can be life threatening.

19. Answers will vary but should include king mackerel, tilefish, swordfish, or shark.

20. Answers will vary but should relate to information about risk fac−tors presented in Table 6.4.

21. According to this information, Bernard has a low risk of CVD because his HDL cholesterol level is high.

22. The liver releases high−sensitivity C−reactive protein in response to infection and inflammation. Elevated CRP may be a marker for atherosclerosis, which means it may be an early warning sign for the condition. A lipoprotein profile can provide information about blood levels of HDL, LDL, and triglycerides.

23. Answers will vary but should include reducing intakes of meats; foods made from whole milk; and crackers, cakes, cookies, pies, and other high−fat processed foods. Increasing intakes of most nuts, fatty fish, and sources of polyunsaturated oils can increase intakes of unsaturated fats.

24. A statin is a prescription drug that reduces elevated blood lipid levels. Statins interfere with the liver's metabolism of cholesterol, effectively reducing LDL cholesterol and/or triglyceride levels as a result.

25. Answers will vary but should include points in Figure 6.25.

26. BAC is "blood alcohol concentration." In August 2014, the legal limit for BAC was 0.8 for people who are 21 years of age or older.

27. Samuel is a heavy drinker.

Chapter 7

1. The amino acid is the chemical unit that makes up a protein.

2. Answers may vary but may include cell development and main−tenance, and the production of enzymes, antibodies, certain hor−mones, structural and contractile components, and blood−clotting factors. Additionally, proteins transport nutrients and oxygen in the bloodstream, help maintain acid−base and fluid balance, and can be used for energy.

3. The three groups that make up an amino acid are the amino or nitrogen−containing group, R group, and acid group.

4. A carbon skeleton is the part of an amino acid that remains after the amino group is removed.

5. Twenty amino acids are needed to make human proteins. Nine of these amino acids are essential.

6. A high−quality or complete protein contains all essential amino acids in amounts that will support protein deposition in muscles

and other tissues or support a young child's growth. A low–quality protein lacks one or more essential amino acids.

7. Most animal proteins are sources of high–quality proteins. Quinoa and processed soy proteins are also good sources of high–quality protein. Other plant foods, particularly fruits, vegetables, and grains, are sources of low–quality proteins.

8. Tryptophan, threonine, lysine, methionine, and cysteine are often the limiting amino acids in foods.

9. Answers will vary but should include key steps noted in Figure 7.6.

10. A protein undergoes denaturation when it is exposed to various conditions that alter the macronutrient's natural folded and coiled shape. Deamination is the removal of the nitrogen–containing group from an amino acid. Transamination is the transfer of an amino group from an amino acid to a receiving compound such as a carbon skeleton.

11. Negative balance occurs during starvation, serious illnesses, and severe injuries. Positive balance occurs during periods of rapid growth such as pregnancy, infancy, and puberty, and when people are recovering from illness or injury. Performing weight–training activities also leads to nitrogen retention.

12. To calculate the answer, convert the woman's weight to kilograms by dividing 143 pounds by 2.2 (65 kg). Multiply her weight in kilograms (65) by 0.8 grams of protein/kg to calculate her RDA for protein (52 g).

13. Answers will vary but should follow the path illustrated in Figure 7.10.

14. The AMDR for adult protein intake is 10 to 35% of energy from protein.

15. Americans generally eat about the same percentage of total calories from protein that they did in the early 1900s. Americans, however, now consume more protein from meat, fish, and poultry than from grains.

16. Answers will vary based on individual food intakes.

17. Answers will vary but should include reading the ingredient list to determine animal, soy, or quinoa sources of protein in the product.

18. Foods that substitute for meat include fish, poultry, eggs, soy products, or protein–rich dairy products such as cheese and yogurt. Extending high–quality protein refers to preparing dishes that incorporate small amounts of animal proteins with much larger amounts of plant proteins. Spaghetti with meat sauce is an example of a dish that extends high–quality protein in meat with more low–quality proteins in pasta.

19. The recipe does not provide a complementary mixture of proteins because fruit is not a good source of plant proteins to combine with peanuts.

20. Answers will vary but should include nuts, dry beans, quinoa, or seeds to complement the cereal protein.

21. Semivegetarians consume small amounts of meat, fish, or poultry, whereas other vegetarians do not eat animal flesh.

22. Plant–based diets may not contain enough energy, high–quality protein, omega–3 fatty acids, vitamins B–12 and D, and minerals zinc, iron, and calcium to meet a person's nutritional needs.

23. Children have higher protein and energy needs per pound of body weight than adults do. Since plant foods add bulk to the diet, vegan children are more likely to eat far less food than adult vegans because they become full sooner during meals. Thus, very young vegans may be unable to eat enough plant foods to meet their protein and energy needs.

24. People suffering from alcoholism, anorexia nervosa, or certain intestinal tract disorders are at risk of protein undernutrition. People with low incomes, especially older adults, are also at risk of protein deficiency.

25. Protein–energy malnutrition results when diets lack sufficient protein as well as energy.

26. According to this information, the child probably suffers from protein–energy malnutrition because of the parental neglect and presence of muscular wasting.

27. Common signs and symptoms of food allergy are hives, swollen or itchy lips, skin flushing, eczema, difficulty swallowing, wheezing and difficulty breathing, and abdominal pain, vomiting, and diarrhea. Common signs and symptoms of celiac disease are abdominal bloating, chronic diarrhea, weight loss, and poor growth in children.

28. They must provide their children with a special diet that is very low in phenylalanine.

29. Information about a patient's genetic makeup could enable physicians to prescribe more effective treatments, including special diets.

30. Answers will vary but may include the points in the "Food & Nutrition Tips" feature in this section.

31. Answers may vary, depending on the person's living situation. Although people can save 50 cents by buying the 5–pound bag of frozen peaches instead of 5 pounds of the fresh fruit, they need to have access to a large freezer if they intend to store the fruit. Buying smaller quantities of the fresh fruit may be a better option for people who do not have a way of storing the frozen fruit.

Chapter 8

1. Vitamins are complex organic compounds that regulate metabolic reactions. The body cannot synthesize most vitamins; vitamins naturally occur in commonly eaten foods; signs and symptoms of deficiency disease eventually occur when a vitamin is missing from the diet; if the deficiency disorder is treated early, good health is restored by supplying the missing vitamin.

2. Foods generally contain much smaller amounts of vitamins than of macronutrients; the body requires vitamins in much smaller amounts than macronutrients; and the body does not use vitamins directly for energy.

3. A provitamin is a vitamin precursor—a substance that does not function as a vitamin until the body converts it into an active form. An antioxidant is a substance that protects other compounds from oxidizing agents. A radical is a substance with an unpaired electron; radicals are highly reactive.

4. The federally regulated enrichment program specifies amounts of thiamin, riboflavin, niacin, folic acid, and iron that manufacturers must add to their refined flour and other milled grain products. Fortification involves the addition of one or more vitamins (and/or other nutrients) to a wide array of commonly eaten foods during manufacturing. The vitamins that are added may or may not be in the food naturally.

5. Answers will vary but should relate to information concerning food preparation, such as cooking methods, and food storage practices.

6. Answers will vary, but the table should include vitamins A, D, E, and K and conform to information provided in Table 8.2.

7. Answers will vary, but the table should include all B vitamins, vitamin C, and choline, and conform to information provided in Table 8.7.

8. Taking megadoses of vitamins can produce druglike effects in the body, including unpleasant and even dangerous side effects.

9. Answers will vary but should include three of the following: flushing of the skin, itchy skin, GI tract upsets, and liver damage (see Table 8.7).

10. High doses of vitamin B–6 have been associated with sensory nerve damage. The damage is usually reversible—after affected people stop taking excessive amounts of the vitamin.

11. Routine vitamin C supplementation does not protect against infection by common cold viruses, but the practice may shorten the duration of cold symptoms.

12. There is no clear scientific evidence that taking antioxidants, such as vitamins C and E, prevents healthy people from developing macular degeneration.

13. Lung cancer is the leading cause of cancer deaths in the United States.

14. *Metastasize* means "spread," so Margaret's breast cancer has spread to her lungs.

15. Answers will vary but should include intakes of alcohol; processed and red meats; fried, grilled, and broiled meats; salted fish; and moldy nuts (see Table 8.15).

16. Answers will vary but should include not smoking, limiting alcohol consumption, and maintaining a healthy body weight.

Chapter 9

1. A mineral nutrient is classified as a major mineral if humans require 100 mg or more per day or a trace mineral if humans require less than 100 mg/day.

2. List should include at least five of the minerals in the trace minerals column of Table 9.1.

3. List should include at least five of the minerals in the major minerals column of Table 9.1.

4. Water is a major solvent, and the nutrient often participates directly in chemical reactions. Water's other physiological roles include transporting substances, removing waste products, lubricating tissues, and regulating body temperature and acid–base balance. Additionally, water is a major component of blood, saliva, sweat, tears, mucus, and the fluid in joints.

5. Osmosis is the diffusion of a solvent, usually water, through a selectively permeable membrane.

6. Extracellular water contains higher concentrations of sodium and chloride ions than intracellular water. Intracellular water contains higher concentrations of potassium and phosphate ions than extracellular water.

7. The body obtains water by consuming various foods and liquids, such as fruit juice, milk, soup, coffee, tea, soft drinks, tap water, and plain or flavored bottled water. Cells also form some water as a metabolic by–product of metabolism. The body loses water in urine, perspiration, exhaled air, feces, vomit, and insensible perspiration.

8. If the body cannot regulate its water balance, cells can shrink, swell, and even die.

9. In response to dehydration, the posterior pituitary gland releases antidiuretic hormone that stimulates kidneys to conserve water. Additionally, the adrenal glands secrete aldosterone, a hormone that signals kidneys to reduce the elimination of sodium in urine. As a result, the kidneys return the mineral to the general circulation. Because water follows sodium, it is conserved as well.

10. The AI for total water intake is approximately 11 cups (2.7 L) for young women and approximately 15.5 cups (3.7 L) for young men.

11. A diuretic is a substance that increases urine production. Alcohol and caffeine have diuretic effects on the body.

12. Signs and symptoms of dehydration include weight loss, fatigue, thirst, loss of muscular strength and endurance, severe weakness, and coma.

13. Signs and symptoms of water intoxication may include dizziness, headache, confusion, inability to coordinate muscular movements, bizarre behavior, seizures, and coma.

14. Answers may vary, but may include inorganic structural components of tissues, such as calcium and phosphorus in bones and teeth. Minerals may also function as inorganic ions, such as calcium ions (Ca^{++}) that participate in blood clotting and sodium ions (Na^+) that help maintain fluid balance. Some ions, such as magnesium (Mg^{++}) and copper (Cu^{++}), are cofactors for chemical reactions. Many minerals are components of various enzymes, hormones, or other organic molecules, such as cobalt in vitamin B–12, iron in hemoglobin, and sulfur in the amino acids methionine and cysteine.

15. Refining foods can result in mineral losses. Minerals are water soluble and can be lost by leaching into watery cooking fluids.

16. The bioavailability of minerals depends largely on the body's need for the micronutrient. Additionally, minerals from animal foods are often better absorbed than minerals in plant foods.

17. The enrichment program requires the addition of iron to grain products.

18. Osteoporosis is a chronic disease characterized by low bone mass and reduced bone structure. People with osteoporosis have weak bones that are susceptible to fractures that can be costly to treat and result in disability and death, particularly among older adults.

19. Answers may vary, but should relate to risk factors listed in Table 9.7.

20. Prehypertension is a condition characterized by persistent systolic blood pressure readings of 120 to 139 mm Hg and diastolic readings of 80 to 89 mm Hg. Hypertension is characterized by persistent systolic values ≥140 mm Hg and diastolic values ≥90 mm Hg. Risk factors for hypertension include advanced age, African–American ancestry, obesity, physical inactivity, smoking cigarettes, and excess alcohol and sodium intakes. Table 9.11 presents major risk factors for hypertension.

21. The Dietary Approaches to Stop Hypertension (DASH) diet is low in sodium, total fat, and saturated fat; and high in fruits, vegetables, and low–fat dairy products. Other lifestyle changes that can reduce blood pressure include losing excess body fat and increasing physical activity.

22. Answers should conform to information in Table 9.5.

23. Iron deficiency is a condition characterized by low blood iron levels that are not low enough to result in severe health problems. Iron deficiency anemia occurs when oxygen transport in

blood is impaired, generally because there are not enough red blood cells to carry the oxygen or because red blood cells do not contain enough hemoglobin. Signs and symptoms of iron deficiency anemia include conditions listed in Table 9.17. People who are likely to develop iron deficiency include those who have lost substantial amounts of blood and young women who exclude meat and enriched bread and cereal products from their diets. Additionally, others at risk of iron deficiency are women of childbearing age (who generally lose some iron during menstruation), pregnant women, and infants born to women who are iron deficient.

24. Hemochromatosis is an inherited disorder in which the body absorbs too much iron. Signs and symptoms include joint pain, fatigue, lack of energy, abdominal pain, loss of sex drive, abnormal bronze skin color, and heart problems. The condition is treated by avoiding iron supplements and periodically having blood removed.

25. In humans, zinc deficiency results in dwarfism, mental retardation, iron deficiency anemia, underdeveloped sexual organs, and delays in sexual maturation.

26. Goiter is an enlarged thyroid gland. Cretinism occurs in infants born to women who were iodine deficient during pregnancy. The condition is characterized by permanent brain damage, reduced intellectual functioning, and growth retardation. Cretinism can be prevented by including a source of iodine in diets of pregnant women.

27. Rich food sources of selenium include Brazil nuts, fish, whole-grain products, and meats (see Table 9.21).

28. Chromium may enhance insulin's action on cell membranes and facilitate the entry of glucose into cells.

29. Answers will vary but should conform to information presented in Table 9.15.

30. Answers will vary but should include arsenic, boron, lithium, nickel, silicon, or vanadium.

31. Answers will vary but should conform to information provided in Table 9.22.

32. According to the FDA, "sparkling water" is treated water that contains the same amount of carbon dioxide it had when it emerged from its source. "Spring water" is from an underground formation from which the water flows naturally to the earth's surface at an identified location.

33. Answers will vary but should include avoiding containers that have the symbol that is shown in Figure 9.25.

Chapter 10

1. Calvin can be "overweight" if he has more muscle and less body fat than other people who are his height.

2. In 2009–2010, 35.7% of adult Americans were obese.

3. Total body fat includes adipose cells and fat in cell membranes, nervous tissue, and certain bones. Fat-free mass is comprised of body water; mineral-rich tissues such as bones and teeth; and protein-rich tissues, including muscles and organs.

4. When food is plentiful, adipose cells remove excess fat from the bloodstream for storage. As the amount of fat stored in adipose cells increases, the size of each cell expands, and the body gains weight. The body can produce more fat cells during periods of rapid growth and in response to overeating.

5. Body fat stores energy. Additionally, fat cells secrete numerous proteins, some of which have roles in regulating food intake, glucose metabolism, and immune responses.

6. Subcutaneous fat helps insulate the body against cold temperatures and protects muscles and bones from bumps and bruises. Subcutaneous fat also provides body contours.

7. Visceral fat is an adipose tissue deposit that lies under abdominal muscles and forms a protective "apron" for abdominal organs.

8. Cellulite is lumpy-appearing skin, but it is not a unique type of fat. Scientists have no clear understanding of why cellulite occurs, but it may simply be subcutaneous fat held in place by irregular bands of connective tissue.

9. Answers will vary but may include "underwater weighing" and measuring dual-energy x-ray absorptiometry, air displacement, bioelectrical impedance, and skinfold thicknesses. For many of the techniques, drawbacks include cost and size of equipment needed to measure body fat.

10. The average healthy young woman has more body fat than the average healthy young man because she needs the extra fat for hormonal and reproductive purposes.

11. He has a healthy percentage of body fat.

12. To estimate daily basal metabolic needs of a 185-pound woman, first convert the woman's weight to kilograms by dividing 185 pounds by 2.2 (approximately 84 kg). Then multiply 84 kg by 0.9 kcal to determine the amount of energy expended for metabolism in an hour (approximately 76 kcal/hr). Multiply 76 kcal/hour by 24 hours to obtain the amount of energy expended for basal metabolic needs in a day (1824 kcal).

13. The four major ways the body uses energy are basal metabolism, physical activity, TEF, and NEAT.

14. For most people, metabolism uses the most energy each day.

15. Answers will vary but may include body composition, thyroid hormone level, sex, body surface area, age, calorie intake, fever, stimulants, pregnancy, milk production after childbirth, and recovery after exercise.

16. Physical activity level can be easily altered.

17. TEF refers to the relatively small amount of energy needed to digest foods and beverages as well as to absorb and further process the macronutrients. TEF increases after meals. Energy needs for physical activity are related to skeletal muscle movements.

18. NEAT is nonexercise activity thermogenesis. NEAT refers to involuntary skeletal muscle activity and includes shivering, fidgeting, maintaining muscle tone, and maintaining body posture when not lying down.

19. A person gains weight when in positive energy balance.

20. Positive energy balance is desirable for pregnant women and during periods of growth, such as during fetal development, infancy, childhood, and puberty.

21. Weight loss is characterized by negative energy balance.

22. This woman is likely to be overweight.

23. Answers will vary but should include conditions listed in Table 10.6.

24. The stigma of obesity is the negative attitude that many people have toward obese persons, such as characterizing overfat people as lazy, stupid, and sloppy.

25. Central–body obesity ("apple shape") is more likely to pose serious health risks than having excess fat below the waist, or a pear-shaped fat distribution. Central–body fat distribution is associated with increased risks of type 2 diabetes and CVD.

26. Measuring a person's waist circumference is a quick and easy way to determine whether body fat distribution is likely to result in serious chronic health problems.

27. Hunger is an uncomfortable feeling that drives a person to consume food. Satiety is the sense that enough food or beverages have been consumed to satisfy hunger.

28. Adipose cells secrete leptin, a hormone that reduces hunger and inhibits fat storage in the body. The stomach secretes ghrelin that stimulates eating behavior.

29. Thrifty genes could benefit people during periods of food deprivation, such as famine.

30. According to the set–point theory, the body's fat content (and, therefore, body weight) is genetically predetermined. The set point acts like a home thermostat, except that it regulates body weight instead of temperature.

31. Hunger is a drive to eat food, whereas appetite is a desire to eat appealing food.

32. Answers will vary but should include food marketing and sensory appeal, such as appearance, taste, and odor. Our work and home environments influence whether we are sedentary or physically active by providing opportunities to be active.

33. Answers will vary but should include genetics, occupations that do not provide enough physical activity, and psychological factors, such as mood and self–esteem.

34. The four key elements necessary for weight loss and maintenance are motivation, calorie reduction, regular physical activity, and behavior modification.

35. Answers will vary but should include points listed in Table 10.7.

36. Before joining a weight–loss group or plan, consumers should find out how much the program costs and how often they will need to pay for the program. Consumers should ask whether they need to sign a contract and the length of the contract. Do special foods or supplements need to be purchased? If nutrition counseling is provided, what are the credentials of the persons providing nutrition counseling and information? Furthermore, does the plan emphasize the importance of making lifestyle changes? Does the program's advertising include questionable weight–loss claims and deceptive testimonials?

37. Answers will vary but should include these: eat a low–calorie diet; eat regular meals, including breakfast almost every day; weigh themselves at least once a week; exercise for an average of 60 minutes daily; and limit television watching.

38. When orlistat is taken along with a meal, the medication reduces fat digestion by about 30%.

39. Roux–en–Y and gastric banding procedures are common forms of bariatric surgery performed in the United States. Bariatric surgeries are effective because they reduce the size of the stomach. As a result, patients can consume only small portions of food at a time. Gastric banding is easier to perform, safer than other types of bariatric surgery, and relatively easy to reverse.

40. Liposuction is a surgical method of reducing the size of local fat deposits by suctioning excess fat out of the body. Risks of liposuction are infection, permanent dimpling of the skin at the suctioning site, and the production of tiny clumps of fat or blood clots that can be deadly, if they enter the bloodstream.

41. A fad diet is a trendy dietary practice that has widespread appeal among a population; after a period, people lose interest in the practice and it becomes no longer fashionable. Fad diets typically promote rapid weight loss without calorie restriction and increased physical activity; limit food selections to be from only a few food groups and dictate specific diet rituals; require buying a book or various gimmicks; use outlandish and unscientific claims to support their usefulness; rely on testimonials from famous people; connect the diet to trendy places; and do not emphasize the need to change eating habits and physical activity patterns.

42. Many overweight and obese people are attracted to fad diets and dietary supplements for weight loss because they believe promoters' claims that the diets or products are "magic bullets" for shedding unwanted weight quickly and effortlessly.

43. Answers will vary but should include supplements presented in Table 10.9.

44. Answers will vary but should include features or claims that the product or service causes rapid and extreme weight loss; requires no need to change dietary patterns or physical activity; results in permanent weight loss; is scientifically proven or doctor endorsed; includes a money–back guarantee; is safe; is supported by satisfied customers; displays before–and–after photos; and provides disclaimers in small print, such as "Results not typical" at the bottom of the ad or with an "after" photo.

45. Chronic diseases such as cancer, tuberculosis, AIDS, inflammatory bowel disease, depression, and hormonal imbalances can result in severe weight loss that is difficult to treat.

46. To gain weight, underweight adults can gradually increase their consumption of calorie–dense foods, especially those high in healthy fats. Eating regular meals and snacks also aids in weight gain and maintenance. If excess physical activity habits contribute to the inability to gain weight, underweight people can find ways to be less active. Furthermore, underweight individuals can add muscle mass by following resistance–training programs regularly, but their calorie intake must support extra energy demands of those programs.

47. Skipping breakfast regularly is a sign of disordered eating, not an eating disorder.

48. The three major types of eating disorders are anorexia nervosa (AN), bulimia nervosa (BN), and binge–eating disorder (BED). Major signs of AN are severely restricted food intake and maintenance of an unhealthy low body weight. People with BN are difficult to recognize, but characteristic signs of the condition are bite marks and scars on the knuckles that result from self–induced vomiting. The major sign of BED is consuming a much larger amount of food than most people would eat under similar circumstances in a brief period of time.

49. Answers will vary but should include the risk factors shown in Table 10.10.

50. Answers will vary but should include the health consequences listed in Table 10.11, as well as death.

Chapter 11

1. Physical activity is any movement that results from skeletal muscle contraction. Exercise refers to physical activities that are usually planned and structured for a particular purpose.

2. Physical fitness is the ability to perform moderate– to vigorous–intensity activities without becoming excessively fatigued.

3. Healthy adults under 65 years of age should engage in at least 150 minutes of moderate–intensity physical activity a week or 75 minutes of vigorous–intensity physical activity a week. Additionally, adults should include eight to 10 strengthening exercises twice a week.

4. Answers will vary but should include benefits indicated in Figure 11.1.

5. Performing resistance exercises regularly can increase muscle mass, strength, and flexibility. Resistance exercises can also increase bone mass.

6. To calculate the target heart rate range of a 24–year–old person performing moderate–intensity activity, subtract the person's age (24) from 220 to obtain 196, the age–related maximum heart rate. Moderate–intensity activity raises the heart rate to 50 to 70% of the age; therefore, multiply 196 × .50 to obtain the lower limit of the range (98 bpm), and 196 × .70 to obtain the upper limit of the range (approximately 137 bpm). Thus, the heart rate range for this individual is 98 to 137 bpm.

7. Muscle cells break down glycogen to provide a source of glucose during exercise.

8. ATP is formed as a result of glycolysis and aerobic respiration. Some ATP is also formed by the breakdown of triglycerides, amino acids, and alcohol. Muscle cells also use phosphocreatine to produce ATP quickly under anaerobic conditions.

9. Muscle cells rely on the PCr–ATP, lactic acid, and oxygen systems to obtain energy. The PCr–ATP system forms ATP by breaking down PCr into creatine and P_i. The energy that is released helps synthesize ATP from ADP and P_i. In anaerobic conditions, muscle cells metabolize glucose to pyruvate and then convert pyruvate to lactic acid. The degradation of glucose to lactic acid produces a small amount of ATP. Lactic acid accumulates in muscles and converts to a related substance, lactate. Although certain muscle cells can use lactate as a fuel, some of the compound enters the bloodstream. The liver removes lactate from blood and can convert the compound into glucose. The oxygen system metabolizes glucose completely to CO_2 and H_2O, resulting in the production of far more ATP–energy than the amount produced by anaerobic systems. The PCr–ATP and lactic acid systems do not need oxygen to produce ATP.

10. Individuals can increase their aerobic exercise capacity by engaging in endurance–training programs that gradually increase the intensity level of activities. Such training improves muscle cells' ability to generate ATP rapidly.

11. Fat is a major energy source for muscles while one is resting or engaged in low– to moderate–intensity physical activities.

12. Practical ways to assess whether an athlete's energy intake is adequate include having the athlete keep accurate food records and use the information to estimate his or her daily calorie intakes. An athlete can also monitor his or her body weight and have skinfold thicknesses measured regularly.

13. Carbohydrate intake contributes to glycogen stores; glycogen depletion is a major cause of fatigue during endurance exercise. To maintain adequate muscle glycogen, athletes should consume 6 to 10 g of carbohydrate per kilogram of body weight daily. By consuming several servings of grains, starchy vegetables, and fruits daily, an athlete can obtain enough carbohydrate to maintain adequate liver and muscle glycogen stores.

14. Answers will vary but should include grains, starchy vegetables, and fruits. Also, see Table 11.4 for high–carbohydrate, low–fat foods.

15. Compared to nonathletes, the typical athlete consumes more food to meet his or her increased energy needs, and, as a result, obtains plenty of dietary protein. Therefore, healthy active Americans who eat varied diets that supply adequate energy do not need to take protein or amino acid supplements. If people consume excess protein from foods or supplements and they do not need the energy, the amino acids in these proteins will not be used for building or repairing muscles. Instead, the body converts the extra amino acids into fat for storage in adipose tissue.

16. Dehydration and overhydration detract from optimal physical performance and can cause serious health problems.

17. Answers will vary but should include signs and symptoms listed in Table 11.8.

18. According to the IMMDA, sports drinks are necessary when workouts or events last longer than 30 minutes. Although electrolytes are lost in sweat, the quantities lost in shorter periods can be easily replaced by consuming foods and beverages, such as water or fruit juice, after the event.

19. The practice of taking antioxidant supplements may not be helpful and could be harmful. Results of studies that examined whether antioxidant vitamin supplements enhanced athletic performance generally concluded that performance was not improved, unless there was a preexisting deficiency of those particular vitamins. Free radicals generated during intense exercise may stimulate the body's natural antioxidant defense system. Thus, the oxidative stress produced during exercise might have benefits, and blocking this process by taking antioxidant vitamin supplements may not be desirable.

20. Iron deficiency can negatively affect athletic performance because the body needs iron to produce red blood cells, transport oxygen, and obtain energy.

21. Female athletes who have irregular or no menstrual cycles may lack adequate amounts of the hormone estrogen. Although weight–bearing exercise, such as jogging, improves bone density, estrogen is necessary for maintaining healthy bones. Female athletes who develop menstrual cycle abnormalities should consult a physician to determine the cause.

22. Athletes often use ergogenic aids to improve their physical performance, because they hope to gain the competitive edge over their sports rivals.

23. Answers will vary but should include ephedra–containing supplements, caffeine (high intakes), anabolic steroids, human growth hormone, and DHEA.

24. Coffee, energy drinks, caffeinated soft drinks, chocolate, and tea (see Table 11.10).

25. Caffeine raises the level of fatty acids in blood, and as a result, exercising muscles can use more fat for energy. Caffeine also enhances the ability of skeletal and heart muscles to contract and increases mental alertness.

26. The three key components of an aerobic workout regimen are warm–up, workout, and cool–down.

27. Answers will vary, but the fitness program should include the principles of exercise variety, balance, and moderation. Furthermore, the person should include activities that are enjoyable and easy to incorporate into his or her routine.

Chapter 12

1. Norovirus is responsible for most cases of food–borne illness in the United States.

2. The illness caused by norovirus is usually the result of a food–borne infection.

3. The FDA regulates nearly all domestic and imported food sold in interstate commerce and enforces federal food safety laws. Additionally, the FDA establishes standards for safe food manufacturing practices, such as Hazard Analysis and Critical Control Point programs. FDA officials can take certain enforcement actions, such as requesting that a food manufacturer recall an unsafe item, so that it is removed from store shelves. The FDA also educates the general public about safe food handling practices. The Food Safety and Inspection Service (FSIS) enforces food safety laws for domestic and imported meat and poultry products. Additionally, FSIS staff collect and analyze food samples to check for the presence of microbial and other unwanted and potentially harmful material in foods. FSIS officials can ask meat and poultry processors to recall unsafe products. FSIS also educates people about proper food handling practices. The EPA oversees drinking water quality and assists state officials in their efforts to monitor water quality. Furthermore, EPA staff regulate toxic substances and wastes to prevent their entry into foods and the environment.

4. Local health departments are responsible for inspecting restaurants, grocery stores, dairy farms, and local food processing companies.

5. Three common ways harmful microbes are transmitted to food are by vermin, poor personal hygiene practices, and improper food handling.

6. Cross–contamination occurs when pathogens in one food are transferred to another food, contaminating it.

7. Pasteurization is a special heating process used by many commercial food producers to kill pathogens.

8. To survive and multiply, most microbes need warmth, moisture, and a source of nutrients, and some also require oxygen.

9. In general, high–risk foods are warm, moist, and protein rich, and they have a neutral or slightly acidic pH (see Table 12.1).

10. Signs and symptoms of food–borne illnesses generally involve the digestive tract and include nausea, vomiting, diarrhea, and intestinal cramps.

11. People who suffer from a food–borne illness should consult a physician when an intestinal disorder is accompanied by one or more of the following signs: fever (oral temperature above 101.5°F), bloody bowel movements, prolonged vomiting that reduces fluid intake, diarrhea that lasts more than 3 days, or dehydration.

12. Food–borne illness generally causes gastrointestinal tract symptoms, whereas influenza is primarily a respiratory tract infection.

13. Answers will vary but should include bacteria listed in Table 12.2.

14. Answers will vary but should include viruses listed in Table 12.3.

15. Answers will vary but should include a protozoan and a parasite listed in Table 12.4.

16. Aflatoxins are poisonous substances produced by certain molds.

17. Answers will vary but should include points under the "Purchasing Food" section of Chapter 12.

18. Answers will vary but should include points under the "Setting the Stage for Food Preparation" and "Preparing Food" sections of Chapter 12.

19. Answers will vary but should include points under the "Storing and Reheating Food" section of Chapter 12.

20. Ground meats and poultry are often sources of food–borne illness because grinding increases the surface area of the protein–rich food, exposing it to contaminants.

21. Raw fish should be frozen for recommended amounts of time before being eaten.

22. The "danger zone" for rapid pathogen multiplication is between 40°F and 140°F.

23. The Check Your Steps program recommends four simplified actions: clean, separate, cook, and chill.

24. Shelf life is the period of time that a food can be stored before it spoils.

25. Answers will vary but should include methods highlighted in Table 12.7.

26. Boiling home–canned, low–acid foods for 10 minutes can make them safe to eat.

27. Answers may vary but can include meats, fresh fruits and vegetables, spices, dry vegetable mixes, seeds, and shell eggs.

28. Answers will vary but should include points made under the "Preparing for Disasters" section of Chapter 12. Table 12.8 lists foods that can be stored safely for emergency situations.

29. Safe sources of drinking water include bottled water, an undamaged water heater, toilet tanks (not bowls), melted water from ice cubes, and fruit juices. Water from pools, spas, radiators, heating systems, and water beds is unsafe to drink.

30. A food additive is a substance added to food that influences the product's characteristics. Direct food additives may maintain the safety of foods, prevent undesirable changes, or improve taste or color of foods. Indirect additives, such as compounds from a food's wrapper or container, can enter food as it is packaged, transported, or stored. Indirect additives have no purpose.

31. Color additives are dyes, pigments, or other substances that provide color to foods, drugs, or cosmetics.

32. Food ingredients that had been in use prior to 1958 were listed as Generally Recognized as Safe (GRAS) when qualified experts generally agreed that the substance was safe for its intended use. Food manufacturers can include substances on the GRAS list as ingredients without testing them for safety or getting prior approval from the FDA.

33. According to the Delaney Clause, food manufacturers cannot add a new compound that causes cancer at any level of intake. Thus, if an additive causes cancer, even though very high doses may be necessary to cause the disease, no amount of the additive is considered to be safe, and none is allowed in food. Evidence for cancer risk could come from either laboratory animal or human studies. The FDA allows very few exceptions to this clause.

34. An unintentional food additive is a substance that accidentally enters food during processing. Common biological and physical food contaminants are insect parts, rodent feces or urine, dust and dirt, and bits of metal or glass from machinery used to process food.

35. A pesticide is any substance that people use to control or kill unwanted insects, weeds, rodents, fungi, or other organisms. Types of pesticides include insecticides, rodenticides, herbicides, and fungicides.

36. Integrated pest management (IPM) involves using a variety of methods for controlling pests while limiting damage to the environment. IPM methods include growing pest−resistant crops, using predatory wasps to control crop−destroying insects, trapping adult insect pests before they can reproduce, and using biologically based pesticides.

37. The EPA regulates the use of pesticides.

38. A pesticide tolerance is the maximum amount of pesticide residue that can be in or on each treated food crop. A pesticide tolerance includes a margin of safety, so the maximum pesticide residue that is allowed to be in or on a food is much lower than amounts that can cause negative health effects.

39. Once a pesticide is applied to cropland, it may remain in the soil, be taken up by plant roots, decompose to other compounds, or enter groundwater and waterways. Winds may carry pesticides in air and dust to distant locations, where the toxic material can land on food crops.

40. Answers will vary but should include using hand sanitizers, drinking only commercially bottled water, boiling water before drinking it, eating foods that are fully cooked and served hot, and not eating locally provided fresh fruits and vegetables that have been washed in unsanitary water.

41. Answers will vary but should include the countries that are colored red in Figure 12.12.

Chapter 13

1. John is an older adult.

2. For women, lactation is the life stage that involves milk production for breastfeeding.

3. Eight weeks after conception, the developing human being is referred to as a fetus.

4. The role of the placenta is to transfer nutrients and oxygen from the mother's bloodstream to the embryo/fetus. Additionally, the placenta transfers wastes from the embryo/fetus to the mother's bloodstream, so her body can eliminate them.

5. Birth weight is a major factor that determines whether a baby is healthy and survives his or her first year of life.

6. Gestational hypertension can be dangerous because it increases the risk of maternal death and premature delivery.

7. Answers will vary but should include enlarged breasts, "morning sickness," tiredness, swollen feet, constipation, and heartburn.

8. Women whose prepregnancy weights were within the healthy range can expect to gain 25 to 35 pounds. Underweight women should gain 28 to 40 pounds; overweight women should gain 15 to 25 pounds during pregnancy. Obese women should gain 11 to 20 pounds during pregnancy. The recommendations are higher for women who are pregnant with more than one fetus.

9. Pregnant women who are folate deficient have a high risk of giving birth to infants with neural tube defects, such as spina bifida. Pregnant women who are iron deficient can develop iron deficiency anemia, a condition that increases the risk of giving birth prematurely and having low−birth−weight (LBW) infants.

10. Women who drink alcohol during pregnancy are at risk of having a child with a fetal alcohol spectrum disorder. Compared to pregnant women who do not smoke cigarettes, expectant mothers who smoke have higher risk of giving birth too early and having LBW babies. Furthermore, expectant mothers who smoke cigarettes may increase the risk of having babies with birth defects or that die of sudden infant death syndrome.

11. In response to an infant sucking on its mother's nipple, the brain releases oxytocin, a hormone that signals breast tissue to "let down" milk. The let−down reflex enables milk to travel in several tubes to the nipple area. When let−down occurs, the infant removes the milk by continued sucking.

12. Lactation increases a new mother's energy needs by about 300 to 400 kcal more than her prepregnancy energy needs.

13. Colostrum is the first secretion of the breasts that occurs after delivery. Colostrum is a very important first food for babies, because the fluid contains antibodies and immune system cells that can be absorbed by the infant's immature digestive tract. Colostrum also contains a substance that encourages the growth of a type of bacteria in the baby's intestinal tract that reduces the risk of infection.

14. New mothers should exclusively breastfeed their babies for the first 6 months of life.

15. Answers will vary but should include points in Table 13.4.

16. Answers will vary but should include points in Table 13.4.

17. Compared to whole cow's milk, human milk provides about the same amount of energy, less protein and calcium, and more carbohydrate and fat.

18. Signs indicating a baby is ready physically to eat solid foods include: loss of the extrusion reflex; physiological maturity to digest, metabolize, and excrete a wider range of foods; and ability to sit up with back support and coordinate muscular control over mouth and neck movements.

19. A healthy infant should triple its birthweight during the first year of life.

20. A food jag is a period in which the child refuses to eat a food that was liked in the past or in which the child wants to eat only a particular food.

21. In children, iron deficiency can lead to decreased physical stamina, learning ability, and resistance to infection.

22. Answers will vary but should include brushing teeth with a pea-sized amount of fluoride−containing toothpaste twice daily; providing routine pediatric dental care; offering fluoridated drinking water; not eating carbohydrate−rich snacks, especially between meals; and offering sugarless chewing gum.

23. Compared to preschoolers, older children often skip breakfast, and they typically consume more foods away from home, larger portions of food, and more fried foods and sweetened beverages. School−age children also tend to consume less milk and fewer fruits and vegetables, except fried potatoes.

24. Answers will vary but should include encouraging children to eat breakfast and other tips from the "Food & Nutrition Tips" feature in the "School—Age Children" section of Chapter 13.

25. Boys usually begin their growth spurt when they are between 12 and 15 years of age. Most girls begin their growth spurt between 10 and 13 years of age.

26. Iron deficiency leads to increased fatigue and decreased ability to concentrate and learn. Inadequate calcium intake during adolescence is associated with decreased bone mass and increased likelihood of bone fractures later in life.

27. Answers should provide the information in Table 13.9. Children and adolescents whose BMI—for—age is greater than or equal to the 85th percentile and less than the 95th percentile are overweight, and youngsters who are at or above the 95th percentile are obese. Although there is no generally accepted definition for *extreme obesity* that applies to children, BMI—for—age at or above the 97th percentile is typically used to identify children who have extreme obesity.

28. Answers will vary but should include elevated blood pressure, cholesterol, and glucose levels and the factors listed in Table 13.10.

29. Answers will vary but should include spending too much time on sedentary activities; consuming too many empty—calorie foods and beverages; and having a family history of obesity, high birth weight, and obese family members.

30. To qualify for bariatric surgery, an adolescent should have extreme obesity, failed to lose weight after 6 months of trying to reduce his or her weight, attained his or her adult height, and developed serious chronic conditions that are associated with obesity.

31. Life expectancy is the length of time a person born in a specific year, such as 1900, can expect to live. Life span refers to the maximum number of years a human can live.

32. Answers will vary but should include points listed in Table 13.12.

33. Compared to younger persons, older adults have greater risk of nutritional deficiencies because of physiological changes associated with the normal aging process. Other factors that can influence an older person's nutritional status include illnesses, medications, low income, and lack of social support.

34. Diets of older adults, particularly older women, often provide inadequate amounts of vitamins D, A, and B—12 and minerals such as calcium and potassium.

35. Caregivers can improve nutrient intakes of older persons by adding more spices to foods, making mealtimes social events, and serving energy—dense snacks between meals, such as cheese, milk—shakes, nuts, or oatmeal cookies. If the elderly person has difficulty chewing, serving soft items such as ground meats, cooked vegetables, pureed fruits, and puddings can increase food intake. The "Food & Nutrition Tips" feature in the "Nutrition for Older Adults" section of Chapter 13 presents more suggestions for improving nutrient intakes of elderly persons.

36. Under certain conditions, calorie restriction extends the life expectancies of organisms that include fruit flies and rodents.

37. Answers may vary but should include adopting healthy lifestyles by consuming a nutritionally adequate diet, obtaining regular moderate— to vigorous—intensity physical activity, maintaining a healthy weight, avoiding tobacco products, limiting alcohol consumption, and having regular physical checkups.

Answers to Practice Test Questions

Chapter 1
1. b	**2.** a	**3.** d	**4.** d	**5.** b
6. a	**7.** c	**8.** c	**9.** b	**10.** a
11. c	**12.** a	**13.** b	**14.** c	**15.** b

Chapter 2
1. d	**2.** b	**3.** a	**4.** d	**5.** c
6. d	**7.** a	**8.** c	**9.** b	**10.** d
11. c	**12.** a			

Chapter 3
1. a	**2.** d	**3.** c	**4.** a	**5.** d
6. a	**7.** d	**8.** d	**9.** b	**10.** a
11. c	**12.** b	**13.** a	**14.** c	**15.** a

Chapter 4
1. a	**2.** d	**3.** b	**4.** c	**5.** d
6. a	**7.** b	**8.** b	**9.** d	**10.** b
11. a	**12.** d	**13.** b	**14.** d	**15.** c
16. b				

Chapter 5
1. b	**2.** c	**3.** a	**4.** b	**5.** b
6. c	**7.** b	**8.** b	**9.** c	**10.** b
11. a	**12.** c	**13.** b	**14.** b	

Chapter 6
1. a	**2.** b	**3.** c	**4.** a	**5.** b
6. d	**7.** b	**8.** c	**9.** b	**10.** c
11. c	**12.** b	**13.** d		

Chapter 7
1. b	**2.** c	**3.** a	**4.** a	**5.** b
6. d	**7.** c	**8.** a	**9.** d	**10.** c
11. d	**12.** c	**13.** a		

Chapter 8
1. d	**2.** c	**3.** a	**4.** d	**5.** d
6. a	**7.** b	**8.** a	**9.** b	**10.** c
11. c	**12.** a	**13.** b	**14.** c	**15.** d
16. a				

Chapter 9

1. c	**2.** b	**3.** d	**4.** d	**5.** a
6. c	**7.** d	**8.** a	**9.** b	**10.** c
11. b	**12.** a			

Chapter 10

1. b	**2.** d	**3.** b	**4.** b	**5.** b
6. c	**7.** a	**8.** b	**9.** a	**10.** b
11. d	**12.** d			

Chapter 11

1. b	**2.** c	**3.** a	**4.** d	**5.** b
6. a	**7.** b	**8.** d	**9.** a	**10.** d
11. b	**12.** c			

Chapter 12

1. a	**2.** a	**3.** c	**4.** d	**5.** c
6. b	**7.** d	**8.** c	**9.** c	**10.** b
11. d	**12.** b			

Chapter 13

1. b	**2.** c	**3.** b	**4.** c	**5.** a
6. c	**7.** c	**8.** d	**9.** a	**10.** d

Appendix H

References

Chapter 1

1. Kant AK and others: Patterns of recommended dietary behaviors predict subsequent risk of mortality in a large cohort of men and women in the United States. *Journal of Nutrition* 139:1374, 2009.

2. U.S. Department of Health and Human Services, U.S. Department of Agriculture. *2015–2020 Dietary Guidelines for Americans*. 2015. www.health.gov/dietaryguidelines/2015/guidelines/executive–summary Accessed: January 21, 2016

3. Dietary Supplement Health and Education Act of 1994. Public Law 103–417, 103rd Congress. http://ods.od.nih.gov/About/DSHEA_Wording.aspx Accessed: July 20, 2014

4. Hoyert DL, Xu J: Deaths: Preliminary data for 2011. *National Vital Statistics Reports* 61 (6):1, 2012. http://www.cdc.gov/nchs/fastats/deaths.htm Accessed: July 20, 2014

5. Editors: Preventable cancer in the USA. *The Lancet* 375 (9727):1665, 2010.

6. Kushi LH and others: American Cancer Society guidelines on nutrition and physical activity for cancer prevention. *CA: A Journal for Clinicians* 62:30, 2012.

7. U.S. Department of Agriculture, Economic Research Service: Food availability (per capita) data system: *Calories: Average daily per capita calories from the U.S. food availability, adjusted for spoilage and other waste*. http://www.ers.usda.gov/data–products/food–availability–%28per–capita%29–data–system.aspx#.Ue8b2W0qmSo Accessed: February 21, 2014

8. Food and Drug Administration and National Institutes of Health. *Healthy People 2020*. http://www.healthypeople.gov/2020/about/new2020.aspx Accessed: July 20, 2014

9. U.S. Department of Agriculture, ChooseMyPlate.gov: *SuperTracker and other tools, empty calories chart*. Last modified: June 2011. http://www.choosemyplate.gov/supertracker–tools/empty–calories–chart.html Accessed: July 20, 2014

10. What is a megadose and why do you recommend against taking mega–doses of vitamins? *Johns Hopkins Medical Letter Health After 50* 13(6):8, 2001.

11. Fletcher RH, Fairfield KM: Vitamins for chronic disease prevention in adults. *Journal of the American Medical Association* 287(23):3127, 2002.

12. Huang H–Y and others: The efficacy and safety of multivitamin and mineral supplement use to prevent cancer and chronic disease in adults: A systematic review for a National Institutes of Health State–of–the–Science Conference. *Annals of Internal Medicine* 145(5):372, 2006.

13. American Dietetic Association: Position of the American Dietetic Association: Functional foods. *Journal of the American Dietetic Association* 109(4):735, 2009.

14. United Nations, UN News Service: *Number of world's hungry to top 1 billion this year—UN food agency*. June 19, 2009. http://www.un.org/apps/news/story.asp?NewsID=31197&Cr=hunger&Cr1=# Accessed: July 20, 2014

15. Black RE and others: Maternal and child undernutrition: Global and regional exposures and health consequences. *The Lancet* 371(9608): 243–60, 2008.

16. Knoll Rajaratnam J and others: Neonatal, postneonatal, childhood and under–5 mortality for 187 countries, 1970–2010: A systematic analysis of progress towards Millennium Development Goal 4. *The Lancet* May 24, 2010 DOI: 10.1016/S0140–6736(10)60703–9

17. World Health Organization, United Nations Children's Fund: *Nutrition security and emergencies*. 2003. http://www.unicef.org/nutrition/index_emergencies.html Accessed: July 20, 2014

18. U.S. Census Bureau: *State and County QuickFacts*. Last revised July 2014. http://quickfacts.census.gov/qfd/states/00000.html Accessed: July 20, 2014

19. U.S. Department of Health and Human Services: *The 2014 HHS Poverty Guidelines*. http://aspe.hhs.gov/poverty/14poverty.cfm Accessed: July 20, 2014

20. Coleman–Jenson A and others: Household food security in the United States in 2011. *Economic Research Report*. (ERR–141). September 2012. http://www.ers.usda.gov/publications/err–economic–research–report/err141.aspx Accessed: July 26, 2013

21. United Nations Children's Fund: *Supply annual report 2013*. 2014. http://www.unicef.org/supply/index_report.html Accessed: July 20, 2014

22. U.S. Food and Drug Administration: *FDA's role in regulating safety of GE foods*. Last updated May 2014. http://www.fda.gov/ForConsumers/ConsumerUpdates/ucm352067.htm Accessed: July 20, 2014

23. Thomson JA: Genetically modified crops—playing a positive role in sustainable development in Africa. *South African Medical Journal* 96(6):509, 2006.

24. Foley JA: Can we feed the world and sustain the planet? *Scientific American* 305(5):60, 2011.

Chapter 2

1. Kraut A: *Dr. Joseph Goldberger & the war on pellagra*. Office of NIH History. http://history.nih.gov/exhibits/Goldberger/index.html Accessed: July 20, 2014

2. Simoni RD and others: Copper as an essential nutrient and nicotinic acid as the anti–black tongue (pellagra) factor: The work of Conrad Arnold Elvehjem. *Journal of Biological Chemistry* 277(34):e22, 2002.

3. Benedetti F and others: How placebos change the patient's brain. *Neuropsychoparmacology* 36(1):339–354, 2011.

4. Centers for Disease Control and Prevention: *National Diabetes Statistics Report, 2014*. 2014. http:www.cdc.gov/diabetes/data/statistics/2014StatisticsReport.html Accessed: July 21, 2014

5. U.S. Federal Trade Commission: Marketers of unproven weight–loss products ordered to pay nearly $2 million. http://www.ftc.gov/opa/2010/01/diet.shtm Accessed: July 21, 2014

6. Bailey RL and others: Dietary supplement use in the United States, 2003–2006. *Journal of Nutrition*. 141 (2):261, 2011.

7. Food and Drug Administration: *Q & A on dietary supplements*. Last updated March 2014. http://www.fda.gov/Food/DietarySupplements/QADietarySupplements/default.htm#what_is Accessed: July 21, 2014

8. National Center for Complementary and Alternative Medicine: *Using dietary supplements wisely*. Updated June 2014. http://nccam.nih.gov/health/supplements/wiseuse.htm Accessed: July 21, 2014

9. Kelly JP and others: Recent trends in use of herbal and other natural products. *Archives of Internal Medicine* 165:281, 2005.

10. National Center for Complementary and Alternative Medicine: *The use of complementary and alternative medicine in the United States.* Last modified February 2013. http://nccam.nih.gov/news/camstats/2007/camsurvey_fs1.htm Accessed: July 21, 2014

11. Hempel S and others: Probiotics for the prevention and treatment of antibiotic–associated diarrhea. *Journal of the American Medical Association* 307(18):1959, 2012.

12. National Institutes of Health, Office of Dietary Supplements: *Background information: dietary supplements.* Reviewed June 2011. http://ods.od.nih.gov/factsheets/DietarySupplements–HealthProfessional/ Accessed: July 21, 2014

13. Food and Drug Administration: *Dietary supplements.* Last updated May 2014. http://www.fda.gov/Food/DietarySupplements/default.htm Accessed: July 21, 2014

14. Food and Drug Administration: *FDA 101: Product recalls.* May 2010. http://www.fda.gov/downloads/ForConsumers/ConsumerUpdates/UCM143332.pdf Accessed: July 21, 2014

15. Enfield S: Market overview 2012: What's driving supplement sales? *Natural Foods Merchandiser*, May 29, 2012 http://newhope360.com/retailing/nfm–market–overview–2012–whats–driving–supplement–sales Accessed: July 21, 2014

16. Liu RH: Potential synergy of phytochemicals in cancer prevention: Mechanism of action. *Journal of Nutrition* 134:3479S, 2004.

Chapter 3

1. Food Marketing Institute: *Supermarket facts: Industry overview 2013.* http://www.fmi.org/ Accessed: July 22, 2014

2. U.S. Department of Agriculture, Economic Research Service: *New products.* Updated February 2013. http://www.ers.usda.gov/topics/food–markets–prices/processing–marketing/new–products.aspx#.U851sLFjnSg Accessed: July 22, 2014

3. Institute of Medicine: *Dietary Reference Intakes for vitamin C, vitamin E, selenium, and carotenoids.* Washington, DC: National Academies Press, 2000.

4. Otten JJ and others (eds): *Dietary Reference Intakes: The essential guide to nutrient requirements.* Institute of Medicine of the National Academies. Washington, DC: National Academies Press, 2006.

5. U.S. Food and Drug Administration: *Draft guidelines: Whole grain label statements.* Updated May 2014. http://www.fda.gov/food/guidanceregulation/guidancedocumentsregulatoryinformation/ucm059088.htm Accessed: July 22, 2014

6. U.S. Department of Agriculture, ChooseMyPlate: *What counts as a cup of fruit?* ND. http://www.choosemyplate.gov/food–groups/ Accessed: July 22, 2014

7. Centers for Disease Control and Prevention: *How to use fruits and vegetables to help manage your weight.* Last updated June 2012. http://www.cdc.gov/healthyweight/healthy_eating/fruits_vegetables.html Accessed: July 22, 2014

8. U.S. Department of Health and Human Services and U.S. Department of Agriculture. *2015–2020 Dietary Guidelines for Americans.* 2015. http://health.gov/dietaryguidelines/2015/guidelines/ Accessed: January 24, 2016

9. U.S. Departments of Agriculture and Health and Human Services: *Scientific report of the 2015 Dietary Guidelines advisory committee* 2015. http://health.gov/dietaryguidelines/2015–scientific–report/PDFs/Scientific–Report–of–the–2015–Dietary–Guidelines–Advisory–Committee.pdf Accessed: January 22, 2016

10. U.S. Department of Agriculture, *ChooseMyPlate.gov.* 2011. http://www.choosemyplate.gov/ Accessed: July 22, 2014

11. U.S. Department of Agriculture, Choose MyPlate: *What are oils?* ND. http://www.choosemyplate.gov/food–groups/oils.html Accessed: July 22, 2014

12. U.S. Department of Agriculture: *Physical activity.* http://www.choosemyplate.gov/physical–activity.html Accessed: July 22, 2014

13. Guenther PM and others: Diet quality of low–income and higher–income Americans in 2003–04 as measured by the Healthy Eating Index–2005. U.S. Department of Agriculture, *Nutrition Insight 42, 2008.* http://www.cnpp.usda.gov/Publications/NutritionInsights/Insight42.pdf Accessed: July 22, 2014

14. American Diabetes Association: Diabetes basics: Tuning up your skills. *Diabetes Forecast* April 2013. http://www.diabetesforecast.org/past–issues–archive.html Accessed: July 22, 2014

15. U.S. Food and Drug Administration, Center for Food Safety and Applied Nutrition: *How to understand and use the Nutrition Facts label.* Updated June 2014. http://www.fda.gov/Food/IngredientsPackagingLabeling/LabelingNutrition/ucm274593.htm Accessed: July 22, 2014

16. U.S. Food and Drug Administration: *Menu & vending machines labeling requirements.* Updated May 2014. http://www.fda.gov/Food/IngredientsPackagingLabeling/LabelingNutrition/ucm217762.htm Accessed: July 22, 2014

17. Urban LE and others: The accuracy of stated energy contents of reduced–energy, commercially prepared foods. *Journal of the American Dietetic Association* 110(1):116, 2010.

18. Earles K: *Sustainable agriculture: An introduction.* National Sustainable Agricultural Service. Page last updated: April 2012. https://attra.ncat.org/attra–pub/viewhtml.php?id=294 Accessed: July 22, 2014

19. U.S. Department of Agriculture, National Organic Program: *What is organic?* Last modified 2012. http://www.ams.usda.gov Accessed: July 22, 2014

20. Comis D: No shortcuts in checking soil health. *Agricultural Research* 55(6):4, 2007. http://www.ars.usda.gov/is/AR/archive/jul07/soil0707.htm Accessed: July 22, 2014

21. U.S. Department of Agriculture, Economic Research Service: *Organic agriculture: Overview.* Updated April 2014. http://www.ers.usda.gov/topics/natural–resources–environment/organic–agriculture.aspx#.U85–Y7FjnSg Accessed: July 22, 2014

22. Organic Trade Association: *Consumer–driven U.S. organic market surpasses $31 billion in 2011.* 2012. http://www.organicnewsroom.com/2012/04/us_consumerdriven_organic_mark.html Accessed: July 22, 2014

23. Dangour AD and others: Nutritional quality of organic foods: A systematic review. *American Journal of Clinical Nutrition* July 29, 2009. DOI: 10.3945/ajcn.2009.28041

24. Smith–Spangler C and others: Are organic foods safer or healthier than conventional alternatives? A systematic review. *Annals of Internal Medicine.* 157(5):348, 2012.

25. Gavrilova NA, Gavrilov LA: Comments on dietary restriction, Okinawa diet and longevity. *Gerontology* 58:221, 2012.

Chapter 4

1. Saladin KS: *Anatomy & physiology.* 7th ed. Boston: McGraw–Hill Publishing Company, 2015.

2. Widmaier E and others: *Vander's human physiology.* 12th ed. Boston: McGraw–Hill Publishing Company, 2010.

3. Seeley RR and others: *Essentials of anatomy & physiology.* 9th ed. Boston: McGraw–Hill Publishing Company, 2011.

4. Prescott LM and others: *Microbiology.* 8th ed. Boston: McGraw–Hill Publishing Company, 2011.

5. Hempel S and others: Probiotics for the prevention and treatment of antibiotic–associated diarrhea: A systematic review and meta–analysis. *Journal of the American Medical Association* 307(18):1959, 2012.

6. American Gastroenterological Association: *Understanding constipation.* January 2013. http://www.gastro.org/patient–center/digestive–conditions/constipation Accessed: July 22, 2014

7. National Institutes of Health, U.S. National Library of Medicine: Nausea and vomiting—adults. *Medline Plus*. Updated 2011. http://www.nlm.nih.gov/medlineplus/ency/article/003117.htm Accessed: July 22, 2014

8. American Gastroenterological Association: Patient center: *Understanding heartburn and reflux disease*. ND. www.gastro.org/patient−center/digestive−conditions/heartburn−gerd Accessed: July 22, 2014

9. American Society for Gastrointestinal Endoscopy: *Understanding upper endoscopy*. ND. www.asge.org/PatientInfoIndex.aspx?id=378 Accessed: July 22, 2014

10. American Gastroenterological Association: Patient center: *A patient's guide to living with irritable bowel syndrome*. ND. http://www.gastro.org/patient−center/digestive−conditions/irritable−bowel−syndrome Accessed: July 22, 2014

Chapter 5

1. Economic Research Service, U.S. Department of Agriculture: *Sugar and sweeteners yearbook tables*. May 2014. http://www.ers.usda.gov/data−products/sugar−and−sweeteners−yearbook−tables.aspx#.U86_arFjnSg Accessed: July 22, 2014

2. Henkel JS and others: Toxins from bacteria. *EXS* 100:1, 2010. PMC3564551.

3. Centers for Disease Control and Prevention, National Center for Emerging and Zoonotic Infectious Diseases. *Botulism*. Updated April 2014. http://www.cdc.gov/nczved/divisions/dfbmd/diseases/botulism/ Accessed: July 22, 2014

4. Academy of Nutrition and Dietetics: Position of the Academy of Nutrition and Dietetics: Use of nutritive and nonnutritive sweeteners. *Journal of the Academy of Nutrition and Dietetics* 112 (5):739, 2012.

5. Swithers SE and others: High−intensity sweeteners and energy balance. *Physiology & Behavior* 100(1):55, 2010.

6. Soffritti M and others: First experimental demonstration of the multi−potential carcinogenic effects of aspartame administered in the feed to Sprague−Dawley rats. *Environmental Health Perspectives* 114(3):379, 2006.

7. U.S. Food and Drug Administration: *FDA Statement on European Aspartame Study*. Updated April 2013. http://www.fda.gov/Food/IngredientsPackagingLabeling/FoodAdditivesIngredients/ucm208580.htm Accessed: July 22, 2014

8. FDA provides guidance on "whole grain" for manufacturers. *FDA News*, P06−23. Updated April 2013. http://www.fda.gov/NewsEvents/Newsroom/PressAnnouncements/2006/ucm108598.htm Accessed: July 22, 2014

9. Otten JJ and others, eds.: *Dietary Reference Intakes: The essential guide to nutrient requirements*. Washington, DC: National Academies Press, 2006.

10. U.S. Department of Agriculture. Agricultural Research Service: NHANES, 2009−2010, *What we eat in America*. Table 1: Nutrient intakes from food: Mean amounts consumed per individual, by gender and age, in the United States, 2009−2010. http://www.ars.usda.gov/Services/docs.htm?docid=13793 Accessed:July 22, 2014

11. U.S. Department of Agriculture, *ChooseMyPlate.gov: Calories: How many can I have?* ND. http://www.choosemyplate.gov/weight−management−calories/calories/empty−calories−amount.html Accessed: July 22, 2014

12. U.S. Department of Agriculture, Agricultural Research Service:What's in the food you eat *search tool*, 5.0. http://www.ars.usda.gov/Services/docs.htm?docid=17032 Accessed: July 22, 2014

13. Malik VS and others: Sugar−sweetened beverages and risk of metabolic syndrome and type 2 diabetes. *Diabetes Care* 33(11):2477, 2010.

14. Sicher J: Special issue: U.S. beverage results for 2013. *Beverage Digest* 65(7):1, 2014. http://www.beverage−digest.com/pdf/top−10_2014.pdf Accessed: July 22, 2014

15. Gaesser GA: Carbohydrate quantity and quality in relation to body mass index. *Journal of the American Dietetic Association* 107(10):1768, 2007.

16. Rosen LA and others: Effects of cereals on postprandial glucose, appetite regulation and voluntary energy intake at subsequent lunch; focusing on rye products. *Nutrition Journal* 10:7, 2011.

17. Saris WH: Sugars, energy metabolism, and body weight control. *American Journal of Clinical Nutrition* 78(Suppl):850S−857S, 2003.

18. Rolls BJ: Plenary lecture 1 dietary strategies for the prevention and treatment of obesity. *Proceedings of the Nutrition Society* 69(1):70, 2010.

19. Aller EEJG and others: Starches, sugars, and obesity. *Nutrients* 3(3): 341, 2011. Published online March 14, 2011. DOI: 10.3390/nu3030341.

20. Jennings A and others: Diet quality is independently associated with weight status in children aged 9−10 years. *Journal of Nutrition* 141(3): 453, 2011.

21. Centers for Disease Control and Prevention: Beverage consumption among high school students—United States, 2010. *Morbidity Mortality Weekly Report* 60(23):778, 2011.

22. Dennis EA and others: Beverage consumption and adult weight management: A review. *Eating Behaviors* 10(4):237, 2009.

23. Yanovski S: Sugar and fat: Cravings and aversions. *Journal of Nutrition*, 133 (3):835S, 2003.

24. Benton D: The plausibility of sugar addiction and its role in obesity and eating disorders. *Clinical Nutrition* 29(3):288, 2010.

25. Hu FB, Malik VS: Sugar−sweetened beverages and risk of obesity and type 2 diabetes: Epidemiologic evidence. *Physiology and Behavior* 100(1):47, 2010.

26. Rizkalla SW: Health implications of fructose consumption: A review of recent data. *Nutrient Metabolism* 4(7):82, 2010.

27. Johnson RK and Yon BA. Weighing in on added sugars and health. *Journal of the American Dietetic Association* 110(9):1296, 2010.

28. U.S. Department of Agriculture, Human Nutrition Information Service: *Nationwide Food Consumption Survey: Food and nutrient intakes by individuals in the United States, 1 day, 1987−88*. Report no. 87−I−1, 1993.

29. Report of the expert committee on the diagnosis and classification of diabetes mellitus. *Diabetes Care* 26(Suppl 1):S5, 2003.

30. Centers for Disease Control and Prevention: *National diabetes statistics report, 2014*. http://www.cdc.gov/diabetes/pubs/statsreport14.htm Accessed: July 22, 2014

31. Hoyert DL, Xu J: Deaths: Preliminary data for 2011. *National Vital Statistics Reports*. 61(6):1, 2012. http://www.cdc.gov/nchs/data/nvsr/nvsr61/nvsr61_06.pdf Accessed: July 22, 2014

32. Yeung WG and others: Enterovirus infection and type 1 diabetes mellitus: Systematic review and meta−analysis of observational molecular studies. *British Medical Journal* 2011;342:d35 DOI: 10.1136/bmj.d35

33. Luopajärvi K and others: Enhanced levels of cow's milk antibodies in infancy in children who develop type 1 diabetes later in childhood. P*ediatric Diabetes* 9(5):434, 2008.

34. Centers for Disease Control and Prevention: *Diabetes & Pregnancy*. 2012. http://www.cdc.gov/Features/DiabetesPregnancy/ Accessed: June 20, 2014

35. Mayo Clinic: *A1C test*. January 2013. http://www.mayoclinic.org/tests−procedures/a1c−test/basics/definition/prc−20012585 Accessed: July 22, 2014

36. American Diabetes Association: *Weight loss*. Last reviewed 2013. http://www.diabetes.org/living−with−diabetes/recently−diagnosed/where−do−i−begin/weight−loss.html Accessed: July 22, 2014

37. National Institutes of Health, National Diabetes Information Clearinghouse: Diabetes prevention program (DPP). Updated 2013. http://diabetes.niddk.nih.gov/dm/pubs/preventionprogram/ Accessed: July 22, 2014

38. Johnson RJ and others: Potential role of sugar (fructose) in the epidemic of hypertension, obesity and the metabolic syndrome, diabetes,

kidney disease, and cardiovascular disease. *American Journal of Clinical Nutrition* 86:899, 2007.

39. Esposito K and others: Prevention of type 2 diabetes by dietary patterns: A systematic review of prospective studies and meta—analysis. *Metabolic Syndrome and Related Disorders* 8(6):471, 2010.

40. Song Y and others: A prospective study of red meat consumption and type 2 diabetes in middle—aged and elderly women: The women's health study. *Diabetes Care* 27(9):2108, 2004.

41. de Munter JSL and others: Whole grain, bran, and germ intake and risk of type 2 diabetes: A prospective cohort study and systematic review. *PLOS Medicine* 4(8):135, 2007.

42. National Institute of Diabetes and Digestive and Kidney Diseases: *Hypo—glycemia*. Publication No. 09–3926. Updated 2012. http://diabetes.niddk.nih.gov/dm/pubs/hypoglycemia/ Accessed: July 22, 2014

43. Ford ES and others: Prevalence and correlates of metabolic syndrome based on a harmonious definition among adults in the US. *Journal of Diabetes* 2(3):180, 2010.

44. National Institutes of Health, National Heart Lung and Blood Institute: *Metabolic syndrome: What is metabolic syndrome?* 2011. http://www.nhlbi.nih.gov/health/health—topics/topics/ms/ Accessed: July 22, 2014

45. National Center for Biotechnology Information: Metabolic syndrome. *PubMed Health*. Last reviewed 2012. http://www.ncbi.nlm.nih.gov/pubmedhealth/PMH0004546/ Accessed: July 22, 2014

46. National Institute of Diabetes and Digestive and Kidney Diseases: *Lactose intolerance*. May 2014. http://digestive.niddk.nih.gov/ddiseases/pubs/lactoseintolerance/index.htm Accessed: July 22, 2014

47. Montalto M and others: Management and treatment of lactose malab—sorption. *World Journal of Gastroenterology* 12(2):187, 2006.

48. National Institute of Mental Health: *Attention deficit hyperactivity disorder*. Revised 2012. http://www.nimh.nih.gov/health/publications/attention—deficit—hyperactivity—disorder/index.shtml Accessed: July 22, 2014

49. Centers for Disease Control and Prevention: *Attention—Deficit/Hyperactivity Disorder (ADHD), Data & statistics*. 2013. http://www.cdc.gov/ncbddd/adhd/data.html Accessed: July 22, 2014

50. World Health Organization: *Cancer*. Last updated February 2014. http://www.who.int/mediacentre/factsheets/fs297/en/index.html Accessed: July 22, 2014

51. National Cancer Institute: *Colorectal cancer prevention (PDQ™) over—view*. Last modified February 2014. http://www.cancer.gov/cancertopics/pdq/prevention/colorectal/HealthProfessional Accessed: July 22, 2014

52. Centers for Disease Control and Prevention: *Colorectal (colon) cancer: What can I do to reduce my risk?* Last updated April 2014. http://www.cdc.gov/cancer/colorectal/basic_info/prevention.htm Accessed: July 22, 2014

53. Webb D: Glycemic index: Gateway to good health or grand waste of time? *Environmental Nutrition* 25(1):1, 6, 2002.

54. Barclay AW and others: Glycemic index, glycemic load, and chronic dis—ease risk—a meta—analysis of observational studies. *American Journal of Clinical Nutrition* 87(3):627, 2008.

55. Foster—Powell K and others: International table of glycemic index and glycemic load values. *American Journal of Clinical Nutrition* 76(1):5, 2002.

56. Denova—Gutierrez E and others: Dietary glycemic index, dietary gly—cemic load, blood lipids, and coronary heart disease. *Journal of Nutrition and Metabolism*. Published online 2010 February 28. DOI: 10.1155/2010/170680

57. Jenkins DJ and others: Effect of low—glycemic index or a high—cereal fiber diet on type 2 diabetes: A randomized trial. *Journal of the American Medical Association* 300(23):2742, 2008.

58. Saul N, Maryniuk MD: Using the glycemic index in diabetes management. *American Journal of Nursing* 110(7):68, 2010.

Chapter 6

1. Shikany JM and others: Is dietary fat "fattening"? A comprehensive research synthesis. *Critical Reviews in Food Science and Nutrition* 50(8):699, 2010.

2. McTiernan A and others: Weight, physical activity, diet, and progno—sis in breast and gynecological cancers. *Journal of Clinical Oncology* 28(26):4074, 2010.

3. Siri—Tarino and others: Saturated fatty acids and risk of coronary heart disease: Modulation by replacement nutrients. *Current Atherosclerosis Reports* 12(6):384, 2010.

4. Hunter JE and others: Cardiovascular disease risk of dietary stearic acid compared with trans, other saturated, and unsaturated fatty acids: A systemic review. *American Journal of Clinical Nutrition* 91(1):46, 2010.

5. Otten JJ and others (eds.): *Dietary Reference Intakes: The essential guide to nutrient requirements*. Washington, DC: National Academies Press, 2006.

6. Remig V and others: Trans fat in America: A review of their use, con—sumption, health implications, and regulation. *Journal of the American Dietetic Association* 110(4):585, 2010.

7. Brouwer IA and others: Effect of animal and industrial trans fatty acids on HDL and LDL cholesterol levels in humans—a quantitative review. *PLoS One* 5(3):e9434, 2010.

8. Hayes KC, Pronczuk A: Replacing trans fat: The argument for palm oil with a cautionary note on interesterification. *Journal of the American College of Nutrition* 29 (3 Suppl):253s, 2010.

9. Astrup A and others: The role of reducing intakes of saturated fat in the prevention of cardiovascular disease: Where does the evidence stand in 2010? *American Journal of Clinical Nutrition* 93(4):684, 2011.

10. Zeisel SH: Nutritional genomics: Defining the dietary requirement and effects of choline. *Journal of Nutrition* 141(3):531, 2011.

11. Penry JT, Manore MM: Choline: An important micronutrient for maxi—mal endurance—exercise performance? *International Journal of Sports Nutrition, Exercise, and Metabolism* 18(2):191, 2008.

12. Rodriguez NR and others: Position of the American Dietetic Associa—tion, Dietitians of Canada, and the American College of Sports Medicine: Nutrition and athletic performance. *Journal of the American Dietetic Association* 109(3):509, 2009.

13. Oregon State University, Linus Pauling Institute: *Choline*. Updated 2009. http://lpi.oregonstate.edu/infocenter/othernuts/choline// Accessed: July 23, 2014

14. U.S. Department of Agriculture: *Nationwide food consumption survey, Food and nutrient intakes by individuals in the United States, 1 day, 1987–88*. http://www.ars.usda.gov/Services/docs.htm?docid=14392 Accessed: July 23, 2014

15. U.S. Department of Agriculture, Agricultural Research Service: *NHANES, 2009—2010, What we eat in America*. Table 1: Nutrient intakes from food: Mean amounts consumed per individual, by gender and age, in the United States, 2009—2010. http://www.ars.usda.gov/SP2User—Files/Place/12355000/pdf/0910/Table_1_NIN_GEN_09.pdf Accessed: July 23, 2014

16. U.S. Departments of Health and Human Services and Agriculture: *2015–2020 Dietary Guidelines for Americans*. 2015. http:health.gov/dietaryguidelines/2015/guidelines/ Accessed: January 23, 2016

17. American Heart Association: AHA statistics update: Heart disease and stroke statistics—2010 update. 2009. http://circ.ahajournals.org/content/early/2009/12/17/CIRCULATIONAHA.109.192667 Accessed: July 23, 2014

18. Hoyert DL, Xu J: Deaths: Preliminary data for 2011. *National Vital Statistics Reports* 61, 2012. http://www.cdc.gov/nchs/data/nvsr/nvsr61/nvsr61_06.pdf Accessed: July 23, 2014

19. Ai M and others: Small dense low density lipoprotein cholesterol and coronary heart disease: Results from the Framingham Offspring Study. *Clinical Chemistry* 56(6):967, 2010.

20. Thanassoulis G and others: Associations of long–term and early adult atherosclerosis risk factors with aortic and mitral valve calcium. *Journal of the American College of Cardiology* 55(22):2491, 2010.

21. National Institutes of Health, National Heart Lung and Blood Institute: *Who is at risk for atherosclerosis?* 2011. http://www.nhlbi.nih.gov/health/health–topics/topics/atherosclerosis/atrisk.html Accessed: July 23, 2014

22. Abraham JM, Cho L: The homocysteine hypothesis: Still relevant to the prevention and treatment of cardiovascular disease? *Cleveland Clinic Journal of Medicine* 77(12):911, 2010.

23. Centers for Disease Control and Prevention: *Diabetes health concerns.* Last reviewed March 2014. http://www.cdc.gov/diabetes/consumer/problems.htm Accessed: July 23, 2014

24. Centers for Disease Control and Prevention: *Smoking & tobacco use: Health effects of cigarette smoking.* Updated February 2014. http://www.cdc.gov/tobacco/data_statistics/fact_sheets/health_effects/effects_cig_smoking/index.htm Accessed: July 23, 2014

25. Centers for Disease Control and Prevention: *Smoking & tobacco use: Health effects of secondhand smoke.* Last updated March 2014. http://www.cdc.gov/tobacco/data_statistics/fact_sheets/secondhand_smoke/health_effects/index.htm Accessed: July 23, 2014

26. Centers for Disease Control and Prevention, National Center for Health Statistics: *FastStats: Cholesterol.* Updated May 2014. http://www.cdc.gov/nchs/fastats/cholesterol.htm Accessed: July 23, 2014

27. Go AS and others: Heart Disease and Stroke Statistics—2013 update: A report from the American Heart Association. *Circulation* 127(1):143, 2013.

28. National Institutes of Health: C–reactive protein. *MedLinePlus.* Last updated July 9, 2014. http://www.nlm.nih.gov/medlineplus/ency/article/003356.htm Accessed: July 23, 2014

29. Fernandez ML, West KL: Mechanisms by which dietary fatty acids modulate plasma lipids. *Journal of Nutrition* 135(9):2075, 2005.

30. De Caterina R: n–3 Fatty acids in cardiovascular disease. *New England Journal of Medicine* 364:2439, 2011.

31. Harris WS and others: Omega–6 fatty acids and risk for cardiovascular disease: A science advisory from the American Heart Association Nutrition Subcommittee of the Council on Nutrition, Physical Activity, and Metabolism; Council on Cardiovascular Nursing; and Council on Epidemiology and Prevention. *Circulation* 119(6):902, 2009.

32. Djoussé L, Gaziano JM: Egg consumption and risk of heart failure in the Physician's Health Study. *Circulation* 117(4):512, 2008.

33. Mayo Clinic: *Butter vs. margarine: Which is better for my heart?* 2012. http://www.mayoclinic.com/print/butter–vs–margarine/AN00835/ Accessed: July 23, 2014

34. National Institutes of Health, National Center for Alternative and Complementary Medicine: *Garlic.* Updated 2012. http://nccam.nih.gov/health/garlic/ataglance.htm Accessed: July 23, 2014

35. American Dietetic Association: Position of the American Dietetic Association: Fat replacers. *Journal of the American Dietetic Association* 105(2):266, 2005.

36. Maji D and others: Safety of statins. *Indian Journal of Endocrinology and Metabolism* 17(4):636, 2013.

37. National Institutes of Health, National Institute on Alcohol Abuse and Alcoholism: *Alcohol: A women's health issue.* 2008. http://pubs.niaaa.nih.gov/publications/brochurewomen/women.htm Accessed: July 23, 2014

38. Substance Abuse and Mental Health Services Administration: *Results from the 2012 National Survey on Drug Use and Health: Summary of National Findings and Detailed Tables.* Last updated 2013. www.samhsa.gov/data/NSDUH/2012SummNatFindDetTables/NationalFindings/NSDUHresults2012.htm#fig3.1 Accessed: July 23, 2014

39. Centers for Disease Control and Prevention: *Alcohol and public health: Fact sheets: Binge drinking.* Updated January 2014. http://www.cdc.gov/alcohol/fact–sheets/binge–drinking.htm Accessed: July 23, 2014

40. Centers for Disease Control and Prevention: *Alcohol and public health: Fact sheets: Excessive alcohol use and risks to men's health.* Last updated January 2014. http://www.cdc.gov/alcohol/fact–sheets/mens–health.htm Accessed: July 23, 2014

41. Centers for Disease Control and Prevention: *Alcohol and public health: Fact sheets: Alcohol use and health.* Updated March 2014. http://www.cdc.gov/alcohol/fact–sheets/alcohol–use.htm Accessed: July 23, 2014

42. American Cancer Society: *Does drinking alcohol increase the risk of cancer?* June 2013. http://www.cancer.org/cancer/news/expertvoices/post/2013/06/26/does–drinking–alcohol–increase–the–risk–of–cancer.aspx Accessed: July 23, 2014

43. American Heart Association: *Alcohol and heart health.* ND. http://www.heart.org/HEARTORG/Conditions/More/MyHeartandStrokeNews/Alcohol–and–Heart–Disease_UCM_305173_Article.jsp Accessed: July 23, 2014

44. Wilsnack SC and others: *Women and the costs of alcohol use. Alcohol Research* 35(2):219, 2014.

Chapter 7

1. Shier D and others: *Hole's human anatomy & physiology.* 12th ed. Boston: McGraw–Hill Publishing Company, 2010.

2. Reeds PJ: Dispensable and indispensable amino acids for humans. *Journal of Nutrition* 130:1835S, 2000.

3. Food and Nutrition Board: *Dietary Reference Intakes for energy, carbohydrate, fiber, fat, fatty acids, cholesterol, protein, and amino acids (macronutrients).* Institute of Medicine of the National Academies, Washington, DC: National Academies Press, 2005.

4. Oelke EA and others: Quinoa. *Alternative Field Crops Manual.* University of Wisconsin–Extension, University of Minnesota: Center for Alternative Plant & Animal Productions, and the Minnesota Extension Service. ND. http://www.hort.purdue.edu/newcrop/afcm/quinoa.html Accessed: July 27, 2014

5. Reinwald S and others: Whole versus the piecemeal approach to evaluating soy. *Journal of Nutrition* 140(12):2335S, 2010.

6. Layman DK: Dietary Guidelines should reflect new understandings about adult protein needs. *Nutrition & Metabolism* 6:12, 2009. DOI: 10.1186/1743–7075–6–12

7. U.S. Department of Agriculture, Agricultural Research Service: *Nutrient intakes from food: Mean amounts consumed per individual, by gender and age, in the United States, 2009–2010.* http://www.ars.usda.gov/SP2UserFiles/Place/12355000/pdf/0910/Table_1_NIN_GEN_09.pdf Accessed: July 25, 2014

8. U.S Department of Agriculture, Center for Nutrition Policy and Promotion: *Nutrient content of the U.S. food supply.* Modified May 2014. http://www.cnpp.usda.gov/USFoodSupply–1909–2010.htm Accessed: July 27, 2014

9. U.S. Department of Agriculture: *ChooseMyPlate.gov: Tips for making wise choices.* http://www.choosemyplate.gov/protein–foods–tips. Accessed: March 17, 2016

10. American Dietetic Association: Position of the American Dietetic Association: Vegetarian diets. *Journal of the American Dietetic Association* 109(7):1266, 2009.

11. Rizzo NC and others: Vegetarian dietary patterns are associated with a lower risk of metabolic syndrome: The Adventist Health Study 2. *Diabetes Care* 34(5):1225, 2011. Published online 2011 April 20. DOI: 10.2337/dc10–1221

12. Craig WJ: Health effects of vegan diets. *American Journal of Clinical Nutrition* 89(5):1627S, 2009.

13. American Dietetic Association: Position of the American Dietetic Association, Dietitians of Canada, and the American College of Sports Medicine: Nutrition and Athletic Performance. *Journal of the American Dietetic Association* 109:509, 2009.

14. Guez S and others: Severe vitamin B12 deficiency in an exclusively breastfed 5—month—old Italian infant born to a mother receiving multi—vitamin supplementation during pregnancy. *BMC Pediatrics* 12:85, 2012. Published online June 24, 2012. DOI: 10.1186/1471—2431—12—85.

15. Bardone—Cone AM and others: The inter—relationships between veg—etarianism and eating disorders among females. *Journal of the Academy of Nutrition and Dietetics* 112(8):1247, 2012.

16. American Cancer Society: *What are the risk factors for colorectal cancer?* Last revised July 2013. http://www.cancer.org/cancer/colonandrectumcancer/detailedguide/colorectal—cancer—risk—factors Accessed: July 28, 2014

17. American Cancer Society: *What are the risk factors for prostate cancer?* Last revised March 2014. http://www.cancer.org/Cancer/ProstateCancer/DetailedGuide/prostate—cancer—risk—factors Accessed: July 28, 2014

18. American Cancer Society: *What are the risk factors for pancreatic cancer?* Last revised June 2014. http://www.cancer.org/cancer/pancreaticcancer/detailedguide/pancreatic—cancer—risk—factors Accessed: July 28, 2014

19. American Cancer Society: *What are the risk factors for stomach cancer?* Last revised May 2014. http://www.cancer.org/cancer/stomachcancer/detailedguide/stomach—cancer—risk—factors Accessed: July 28, 2014

20. Campbell WW, Tang M: Protein intake, weight loss, and bone mineral density in postmenopausal women. *Journal of Gerontology*, Series A 65A(10):1115, 2010. DOI: 10.1093/gerona/glq083. Advance access published on July 6, 2010.

21. Halford JCG, Harrold JA: Satiety—enhancing products for appetite control: Science and regulation of functional foods for weight management. *Proceedings of the Nutrition Society 71*, 350; 2012. DOI: 10.1017/S0029665112000134.

22. World Health Organization: *Global health observatory: Underweight in children.* ND. http://www.who.int/gho/mdg/poverty_hunger/under—weight_text/en/index.html Accessed: July 28, 2014

23. Vally H, Misso NLA: Adverse reactions to the sulphite additives. *Gastroenterology and Hepatology from Bed to Bench* 5(1):16; 2012.

24. National Institutes of Health, National Institute of Allergy and Infectious Diseases: *Food Allergy: Guidelines for the diagnosis and management of food allergy in the United States.* Last updated August 2013. http://www.niaid.nih.gov/topics/foodAllergy/clinical/Pages/patients.aspx Accessed: July 28, 2014

25. Gerez IFA and others: Diagnostic tests for food allergy..*Singapore Medical Journal* 51(1):4, 2010.

26. Center for Food Safety and Applied Nutrition: *Food Allergen Labeling and Consumer Protection Act of 2004. Questions and answers.* Updated 2013. http://www.fda.gov/food/guidanceregulation/guidancedocumentsregulatoryinformation/allergens/ucm106890.htm Accessed: July 28, 2014

27. National Institutes of Health, National Digestive Diseases Information Clearinghouse: *Celiac disease.* Updated 2012. http://digestive.niddk.nih.gov/ddiseases/pubs/celiac/index.aspx Accessed: July 28, 2014

28. National Institutes of Health, U.S. Department of Health and Human Services, National Human Genome Research Institute: *Learning about phenylketonuria (PKU).* Last updated August 2012. http://www.genome.gov/pfv.cfm?pageID=25020037 Accessed: July 28, 2014

29. Centers for Disease Control and Prevention: *After the baby arrives: Health: Newborn screening.* Last updated July 2014. http://www.cdc.gov/pregnancy/after.html Accessed: July 28, 2014

30. Prasad C and others: Introducing nutritional genomics teaching in under—graduate dietetic curricula. *Journal of Nutrigenetics and Nutrigenomics* 4(3):165, 2011.

31. Saukko PM and others: Negotiating the boundary between medicine and consumer culture: Online marketing of nutrigenetic tests. *Social Science and Medcine* 70:744, 2010.

32. U.S. Department of Agriculture, Food Safety and Inspection Service: *Food product dating.* Last modified August 2013. http://www.fsis.usda.gov/wps/portal/fsis/topics/food—safety—education/get—answers/food—safety—fact—sheets/food—labeling/food—product—dating/food—product—dating Accessed: July 28, 2014

Chapter 8

1. Bartholomew, M: James Lind's *Treatise of the Scurvy* (1753). *Postgraduate Medicine* 78:695, 2002.

2. Corbin KD, Zeisel SH: Choline metabolism provides novel insights into non—alcoholic fatty liver disease and its progression. *Current Opinions in Gastroenterology* 28(2):159, 2012. DOI: 10.1097/MOG.0b013e32834e7b4b. PMCID: PMC3601486.

3. What is a megadose and why do you recommend against taking megadoses of vitamins? *Johns Hopkins Medical Letter Health After 50*, p. 8, August 2001.

4. Food and Nutrition Board: *Dietary Reference Intakes for vitamin C, vitamin E, selenium, and carotenoids.* Washington, DC: National Academy Press, 2000.

5. Vandamme EJ: Production of vitamins, coenzymes and related biochemicals by biotechnological processes. *Journal of Chemical Technology & Biotechnology* 53(4):313, 1992.

6. Gahche J and others: Dietary supplement use among U.S. adults has increased since NHANES III (1988—1994). *NCHS Data Brief* 61:1, 2011.

7. U.S. Food and Drug Administration: *Food: Overview of food ingredients, additives & colors.* Updated March 2013. http://www.fda.gov/food/ingredientspackaginglabeling/foodadditivesingredients/ucm094211htm Accessed: July 28, 2014

8. U.S. Department of Agriculture, Agricultural Research Service: *Nutrient intakes from food: Mean amounts consumed per individual, by gender and age, in the United States, 2009–2010.* http://ars.usda.gov/Services/docs.htm?docid=13793 Accessed: July 28, 2014

9. Office of Dietary Supplements: *Dietary supplement fact sheet: Vitamin C.* Last reviewed June 2013. http://ods.od.nih.gov/factsheets/VitaminC—HealthProfessional/ Accessed: July 28, 2014

10. Food and Drug Administration, Center for Devices and Radiological Health, CDRH Consumer Information: *Microwave oven radiation.* Updated 2011. http://www.fda.gov/Radiation—EmittingProducts/ResourcesforYouRadiationEmittingProducts/ucm252762.htm Accessed: July 28, 2014

11. Office of Dietary Supplements: *Dietary supplement fact sheet: Vitamin A and carotenoids.* 2013. http://ods.od.nih.gov/factsheets/VitaminA—HealthProfessional/ Accessed: July 28, 2014

12. World Health Organization: *Micronutrient deficiencies: Vitamin A deficiency.* ND. http://www.who.int/nutrition/topics/vad/en/ Accessed: July 28, 2014

13. Holick MF: Vitamin D deficiency. *New England Journal of Medicine* 357:266, 2007.

14. National Institutes of Health, Office of Dietary Supplements: *Dietary supplement fact sheet: Vitamin D.* 2011. http://ods.od.nih.gov/fact—sheets/VitaminD—HealthProfessional/ Accessed: July 28, 2014

15. Bischoff—Ferrari HA and others: Benefit—risk assessment of vitamin D supplementation. *Osteoporosis International* 21(7):1121, 2010. DOI: 10.1007/s00198—009—1119—3

16. National Institutes of Health, Office of Dietary Supplements: *Dietary supplement fact sheet: Vitamin E.* 2013. http://ods.od.nih.gov/factsheets/VitaminE—HealthProfessional/Accessed: July 28, 2014

17. Linus Pauling Institute, Oregon State University, Micronutrient Information Center: *Vitamin K.* Updated 2011. http://lpi.oregonstate.edu/infocenter/vitamins/vitaminK/Accessed: January 2, 2014

18. Food and Nutrition Board: *Dietary Reference Intakes for thiamin, riboflavin, niacin, vitamin B−6, folate, vitamin B−12, pantothenic acid, biotin, and choline.* Washington, DC: National Academy Press, 1998.

19. National Institutes of Health, Office of Dietary Supplements: *Dietary supplement fact sheet: Vitamin B6.* Updated 2011. http://ods.od.nih.gov/factsheets/VitaminB6−HealthProfessional/ Accessed: July 28, 2014

20. Office of Dietary Supplements: *Dietary supplement fact sheet: Folate.* Reviewed 2012. http://ods.od.nih.gov/factsheets/Folate−HealthProfessional/ Accessed: July 28, 2014

21. Centers for Disease Control and Prevention: *Spina bifida homepage: Facts.* 2013. http://www.cdc.gov/ncbddd/spinabifida/facts.html Accessed: July 28, 2014

22. Centers for Disease Control and Prevention: *Anencephaly.* Last reviewed July 2013. http://www.cdc.gov/ncbddd/birthdefects/Anencephaly.html Accessed: July 28, 2014

23. Centers for Disease Control and Prevention: Spina bifida: Data and statistics. Reviewed 2013. http://www.cdc.gov/ncbddd/spinabifida/data.html Accessed: July 28, 2014

24. Centers for Disease Control and Prevention: *Folic acid: Data and statistics.* 2010. http://www.cdc.gov/ncbddd/folicacid/data.html Accessed: July 28, 2014

25. Dali−Youcef N, Andrès R: An update on cobalamin deficiency in adults. *Quarterly Journal of Medicine* 102(1):17, 2008.

26. National Institutes of Health, Office of Dietary Supplements: *Dietary supplement fact sheet: Vitamin B 12.* Last reviewed June 2011. http://ods.od.nih.gov/factsheets/VitaminB12−HealthProfessional/ Accessed: July 28, 2014

27. Rodrigues V and others: Severe megaloblastic anaemia in an infant. *BMJ Case Reports* 2011:bcr0220113835. Published online May 17, 2011. DOI: 10.1136/bcr.02.2011.3835. PMCID: PMC3097362.

28. The HPS2−THRIVE Collaborative Group: *Effects of extended−release niacin with Laropiprant in high−risk patients. New England Journal of Medicine* 371(3):203, 2014.

29. U.S. Preventive Services Task Force: *Routine vitamin supplementation to prevent cancer and cardiovascular disease: Recommendations and rationale.* Agency for Healthcare Research and Quality, Rockville, MD, June 2003. http://www.uspreventiveservicestaskforce.org/3rduspstf/vitamins/vitaminsrr.htm#discussion Accessed: July 25, 2014

30. Liu RH: Health benefits of fruits and vegetables are from additive and synergistic combinations of phytochemicals. *American Journal of Clinical Nutrition* 78:517S, 2003.

31. American Cancer Society: *Cancer Facts & Figures 2014.* http://www.cancer.org/research/cancerfactsstatistics/cancerfactsfigures2014/index Accessed: July 28, 2014

32. American Cancer Society: *Cancer facts and statistics: Current cancer prevention & early detection facts & figures.* http://www.cancer.org/research/cancerfactsstatistics/index Accessed: July 28, 2014

33. American Cancer Society: *ACS guidelines on nutrition and physical activity for cancer prevention: Common questions about diet and cancer.* Last revised August 2012. http://www.cancer.org/healthy/eathealthygetactive/acsguidelinesonnutritionphysicalactivityforcancerprevention/index Accessed: July 25, 2014

34. American Cancer Society: *Bladder cancer.* Revised February 2014. http://www.cancer.org/cancer/bladdercancer/detailedguide/bladder−cancer−prevention Accessed: July 28, 2014

Chapter 9

1. Centers for Disease Control and Prevention: Hyperthermia and dehydration−related deaths associated with intentional rapid weight loss in three collegiate wrestlers—North Carolina, Wisconsin, and Michigan, November−December 1997. *Morbidity and Mortality Weekly Report* 47:105, 1998. http://www.cdc.gov/mmwr/preview/mmwrhtml/00051388.htm

2. Saladin KS: *Anatomy & physiology.* 7th ed. Boston: McGraw−Hill Publishing Company, 2015.

3. Negoianu D, Goldfarb S: Just add water. *Journal of the American Society of Nephrology* 19(6):1041, 2008.

4. Food and Nutrition Board, Institute of Medicine: *Dietary Reference Intakes for water, potassium, sodium, chloride, and sulfate.* Washington, DC: National Academy Press, 2004.

5. Valtrin H: "Drink at least eight glasses of water a day." Really? Is there evidence for "8 × 8"? *American Journal of Physiological Regulation and Integrative Comparative Physiology* 283:R993, 2002.

6. Verster JC, Berthélemy O: Consumer satisfaction and efficacy of the hangover cure After−Effect©. *Advances in Preventive Medicine* 2012. Article ID 617942. http://dx.doi.org/10.1155/2012/617942

7. Casa DJ and others: American College of Sports Medicine roundtable on hydration and physical activity: Consensus statements. *Current Sports Medicine Reports* 4:115, 2005.

8. Yeates KE and others: Salt and water: A simple approach to hyponatremia. *Canadian Medical Association Journal* 170:365, 2004.

9. U.S. Department of Health and Human Services: *Bone health and osteoporosis: A report of the Surgeon General.* Rockville, MD: U.S. Department of Health and Human Services, Office of the Surgeon General, 2004. http://www.surgeongeneral.gov/library/bonehealth/content.html Accessed: July 25, 2014

10. Office of Dietary Supplements, National Institutes of Health: *Calcium.* Reviewed November 2013. http://ods.od.nih.gov/factsheets/Calcium−HealthProfessional/ Accessed: August 31, 2014

11. Guéguen L, Pointillart A: The bioavailability of dietary calcium. *Journal the American College of Nutrition* 19:119S, 2000.

12. Linus Pauling Institute, Micronutrient Information Center: *Calcium.* Updated 2010. http://lpi.oregonstate.edu/infocenter/minerals/calcium/ Accessed: August 31, 2014

13. National Institutes of Health, Office of Dietary Supplements: *Dietary supplements: What you need to know.* 2011. http://ods.od.nih.gov/HealthInformation/DS_WhatYouNeedToKnow.aspx Accessed: August 31, 2014

14. U.S. Department of Agriculture. Agricultural Research Service: *NHANES, 2009−2010, What we eat in America.* Table 1: Nutrient intakes from food: Mean amounts consumed per individual, by gender and age, in the United States, 2009−2010. http://www.ars.usda.gov/SP2User−Files/Place/12355000/pdf/0910/Table_1_NIN_GEN_09.pdf Accessed: January 10, 2014

15. National Osteoporosis Foundation: *What is osteoporosis?* ND. http://nof.org/articles/7 Accessed: August 31, 2014

16. National Osteoporosis Foundation: *Bone basics.* ND. http://nof.org/learn/bonebasics Accessed: August 31, 2014

17. National Institutes of Health: NIH SeniorHealth: *Osteoporosis: Frequently asked questions* http://nihseniorhealth.gov/osteoporosis/faq/faq12.html Accessed: August 31, 2014

18. U.S. National Library of Medicine: PubMed Health: *Osteoporosis—overview.* 2013. http://www.ncbi.nlm.nih.gov/pubmedhealth/PMH0001400/ Accessed: August 31, 2014

19. National Library of Medicine: PubMed Health: *Fact sheet: Preventing osteoporosis.* 2012. http://www.ncbi.nlm.nih.gov/pubmedhealth/PMH0004996/ Accessed: August 31, 2014

20. Bolívar JJ: Essential hypertension: An approach to its etiology and neurogenic pathophysiology. *International Journal of Hypertension* 2013; 2013: 547809. Published online December 9, 2013. DOI: 10.1155/2013/547809

21. Centers for Disease Control and Prevention: *High blood pressure.* Last updated July 2014. http://www.cdc.gov/bloodpressure/ Accessed: August 31, 2014

22. Stephens MM and others: Therapeutic options for the treatment of hypertension in children and adolescents. *Clinical Medicine Insights*:

Circulatory, Respiratory, and Pulmonary Medicine 6:13, 2012. Published online February 29, 2012. DOI: 10.4137/CCRPM.S7602

23. Centers for Disease Control and Prevention: Salt: *Most Americans should consume less salt*. Last updated February 2014. http://www.cdc.gov/salt/ Accessed: August 31, 2014

24. National Heart, Lung, and Blood Institute: *Explore DASH eating plan*. 2015. http://www.nhlbi.nih.gov/health/health–topics/topics/dash Accessed: January 24, 2016

25. National Heart, Lung, and Blood Institute, National Institutes of Health: *Your guide to lowering high blood pressure with DASH*. 2006. http://www.nhlbi.nih.gov/health/resources/heart/hbp–dash–index.htm Accesssed: August 31, 2014

26. Doorenbos CJ, Vermeij CG: Danger of salt substitutes that contain potassium in patients with renal failure. *British Medical Journal* 325:35, 2003.

27. Office of Dietary Supplements, National Institutes of Health: *Magnesium*. 2013. http://ods.od.nih.gov/factsheets/Magnesium–HealthProfessional/ Accessed: August 31, 2014

28. Food and Nutrition Board: *Dietary Reference Intakes for vitamin A, vitamin K, arsenic, boron, chromium, copper, iodine, iron, manganese, molybdenum, nickel, silicon, vanadium, and zinc*. Washington, DC: National Academy Press, 2000.

29. Ghosh K: Non–haematological effects of iron deficiency—A perspective. *Indian Journal of Medical Sciences* 60:30, 2006.

30. World Health Organization: *Miconutrient deficiencies: Iron deficiency anemia*. ND. http://www.who.int/nutrition/topics/ida/en/ Accessed: August 31, 2014

31. Centers for Disease Control and Prevention: *Iron and iron deficiency*. Last updated February 2011. http://www.cdc.gov/nutrition/everyone/basics/vitamins/iron.html Accessed: August 31, 2014

32. American Red Cross: *Blood donors step up; urgent need remains*. 2014. http://www.redcross.org/news/article/Blood–Shortage–Looms–Red–Cross–Issues–Urgent–Call–for–Donors Accessed: August 1, 2014

33. Office of Dietary Supplements, National Institutes of Health: *Dietary supplement fact sheet: Iron*. Reviewed April 2014. http://ods.od.nih.gov/factsheets/Iron–HealthProfessional/ August 31, 2014

34. Tenebein M: Unit–dose packaging of iron supplements and reduction of iron poisoning in young children. *Archives of Pediatric and Adolescent Medicine* 159: 557, 2005.

35. National Institute of Diabetes and Digestive and Kidney Diseases: *Hemochromatosis*. NIH Publication No. 07–4621, National Digestive Diseases Information Clearinghouse. Last updated March 2014. http://digestive.niddk.nih.gov/ddiseases/pubs/hemochromatosis/ Accessed: August 31, 2014

36. Prasad A: Zinc deficiency. *British Medical Journal* 326:409, 2003.

37. Prasad AS and others: Zinc deficiency in sickle cell disease. *Clinical Chemistry* 21:582, 1975.

38. Office of Dietary Supplements, National Institutes of Health: *Dietary supplement fact sheet: Zinc*. Reviewed June 2013. http://ods.od.nih.gov/factsheets/Zinc–HealthProfessional/ Accessed: August 31, 2014

39. Carpenter KJ: David Marine and the problem of goiter. *Journal of Nutrition* 135:675, 2005.

40. Office of Dietary Supplements, National Institutes of Health: *Dietary supplement fact sheet: Iodine*. Updated June 2011. http://ods.od.nih.gov/factsheets/Iodine–HealthProfessional/ Accessed: August 31, 2014

41. Office of Dietary Supplements, National Institutes of Health: *Selenium*. Updated July 2013 http://ods.od.nih.gov/factsheets/Selenium–Health–Professional/ Accessed: August 31, 2014

42. Office of Dietary Supplements, National Institutes of Health: *Chromium*. 2013 http://ods.od.nih.gov/factsheets/Chromium–HealthProfessional/ Accessed: August 31, 2014

43. Oregon State University, Linus Pauling Institute, Micronutrient Information Center: Manganese. 2010. http://lpi.oregonstate.edu/infocenter/minerals/manganese/ Accessed: August 31, 2014

44. Oregon State University, Linus Pauling Institute, Micronutrient Information Center: *Molybdenum*. 2013. http://lpi.oregonstate.edu/infocenter/minerals/molybdenum/ Accessed: August 31, 2014

45. International Bottled Water Association: *U.S. Consumption of Bottled Water Shows Continued Growth, Increasing* 6.2 *Percent in* 2012; *Sales up* 6.7 *Percent*. 2013. http://www.bottledwater.org/us–consumption–bottled–water–shows–continued–growth–increasing–62–percent–2012–sales–67–percent Accessed: August 31, 2014

46. Environmental Protection Agency: *Water health series: Bottled water basics*. 2005. http://water.epa.gov/drink/info/ Accessed: January 11, 2014

47. U.S. Food and Drug Administration: *Food facts from the U.S. Food and Drug Administration*. Last updated May 2014. http://www.fda.gov/Food/ResourcesForYou/Consumers/ucm046894.htm Accessed: August 31, 2014

48. National Institute of Environmental Health Sciences: *Bisphenol A (BPA)*. Last reviewed August 28, 2014. http://www.niehs.nih.gov/health/topics/agents/sya–bpa/index.cfm Accessed: August 31, 2014

Chapter 10

1. National Institutes of Health, National Heart Lung and Blood Institute: *Aim for a healthy weight: What is overweight and obesity?* ND. http://www.nhlbi.nih.gov/health/educational/lose_wt/ Accessed: September 6, 2014

2. Flegal M and others: Prevalence of obesity and trends in the distribution of body mass index among US adults, 1999–2010. *Journal of the American Medical Association* 307(5):491, 2012.

3. National Center for Health Statistics: *Health, United States, 2011: With Special Features on Socioeconomic Status and Health*. Hyattsville, MD; U. S. Department of Health and Human Services; 2012.

4. Fryar CD and others: Prevalence of overweight, obesity, and extreme obesity among adults: United States, trends 1960–1962 through 2009–2010. *NCHS Health E–Stat*. Last updated September 2012. http://www.cdc.gov/nchs/data/hestat/obesity_adult_09_10/obesity_adult_09_10.htm#table2 Accessed: September 6, 2014

5. Ogden CL and others: Prevalence of obesity and trends in body mass index among US children and adolescents, 1999–2010. *Journal of the American Medical Association* 307(5):483, 2012.

6. World Health Organization: *Obesity and overweight*. Updated August 2014. http://www.who.int/mediacentre/factsheets/fs311/en/ Accessed: September 6, 2014

7. U.S. Department of Health and Human Services: *Healthy People 2020: Nutrition and weight status*. http://healthypeople.gov/2020/topicsobjectives2020/objectiveslist.aspx?topicId=29 Accessed: September 6, 2014

8. Williams MH: *Nutrition for health, fitness, and sport*. 9th ed. New York: McGraw–Hill, 2010.

9. Naaz A and others: Loss of cyclin–dependent kinase inhibitors produces adipocyte hyperplasia and obesity. *The FASEB Journal* 18:1925, 2004.

10. Trayhurn P: Adipose tissue in obesity—An inflammatory issue. *Endocrinology* 146:1003, 2005.

11. McBean JC, Katz BE: Laser lipolysis: An update. *Journal of Clinical Aesthetic Dermatology* 4(7):25, 2011. PMCID: PMC3140909

12. Saladin KS: *Anatomy & Physiology*. 7th ed. Boston: McGraw–Hill Publishing Company, 2015.

13. Cannon B, Nedergaard J: Yes, even human brown fat is on fire! Commentary *Journal of Clinical Investigation* 122(2):486, 2012.

14. Bray GA, Champagne CM: Dietary patterns may modify central adiposity. *Journal of the American Dietetic Association* 109:1354, 2009.

15. Food and Nutrition Board, National Institute of Health: *Dietary Reference Intakes for energy, carbohydrate, fiber, fat, fatty acids, cholesterol, protein, and amino acids (macronutrients)*. Washington, DC: National Academies Press, 2005.

16. Roberts SB, Dallal GE: Energy requirements and aging. *Public Health Nutrition* 8:1028, 2005.

17. Haugen HA and others: Variability of measured resting metabolic rate. *American Journal of Clinical Nutrition* 78:1141, 2005.

18. Garland T Jr. and others: The biological control of voluntary exercise, spontaneous physical activity and daily energy expenditure in relation to obesity: human and rodent perspectives. *The Journal of Experimental Biology* 214(2):206, 2011. DOI. 10.1242/jeb.048397

19. Gropper SS and others: Weight and body composition changes during the first three years of college. *Journal of Obesity* 2012; 2012: 634048. Published online September 25, 2012. DOI: 10.1155/2012/634048 PMCID: PMC3463803

20. National Institutes of Health, National Heart Lung and Blood Institute: *Assessing your weight and health risk.* ND. http://www.nhlbi.nih.gov/health/educational/lose_wt/risk.htm Accessed: September 6, 2014

21. Berrington de Gonzalez A and others: Body–mass index and mortal–ity among 1.46 million white adults. *New England Journal of Medicine* 363(23):2211, 2010.

22. Schvey NA and others: The impact of weight stigma on caloric consump–tion. *Obesity* 19(10):1957, 2011. DOI: 10.1038/oby.2011.204

23. Hamdy O and others: Metabolic obesity: The paradox between visceral and subcutaneous fat. *Current Diabetes Review* 2(4):367, 2006.

24. Romaguera D and others: Dietary determinants of changes in waist circumference adjusted for body mass index–a proxy measure of vis–ceral adiposity. *PLoS ONE*5(7):e11588, 2010. DOI: 10.1371/journal.pone.0011588

25. Jensen MD and others: 2013 AHA/ACC/TOS Guideline for the manage–ment of overweight and obesity in adults: A report of the American Col–lege of Cardiology/American Heart Association Task Force on Practice Guidelines and The Obesity Society. *Circulation* 2013 Nov 12. [Epub ahead of print] PMID:24222017

26. Mantzoros CS and others: Leptin in human physiology and pathophysiol–ogy. *American Journal of Physiology–Endocrinology and Metabolism* 301(4):E567, 2011. PMCID: PMC3191548

27. Rolls BJ: Plenary Lecture 1: Dietary strategies for the prevention and treatment of obesity. *Proceedings of the Nutrition Society* 69(1):70, 2010. DOI: 10.1017/S0029665109991674.

28. Aller EEJG and others: Starches, sugars, and obesity. *Nutrients* 3(3): 341, 2011. Published online March 14, 2011. DOI: 10.3390/nu3030341

29. McNay DEG, Speakman JR: High fat diet causes rebound weight gain. *Molecular Metabolism* 2 (2):103, 2013. Published online November 2, 2012. DOI: 10.1016/j.molmet.2012.10.003 PMCID: PMC3817395

30. Duffey KJ, Popkin BM: Energy density, portion size, and eating occa–sions: Contributions to increased energy intake in the United States, 1977–2006. *PLoS Med*8(6):e1001050, 2011. Published online June 28, 2011. DOI: 10.1371/journal.pmed.1001050

31. U.S. Department of Agriculture, Agricultural Research Service: *Nutrient intakes from food: Mean amounts consumed per individual, by gen–der and age, in the United States, 2009–2010.* http://www.ars.usda.gov/main/main.htm Accessed: July 25, 2014

32. Centers for Disease Control and Prevention: *Physical activity: Facts about physical activity.* Last updated May 2014. http://www.cdc.gov/physicalactivity/data/facts.html Accessed: September 6, 2014

33. Centers for Disease Control and Prevention: *Physical activity: How much physical activity do adults need?* Updated March 2014. http://www.cdc.gov/physicalactivity/everyone/guidelines/adults.html Accessed: September 6, 2014

34. Morandi A and others: Estimation of newborn risk for child or adoles–cent obesity: Lessons from longitudinal birth cohorts. *PLoS One* 7(11): e49919, 2012. Published online November 28, 2012. DOI: 10.1371/journal.pone.0049919

35. Ino T: Maternal smoking during pregnancy and offspring obesity: Meta–analysis. *Pediatrics International* 52(1):94, 2010. DOI: 10.1111/j.1442–200X.2009.02883.x. Epub April 27, 2009.

36. Gavin AR and others: Racial/ethnic differences in the association between obesity and major depressive disorder: Findings from the Comprehensive Psychiatric Epidemiology Surveys. *Public Health Reports* 125(5):698, 2010. PMCID: PMC2925006

37. Bish CL and others: Diet and physical activity behaviors among Americans trying to lose weight: 2000 Behavioral Risk Factor Surveillance System. *Obesity Research* 13:596, 2005.

38. Kruger J and others: Attempting to lose weight: Specific practices among U.S. adults. *American Journal of Preventive Medicine* 269:402, 2004.

39. U.S. Department of Agriculture: *Weight management: why is weight management important?* (ND). http://www.choosemyplate.gov/weight–management Accessed: January 24, 2016

40. Chapman CD and others: Lifestyle determinants of the drive to eat: A meta–analysis. *American Journal of Clinical Nutrition* 96(3):492, 2012. Published online July 25, 2012. DOI: 10.3945/ajcn.112.039750

41. Hall KD and others: Energy balance and its components: Implications for body weight regulation. *American Journal of Clinical Nutrition* 95(4): 989, 2012. DOI: 10.3945/ ajcn.112.036350 PMCID: PMC3302369

42. Irwin ML and others: Estimation of energy expenditure from physical activity measures: Determinants of accuracy. *Obesity Research* 9:517, 2001.

43. National Weight Control Registry. http://www.nwcr.ws/ Accessed: September 6, 2014

44. Hollywood A, Ogden J: Taking orlistat: Predicting weight loss over 6 months. *Journal of Obesity*, 2011: DOI: 10.1155/2011/806896.

45. American Society for Metabolic & Bariatric Surgery: *Benefits of bar–iatric surgery.* http://asmbs.org/patients/benefits–of–bariatric–surgery Accessed: September 6, 2014

46. Neff KJ and others: Bariatric surgery: The challenges with can–didate selection, individualizing treatment and clinical outcomes. *BMC Medicine* 11:8, 2013. Published online January 10, 2013. DOI: 10.1186/1741–7015–11–8

47. Hession M and others: Systematic review of randomized controlled trials of low–carbohydrate vs. low–fat/low–calorie diets in the management of obesity and its comorbidities. *Obesity Reviews* 10:36, 2009.

48. Federal Trade Commission, Bureau of Consumer Protection: Weighing the claims in diet ads. 2012. http://www.consumer.ftc.gov/articles/0061–weighing–claims–diet–ads Accessed: September 6, 2014

49. Fryar CD, Ogden CL: *Prevalence of underweight among adults aged 20 years and over: United States, 1960–1962 through 2007–2010.* September 2012. http://www.cdc.gov/nchs/data/hestat/underweight_adult_07_10/underweight_adult_07_10.htm Accessed: September 6, 2014

50. American Psychiatric Association: Feeding and eating disorders. In *Diagnostic and Statistical Manual of Mental Disorders.* 5th ed. DOI: 10.1176/appi.books.9780890425596.323864, 2013.

51. Ozier AD, Henry BW: Position of the American Dietetic Association: Nutrition intervention in the treatment of eating disorders. *Journal of the American Dietetic Association* 111(8):1236, 2011.

52. Stice E and others: Prevalence, incidence, impairment, and course of the proposed DSM–5 eating disorder diagnoses in an 8–year prospective community study of young women. *Journal of Abnormal Psychology* 122(2):455, 2013.

53. Pinheiro AP and others: The genetics of anorexia nervosa: Current find–ings and future perspectives. *International Journal of Child and Ado–lescent Health* 2(2):153, 2009.

54. Dimitropoulos G and others: Inpatients with severe anorexia nervosa and their siblings: Non–shared experiences and family functioning. *European Eating Disorders Review* 21:284, 2013.

55. Quiles–Marcos Y and others: Peer and family influence in eating disor–ders: A meta–analysis. *European Psychiatry* 28:199, 2013.

56. Helfert S, Warschburger P: The face of appearance–related social pressure: Gender, age and body mass variations in peer and parental pressure during adolescence. *Child and Adolescent Psychiatry and Mental Health* 7(16):1, 2013.

57. Centers for Disease Control and Prevention: *Healthy diet—it's not a diet, it's a lifestyle: About BMI for adults*, 2011. http://www.cdc.gov/healthyweight/assessing/bmi/adult_bmi/index.html Accessed: July 25, 2014

58. Rosen DS and others: Clinical report—identification and management of eating disorders in children and adolescents. *Pediatrics* 126(6):1240, 2010.

59. Hudson JI and others: The prevalence and correlates of eating disorders in the national comorbidity survey replication. *Biological Psychiatry* 61:348, 2007.

60. Smink FR and others: Epidemiology of eating disorders: Incidence, prevalence, and mortality rates. *Current Psychiatry Reports* 14:406, 2012.

61. Arcelus J and others: Mortality rates in patients with anorexia nervosa and other eating disorders: A meta–analysis of 36 studies. *Archives of General Psychiatry* 68(7):724, 2011.

62. Crow SJ and others: Increased mortality in bulimia nervosa and other eating disorders. *American Journal of Psychiatry* 66(12):1342, 2009. DOI: 10.1176/appi.ajp.2009.09020247. E–pub October 15, 2009.

63. Fischer S and others: Night eating syndrome in young adults: Delineation from other eating disorders and clinical significance. *Psychiatry Research* 200:494, 2012.

64. Allison KC and others: An open–label efficacy trial of escitalopram for night eating syndrome. *Eating Behaviors* 14:199, 2013.

65. Gagnon C and others: Comorbid diabetes and eating disorders in adult patients: Assessment and considerations for treatment. *Diabetes Educator* 35:537, 2012.

66. Matheiu J: What is diabulimia? *Journal of the American Dietetic Association* 108(5):769, 2008.

67. Murray SB and others: Muscle dysmorphia and the DSM–V conundrum: Where does it belong? A review paper. *International Journal of Eating Disorders* 43:483, 2010.

68. Gibbs, JC and others: Prevalence of individual and combined components of the female athlete triad. *Medicine and Science in Sports and Exercise* 45(5):985, 2013.

69. Nazem TH, Ackerman KE: The female athlete triad. *Sports Health* 4(4):302, 2012.

70. Thein–Nissenbaum, J: Long–term consequences of the female athlete triad. *Maturitas* 75:107, 2013.

71. National Eating Disorder Association: *What Should I Say?* http://www.nationaleatingdisorders.org/what–should–i–say Accessed: July 25, 2014

Chapter 11

1. Centers for Disease Control and Prevention: *Physical activity: Facts about physical activity*. Last updated May 2014. http://www.cdc.gov/physicalactivity/data/facts.html Accessed: September 7, 2014

2. Centers for Disease Control and Prevention: *Physical activity: How much physical activity do adults need?* Last updated March 2014. http://www.cdc.gov/physicalactivity/everyone/guidelines/index.html Accessed: September 7, 2014

3. Centers for Disease Control and Prevention: *Physical activity and health: The benefits of physical activity*. Last updated February 2011. http://www.cdc.gov/physicalactivity/everyone/health/index.html Accessed: September 7, 2014

4. U.S. Department of Health and Human Services: *2008 Physical activity guidelines for Americans summary*. 2008. http://www.health.gov/paguidelines/guidelines/summary.aspx Accessed: September 7, 2014

5. Centers for Disease Control and Prevention: *Target heart rate and estimated maximum heart rate*. 2011. http://www.cdc.gov/physicalactivity/everyone/measuring/heartrate.html Accessed: September 7, 2014

6. Williams MH and others: *Nutrition for health, fitness, and sport*. 10th ed. New York: McGraw–Hill, 2013.

7. Saladin KS: *Anatomy and physiology*. 7th ed. New York: McGraw–Hill, 2015.

8. Jeppesen J, Kiens B: Regulation and limitations to fatty acid oxidation during exercise. *Journal of Physiology* 590:1059, 2012.

9. Yeo WK and others: Fat adaptation in well–trained athletes: Effects on cell metabolism. *Applied Physiology, Nutrition, and Metabolism* 36:12, 2011.

10. American Dietetic Association: Position of the American Dietetic Association, Dietitians of Canada, and the American College of Sports Medicine—Nutrition and athletic performance. *Journal of the American Dietetic Association* 109:509, 2009.

11. Economos CD and others: Nutritional practices of elite athletes: Practical recommendations. *Sports Medicine* 16:381, 1993.

12. Otten JJ and others (eds.): Institute of Medicine of the National Academies: *Dietary Reference Intakes: The essential guide to nutrient requirements*. National Academies Press: Washington, DC, 2006.

13. Lambert EV and others: High–fat diet versus habitual diet prior to carbohydrate loading: Effects of exercise metabolism and cycling performance. *International Journal of Sports Nutrition and Exercise Metabolism* 11:209, 2001.

14. Wismann J, Willoughby D: Gender differences in carbohydrate metabolism and carbohydrate loading. *Journal of the International Society of Sports Nutrition* 3(1):28, 2006.

15. Hulmi JJ and others: Effect of protein/essential amino acids and resistance training on skeletal muscle hypertrophy: A case for whey protein. *Nutrition and Metabolism* 7:51, 2010.

16. Joy JM and others: The effects of 8 weeks of whey or rice protein supplementation on body composition and exercise performance. *Nutrition Journal* 12:86, 2013.

17. Poole C and others: The role of post–exercise nutrient administration on muscle protein synthesis and glycogen synthesis. *Journal of Sports Science and Medicine* 9:354, 2010.

18. A guide to the best and worst drinks. *Consumer Reports on Health*, p. 8, July 2006.

19. Coyle EF: Fluid and fuel intake during exercise. *Journal of Sports Science* 22:39, 2004.

20. MayoClinic.com: *Heat cramps: First aid*. 2012. http://www.mayoclinic.org/first–aid/first–aid–heat–cramps/basics/art–20056669 Accessed: September 7, 2014

21. MayoClinic.com: *Heat exhaustion: First aid*. 2012. http://www.mayoclinic.org/first–aid/first–aid–heat–exhaustion/basics/art–20056651 Accessed: September 7, 2014

22. MayoClinic.com: *Heat stroke: First aid*. 2012. http://www.mayoclinic.org/first–aid/first–aid–heatstroke/basics/art–20056655 Accessed: September 7, 2014

23. Association of International Marathons and Road Races: *IMMDA's revised fluid recommendations for runners & walkers*. 2006. http://www.aims–association.org/guidelines_fluid_replacement.htm Accessed: September 7, 2014

24. Powers SK and others: Dietary antioxidants and exercise. *Journal of Sports Sciences* 22:81, 2004.

25. Nieman DC and others: Vitamin E and immunity after the Kona Triathlon World Championship. *Medicine and Science in Sports and Exercise* 36:1328, 2004.

26. National Collegiate Athletic Association: *NCAA 2013–2014 banned drugs*. http://www.ncaa.org/health–and–safety/policy/2013–14–ncaa–banned–drugs Accessed: September 7, 2014

27. U.S. Anti–doping Agency: *WADA prohibited list*. http://www.usada.org/substances/prohibited–list/ Accessed: September 7, 2014

28. U.S. Food and Drug Administration: *FDA consumer advice on pure powdered caffeine*. July 2014. http://www.fda.gov/food/recallsoutbreaksemergencies/safetyalertsadvisories/ucm405787.htm Accessed: September 7, 2014

Chapter 12

1. Centers for Disease Control and Prevention: *Norovirus: Overview*. 2013. http://www.cdc.gov/norovirus/about/overview.html Accessed: February 6, 2014

2. Centers for Disease Control and Prevention: *Norovirus*. Updated October 2013. http://www.cdc.gov/norovirus/index.html Accessed: February 6, 2014

3. Food and Drug Administration: *Frequently asked questions*. Last updated February 3, 2104. http://www.fda.gov/Food/GuidanceRegulation/FSMA/ucm247559.htm Accessed: February 5, 2014

4. Centers for Disease Control and Prevention: *Food safety: Foodborne illness, foodborne disease, (sometimes called "food poisoning"): Diagnosing and treating foodborne illness*. Updated 2012. http://www.cdc.gov/foodsafety/facts.html Accessed: February 5, 2014

5. USDA Food Safety and Inspection Service: *Molds on food: Are they dangerous?* 2013. http://www.fsis.usda.gov/wps/portal/fsis/topics/food-safety-education/get-answers/food-safety-fact-sheets/safe-food-handling/molds-on-food-are-they-dangerous-/CT_Index Accessed: February 9, 2014

6. Food and Drug Administration: *Bad bug book*. 2nd ed. 2012. http://www.fda.gov/Food/FoodborneIllnessContaminants/CausesOfIllnessBadBugBook/default.htm Accessed: February 5, 2014

7. U.S. Department of Health and Human Services: *Keep foods safe: Cook*. ND. http://www.foodsafety.gov/keep/basics/cook/index.html Accessed: February 9, 2014

8. U.S. Department of Agriculture, Food Safety and Inspection Service: *Appliances and thermometers: Cooking safely in the microwave oven*. Last modified August 2013. http://www.fsis.usda.gov/wps/portal/fsis/topics/food-safety-education/get-answers/food-safety-fact-sheets/appliances-and-thermometers/cooking-safely-in-the-microwave/cooking-safely-in-the-microwave-oven Accessed: February 9, 2014

9. University of Illinois, College of Agricultural, Consumer and Environmental Sciences: If you drop it, should you eat it? Scientists weigh in on the 5-second rule. *ACES News*. University of Illinois at Champaign-Urbana, College of Agricultural, Consumer and Environmental Sciences, 2003. www.news.aces.illinois.edu/news/if-you-drop-it-should-you-eat-it-scientists-weigh-5-second-rule Accessed: February 9, 2014

10. U.S. Department of Agriculture, Food Safety and Inspection Service: *Food safety information: Basics for handling food safely*. Revised June 2011. http://www.fsis.usda.gov/PDF/Basics_for_Safe_Food_Handling.pdf Accessed: February 9, 2014

11. U.S. Department of Agriculture, Food Safety and Inspection Service: *Keeping food safe during an emergency*. 2013. http://www.fsis.usda.gov/wps/portal/fsis/topics/food-safety-education/get-answers/food-safety-fact-sheets/emergency-preparedness/keeping-food-safe-during-an-emergency/CT_Index Accessed: July 24, 2014

12. Centers for Disease Control and Prevention, National Center for Emerging and Zoonotic Infectious Diseases: *Irradiation of food: Frequently asked questions*. 2009. http://www.cdc.gov/nczved/divisions/dfbmd/diseases/irradiation_food/ Accessed: February 9, 2014

13. Casey-Lockyer M and others: Deaths associated with Hurricane Sandy—October-November 2012. *Morbidity and Mortality Weekly Report* 62(20):393, 2013.

14. Federal Emergency Management Agency: *Hurricane Sandy: timeline*. 2013. http://www.fema.gov/hurricane-sandy-timeline Accessed: February 7, 2014

15. U.S. Food and Drug Administration: *Food: Overview of food ingredients, additives & colors*. Last updated March 2013. http://www.fda.gov/food/ingredientspackaginglabeling/foodadditivesingredients/ucm094211.htm Accessed: February 10, 2014

16. U.S. Environmental Protection Agency: *Pesticides: Topical & chemical fact sheets: Assessing health risks from pesticides*. Updated January 2014. http://www.epa.gov/pesticides/factsheets/riskassess.htm Accessed: February 10, 2014

17. U.S. Food and Drug Administration: *Food: Defect levels handbook*. Last updated November 2013. http://www.fda.gov/food/guidanceregulation/guidancedocumentsregulatoryinformation/sanitationtransportation/ucm056174.htm Accessed: February 10, 2014

18. Environmental Protection Agency: *Pesticides: Topical & chemical fact sheets: The EPA and food security*. Last updated May 2012. http://www.epa.gov/pesticides/factsheets/securty.htm Accessed: February 10, 2014

19. Centers for Disease Control and Prevention: *Fourth national report on human exposure to environmental chemicals*. Updated June 2011. http://www.cdc.gov/exposurereport/pdf/FourthReport.pdf Accessed: July 24, 2014

20. National Institutes of Health, National Cancer Institute: *Agricultural health study*. Last reviewed 2011. http://www.cancer.gov/cancertopics/factsheet/risk/ahs Accessed: February 10, 2014

21. Connor BA: Chapter 2: The pre-travel consultation: Self-treatable conditions. *CDC health information for international travel 2014;* http://wwwnc.cdc.gov/travel/yellowbook/2014/chapter-2-the-pre-travel-consultation/travelers-diarrhea Accessed: September 25, 2014

22. Centers for Disease Control and Prevention: *Water disinfection*. 2013. http://wwwnc.cdc.gov/travel/page/water-disinfection Accessed: February 7, 2014

23. Centers for Disease Control and Prevention: *Water-related emergencies & outbreaks: Personal preparation and storage of safe water*. 2013. http://www.cdc.gov/healthywater/emergency/safe_water/personal.htm Accessed: February 10, 2014

Chapter 13

1. Otten JJ and others (eds.): Institute of Medicine: *Dietary Reference Intakes: The essential guide to nutrient requirements*. Washington, DC: National Academies Press, 2006.

2. Centers for Disease Control and Prevention: *Unintended pregnancy prevention*. Last update: 2013. http://www.cdc.gov/reproductivehealth/UnintendedPregnancy/index.htm Accessed: February 20, 2014

3. Thame M and others: Fetal growth is directly related to maternal anthropometry and placental volume. *European Journal of Clinical Nutrition* 58:894, 2004.

4. U.S. Department of Health and Human Services: *Child health USA 2011*. 2011. http://mchb.hrsa.gov/chusa11/hstat/hsi/pages/201lbw.html Accessed: February 20, 2014

5. Centers for Disease Control and Prevention: FastStats: *Births and natality*. Last updated: June 2014. http://www.cdc.gov/nchs/fastats/births.htm Accessed: September 12, 2014

6. U.S. Department of Health and Human Services: *The health consequences of smoking—50 years of progress: A report of the Surgeon General*. 2014. http://www.surgeongeneral.gov/library/reports/50-years-of-progress/fact-sheet.html Accessed: September 12, 2014

7. Martin JA, Osterman MJK: Preterm births—United States, 2006 and 2010. *Morbidity and Mortality Weekly Report* 63(3):136, 2013.

8. Kharrazia M and others: California very preterm birth study: Design and characteristics of the population- and biospecimen bank-based nested case control study. *Paediatric and Perinatal Epidemiology* 26(3): 250, 2012. DOI: 10.1111/j.1365-3016.2011.01252.x

9. Neville MC, McManaman JL: Milk secretion and composition. In *Neonatal nutrition and metabolism*. 2nd ed. Thureen P, Hay W (eds.) New York, New York: Cambridge University Press, 2006.

10. U.S. National Library of Medicine and National Institutes of Health: Morning sickness. *MedLinePlus*. Updated 2012. http://www.nlm.nih.gov/medlineplus/ency/article/003119.htm Accessed: September 12, 2014

11. Centers for Disease Control and Prevention: *Nutrition for everyone*: *Iron and iron deficiency*: *What is iron and why do we need it?* 2011. http://www.cdc.gov/nutrition/everyone/basics/vitamins/iron.html Accessed: September 12, 2014

12. U.S. Food and Drug Administration: *Food safety for moms–to–be*: *At a glance*. Last updated June 2014. http://www.fda.gov/food/foodborneillnesscontaminants/peopleatrisk/ucm081819.htm Accessed: September 12, 2014

13. Centers for Disease Control and Prevention: *2011 Pregnancy Nutrition Surveillance*. 2012. http://www.cdc.gov/pednss/pnss_tables/tables_health_indicators.htm#Maternal%20Health Accessed: September 12, 2014

14. Academy of Nutrition and Dietetics: *Weight gain during pregnancy*. 2013. http://www.eatright.org/Public/content.aspx?id=10933 Accessed: September 12, 2014

15. Mayo Clinic Staff: *Diseases and conditions*: *Fetal macrosomia*. 2012. http://www.mayoclinic.org/diseases–conditions/fetal–macrosomia/basics/definition/CON–20035423?p=1 Accessed September 12, 2014

16. U.S. Department of Health and Human Services, Office on Women's Health: Publications: *Prenatal care fact sheet*. Last updated 2012. http://womenshealth.gov/publications/our–publications/fact–sheet/prenatal–care.html Accessed: September 12, 2014

17. Centers for Disease Control and Prevention, Department of Health and Human Services: *Gestational diabetes and pregnancy*: *Diabetes in pregnancy*. ND. http://www.cdc.gov/pregnancy/diabetes–gestational.html Accessed: September 12, 2014

18. National Institutes of Health: *Preeclampsia and eclampsia*: *Condition information*. Last reviewed 2013. http://www.nichd.nih.gov/health/topics/preeclampsia/conditioninfo/Pages/default.aspx Accessed: September 12, 2014

19. National Heart Lung and Blood Institute: *High blood pressure in pregnancy*. ND. http://www.nhlbi.nih.gov/health/public/heart/hbp/hbp_preg.htm Accessed: September 12, 2014

20. National Institutes of Health: *Sudden infant death syndrome (SIDS)*: *Overview*. Updated 2103. http://www.nichd.nih.gov/health/topics/sids/Pages/default.aspx Accessed: September 12, 2014

21. March of Dimes: *Physical activity, Exercise during pregnancy (video)*. ND. http://www.marchofdimes.org/pregnancy/physical–activity.aspx Accessed: September 12, 2014

22. Neville MC: Personal communication. November 2006.

23. American Dietetic Association: Position paper: Promoting and supporting breastfeeding. *Journal of the American Dietetic Association* 109:1926, 2009.

24. Hurst N: Breastfeeding after breast augmentation. *Journal of Human Lactation* 19:70, 2003.

25. American Academy of Pediatrics: Policy Statement: Breastfeeding and the use of human milk. *Pediatrics* 129 (3):e827, 2012. DOI: 10.1542/peds.2011–3552

26. Centers for Disease Control and Prevention: *Breastfeeding Among U.S. Children Born 2001–2011, CDC National Immunization Survey*. Last reviewed July 2014. http://www.cdc.gov/breastfeeding/data/NIS_data/index.htm Accessed: September 12, 2014

27. Saarela T and others: Macronutrient and energy contents of human milk fractions during the first six months of lactation. *Acta Paediatricia* 94(9):1176, 2005.

28. Fomon SJ: Infant feeding in the 20th century: Formula and beikost. *Journal of Nutrition* 131:409S, 2001.

29. American Academy of Pediatrics: Expert panel on integrated guidelines for cardiovascular health and risk reduction in children and adolescents: Summary report. *Pediatrics* 128 (S5):S213, 2011, pp. S213, 2011. DOI: 10.1542/peds.2009–2107C

30. Academy of Nutrition and Dietetics: *Introducing solid foods to toddlers*. Reviewed 2012. http://www.eatright.org/Public/content.aspx?id=8049 Accessed: September 12, 2014

31. Centers for Disease Control and Prevention: *Basics about childhood obesity*. Last updated April 2012. http://www.cdc.gov/obesity/childhood/basics.html Accessed: September 12, 2014

32. U.S. Department of Agriculture: ChooseMyPlate.gov: *Daily food plan for preschoolers*: *Learn about beverages*. ND. http://www.choosemyplate.gov/preschoolers/daily–food–plans/about–beverages.html Accessed: September 12, 2014

33. American Dental Association: *Diet and dental health*. ND. http://www.mouthhealthy.org/en/az–topics/d/diet–and–dental–health Accessed: September 12, 2014

34. American Dental Association: *Chewing gum*. ND. http://www.mouthhealthy.org/en/az–topics/c/chewing–gum Accessed: September 12, 2014

35. Reeding J, Krebs–Smith S: Dietary sources of energy, solid fats, and added sugars among children and adolescents in the United States. *Journal of the American Dietetic Association* 110(10):1477, 2010.

36. U.S. Department of Agriculture, Agricultural Research Service: *What We Eat in America, NHANES 2009–2010*: *Nutrient Intakes from food by gender and age*. http://www.ars.usda.gov/Services/docs.htm?docid=18349 Accessed: September 12, 2014

37. Kranz S: What do we know about dietary fiber intake in children and health? The effects of fiber intake on constipation, obesity, and diabetes in children. *Advances in Nutrition* 3 (1):47, 2012.

38. Rampersaud GC and others: Breakfast habits, nutritional status, body weight, and academic performance in children and adolescents. *Journal of the American Dietetic Association* 105:743, 2005.

39. Saladin KS: *Anatomy & Physiology*. 7th ed. Boston: McGraw–Hill Publishing Company, 2015.

40. American Academy of Dermatologists: *Frequently asked questions about acne*. ND. http://www.skincarephysicians.com/acnenet/FAQ.html#1 Accessed: February 22, 2014

41. Centers for Disease Control and Prevention: *Adolescent and Youth Risk Behavior Surveillance System (YRBSS)*. 2014. http://www.cdc.gov/healthyyouth/yrbs/index.htm Accessed: September 12, 2014

42. Position of the American Dietetic Association and Dietitians of Canada: Vegetarian diets. *Journal of the American Dietetic Association* 109:748, 2009.

43. Centers for Disease Control and Prevention: *Overweight and obesity*: *Data and statistics*. Updated September 3, 2014. http://www.cdc.gov/obesity/data/childhood.html Accessed: September 12, 2014

44. Ogden C, Carroll M: Prevalence of obesity among children and adolescents: United States, trends 1963–1965 through 2007–2008. *NCHS Health E–Stat*. Updated 2010. http://www.cdc.gov/nchs/data/hestat/obesity_child_07_08/obesity_child_07_08.htm Accessed: September 12, 2014

45. Centers for Disease Control and Prevention: Progress on childhood obesity. *CDC Vital Signs*. Updated August 2013. http://www.cdc.gov/VitalSigns/ChildhoodObesity/ Accessed: September 12, 2014

46. Pan L and others: Trends in the prevalence of extreme obesity among US preschool–aged children living in low–income families, 1998–2010. *Journal of the American Medical Association* 308 (24):2563, 2012.

47. Centers for Disease Control and Prevention: *Overweight and obesity*: *A growing problem*: *What causes childhood obesity?* Updated April 2013. http://www.cdc.gov/obesity/childhood/problem.html Accessed: September 12, 2014

48. Dattilo AM and others: Need for early interventions in the prevention of pediatric overweight: A review and upcoming directions. *Journal of Obesity* 2012:123023. Published online May 7, 2012. DOI: 10.1155/2012/123023 PMCID: PMC3362946

49. White House Task Force on Childhood Obesity: *A report to the President*: *Solving the problem of childhood obesity within a generation, 2010*. http://www.letsmove.gov/sites/letsmove.gov/files/TaskForce_on_Childhood_Obesity_May2010_FullReport.pdf Accessed: February 20, 2014

50. Let's Move! America's move to raise a healthier generation of kids. ND. http://www.letsmove.gov/ Accessed: February 20, 2014

51. Institute of Medicine, Committee on Obesity Prevention Policies for Young Children: *Early childhood obesity prevention policies*. 2011. Washington, DC: The National Academies Press www.nap.edu Accessed: February 20, 2014

52. Centers for Disease Control and Prevention: *Healthy weght—it's not a diet, it's a lifestyle! Tips for parents—ideas to help children maintain a healthy weight*. 2011. http://www.cdc.gov/healthyweight/children/index.html Accessed: September 12, 2014

53. National Institute of Diabetes and Digestive and Kidney Diseases, Weight Control Information Network: *Bariatric surgery for severe obesity*: *Bariatric surgery for youth*. Last modified January 2014. http://win.niddk.nih.gov/publications/gastric.htm Accessed: September 12, 2014

54. Centers for Disease Control and Prevention: *FastStats*: *Life expectancy*. Last updated November 2013. http://www.cdc.gov/nchs/fastats/life−expectancy.htm Accessed: September 12, 2014

55. U.S. Census Bureau: *Facts for features: Older Americans month: May 2014*. http://www.census.gov/newsroom/facts−for−features/2014/cb14−ff07.html Accessed: September 12, 2014

56. U.S. Census Bureau: *U.S. Census Bureau projections show a slower growing, odder, more diverse nation a half century from now*. December 2012. http://www.census.gov/newsroom/releases/archives/population/cb12−243.html Accessed: September 12, 2014

57. Mokdad AH and others: Actual causes of death in the United States, 2000. *Journal of the American Medical Association* 291:1238, 2004.

58. Centers for Disease Control and Prevention, US Department of Health and Human Services: *The state of aging and health in America 2013*. 2013. http://www.cdc.gov/aging/help/DPH−Aging/state−aging−health.html Accessed: September 12, 2014

59. Krebs−Smith SM and others: Americans do not meet federal dietary rec−ommendations. *Journal of Nutrition* 140 (10):1832, 2010.

60. Pesonen J and others: High bone mineral density among perimenopausal women. *Osteoporosis International* 16:1899, 2005.

61. Manini TM and others: Daily activity energy expenditure and mortal−ity among older adults. *Journal of the American Medical Association* 296(2):171, 2006.

62. Centers for Disease Control and Prevention: Edentulism. *health data interactive*. http://205.207.175.93/HDI/TableViewer/tableView.aspx?ReportId=110 Accessed: September 12, 2014

63. Savoca MR and others: Severe tooth loss in older adults as a key indicator of compromised diet quality. *Public Health Nutrition* 13(4):466, 2010.

64. Bailey RL and others: Dietary supplement use in the United States, 2003−2006. *Journal of Nutrition* 141(2):261, 2011.

65. Federal Interagency Forum on Aging Related Statistics: *Older Americans 2012*: *Key indicators of well being*. 2012. http://agingstats.gov/Agingstatsdotnet/Main_Site/default.aspx Accessed: September 12, 2014

66. National Institutes of Health, National Institute on Aging: *Can we pre−vent aging: Tips from the National Institute on Aging*. Last updated August 2014. http://www.nia.nih.gov/health/publication/can−we−prevent−aging Accessed: September 12. 2014

Glossary

A

absorption process by which substances are taken up from the GI tract and enter the bloodstream or the lymph

Acceptable Macronutrient Distribution Ranges (AMDRs) macronutrient intake ranges that are nutritionally adequate and may reduce the risk of diet-related chronic diseases

acid-base balance maintaining the proper pH of body fluids

acid group acid portion of a compound

acids substances that donate hydrogen ions

added sugars sugars added to foods during processing or preparation

adenosine diphosphate (ADP) high-energy compound; by-product of ATP use

adenosine triphosphate (ATP) molecule that stores energy

Adequate Intakes (AIs) dietary recommendations that assume a population's average daily nutrient intakes are adequate because no deficiency diseases are present

adipose cells fat cells

adolescence life stage in which a child matures physically into an adult

aerobic conditions that require free oxygen

aerobic exercise physical activities that involve sustained, rhythmic contractions of large muscle groups

air displacement method of estimating body composition by determining body volume

aldosterone hormone that participates in sodium and water conservation

alpha-linolenic acid an essential fatty acid

alpha-tocopherol vitamin E

alternative sweeteners substances that sweeten foods while providing few or no kilocalories

amino acids nitrogen-containing chemical units that comprise proteins

amino or nitrogen-containing group portion of an amino acid that contains nitrogen

anaerobic conditions that lack free oxygen

anatomy scientific study of cells and other body structures

anecdotes reports of personal experiences

anemia disorder characterized by a reduction in the oxygen-carrying ability of red blood cells

anencephaly type of neural tube defect in which the brain does not form properly or is missing

anorexia nervosa (AN) severe psychological disturbance characterized by self-imposed starvation

antibodies infection-fighting proteins

antidiuretic hormone (ADH) hormone that participates in water conservation

antioxidant substance that protects other compounds from being damaged or destroyed by certain factors

appetite desire to eat appealing food

arterial plaque lipid-filled deposits that form under the lining of certain arteries

arteries vessels that carry blood away from the heart

arteriosclerosis condition that results from atherosclerosis and is characterized by loss of arterial flexibility

ascorbic acid vitamin C

atherosclerosis long-term disease process in which plaques build up inside arterial walls

B

bacteria simple single-celled microorganisms

bariatric medicine medical specialty that focuses on the treatment of obesity

basal metabolism minimal number of kilocalories the body uses to support vital activities after fasting and resting for 12 hours

bases substances that accept hydrogen ions

beriberi thiamin deficiency disease

beta-carotene carotenoid that the body can convert to vitamin A

bile substance that is produced by the liver to prepare fat and fat-soluble vitamins for digestion and absorption

bile salts components of bile that enhance lipid digestion and absorption

binge eating consuming a much larger amount of food than is normally eaten in a brief period

binge-eating disorder (BED) eating disorder featuring recurrent episodes of binge eating that are not followed by purging behaviors

bioavailability extent to which the digestive tract absorbs a nutrient and how well the body uses it

bioelectrical impedance technique of estimating body composition in which a device measures the conduction of a weak electrical current through the body

biological activity describes vitamin's degree of potency or effects in the body

biotechnology using living things to manufacture new products

body mass index (BMI) numerical value of relationship between body weight and risk of certain chronic health problems associated with excess body fat

buffer substance that can protect the pH of a solution

bulimia nervosa (BN) severe psychological condition characterized by repeated episodes of binge eating followed by unhealthy behaviors to prevent weight gain

C

caffeine naturally occurring stimulant drug

calcitonin hormone secreted by the thyroid gland when blood calcium levels are too high

capillaries smallest blood vessels

carbohydrate (glycogen) loading practice of manipulating physical activity and dietary patterns to increase muscle glycogen stores

carbohydrates class of nutrients that includes glucose, a major source of energy for the body

carcinogen factor that triggers cancer

cardiovascular disease (CVD) group of diseases that affect the heart and blood vessels

carotenemia yellowing of the skin that results from excess beta-carotene in the body

carotenoids yellow-orange pigments in fruits and vegetables

case-control study study in which individuals who have a health condition are compared with individuals with similar characteristics who do not have the condition

casein major protein in cow's milk

cell smallest living functional unit in an organism

central-body obesity condition characterized by excessive visceral fat

chemical bond attraction that holds atoms together

chemical reactions processes that change the atomic arrangements of molecules

chemistry study of the composition and characteristics of matter and changes that can occur to it

cholecystokinin (CCK) hormone that stimulates the gallbladder to release bile and pancreas to secrete digestive enzymes

cholesterol sterol in animal foods and precursor for steroid hormones, bile, and vitamin D

choline water-soluble compound in lecithin

chylomicron particle formed by small intestinal cells that transports lipids in the bloodstream

chyme mixture of gastric juice and partially digested food

coenzyme ion or small molecule that interacts with enzymes, enabling the enzymes to function

cofactor ion or molecule that activates certain chemical reactions

cognitive behavioral therapy (CBT) psychological therapy approaches that address unhealthy emotions and behaviors

cohort study study that measures variables of a group of people over time

collagen   fibrous protein that gives strength to connective tissue

color additives   dyes, pigments, or other substances that provide color to food

colostrum   initial form of breast milk that contains anti-infective properties

complementary and alternative medicine (CAM)   variety of health care practices that are not accepted by the majority of conventional medical practitioners

complementary combinations   mixing certain plant foods to provide all essential amino acids without adding animal protein

complex carbohydrates (polysaccharides)   compounds comprised of 10 or more monosaccharides bonded together

compounds   molecules that contain two or more different elements in specific proportions

conception   moment when a sperm enters an egg (fertilization)

contaminated food   item that is impure or unsafe for human consumption

control group   group being studied that does not receive a treatment

coronary artery disease (CAD)   a major form of CVD

correlation   relationship between two variables

cretinism   condition affecting infants of women who were iodine deficient during pregnancy

cross-contamination   unintentional transfer of pathogenic microbes from one food to another

cytochromes   group of proteins involved in the release of energy from macronutrients

D

Daily Values (DVs)   set of nutrient intake standards developed for labeling purposes

deamination   removal of the nitrogen-containing group from an amino acid

deficiency disease   state of health that occurs when a nutrient is missing from the diet

dehydration   body water depletion

Delaney Clause   component of the 1958 Food Additives Amendment that prevents manufacturers from adding carcinogenic compounds to food

denaturation   altering a protein's natural shape and function by exposing it to conditions such as heat, acids, and physical agitation

diabetes mellitus (diabetes)   group of serious chronic diseases characterized by abnormal glucose, fat, and protein metabolism

diabulimia   popular term used to describe people with type I diabetes who skip insulin injections or use less insulin than prescribed to control their body weight

diastolic pressure   pressure in an artery that occurs when the ventricles relax between contractions

diet   usual pattern of food choices

dietary fiber (fiber)   nondigestible plant material; most types are polysaccharides

Dietary Reference Intakes (DRIs)   various energy and nutrient intake standards for Americans

dietary supplements   nutrient preparations, certain hormones, and herbal products

digestion   process by which large food molecules are mechanically and chemically broken down

disaccharide   simple sugar comprised of two monosaccharides

disordered eating   chaotic and abnormal food-related practices

diuretic   substance that increases urine production

diverticula   abnormal, tiny sacs that form in wall of colon

DNA   hereditary material that provides instructions for making proteins

double-blind study   experimental design in which neither the participants nor the researchers are aware of each participant's group assignment

dual-energy x-ray absorptiometry (DXA)   technique of estimating body composition that involves scanning the body with multiple low-energy x-rays

duodenum   first segment of the small intestine

E

eating disorders   psychological disturbances that lead to certain physiological changes and serious health complications

edema   accumulation of fluid in tissues

electrolytes   ions of minerals that conduct electricity when they are dissolved in water

electrons   small, negatively charged particles that surround the nucleus of an atom

element   each type of atom; substance that cannot be separated into simpler substances by ordinary chemical or physical means

embolus   thrombus or part of a plaque that breaks free and travels through the bloodstream

embryo   human organism from 14 days to 8 weeks after conception

empty calorie   describes food or beverage that supplies excessive amounts of unhealthy solid fat, added sugars, and/or alcohol

emulsifier   substance that helps water-soluble and water-insoluble compounds mix with each other

energy   capacity to perform work

energy density   energy value of a food in relation to the food's weight

energy equilibrium   calorie intake equals calorie output

energy intake   calories from foods and beverages that contain macronutrients and alcohol

energy output   calories cells use to carry out their activities

enrichment   addition of specific amounts of iron and certain B vitamins to cereal grain products

enterohepatic circulation   process that recycles cholesterol in the body

enzyme   molecule (usually a protein) that speeds up a particular chemical reaction

epidemiology   study of the occurrence, distribution, and causes of health problems in populations

epiglottis   flap of tissue that folds down over the windpipe to keep food from entering the respiratory system during swallowing

epithelial cells   cells that form protective tissues that line the body

ergogenic aids   foods, devices, dietary supplements, or drugs used to improve physical performance

esophagus   tubular structure of the GI tract that connects the pharynx with the stomach

essential amino acids   amino acids the body cannot make or make enough of to meet its needs

essential fatty acids   lipids that must be supplied by the diet

essential nutrient   nutrient that must be supplied by food

Estimated Average Requirement (EAR)   amount of a nutrient that meets the needs of 50% of healthy people in a life stage/sex group

Estimated Energy Requirement (EER)   average daily energy intake that meets the needs of a healthy person maintaining his or her weight

estrogen   hormone that plays a role in normal bone development and maintenance

evidence based   information that is based on results of scientific studies

Exchange System   method of classifying foods into lists based on macronutrient composition

exercise   physical activities that are usually planned and structured for a purpose

extracellular water   water that surrounds cells or is in liquid portion of blood

extrusion reflex   involuntary response in which a young infant thrusts its tongue forward when a solid or semisolid object is placed in its mouth

F

fad   trendy practice that has widespread appeal for a period, then becomes no longer fashionable

fat-free mass   body compartment that is comprised of body water, mineral-rich tissues, and protein-rich tissues

fat-soluble vitamins   vitamins A, D, E, and K

female athlete triad   condition that is characterized by low energy availability, menstrual problems, and reduced bone mineral density in female athletes

fermentation   process used to preserve or produce a variety of foods, including pickles and wine

fetus   human organism from 8 weeks after conception until birth

folic acid   form of folate

food additive   any substance that becomes incorporated into food during production, packaging, transport, or storage

Food Additives Amendment   U.S. legislation that requires evidence that a new food additive is safe before it can be marketed for use

Food and Nutrition Board (FNB)   group of nutrition scientists who develop DRIs

food-borne illness   disorder that is caused by consuming disease-causing agents in food or water

food-borne infection   illness that results when a pathogen in food inflames the intestinal tract or other body tissues

food insecurity   situation in which individuals or families are concerned about running out of food or not having enough money to buy more food

food intoxication   illness that results when poisons produced by certain microbes contaminate food and irritate the intestinal tract

fortification   addition of any of nutrient to food

fructose   monosaccharide in fruits, honey, and certain vegetables; "levulose" or "fruit sugar"

fungi   simple organisms that live on dead or decaying organic matter

fungicides   substances used to limit the spread of fungi

G

galactose   monosaccharide that is a component of lactose

gastroesophageal reflux disease (GERD)   condition that can result when acid reflux damages the wall of the lower esophagus and causes ulcers

gastroesophageal sphincter   section of esophagus next to the stomach that controls the opening to the stomach

gastrointestinal (GI) tract   muscular tube that extends from the mouth to the anus

gene   portion of DNA

Generally Recognized as Safe (GRAS)   ingredients considered to be safe

genetic endowment   inherited physical characteristics that can affect physical performance

genetic modification   techniques that alter an organism's DNA

gestational diabetes   form of diabetes that pregnant women can develop

gestational hypertension   type of hypertension that can develop during pregnancy

ghrelin   protein that stimulates eating behavior

glucagon   hormone that helps regulate blood glucose levels

glucose   monosaccharide that is a primary fuel for muscles and other cells; "dextrose" or "blood sugar"

glycogen   storage polysaccharide in animals

glycogenolysis   glycogen breakdown

glycolysis   first stage of glucose oxidation

goitrogens   compounds that inhibit iodide metabolism by the thyroid gland

H

H^+ chemical symbol for hydrogen ion

heartburn   backflow of irritating stomach contents into the esophagus

heat cramps   heat-related illness characterized by painful muscle contractions

heat exhaustion   heat-related illness that can occur after intense exercise

heatstroke   most dangerous form of heat-related illness

heme iron   form of iron in hemoglobin and myoglobin

hemoglobin   iron-containing protein in red blood cells that transports oxygen to tissues and some carbon dioxide away from tissues

herbicides   substances used to destroy weeds

hereditary hemochromatosis   most common type of iron overload disease

high-birth-weight (HBW)   describes baby who weighs more than 8.8 pounds at birth

high-density lipoprotein (HDL)   lipoprotein that transports cholesterol away from tissues and to the liver, where it can be eliminated

high-fructose corn syrup (HFCS)   caloric sweetener that is often added to food

high-quality (complete) protein   protein that contains all essential amino acids in amounts that support the deposition of protein in tissues and the growth of a young person

high-sensitivity C-reactive protein (hs-CRP)   protein produced primarily by the liver in response to inflammation

homeostasis   maintenance of an internal chemical and physical environment that is critical for good health and survival

homocysteine   amino acid that may play a role in the development of atherosclerosis

hunger   uncomfortable feeling that drives a person to consume food

hydration   water status

hydrocarbon chain   chain of carbon atoms bonded to each other and to hydrogen atoms

hydrogenation   food manufacturing process that adds hydrogen atoms to liquid vegetable oil, forming trans fats

hydrophilic   part of molecule that attracts water

hydrophobic   part of molecule that avoids water and attracts lipids

hypercalcemia   condition characterized by higher-than-normal concentration of calcium in blood

hyperglycemia   abnormally high blood glucose level

hypertension   abnormally high blood pressure levels that persist

hyperthermia   very high body temperature

hypoglycemia   condition that occurs when the blood glucose level is abnormally low

I

ileum   last segment of the small intestine

infant formula   synthetic food that simulates human milk

insecticides   substances used to control or kill insects

insoluble fiber   forms of dietary fiber that generally do not dissolve in water

insulin   hormone that helps regulate blood glucose levels

intracellular water   water that is inside cells

intrinsic factor (IF)   substance produced in the stomach that facilitates intestinal absorption of vitamin B-12

ion   atom or group of atoms that has a positive or negative charge

iron deficiency   condition characterized by low body stores of iron

J

jejunum   middle segment of the small intestine

K

keratin   tough protein found in hair, nails, and the outermost layers of skin

ketoacidosis   condition that occurs when the body forms excessive ketone bodies

ketone bodies   chemicals that result from incomplete fat breakdown

kilocalorie or **Calorie**   heat energy needed to raise the temperature of 1 liter of water $1°$ Celsius; measure of food energy

kwashiorkor   form of undernutrition that results from consuming adequate energy and insufficient high-quality protein

L

lactase   enzyme that splits lactose molecule

lactation   milk production

lacteal   lymph vessel in villus that absorbs most lipids

lactic acid   compound formed from pyruvate during anaerobic metabolism

lactoovovegetarian   vegetarian who consumes milk products and eggs for animal protein

lactose   disaccharide comprised of a glucose and a galactose molecule; "milk sugar"

lactose intolerance   inability to digest lactose properly

lactovegetarian   vegetarian who consumes milk and milk products for animal protein

lecithin   major phospholipid in food

legumes   plants that produce pods with a single row of seeds

leptin   hormone that reduces hunger and inhibits fat storage in the body

life expectancy   length of time an average person born in a specific year can expect to live

life span   maximum number of years an organism can live

lifestyle   usual way of living, including dietary practices and physical activity habits

linoleic acid   an essential fatty acid

lipases   enzymes that break down lipids

lipids   class of nutrients that generally do not dissolve in water

lipolysis   fat breakdown

lipoprotein   water-soluble structure that transports lipids through the bloodstream

lipoprotein lipase   enzyme in capillary walls that breaks down triglycerides

liposuction   surgical method of reducing the size of local fat deposits

low-birth-weight (LBW)   describes baby generally weighing less than 5½ pounds at birth

low-density lipoprotein (LDL)   lipoprotein that carries cholesterol into tissues

low energy availability   state of negative energy balance

low-quality (incomplete) protein   protein that lacks or has inadequate amounts of one or more of the essential amino acids

lumen   open space within a structure such as the small intestine

lymph   fluid in the lymphatic system

M

macronutrients   nutrients needed in gram amounts daily and that provide energy; carbohydrates, proteins, and fats

major minerals   essential mineral elements required in amounts of 100 mg or more per day

malignant tumor   mass of cancerous cells

malnutrition   state of health that occurs when the body is improperly nourished

maltase   enzyme that splits maltose molecule

maltose   disaccharide comprised of two glucose molecules; "malt sugar"

marasmus   starvation

megadose   generally defined as 10 times the recommended amount of a vitamin or mineral

metabolic syndrome   condition that increases risk of type 2 diabetes and CVD

metabolic water   water formed by cells as a metabolic by-product

metabolism   total of all chemical processes that take place in living cells

metastasized   spread to other tissues

micelle   lipid-rich particle that is surrounded by bile salts; transports lipids to absorptive cells

micronutrients   vitamins and minerals

minerals   elements that are found in the Earth's crust

mitochondria   cellular structures that release energy from macronutrients

moderation   obtaining adequate amounts of nutrients while balancing calorie intake with calorie expenditure

molecule   matter that forms when two or more atoms interact and are held together by a chemical bond

monoglyceride   single fatty acid attached to a glycerol backbone

monosaccharide   simple sugar that is the basic chemical unit of carbohydrates

monounsaturated fatty acid (MUFA)   fatty acid that has one double bond within the carbon chain

morning sickness   nausea and vomiting associated with pregnancy

mucus   fluid that lubricates and protects certain cells

multivitamin/mineral (MV/M)   describes a dietary supplement that contains vitamins and minerals

muscle dysmorphia   unhealthy preoccupation with the body being too small or not muscular enough

myocardial infarction   heart attack

myoglobin   iron-containing protein in muscle cells that controls oxygen uptake from red blood cells

MyPlate   USDA's interactive Internet dietary and menu planning guide

N

negative energy balance   calorie intake is less than calorie output

negative nitrogen balance   state in which the body loses more nitrogen than it retains

neural tube   embryonic structure that eventually develops into the brain and spinal cord

night eating syndrome (NES)   episodic food binges that are not followed by purging; binges take place after the evening meal and when the person wakens from sleep during the night

nitrogen balance (equilibrium)   balancing nitrogen intake with nitrogen losses

nonessential amino acids   group of amino acids that the body can make

nonexercise activity thermogenesis (NEAT)   involuntary skeletal muscular activities such as fidgeting

nonheme iron   form of iron that is primarily in vegetables, grains, meats, and supplements

nonnutritive sweeteners   group of synthetic compounds that are intensely sweet tasting compared to sugar

nutrient-dense   describes food or beverage that has more vitamins and minerals in relation to its unhealthy fat, added sugar, and/or alcohol contents

nutrients   chemicals necessary for proper body functioning

nutrigenetics   study of how a person's genetic makeup affects the way his or her body responds to food

nutrigenomics   study of how nutrients and other food components can affect one's genetic expression

nutrition   scientific study of nutrients and how the body uses these substances

nutritional genomics   science that investigates the complex interactions among gene functioning, dietary choices, and the environment

nutritive sweeteners   substances that sweeten and contribute energy to foods

O

obesity   condition characterized by excessive and unhealthy amounts of body fat

omega-3 fatty acid   type of polyunsaturated fatty acid

omega end   first carbon of a fatty acid chain that has three hydrogen atoms attached to it

omnivore   organism that can digest and absorb nutrients from plants, animals, fungi, and bacteria

organ   collection of tissues that function in a related fashion

organ system   group of organs that work together for a similar purpose

organelles   structures in cells that have specific functions

organic foods   foods produced without the use of antibiotics, hormones, synthetic fertilizers and pesticides, genetic improvements, or spoilage-killing radiation

osmosis   diffusion of a solvent, such as water, through a selectively permeable membrane

osteoblasts   bone cells that add bone to where the tissue is needed

osteoclasts   bone cells that tear down bone tissue

osteomalacia   adult rickets; condition characterized by poorly mineralized (soft) bones

osteoporosis   chronic disease characterized by loss of bone mass and reduced bone structure

overweight   having extra weight from bone, muscle, body fat, and/or body water

ovovegetarian   vegetarian who eats eggs for animal protein

oxidizing agent   substance that removes electrons from atoms or molecules

oxytocin   hormone that elicits the "let-down" response and causes the uterus to contract

P

pancreatic amylase enzyme secreted by pancreas that breaks down starch into maltose molecules

pancreatic lipase digestive enzyme that removes two fatty acids from each triglyceride molecule

parasite organism that lives in or on another organism, often deriving nourishment from its host

parathyroid hormone (PTH) hormone secreted by parathyroid glands when blood calcium levels are too low

pasteurization process that kills the pathogens in foods and beverages as well as many microbes responsible for spoilage

pathogens disease-causing microbes

peer review expert critical analysis of a research article before it is published

pellagra niacin deficiency disease

pepsin gastric enzyme that breaks down proteins into smaller polypeptides

peptide bond chemical attraction that connects two amino acids together

peptides small chains of amino acids

peristalsis type of muscular contraction of the gastrointestinal tract

pernicious anemia condition caused by the lack of intrinsic factor and characterized by vitamin B-12 deficiency, nerve damage, and megaloblastic RBCs

pesticide substance that people use to kill or control unwanted insects, weeds, or other organisms

pH measure of the acidity or alkalinity of a solution

phosphocreatine (PCr) high-energy compound used to reform ATP under anaerobic conditions

phospholipid type of lipid needed to make cell membranes and for proper functioning of nerve cells

physical activity movement resulting from contraction of skeletal muscles

physical fitness ability to perform moderate-to vigorous-intensity activities without becoming excessively fatigued

physiological dose amount of a nutrient that is within the range of safe intake and enables the body to function optimally

physiology scientific study of the functioning of cells and other body structures

phytochemicals compounds made by plants that are not nutrients

pica craving nonfood items

placebo fake treatment, such as a sham pill, injection, or medical procedure

placebo effect response to a placebo

placenta organ of pregnancy that connects the uterus to the embryo/fetus via the umbilical cord

polypeptide protein comprised of two or more amino acids

polyunsaturated fatty acid (PUFA) fatty acid that has two or more double bonds within the carbon chain

positive energy balance calorie intake is greater than calorie output

positive nitrogen balance state in which the body retains more nitrogen than it loses

pre-diabetes condition characterized by fasting blood glucose levels that are 100 to 125 mg/dl

prehypertension persistent systolic blood pressure readings of 120 mm Hg to 139 mm Hg and diastolic readings of 80 mm Hg to 89 mm Hg

prenatal care specialized health care for pregnant women

prenatal period time between conception and birth; pregnancy

prolactin hormone that stimulates milk production after delivery

prooxidant substance that promotes free radical production

protein-energy malnutrition (PEM) condition that results from diets that provide inadequate amounts of protein and energy

protein turnover cellular process of breaking down proteins and recycling their amino acids

proteins large, complex organic molecules made up of amino acids

protons positively charged particles in the nucleus of an atom

protozoans single-celled microorganisms that have complex cell structures

pseudoscience presentation of information masquerading as factual and obtained by scientific methods

purging activities that limit calorie intake or increase calorie output

pyruvate compound that results from anaerobic breakdown of glucose

Q

quackery promotion of useless medical treatments

R

R group part of amino acid that identifies the molecule as a particular amino acid

radical substance with an unpaired electron

Recommended Dietary Allowances (RDAs) standards for recommending daily intakes of several nutrients

rectum lower section of the large intestine

registered dietitian (RD), registered dietitian nutritionist (RDN), or licensed dietitian nutritionist (LDN) college-trained health care professional who has extensive knowledge of foods, nutrition, and dietetics

requirement smallest amount of a nutrient that maintains a defined level of nutritional health

resting metabolic rate (RMR) body's rate of energy use a few hours after resting and eating

retinol (preformed vitamin A) most active form of vitamin A in the body

rhodopsin vitamin A–containing protein that is needed for vision in dim light

rickets vitamin D deficiency disorder in children

risk factor personal characteristic that increases a person's chances of developing a disease

rodenticides substances used to kill mice and rats

S

salivary amylase enzyme secreted by salivary glands that begins starch digestion

salt substance that forms when an acid combines with a base

satiety sense that enough food or beverages have been consumed to satisfy hunger

saturated fatty acid fatty acid that has each carbon atom within the chain filled with hydrogen atoms

scurvy vitamin C–deficiency disease

selectively permeable membrane barrier that allows the passage of certain substances and prevents the movement of other substances

semivegetarian (or flexitarian) vegetarian who eats animal products, except red meat

senescence declining organ functioning and increased vulnerability

set-point theory scientific notion that body fat content is genetically predetermined

shelf life period of time that a food can be stored before it spoils

simple carbohydrates group of carbohydrates that includes sugars

simple diffusion movement of substances from a region of higher to lower concentration

skinfold thickness measurements technique of estimating body composition in which calipers are used to measure the width of skinfolds at multiple body sites

solid fats fats that are fairly hard at room temperature

solubility describes a substance's ability to dissolve and form a solution

soluble fiber forms of dietary fiber that dissolve or swell in water

solute lesser component of a solution that dissolves in solvent

solution evenly distributed mixture of two or more compounds

solvent primary component of a solution

spina bifida type of neural tube defect in which the spine does not form properly before birth, and it fails to enclose the spinal cord

starch storage polysaccharide in plants

sterilization process that kills or destroys all microorganisms and viruses

sucrase   enzyme that splits sucrose molecule

sucrose   disaccharide comprised of a glucose and a fructose molecule; "table sugar"

sustainable agriculture   farming methods that do not deplete natural resources or harm the environment while meeting the demand for food

syndrome   group of signs and symptoms that occur together and indicate a specific health problem

systolic pressure   maximum blood pressure within an artery that occurs when the ventricles contract

T

target heart rate zone   heart rate range that reflects intensity of physical exertion

teratogen   agent that causes birth defects

testimonial   personal endorsement of a product

testosterone   hormone needed for normal bone development and maintenance

tetrahydrofolic acid (THFA)   folate coenzyme

thermic effect of food (TEF)   energy used to digest foods and beverages as well as absorb and further process the macronutrients

thrombus   fixed bunch of clots that remains in place

thyroid hormone   hormone that regulates the body's metabolic rate

tissues   masses of cells that have similar characteristics and functions

Tolerable Upper Intake Level (Upper Level or UL)   standard representing the highest average amount of a nutrient that is unlikely to be harmful when consumed daily

tolerances   maximum amounts of pesticide residues that can be in or on each treated food crop

total body fat   essential fat and adipose tissue

total water intake   water in beverages and foods

trace minerals   essential mineral elements required in amounts that are less than 100 mg per day

trans fats   unsaturated fatty acids that have a *trans* double bond

transamination   transfer of the nitrogen-containing group from an unneeded amino acid to a carbon skeleton to form an amino acid

treatment group   group being studied that receives a treatment

triglyceride   lipid that has three fatty acids attached to a three-carbon compound called glycerol

U

underwater weighing   technique of estimating body composition that involves comparing weight on land to weight when completely submerged in a tank of water

underweight   describes person with a BMI of less than 18.5

unintentional food additives   substances that are accidentally in foods

unsaturated fatty acid   fatty acid that is missing hydrogen atoms and has one or more double bonds within the carbon chain

urea   waste product of amino acid metabolism

uterus   female reproductive organ that protects the developing organism during pregnancy

V

variable   personal characteristic or other factor that changes and can influence an outcome

vegan   vegetarian who eats only plant foods

vegetarians   people who eat plant-based diets

veins   vessels that return blood to the heart

very-low-density lipoprotein (VLDL)   lipoprotein that carries much of the triglycerides in the bloodstream

villi   (singular, villus) tiny, fingerlike projections of the small intestinal lining that participate in digesting and absorbing food

virus   microbe consisting of a piece of genetic material coated with protein

vitamin   complex organic molecule that regulates certain metabolic processes

W

water intoxication   condition that occurs when too much water is consumed in a short time period or the kidneys have difficulty filtering water from blood

water-soluble vitamins   thiamin, riboflavin, niacin, vitamin B-6, pantothenic acid, folate, biotin, vitamin B-12, and vitamin C

weaning   gradual process of shifting from breastfeeding or bottle-feeding to drinking from a cup and eating solid foods

Wernicke-Korsakoff syndrome   degenerative brain disorder resulting from thiamin deficiency that occurs primarily among alcoholics

X

xerophthalmia   condition affecting the eyes that results from vitamin A deficiency

Photo Credits

Front Matter

Page v(top): © Burke/Triolo Productions/ Getty Images RF; p. v(bottom): © C. Squared Studios/Getty Images RF; p. vii(top): © bdspn/ iStockphoto.com RF; p. vii(bottom): © Anna Verdina/Getty Images RF; p. xiii(top): © M. Freeman/PhotoLink/Getty Images RF; p. xiii(Lemon), p. xiii(Wine): © Burke/Triolo Productions/Getty Images RF; p. xiii(Cola): © Royalty-Free/Corbis RF; p. xiii(Tomato), p. xiii(Banana): © Stockdisc/PunchStock RF; p. xiii(Coffee): © Royalty-Free/Corbis RF; p. xiii(Milk): © McGraw-Hill Education. Bob Coyle, photographer; p. xiii(Egg): © Siede Preis/Getty Images RF; p. xiii(Baking Soda): © McGraw-Hill Education. Stephen Frisch, photographer; p. xiii(Ammonia): © McGraw-Hill Education. Jacques Cornell, photographer; p. xiii(Oven cleaner): © McGraw-Hill Education. Ken Karp, photographer; p. xiv(Strawberry): © Burke/Triolo Productions/Getty Images RF; p. xiv(Bottle): © Wendy Schiff; p. xiv(Pills): © McGraw-Hill Education. Jill Braaten, photographer; p. xvi(left): © Wendy Schiff; p. xvi(top): © C. Squared Studios/Getty Images RF; p. xvi(middle right), p. xvii(both): © Wendy Schiff; p. xviii: © McGraw-Hill Education. Jacques Cornell, photographer; p. xx(middle): U.S. Department of Health and Human Services; p. xxi(Helix): © Digital Vision/Getty Images RF; p. xxi(Vitamin): © McGraw-Hill Education. John Flournoy, photographer; p. xxi(Wine): © FoodCollection/StockFood RF; p. xxi(Bread): © Ingram Publishing RF; p. xxiii: © Photodisc/Punch-Stock RF; p. xxiv: © C. Squared Studios/Getty Images RF; p. xxv: © Photodisc/PunchStock RF; p. xxvi: © Ingram Publishing/Alamy RF; p. xxvii, p. xxviii, p. xxix: © C. Squared Studios/Getty Images RF.

Design Elements

Fruit Salad: © Anna Verdina/Getty Images RF; Spondias: © bdspn/iStockphoto.com RF; MyPlate: U.S. Dept. of Agriculture; Blueberries: © PhotoAlto/PunchStock RF; Stacked Books: © Stockdisc/Getty Images RF; Nuts: © C. Squared Studios/Getty Images RF; Recipe Box: © C. Squared Studios/Getty Images RF; Raspberry: © Digital Vision/Getty Images RF; Pineapple: © Stockdisc/Punch-Stock RF; Radish: © Stockdisc/PunchStock RF; Brass Weights: © Hermera Technologies/ Alamy RF.

Chapter 1

Opener: © Blend Images/Getty Images RF; 1.1: © Wendy Schiff; 1.3: © McGraw-Hill Education. Aaron Roeth Photography; Page 6: © Greg Kuchik/Getty Images RF; p. 7(Kale): © Stockdisc/PunchStock RF; p. 7(Red Onion): © C. Squared Studios/Getty Images RF; p. 7(Garlic): © Stockdisc/Punch-Stock RF; p. 7(Carrots): © Photodisc/Getty Images RF; p. 8(Apple): © Burke/Triolo Pro-ductions/Getty Images RF; p. 8(Plums): Scott Bauer/ARS/USDA; p. 8(Red Grapes): © Jules Frazier/Getty Images RF; p. 8(Strawberry), p. 8(Raspberry): © Burke/Triolo Productions/ Getty Images RF; p. 8(Almonds): © C. Squared Studios/Getty Images RF; p. 8(Chili Pepper): © Royalty-Free/Corbis RF; p. 9: © Pixtal/PunchStock RF; p. 10(Graph): Economic Research Service, U.S. Depart-ment of Agriculture; p. 10(Healthy People): U.S. Department of Health and Human Services. Office of Disease Prevention and Health Promotion. Healthy People 2020. Washington, DC.; p. 10(Pastries): © Food-Collection/StockFood RF; p. 11: © Royalty-Free/Corbis RF; p. 12(Scales): © Burke/ Triolo/Brand X Pictures/JupiterImages RF; 1.6(Bread): © Ed Carey/Cole Group/Getty Images RF; 1.6(Milk), 1.6(Potato): © McGraw-Hill Education. Christopher Kerrigan, photographer; 1.6(Donut): © Wendy Schiff; 1.7: U.S. Dept. of Agricul-ture; p. 14(Pumpkin Pie): © Royalty-Free/ Corbis RF; 1.8(Milk): © Sandy Jones/Getty Images RF; 1.8(Soda): © Royalty-Free/Corbis RF; p. 16(Brownies): © Michael Lamotte/ Cole Group/Getty Images RF; 1.9(Burger), 1.9(Peanuts): © Wendy Schiff; 1.9(Straw-berries): © Burke/Triolo Productions/Getty Images RF; p. 17(Supplements): © Nancy R. Cohen/Getty Images RF; p. 18(Spread): © Wendy Schiff; p. 18(Wheat): © PhotoDisc/ PunchStock RF; p. 18(Flour): © McGraw-Hill Education. Michael Scott, photographer; 1.12: © Lars A. Niki RF; p. 19(Locusts): © IT Stock/Alamy RF; 1.14: © Digitial Vision/ PunchStock RF; 1.15: Centers for Disease Control/Dr. Lyle Conrad; 1.16: © Getty Images RF; p. 22: USDA Photo by Ken Hammond; 1.17: © Comstock/Alamy RF; p. 23(Kernels): © Don Farrall/Getty Images RF; p. 24-25(Strawberries): © Burke/Triolo Productions/Getty Images RF; p. 28(Muffin): © Wendy Schiff; p. 29: © Photodisc/Getty Images RF; p. 31(Peas): © Burke/Triolo Pro-ductions/Getty Images RF; p. 31(Eggs): © Image Source/PunchStock RF; p. 31(Pickles): © Kevin Sanchez/Cole Group/ Getty Images RF; p. 31(Raspberries): © PhotoAlto/PunchStock RF; p. 31(Kale), p. 30(Broccoli): © Stockdisc/PunchStock RF; p. 31(Cabbage): © Burke/Triolo Productions/ Getty Images RF.

Chapter 2

Opener: © McGraw-Hill Education. Aaron Roeth Photography; 2.2: © Adam Gault/ Getty Images RF; Page 36(Pellagra): Centers for Disease Control; p. 36(Cabbage): © Burke/Triolo Productions/Getty Images RF. p. 36(Potatoes): © Ingram Publishing/Alamy RF; p. 36(Goldberger): Centers for Disease Control; p. 40: © Getty Images RF; p. 41, 2.6, p. 44: © Wendy Schiff; p. 45: © Stockdisc/ Punchstock RF; 2.7: © Wendy Schiff; p. 48: © McGraw-Hill Education. David Moyer, photographer; p. 49, p. 50(Label): © Wendy Schiff; p. 50(Pills): © McGraw-Hill Education. Jill Braaten, photographer; p. 52(Echinacea): © Brand X Pictures/PunchStock RF; p. 52(Ginger): © Stockbyte/Getty Images RF; p. 53(Tea): © Mitch Hrdlicka/Getty Images RF; p. 53(Plant): Jennifer Anderson/USDA-NRCS Plants Database; p. 55: © Photodisc/ Getty Images RF; p. 57(Soup): © Wendy Schiff; p. 58: © G.K & Vikki Hart/Getty Images RF; p. 59: © Wendy Schiff.

Chapter 3

Opener: © Digital Vision/Getty Images RF; Page 61: © Digitial Vision/PunchStock RF; 3.1: © Ryan McVay/Getty Images RF;

p. 65(Breads): © Wendy Schiff; p. 65(Dairy): © D. Hurst/Alamy RF; p. 66(middle), p. 66(Tomatillo), p. 67(Fats): © Wendy Schiff; 3.4: © McGraw-Hill Education. Christopher Kerrigan, photographer; p. 68(Salt): © C. Squared Studios/Getty Images RF; p. 68(Wine), p. 68(Bread): © Jules Frazier/Getty Images RF; p. 69: U.S. Department of Health and Human Services; p. 72(Cake): © FoodCollection/StockFood RF; p. 72(Apple): © Photodisc/Getty Images RF; p. 73: © Wendy Schiff; p. 74(top): © C. Squared Studios/Getty Images RF; 3.8(Dice): © McGraw-Hill Education. Christopher Kerrigan, photographer; 3.8(Mouse): © Royalty-Free/Corbis RF; 3.8(Ball): © Radlung & Associates/Getty Images RF; 3.8(Baseball): © Ryan McVay/Getty Images RF; 3.8(Yo yo): © PhotoDisc/Getty Images RF; 3.8(Soap): © McGraw-Hill Education. Christopher Kerrigan, photographer; p. 75(middle), p. 77, 3.11, 3.12, p. 82, 3.13, 3.14, 3.15: © Wendy Schiff; p. 86: © Royalty-Free/Corbis RF; p. 89(Sushi): © Burke/Triolo Productions/Getty Images RF; p. 90, p. 93(Lassi): © Wendy Schiff; p. 95(MyPlate): U.S. Dept. of Agriculture, Center for Nutrition Policy and Promotion; p. 95(Seeds): © Royalty-Free/Corbis RF; p. 96: © D. Hurst/Alamy RF.

Chapter 4

Opener: © Comstock Images RF; 4.3: © Wendy Schiff; 4.5(Lemon), 4.5(Wine): © Burke/Triolo Productions/Getty Images RF; 4.5(Cola): © Royalty-Free/Corbis RF; 4.5(Tomato), 4.5(Banana): © Stockdisc/PunchStock RF; 4.5(Coffee): © Royalty-Free/Corbis RF; 4.5(Milk): © McGraw-Hill Education. Bob Coyle, photographer; 4.5(Egg): © Siede Preis/Getty Images RF; 4.5(Baking Soda): © McGraw-Hill Education. Stephen Frisch, photographer; 4.5(Ammonia): © McGraw-Hill Education. Jacques Cornell, photographer; 4.5(Oven cleaner): © McGraw-Hill Education. Ken Karp, photographer; Page 102(Cleaners): © McGraw-Hill Education. Stephen Frisch, photographer; 4.6, 4.8: © Wendy Schiff; p. 112(Ice Cream): © Royalty-Free/Corbis RF; p. 112(bottom): © Brand X Pictures/PunchStock RF; 4.28: © Biophoto Associates/Science Source; p. 118, p. 119: © Wendy Schiff; p. 120: © Lars A. Niki RF; 4.32: © David M. Martin, M.D./Science Source; p. 122(right): © McGraw-Hill Education. Pat Watson, photographer; p. 125(right): © Jonelle Weaver/Getty Images RF; p. 126: © Wendy Schiff.

Chapter 5

Opener: © Ryan McVay/Getty Images RF; Page 131: © Allan & Sandy Carey/Getty Images RF; p. 132, p. 133(Sugar): © Wendy Schiff; p. 133(Honey): © Brand X Pictures/Getty Images RF; p. 134(Sweeteners), p. 134(Dr. Pepper), p. 135, 5.6: © Wendy Schiff; p. 137(bottom): © Cole Group/Getty Images RF; p. 138(Carrots): © C. Squared Studios/Getty Images RF; p. 138(Lettuce), p. 138(Raspberries): © Burke/Triolo Productions/Getty Images RF; p. 138(Potato): © McGraw-Hill Education. Christopher Kerrigan, photographer; p. 138(Banana): © Stockdisc/PunchStock RF; p. 138(Soy): © Siede Preis/Getty Images RF; p. 138(Strawberries): © Burke/Triolo Productions/Getty Images RF; p. 140: © PhotoLink/Getty Images RF; p. 144: © Pixtal/AGE fotostock RF; p. 145: © PhotoLink/Getty Images RF; 5.13: © Wendy Schiff; p. 148: © Brand X Pictures/JupiterImages RF; p. 149(left): © FoodCollection/StockFood RF; p. 149(right), p. 150: © Wendy Schiff; p. 151: © Lars A. Niki RF; p. 152(Bran): © Wendy Schiff; p. 152(Yogurt): © McGraw-Hill Education. Bob Coyle, photographer; 5.14: © Wendy Schiff; 5.15: © Du Cane Medical Imaging Ltd/Science Source; p. 154: Scott Bauer/ARS/USDA; 5.17: © Wendy Schiff; p. 155(Bread), p. 155(Cereal): © Photodisc/Getty Images RF; p. 156(Lentils): © Wendy Schiff; p. 156(Cookies): © Comstock/PunchStock RF; p. 157: © Burke/Triolo Productions/Getty Images RF; p. 158: © Photodisc/Getty Images RF; p. 159(Grains): © Royalty-Free/Corbis RF; p. 159(Blueberries), p. 160: © C. Squared Studios/Getty Images RF; p. 162: © Royalty-Free/Corbis RF; p. 163: © Burke/Triolo Productions/Getty Images RF.

Chapter 6

Opener: © Fuse/Getty Images RF; Page 165: © Photodisc/Getty Images RF; p. 169: © Photodisc/Getty Images RF; p. 170: © McGraw-Hill Education. Elite Images, photographer; p. 172: © Pixtal/AGE fotostock RF; p. 173(top): © McGraw-Hill Education. Bob Coyle, photographer; p. 173(bottom): © Wendy Schiff; p. 179: © BananaStock/JupiterImages RF; 6.14: © Wendy Schiff; 6.16a: © McGraw-Hill Education. Al Telser, photographer; 6.16b: © Image Source/Getty Images RF; p. 185: © Photodisc/Getty Images RF; p. 186: © McGraw-Hill Education. Gary He, photographer; p. 187: © Comstock/PunchStock RF; p. 188: © Wendy Schiff; p. 189(top): © Adam Crowley/Getty Images RF; p. 189(bottom): © C. Squared Studios/Getty Images RF; p. 190: © Wendy Schiff; p. 191(top): © McGraw-Hill Education. Ken Cavanagh, photographer; p. 191(bottom): © FoodCollection/StockFood RF; p. 192(top): © Ingram Publishing/Alamy RF; p. 192(bottom): © C. Squared Studios/Getty Images RF; p. 193: © Wendy Schiff; p. 194: © Royalty-Free/Corbis RF; p. 195: © Photodisc/Punchstock RF; p. 196(top): © Ryan McVay/Getty Images RF; 6.22: © Wendy Schiff; p. 199: Centers for Disease Control/Gwinnet County Police Department; 6.26: © Arthur Glauberman/Science Source; p. 205: © Photodisc/PunchStock RF; p. 206(top): © Burke/Triolo Productions/Getty Images RF; p. 206(bottom): © Burke/Triolo Productions/Getty Images RF; p. 207: © Wendy Schiff; p. 208: © John A. Rizzo/Getty Images RF; p. 209: © McGraw-Hill Education. Elite Images, photographer; p. 210: © Spike Mafford/Getty Images RF; p. 211, p. 213: © Burke/Triolo Productions/Getty Images RF.

Chapter 7

Opener: © Ingram Publishing/SuperStock RF; Page 218(Jell-O): © Wendy Schiff; p. 218(Soup): © John A. Rizzo/Getty Images RF; p. 218(Peas): © Getty Images RF; p. 218(Beans): © Royalty-Free/Corbis RF; p. 218(Ham): © Burke/Triolo Productions/Getty Images RF; p. 218(Tofu): © C. Squared Studios/Getty Images RF; p. 218(Bagel): © Photodisc/Getty Images RF; p. 218(Pizza): © C. Squared Studios/Getty Images RF; 7.3(left): © Photodisc/PunchStock RF; 7.3(right): © C. Squared Studios/Getty Images RF; p. 219(bottom): © Wendy Schiff; 7.8: CDC/Sickle Cell Foundation of Georgia: Jackie George, Beverly Sinclair/Photo by Janice Haney Carr; p. 223: © McGraw-Hill Education. Joe DeGrandis, photographer; p. 226(top): © liquidllibrary/PictureQuest RF; p. 226(bottom): Scott Bauer/ARS/USDA; p. 227(Beef), p. 227(Fish): © Photodisc/PunchStock RF; p. 227(Turkey): © Paul Poplis/StockFood Creative/Getty Images; p. 227(Rice): © McGraw-Hill Education. Jacques Cornell, photographer; p. 227(Bread): © C. Squared Studios/Getty Images RF; p. 227(Beans): © Burke/Triolo Productions/Getty Images RF; p. 227(Dairy): © Photodisc/Getty Images RF; p. 227(Egg): © Siede Preis/Getty Images RF; p. 227(Nuts): © C. Squared Studios/Getty Images RF; p. 227(Tripe): © Wendy Schiff; 7.15: © Ingram Publishing/Alamy RF; p. 229: © PhotoLink/

Chapter 8

Chapter 9

© PhotoLink/Getty Images RF; p. 466(top): Centers for Disease Control; p. 466(Mushrooms): © McGraw-Hill Education. Stephen P. Lynch, photographer; p. 466(Cheese): © Stockbyte/PunchStock RF; p. 467: © Royalty-Free/Corbis RF; p. 468: © McGraw-Hill Education. Rick Brady, photographer; p. 469: Centers for Disease Control/James Gathany; 12.5, 12.6: © Wendy Schiff; p. 471(middle): © Royalty-Free/Corbis RF; p. 471(bottom): U.S. Department of Agriculture, Food Safety and Inspection Service; p. 472: © C. Squared Studios/Getty Images RF; p. 473(top): © BananaStock/PunchStock RF; 12.7: U.S. Department of Agriculture, Food Safety and Inspection Service; p. 475(Dried Fruits): © C. Squared Studios/Getty Images RF; p. 475(Pickles): © Kevin Sanchez/Cole Group/Getty Images RF; p. 475(Spam): © McGraw-Hill Education. Elite Images, photographer; p. 475(Cheese): © Burke/Triolo Productions/Getty Images RF; 12.8: Photo by Stephen Ausmus/ARS/USDA; 12.9: U.S. Department of Agriculture, Food Safety and Inspection Service; p. 477: Photo by Liz Roll/FEMA; p. 479: © Wendy Schiff; p. 480: © Photodisc/Getty Images RF; 12.10: ARS/USDA; p. 483: © Brand X Pictures/PunchStock RF; 12.13: Courtesy of Katadyn North America; p. 486: © FoodCollection/

StockFood RF; p. 488: Courtesy of National Cancer Institute; p. 489: © Comstock Images/PictureQuest RF; p. 490: © Kevin Sanchez/Cole Group/Getty Images RF; p. 491: Historicus/Library of Congress.

Chapter 13

Opener: © Karena Rigby; Page 493: © Brand X Pictures/PunchStock RF; 13.2: © Royalty-Free/Corbis RF; p. 496(bottom): © Mike Marsland/WireImage/Getty Images; p. 498(Cereal): © McGraw-Hill Education. John Flournoy photographer; p. 498(Juice): © McGraw-Hill Education. Emily & David Tietz, photographers; p. 498(Beans): © Royalty-Free/Corbis RF; p. 499: © Stockbyte RF; p. 502, 13.4a: © Photodisc/Getty Images RF; 13.4b: © Brand X Pictures/PunchStock RF; p. 504: © Jiang Jin/Purestock/SuperStock RF; 13.5: © Royalty-Free/Corbis RF; 13.6: © Keith Eng 2007 RF; p. 507, 13.7, p. 508(all), p. 509(top): © Wendy Schiff; p. 509(bottom): © Sky View/Digital Vision/Getty Images RF; 13.8: © Creatas/PictureQuest RF; p. 510(bottom): © Nancy Ney/Getty Images RF; p. 511: © Creatas/PictureQuest RF; 13.9, p. 513: © BananaStock/PunchStock RF; p. 514: © Image Source/PunchStock RF; p. 516(top): U.S.

Department of Agriculture, Center for Nutrition Policy and Promotion; p. 516(middle): © BananaStock/PunchStock RF; 13.10: © Purestock/Getty Images RF; p. 518: © Royalty-Free/Corbis RF; p. 520: © Image Source/Corbis RF; p. 523: © Wendy Schiff; p. 525: © Steve Mason/Getty Images RF; p. 526: © Steve Cole/Getty Images RF; p. 527: © Kieth Brofsky/Getty Images RF; p. 528: USDA Photo by Ken Hammond; p. 529: Library of Congress, Prints and Photographs Division; p. 532: © Royalty-Free/Corbis RF; p. 533: © Wendy Schiff; p. 535: © Royalty-Free/Corbis RF.

Appendix:

A-1: © Hermera Technologies/Alamy RF; A-2: © Wendy Schiff; A-5: © McGraw-Hill Education. Ken Karp, photographer; A-6(Ham): © Royalty-Free/Corbis RF; A-6(Dairy): © D. Hurst/Alamy RF; A-6(Egg): © McGraw-Hill Education. Ken Karp, photographer; A-7: © Royalty-Free/Corbis RF; A-23: © Burke/Triolo Productions/Getty Images RF; A-24: © Wendy Schiff.

A

Absorption
bioavailability and, 111
carbohydrates, 139–140, 139f
cystic fibrosis, 117
defined, 111
inflammatory bowel disease, 118
of protein, 222–223, 223f
small intestines, 114, 116f
vitamin B-12, 291, 292f
vitamins, 262–263
Academy of Nutrition and Dietetics website, 48t
Acai berry, 407t
Acceptable Macronutrient Distribution Ranges (AMDRs), 64t
defined, 63
fat, 179
protein consumption and, 226
weight-loss diet and, 395
Accessory organs, 111
Accident, as cause of death in U.S., 4f
Acesulfame-K, 134, 134t
Acetaldehyde dehydrogenase, 197, 197f
Acid-base balance
defined, 216
proteins and, 216
Acid group, 217
Acidosis, 102
Acids
defined, 101
hydrogen ions, 101
pH scale, 102, 102f
ADA Guide to Eating Right When You Have Diabetes, 76
Added sugars, 15, 68–69, 132, 133t
average American consumption of, 142
calories and, 142
MyPlate and, 142
soft drinks and, 142, 144
Additives, 478–483
antioxidant, 478
benzene, 480
chemical contaminants, 480
color, 478
common types of direct, 479t
defined, 478
Delaney Clause, 480

FDA and safety of, 478–480
flavors/flavor enhancers, 479t
food safety legislation on, 479–480
Generally Recognized as Safe (GRAS), 479
pesticides, 481–482
sulfites, 478
unintentional food additives, 480
Adenosine diphosphate (ADP)
defined, 430
energy from ATP and, 430, 432f
Adenosine triphosphate (ATP)
defined, 377, 430
energy for cells from, 430, 432f
energy for muscles, 435t
formation of, 430, 430f, 432f
lactic acid energy system, 433–434, 434f
oxygen energy system, 435
PCr-ATP energy system, 432–433, 433f
Adequate Intakes (AIs), 64t
applying, 63
defined, 63
establishing, 63, 63f
ADHD, 153
Adipose cells, 178, 178f
defined, 373
function of, 373
maintaining blood glucose levels, 140f
Adipose tissue, 373
brown fat, 374
leptin, 389
regulating food intake, 389
Adjustable gastric banding, 402, 403f
Adolescents
calcium, 518
defined, 517
growth spurt, 517
iron, 518
nitrogen balance, 225, 225f
nutrition-related concerns of, 517–519
osteoporosis, 518
overweight, 372, 518
peer pressure, 517
physical activity, 518
positive energy balance, 384
puberty, 517
vegetarianism, 233–234, 518

Adolsterone, vitamin C and, 295
ADP. *See* Adenosine diphosphate (ADP)
Adrenaline, 150
Advertising hype, 407–408
Aerobic capacity, 435
Aerobic condition, 430, 431f
oxygen energy system, 435
Aerobic exercise, 435t
defined, 429
in physical activity pyramid, 428–429, 428f
Aerobic respiration, 431
Aflatoxin, 304, 305t, 465
African Americans, risk for hypertension, 338
African heritage diets, 88
Age. *See also* Life stages and nutritional needs
hypertension and, 338
metabolism and, 380
number of taste buds and, 112
Age-related macular degeneration (AMD), carotenoids, 300–301
Age-related maximum heart rate, 426–427
Aging process, 523–524, 523t
Agriculture
comparing organic/nonorganic farming systems, 84t
sustainable, 23
Air displacement, 375, 375f
Alanine, 217f, 217t, A5
Albumin, 216
Alcohol, 195–204
abuse and dependence, 199t, 200, 204
binge drinking, 198–199
body's processing of, 196–198
body water and, 202–203
brain, effect on, 201
breastfeeding and, 506
cancer and, 202, 304, 305t
carbohydrate/alcoholic content of various beverages, 196t
cardiovascular system, effect on, 202
chemical structure of, 195, 195f
classification of drinkers, 198–199, 198t
congeners, 322–323
consumption as risk factor, 9

dehydration and, 323
2015–2020 Dietary Guidelines for Americans, 69
as diuretic, 322–323
drug interaction with, 202
as empty-calorie food, 67
energy and, 12
fetal alcohol syndrome, 203
gastrointestinal tract and, 200–201
health benefits of, 203
hypertension and, 338
kcal in gram of, 12
liver, effect on, 201–202
metabolism of, 197
nutritional status, 202
people who should avoid, 203t
physical performance and, 203–204
physiological effect of, 200–203, 200f
pregnancy and, 203, 501
production of, 195–196
raising HDL and, 193
tolerance, 200
triglycerides synthesis, 179
Alcoholism
magnesium deficiency, 343
niacin deficiency, 285
signs of, 199t
thiamin deficiency, 202
vitamin B-6 deficiency, 287
Wernicke-Korsakoff syndrome, 284
zinc deficiency, 352
Alcohol poisoning, 199
Aldosterone, 322, 322f
Alfalfa claims/benefits/risks, 52t
Algae, 189t, 233
Allergen, 238–239
Allergies
cow's milk and infants, 509
introducing solid foods to infants, 509–510
preschool children, 514
Alli, 401
Allicin, 192
Allkaloids, sources/biological effect of, 8t
Allylic sulfur compounds, sources/biological effect of, 8t
Alpha-carotene, sources/biological effect of, 8t

Alpha-linolenic acid, 167, 168f
Alpha-tocopherol, 259t, 277. See also Vitamin E
Alternative sweeteners, 133–135, 134t
Alzheimer's disease
    as cause of death in U.S., 4f
    folate, vitamin B-6 and B-12 and, 298
    vitamin C and, 299
    vitamin E and, 299
American Academy of Pediatrics (AAP)
    breastfeeding recommendations, 506
    iron-fortified infant formula, 508
American College of Sports Medicine (ACSM), 437
    athletes' protein consumption, 442
    daily moderate-intensity physical activity, 392, 425
American Diabetes Association (ADA), 75
American Gastroenterological Association, 120
American Heart Association
    daily moderate-intensity physical activity, 425
    website, 48t
American Journal of Clinical Nutrition, 41
Amino acids, 141, A5
    chemical structure of, 216–217, 217f, A5
    classifying, 217
    deamination, 224
    defined, 216
    denaturation, 222f
    essential, 217, 217t
    limiting, 219
    nonessential, 217, 217t
    peptide bond, 220, 220f
    protein digestion and absorption, 222–223, 223f
    protein supplements and, 441
    protein turnover, 222–223
    transamination, 224, 224f
    umami taste, 112
Amino group, 217
Amylase
    pancreatic, 139, 139f
    in saliva, 112, 139, 139f
Amylopectin, 136f
Amylose, 136f
Anabolic reaction, 103
Anabolic steroids, 448t
Anaerobic condition, 430, 431f
    lactic acid energy system, 433–434, 434f
    PCr-ATP energy system, 432–433, 433f
Anaerobic exercise, 435t

Anal sphincter, 117, 117f
Anaphylaxis, food allergy, 239
Anatomy, 104
Anecdotes, 33
Anemia
    folate, 289
    iron deficiency anemia, 349
    megaloblastic, 289
    older adults and, 526
    pernicious anemia, 293
    physiological, 497
    sports anemia, 445
    vitamin B-6 and, 286
Anencephaly, 290
Animal cloning, 85
Anisakis, 465, 465f, 466t
Anorexia nervosa
    common health consequences of, 412t
    signs and symptoms of, 412
    treatment of, 412
    vegetarian teens and, 234
Anthocyanin, 8t, 102
Antibodies, 216
Antidiuretic hormone (ADH), 322, 322f
Antimotility agents, 485
Antioxidant additives, 478
Antioxidants. See also specific antioxidants
    beer and wine, 203
    defined, 6, 259
    dietary advice for athletes, 445
    function of, 7, 259, 261f
    as nonnutrient, 7
    selenoproteins, 357
    vitamin C as, 295
Anus, lipid digestion, 177f
Appetite, 391
Apple shape, 387, 387f
Arachidonic acid (AA), 167, 168f, 504
Arginine, 217t, A5
Arsenic
    as essential nutrient, 100t
    summary of, 360t
Arterial plaque, 181f, 182
Arteries
    from atherosclerosis to cardiovascular disease, 181–183, 181f, 182f
    function of, 107, 107f
    hardening of, 181f
Arteriosclerosis, 183
Artesian water, 362, 362t
Artificial sweeteners, 133
Ascorbic acid, 101, 259t, 282t, 294. See also Vitamin C
Aseptic processing, 474
Asian Diet Pyramid, 88–89, 89f
Asian influences on diet, 88–89
Asparagine, 217t, A5
Aspartame, 134–135, 134t, 135
    PKU and, 242

Aspartic acid, 134, 217t, A5
Atherosclerosis
    assessing your risk for, 184–188, 187t
    characteristics and development of, 181–182, 181f
    cholesterol, HDL, LDL and triglyceride levels and, 187, 187t
    coronary calcium, 188
    C-reactive protein, 188
    defined, 181
    dietary changes to reduce risk of, 188–194, 194t
    homocysteine and, 185
    lipoproteins and, 183–184, 184f
Athletes
    alcohol consumption and physical performance, 203–204
    antioxidant vitamins and, 445
    benefits of regular exercise, 426, 427f
    caffeine and, 447
    calcium and, 446
    carbohydrates and, 438–441, 439t, 440t
    dehydration, 323
    dietary fat and, 438
    energy for athletic performance, 436t, 437–438
    energy for muscular work, 429–432–6
    energy or sports bars, 442, 442f, 443t
    ergogenic aids, 446–449
    female athlete triad, 446
    fiber and, 439
    fluids and, 443–445
    genetic endowment, 437
    heat-related illness in, 443, 444, 444t
    iron and, 445
    pre-event meals and snacks, 438–441
    protein and, 441–442
    sports anemia, 445
    sports drinks, 444–445
    water and, 443–445
    water intoxication, 324, 444
Atkins diet, 144, 236
Atom, 99f
ATP. See Adenosine triphosphate (ATP)
Attention deficit hyperactivity disorder (ADHD), 153

B

Baby bottle caries, 511
Bacillus cereus, 464t

Bacteria
    as food-borne illness pathogen, 463, 464t
    in small and large intestine, 118
Baking soda, 101
    acid-base reaction, 103
    used in baking, 103
Balanced diet, 14
Bariatric medicine, 402
Bariatric surgery, 402–403, 403f, 522
Basal metabolism
    calculating, 380
    defined, 378
Bases
    defined, 101
    hydrogen ions, 101
    pH scale, 102, 102f
Basic Four, 71
Beano®, 155
Beans, 138t. See also Legumes
Bee pollen, 448t
Behavior modification, weight-loss plans, 396–399
Belviq, 401
Benign tumor, 303
Benzene, 480
Beriberi, 257, 283, 284f
Beta-carotene
    age-related macular degeneration (AMD), 300–301
    cancer and, 300
    defined, 270
    food sources of, 269–270
    as precursor to vitamin A, 259
    sources/biological effect of, 8t
Beta-cryptoxanthin, 300
Beta-hydroxy-beta-methylbutyrate, 407t, 448t
Beverages, fortified, 262
BHA, 261
BHT, 261
Bicarbonate, pancreas, 115
Bile
    body production of, 172
    dietary fiber, cholesterol and, 154
    role in digestion, 115, 174
    vitamin absorption and, 262
Bile salts, 174, 178, 178f
Binge drinking, 198–199, 198t
Binge-eating disorder
    signs and symptoms of, 413
    treatment of, 413
Bioavailability, 111
Bioelectrical impedence, 376, 376f
Biogerontologists, 529
Biological activity, 261
Biotechnology, 22
Biotin, 259t, 294
    body's production of, 262
    Daily Value, A1

Biotin, *(continued)*
  energy metabolism, A6
  as essential nutrient, 7t
  function of, 260f
  summary of, 282t
Bismuth subsalicylate (BSS), 485
Bitter orange, claims/benefits/
  risks, 52t
Bitter taste, benefit of, 112
Bladder, function of, 108, 108f
Blood
  blood sugar, 131, 140
  function of, 107
  pH of, 102, 102f
  during pregnancy, 496–497
  vitamin E and, 278
  vitamin K and clotting, 278, 279f
Blood alcohol concentration
  (BAC), 197, 198f, 201t
Blood clotting
  atherosclerosis and, 182
  omega-6 and, 189
  vitamin K and, 278, 279f
Blood glucose
  diabetes, 146
  hyperglycemia, 146
  hypoglycemia, 150
  maintaining, 140–141, 140f
  metabolic syndrome, 151t
Blood pressure. *See also*
  Hypertension
  blood proteins and, 216, 216f
  diastolic, 337
  metabolic syndrome, 151t
  potassium and, 341
  sodium and, 336, 338
  systolic, 336
BOD POD, 375f
Body composition, 372–377
  adipose tissue, 373
  apple shape, 387, 387f
  central-body obesity, 387–388,
    387f
  fat-free mass, 372
  gender differences, 5f
  measuring, 374–376,
    374f–376f
  metabolism, 379
  of nutrients, 5f
  pear shape, 387, 387f
  weight classification and, 376,
    377t, 386t
Body fat. *See* Fat, body
Body mass index (BMI)
  boys 2 to 20 years, A7
  calculating, 386
  deciding on weight loss, 394,
    394f
  defined, 371
  education and, 393
  for-age, 512
  girls 2 to 20 years, A8
  health risks of high, 386, 387t

uses of, 371
  weight classifications based on,
    386, 386t, 394, 394f
Body surface area, metabolism
  and, 379
Bok choy, 333
Bones
  calcium and, 329, 330f
  function of, 109f, 110
  osteoporosis, 330, 330f, 332–335
  rickets, 272, 272f
  vitamin A and, 268
  vitamin D and, 272–273, 272f
  vitamin K and, 279
Boron
  as essential nutrient, 100t
  summary of, 360t
Botanicals, 50
Bottled water, 361–362
Botulism, 133, 475
Bowel movements
  constipation, 120
  diarrhea, 120
  fiber and, 140, 153
  frequency of, 120
BPA, 362
Brain, 109f
  alcohol's effect on, 201
  function of, 109
  iodine deficiency and, 356
Branched chain amino
  acids, 448t
Breakfast, school-age children,
  516
Breast cancer
  alcohol consumption and, 202
  breastfeeding and, 504
Breastfeeding
  advantages of, 503–504, 504t
  alcohol and, 506
  calorie needs for, 506
  colostrum, 503
  fat in, 508
  iron and, 507
  length of time recommended,
    506, 507
  let-down reflex, 504, 505f
  milk production process,
    504–506, 505f
  mother's fluid intake when, 506
  supplements for infants, 507
  undernutrition and
    recommendations for,
    20–21
  vegetarians and, 233, 507
  vitamin B-12 and, 293, 507
  vitamin D and, 276, 506
  weaning, 509–510
  zinc deficiency, 352
Breasts, changes during
  pregnancy, 496
Brown fat (BAT), 374
Buffer, 216

Bulimia nervosa, 412–413, 415
  real story of, 415

C
Cadaver, 111
Caffeine
  athletes and, 447
  defined, 442
  as diuretic, 322
  in energy drink, 442–443, 447
  as ergogenic aid, 447, 448t
  as phytochemical, 6
  of selected beverages, 449t
  sources/biological effect of, 8t
Calcitonin, 329
Calcium, 329–332
  adolescents, 518
  AI, 332
  bioavalibility of, 330, 330f
  bone development and
    maintenance, 329, 330f
  characteristics of, 329
  Daily Value, A1
  deficiency, 332–335
  dietary adequacy, 332
  dietary advice for athletes, 446
  as essential nutrient, 7t, 100t
  food sources, 330–331, 330t,
    331f, 334
  function of, 325f, 329
  health claim, 81t
  high-protein diet, 235
  hypercalcemia, 332
  maintaining blood calcium
    levels, 329
  MyPlate, 326f, 331f
  osteoporosis, 332–335
  structure/function claim, 81
  summary of, 328t
  supplements, 331–332
  thyroid and parathyroid, 329,
    329f
  toxicity, 332
  vitamin D and metabolism of,
    273, 274f
Calcium phosphate, 273
Calories
  added sugars and, 142
  "calorie free" legal definition, 82t
  defined, 12
  dietary advice for athletes,
    436t, 437–438
  Dietary Guidelines, 67–69
  energy balance, 384
  estimating energy need for, 384
  nutrient content claims, 82t
Calorie intake
  breastfeeding and, 506
  metabolism and, 380
  during pregnancy, 498
Calorie reduction
  calorie restriction and aging
    process, 529

fad diets, 404–405
  in medically sound weight-loss
    plans, 395–396
  unreliable methods of weight
    loss, 404–409
  very-low-calorie diet and
    metabolism, 380
Calorie restriction (CR), longevity
  and, 529
Campylobacter jejuni, 464t
Cancer
  alcohol consumption and,
    202, 304
  body fat and, 304–305
  breastfeeding and, 504
  as cause of death in U.S.,
    4f, 9
  causes of, 304
  death from, 302
  defined, 303
  development and progression
    of, 302f–303f
  diet and, 3, 304–305
  leading sites for, 302
  lowering risk for, 275, 299, 300,
    304, 306
  mechanism of, 302–303
  pesticides and, 482
  risk factors for, 9
  selenium intake and, 357
Capillaries, function of,
  107, 107f
Capsaicin, sources/biological
  effect of, 8t
Capsaicinoids, sources/biological
  effect of, 8t
Carbohydrates, 129–161. *See also*
  Complex carbohydrates;
  Simple carbohydrates
  added sugar, 68–69, 143
  in alcoholic beverages, 196t
  AMDR for, 63, 64t
  athletes and, 438–441, 439t,
    440t
  ATP formation, 431, 431f
  body composition of, 5f
  body fat and, 144
  carbohydrate loading,
    439–441
  consumption patterns,
    142–143, 142f
  counting, 76
  Daily Value, A1
  defined, 129
  diabetes and, 141, 146
  digestion and absorption of,
    139–140, 139f
  Exchange System, 76
  for fueling exercise, 436
  functions of, 5t
  glucose for energy, 141–142
  glycemic index, 156–157
  hyperactivity and sugar, 153

hypoglycemia and health, 150–151
kcal in gram of, 12
lactose intolerance and, 152
low-carbohydrate diet, 405–406, 405t
as macronutrient, 12
maintaining blood glucose levels, 140–141, 140f
metabolic syndrome and, 151–152
as nutrient, 5
Nutrition Facts panel, 143, 144f
plants as source of, 129, 129f
RDA, 78, 141
reactive hypoglycemia and, 151
refined, reducing intake of, 142, 143
tooth decay and, 152
triglycerides synthesis, 179
Carbon, as essential element, 100t
Carbon dioxide
    in acid-base reaction, 102, 103f
    ATP formation, 431, 431f
    in baking, 103
Carbon skeleton, 217, 217f
Carcinogens, 303, 305t, 480
Cardiorespiratory system, 435
Cardiovascular disease (CVD), 181–195
    alcohol consumption and, 203
    arteriosclerosis, 183
    assessing risk for, 184–188
    atherosclerosis, 181–184, 181f
    body fat distribution and, 386, 387
    defined, 181
    diabetes and, 186
    dietary changes to reduce risk of atherosclerosis, 188–194, 194t
    dietary fat, reducing, 191–192, 194t
    fiber and, 154
    folate, vitamin B-6 and B-12 and, 298
    homocysteine and, 185
    hypertension and, 186
    incidence of, 181
    metabolic syndrome and, 152
    modifiable risk factors, 186
    omega-3 fatty acids, 189–190
    risk factors for, 184–185, 185t
    saturated fats and, 67, 168, 169
    smoking and, 186
    statins, 194
    stress and, 186
    vitamin B-6, 286, 298
    vitamin C, 299
    weight loss and exercise, 191
Cardiovascular system
    alcohol's effect on, 202
    overview of, 106f, 107, 107t

Carotenemia, 271
Carotenoids
    age-related macular degeneration (AMD), 300–301
    beta-carotene, 269–270
    cancer and, 300
    defined, 267
    function of, 260f
    lutein, 270
    lycopene, 270
    sources/biological effect of, 8t
    Vitamin A and, 267
    vitamin supplements, 300–301
    zeaxanthin, 270
Carotid arteries, 182, 182f
Case-control study, 38
Casein, 508
Catabolic reaction, 103
Catabolize, 429
Catechins, sources/biological effect of, 8t
Celiac disease, 240, 240t, 241
Cells
    defined, 5
    structure and function, 105, 105f
    tissue, 106, 106f
Cellulite, 373
Cellulose, 136, 137t
Centers for Disease Control and Prevention (CDC), 437
    on irradiated food, 476
    role in food safety, 458
    website, 48t
Centi, 12
Central-body obesity, 387–388, 387f
Cereal, fiber content, 138t
Chemical bond, 100, 100f
Chemical contaminants, 480
Chemical digestion, 112
Chemical formula, 100
Chemical reactions
    anabolic reaction, 103
    catabolic reaction, 103
    decomposition reaction, 102–103
    defined, 102
    enzymes, 103–104
    hydrolytic, 114
    synthetic reaction, 103
Chemistry
    acids and bases, 101–102, 102f
    atoms, 99–100
    chemical reaction, 102–103
    compounds, 100
    defined, 4
    elements, 99, 100t
    enzymes, 103–104
    ions, 100–101
    molecules, 100

Chia seed, 407t
Child and Adult Care Food Program, 22t
Childhood obesity, 519–522, 519f
    bariatric surgery for, 522
    contributing factors, 519–520
    defining, 519
    environmental factors, 392, 521, 521t
    genetics and biological factors, 520
    health problems associated with, 519, 520t
    incidence of, 372
    preventing, 521
    sugar and soft drinks, 145–146
    treating, 521–522
    weight status classifications, 519t
Children. See also Adolescents; Childhood obesity; Infants
    body mass index (BMI), 512
    childhood nutrition, 512–514
    food allergies, 239
    growth rate for, 512–513
    honey and, 133
    iron deficiency anemia, 350
    kwashiorkor, 237, 237f
    marasmus, 237–238, 237f
    overweight, 372, 514, 518–522, 519f
    positive energy balance, 384
    preschool, 512–514, 513t, 514
    protein-energy malnutrition, 236–237, 237f
    school-age children, 515–516, 519–522, 519f
    tooth decay, 152
    undernutrition and, 20–21
    vegetarian, 233, 518
    zinc deficiency, 352–353
Chinese diet pills, 407t
Chitosan, 407t
Chloride, 344–345
    Daily Value, A1
    deficiency and toxicity, 344–345
    as essential element, 7t, 100t
    extracellular water, 319
    function of, 325f
    summary of, 328t
Chlorophyll, 270
Chocolate, 13
Cholecystokinin (CCK), 115
    appetite and, 389, 390f
    defined, 174
    role of, 174
Cholesterol
    atherosclerosis and, 183
    body's need for, 172
    body's production of, 172
    cardiovascular disease and, 185t

"cholesterol free," legal definition, 82t
chromium deficiency and, 359
content of, in common foods, 173f
Daily Value, A1
defined, 172
Dietary Guidelines, 69
during digestion, 172
eggs and, 190
enterohepatic circulation, 178, 178f
fat replacers, 192
fiber and, 154–155, 193–194
on food label, 180, 180f
gallstones and, 115
health claims and, 80
healthy/unhealthy levels of, 187–188, 187t
high-density lipoprotein (HDL), 183–184
interesterified oil and, 169
low-carbohydrate diets, 406
low-density lipoprotein (LDL), 183
nutrient content claims, 82t
reducing by food selection and preparation, 191–192, 194t
statins, 194
sterols/stanols reducing absorption of, 172
structure of, 172f
trans fat and, 168–169
very-low-density lipoproteins (VLDL), 184
Choline, 7t, 171, 259t, 297
    body's need for, 258
    function of, 260f
    summary of, 282t
    supplements, 172
Chondroitin, 52t
Choose MyPlate, 14
Chromium, 358–359, 448t
    AI, 359
    Daily Value, A1
    deficiency, 359
    dietary adequacy, 359
    as essential nutrient, 7t, 100t
    food sources of, 348
    function of, 325f, 358
    insulin and, 358
    summary of, 346t
    toxicity, 359
Chromium picolinate, 407t
Chronic diseases, 9
Chylomicron, 117, 175, 177f, 183f
Chyme, 113, 114
Chymotrypsin, protein digestion, 222, 223f
Cigarette smoking
    beta-carotene and, 300, 301
    cardiovascular disease and, 186

Cigarette smoking *(continued)*
  coronary calcium, 188
  oxidation of LDL and, 184
  during pregnancy, 501
  as risk factor, 9
  vitamin C and, 296
Circulatory changes, in aging, 523t
Cirrhosis, 202
Citric acid cycle, A3
Clinical dietitians, 49
Cloning, 85
Clostridium botulinum, 464t
  home-canned foods and, 475
  honey and, 133
Clostridium perfringens, 464t
Cobalamin, 259t
Cobalamine, 259t
Cobalt, as essential element, 100t
Coenzyme, 281, 281f
Coenzyme Q10, 52t
Cofactor, 325
Cognitive behavioral therapy, 416
Cohort study, 38
Cold, common
  chicken soup and, 57
  vitamin C and, 298–299
Collagen, 215, 295
Colon. *See* Intestine, large
Color additives, 478, 479t
Colorectal cancer, 304
Colostrum, 503
Commodity Distribution
    Program, 22t
Community nutritionists, 49
Complementary and alternative
    medicine (CAM), 51
Complementary combinations,
    230–231
Complete protein, 219
Complex carbohydrates, 136–137
  fiber and, 136, 136f, 136t,
    153–155
  starch and glycogen, 136, 136f
Compounds, 100
Computerized tomography (CT)
    scans, coronary calcium and,
    188
Conception, 494, 494f
Cones, 268
Congeners, 322–323
Conjugated linoleic acid, 407t
Connective tissue, 106
Constipation, 153
  causes and treatment for, 120
  older adults and, 526
  during pregnancy, 497
Contaminated food, 460
Control group, 34, 35
Conversions, A0
Cooking methods. *See* Food
    preparation
Copper
  Daily Value, A1
  as essential nutrient, 7t, 100t

function of, 325f
  summary of, 346t
Corn syrup, 131, 132t
Coronary artery disease (CAD)
  defined, 181
  eggs and, 190
Coronary calcium, 188
Correlation
  defined, 39
  direct/inverse, 39
  negative/positive, 39
Cortisol, vitamin C and, 295
Country of origin, 76
Cravings, during pregnancy, 499
C-reactive protein, 188
Creatine, 433, 433f, 448t
Creatinine, 224
Cretinism, 356
Crohn's disease, 118
Cross-contamination, 460, 472
Cryptosporidium, 465, 466t
Cultural food traditions, 74
Cyclamate, 134
Cysteine, 217t, 219, A5
Cystic fibrosis
  digestion and, 117
  overview of, 117
  vitamin absorption and, 263
  vitamin K deficiency and, 280
Cytochromes, 347
Cytoplasm, 105, 105f

D

Daily Values (DVs)
  carbohydrate, 78
  compared to RDAs, 78
  defined, 78
  development of, 64
  fat, 79
  percents of, 79
  Table, A1
Dairy foods. *See also* Milk
  as calcium source, 330
  fat content, 66
  food allergy and, 239
  fortification, 262
  as high-risk foods, 461, 461t
  lactose intolerance, 152
  as major food group, 65–66
  micronutrients in, 66
  as MyPlate food group, 71, 71f
  reducing dietary fat and, 192
  riboflavin and, 284
  serving size, 66
  storage tips, 472, 472t
Deamination, 224, 224f
Deci, 12
Decomposition reaction,
    digestion as, 103
Deficiency and deficiency
    diseases, 263
  anemia, 349
  beriberi, 283, 284f
  calcium, 332–335

chromium, 359
  defined, 6
  essential fatty acid, 167–168
  folate, 288–289
  historical perspective on, 36
  iodine, 356
  iron, 349
  magnesium, 343
  neural tube defects, 290
  niacin, 285–286, 286f
  osteomalacia, 276
  osteoporosis, 332–335
  pellagra, 286, 286f
  pernicious anemia, 293
  physiological dose, 16
  populations at risk for, 263
  protein, 236–237, 237f
  rickets, 272, 272f, 276
  scurvy, 257
  selenium, 357
  sodium, 335
  thiamin, 284
  vitamin A, 270–271
  vitamin B-12, 293
  vitamin D, 276
  vitamin E, 278
  vitamin K, 280
  Wernicke-Korsakoff syndrome,
    284
  xerophthalmia (dry eye), 271
  zinc, 352
Dehydration, 323
  alcohol, 323
  athletes and, 443–445
  avoiding, 321–322
  defined, 315
  diarrhea and, 121, 485
  high-protein diet, 235
  rapid weight loss and, 315
  vomiting and, 121
  weight loss and, 323
Delaney Clause, 480
Denaturation, 222, 222f
Dental caries
  baby bottle caries, 511
  in preschool children, 514
Dental fluorosis, 357, 357f
Depression, older adults, 527
Dextrin, 136
Dextrose, 131
DHE and androstenedione,
    448t
Diabetes mellitus (diabetes),
    64, 146
  adult-onset, 146
  body fat and, 148, 386, 387
  cardiovascular disease
    and, 186
  chromium and, 358
  controlling, 149
  counting carbohydrates, 76
  deaths per year from, 147
  Exchange System, 75–76
  gestational, 500

glycemic index, 149, 157
  incidence of, 146–147, 146f
  juvenile, 146
  metabolic syndrome, 151
  physical activity and, 149
  pre-diabetes, 146
  preventing, 149–150
  race/ethnicity and, 37
  real story of, 155
  risk factors for, 9, 147
  signs and symptoms,
    146, 147f
  type 1, 146, 147–148
  type 2, 3, 146, 148–149
Diabulimia, 414
Diarrhea, causes and treatment
    for, 120–121
Diastolic pressure, 337
Diet
  changes in American, 9
  defined, 3
  preventable deaths and, 3–4
Diet, weight loss
  fad, 404–405
  low-carbohydrate, 144,
    405–406, 405t
  very-low-calorie and
    metabolism, 380
Dietary analysis software, 85–86
Dietary Approaches to
    Stop Hypertension (DASH),
    339
Dietary fiber. *See* Fiber
*Dietary Guidelines for Americans
    2005,* 71
*2015–2020 Dietary Guidelines for
    Americans,* 67–70
  applying to usual food
    choices, 70t
  fats, 68–69, 189
  focus on variety, nutrient
    density, and amounts of
    foods, 68
  follow a healthy eating
    pattern, 68
  key recommendations of, 68t
  limit calories from added
    sugars and saturated fats
    and reduce sodium
    intake, 69
  MyPlate based on, 71
  overarching guidelines, 68t
  physical activity, 68–69, 426
  recommendations for specific
    population groups, 69
  selected messages for
    consumers, 69t
  shift to healthier food and
    beverage choices, 69
  support healthy eating patterns
    for all, 69
  sodium, 68–69, 338
  weight management, 68–69

Dietary guides
 Asian Diet Pyramid, 88–89, 89f
 Exchange System, 75–76
 Food Guide Pyramid, 71
 historical perspective, 71
 Mediterranean Diet Pyramid,
   88, 88f
 MyPlate, 71–72
 MyPyramid Plan, 71
Dietary Reference Intakes (DRIs),
   62–64, 62f, 64t
 Adequate Intakes (AIs), 63
 applying, 64
 defined, 62
 Estimated Average
   Requirement (EAR), 62
 Estimated Energy Requirement
   (EER), 62–63
 pregnancy, 497t
 purpose of, 62
 Recommended Dietary
   Allowances (RDAs), 62–63
 Tolerable Upper Intake Level
   (UL), 63
Dietary Supplement and Health
   Education Act of 1994
   (DSHEA), 7, 50
Dietary supplements. See also
   Vitamin supplements
 defined, 7, 50
 disadvantages of using, 18
 health claims, 82–83
 labeling, 51, 82–83, 83f
 as mineral source, 327
 older adults and prescription
   drugs, 526–527
 pseudoscience, 44
 regulation of, 51, 54
 Supplement Facts label, 82–83,
   83f
 tips for using wisely, 54
 use of, by Americans, 50–51
Dietitian. See Registered
   dietitian (R.D.)
Diffusion, 317–318, 317f
Digestion
 bioavailability, 111
 carbohydrates, 139–140, 139f
 chemical digestion, 112
 as decomposition reaction, 103
 esophagus, 112–113
 large intestines, 117–118
 lipids, 174–179
 liver, pancreas, gallbladder, 115
 mechanical digestion, 111
 mouth, 111–112
 of protein, 222–223, 223f
 small intestines, 114, 116f
 stomach, 113–114
Digestion problems
 constipation, 120
 Crohn's disease, 118
 cystic fibrosis, 117
 diarrhea, 120–121

heartburn, 121
inflammatory bowel disease, 118
irritable bowel syndrome, 123
older adults and, 526
peptic ulcer, 122
during pregnancy, 497
vomiting, 121
Digestive system
 absorbing nutrients, 116–117
 adaptability of, 118
 esophagus, 111f, 112–113, 113f
 gastrointestinal (GI) tract,
   111–119, 111f
 large intestines, 111f, 117–118
 liver, pancreas and gallbladder,
   111f, 115
 microbes in, 118
 mouth, 111–112, 111f, 113f
 normal aging changes, 523t
 overview of, 107t, 111, 111f
 small intestines, 111f, 114,
   114f, 116f
 stomach, 111f, 113–114, 114f
Digestive tract. See
   Gastrointestinal (GI) tract
Direct additives, 478, 479t
Disaccharides, 130
 lactose, 131
 maltose, 131
 sucrose, 131
Disaster preparation, 476–478
Disclaimers, label, 47, 47f
Disordered eating, 410
Dispensable amino acids, 217
Diuretics
 alcohol, 322–323
 caffeine, 322
 defined, 322
Diverticula, 120, 153, 154f
Diverticulitis, 120, 154, 154f
DNA, 221f
 defined, 105, 220
 genetic defects, 221, 222
 protein synthesis, 220–222, 221f
Docosahexaenoic acid (DHA), 167,
   168f, 504
Double-blind studies, 37
DRI. See Dietary Reference Intakes
   (DRIs)
Drug interaction, alcohol
   consumption and, 202
Drugs
 pregnancy and, 501
 for weight loss, 401
Dual-energy X-ray absorptiometry
   (DXA), 375, 37ç5f
Duodenum, 114

E
E. coli (Escherichia coli), 464t
 cooking temperature, 469
 irradiation, 476
Eating cues, 396

Eating disorders, 410–416
 anorexia nervosa, 412
 binge-eating disorder, 413
 bulimia nervosa, 412–413
 defined, 410
 female athlete triad, 414
 incidence of, 410, 412
 major types of, 410
 night eating syndrome,
   413–414
 preventing, 415
 risk factors for, 410–411, 411t
 treating, 415
Eating habits
 changes in American diet, 9
 weight loss and behavior
   modification, 396
Eating Healthy with Diabetes, 76
Echinacea
 claims/benefits/risks, 52t
 scientific testing of, 50
Eclampsia, 501
Edema, 319
 blood pressure and blood
   proteins, 216, 216f
 defined, 216
 intracellular water and, 319
 kwashiorkor, 237, 237f
 during pregnancy, 497
Eggs, 190, 219
 primary pathogens, 461t
Eicosapentaenoic acid (EPA), 167,
   168f
Elderly. See Older adults
Elderly Nutrition Program, 22t
Electrolytes, 318
 defined, 101
 sports drinks, 441, 444–445
Electrons, 99f
 antioxidants, 259, 260, 261f
 defined, 99
 ions, 100–101
 radicals, 259, 261f
Electron transfer, A4
Element, 100t
Elements, 99
Ellagic acid, sources/biological
   effect of, 8t
Elvehjem, Conrad, 36
Embolus, 182, 182f
Embryo, 494, 494f
Emergency food supply,
   476–478
Empty-calorie foods, 15
 characteristics of, 67
 as food group, 67
 fortification of, 262
 MyPlate and, 71, 72, 142
 in personal dietary plans, 142
Emulsifiers, 171, 479t
Endocrine system
 normal aging changes, 523t
 overview of, 107t, 109, 109f
Endogenous source, 223

Energy
 defined, 377
 energy metabolism, 429–432
Energy balance
 concept of, 383–385, 384f–385f
 energy intake, 377
 energy output, 378
Energy bars, 442, 442f, 443t
Energy dense foods, 15
Energy drinks, 143, 442–443, 447
Energy equilibrium, 383–385,
   384f–385f
Energy intake. See also Calories
 adenosine triphosphate, 377
 defined, 377
 environmental influences,
   391–392
 physiological factors, 388–391
Energy metabolism, A2–A4, A6
Energy output, 378
 basal and resting metabolism,
   378–380
 defined, 378
 estimating energy requirement,
   384
 factors influencing metabolic
   rate, 379–380
 nonexercise activity
   thermogenesis, 382
 for physical activity, 381–382,
   381t
 thermic effect of food, 381
 thyroid hormone and, 378–379
Enrichment, defined, 65, 262
Enterohepatic circulation, 178, 178f
Environmental influences
 obesity and overweight,
   391–392
 weight loss and behavior
   modification, 396–399
Environmental Protection Agency
   (EPA)
 pesticides, 481
 regulation of tap water,
   361–362, 459
 role in food safety, 458
Enzymes
 characteristic and function of,
   103–104, 104f
 defined, 103, 216
 function of, 216
 pancreas, 115
 protein digestion, 222, 223f
 in saliva, 112
Ephedra, 406, 407t, 447
Ephedrine, 407t, 447
Epidemiological studies, 37–40
 analyzing data, drawing
   conclusions, reporting
   findings, 40–42
 case-control study, 38
 cohort study, 38
 confusing and conflicting
   findings, 42

Epidemiological studies,
    (continued)
  defined, 37
  designing, 40–41
  developing hypothesis, 40
  double-blind studies, 37
  experimental (intervention),
      35–36
  federal guidelines for human
      research, 41
  follow-up research, 42
  limitations of, 39–40
  observational studies, 38
  physical examination to obtain
      health information, 37–38
  placebo effect, 37
  prospective study, 38
  research bias, 41
  results in media, 41–42
  retrospective study, 38
  review of scientific literature,
      40
Epiglottis, 112, 113f
Epinephrine, hypoglycemia, 150
Epithelial cells, vitamin A and,
    267–268, 267f, 270
Epithelial tissue, 106
Equal, 134
Ergogenic aids, 446–449
  caffeine as, 447, 448t
  evaluation of popular, 448t
Esophagus
  gastroesophageal reflux
      disease, 121
  peristalsis, 112, 113f
  structure and function of, 111f,
      112–113, 113f, 114f
Essential amino acids, 217, 217t
  complete proteins, 219
  incomplete proteins, 219
Essential fatty acids
  alpha-linolenic acid, 167, 168f
  deficiency, 167–168
  linoleic acid, 167–168, 168f
  omega-3 fatty acid, 167, 168f
  omega-6 fatty acid, 167, 168f
Essential nutrients, 6
  deficiency disease, 6
  defined, 6
  key features of, 6
Estimated Average Requirement
    (EAR), 64t
  applying, 64
  defined, 62
  establishing, 62
  protein, 225
Estimated Energy Requirement
    (EER)
  calculating, 384
  defined, 62
  pregnancy, 498
Estrogen, osteoporosis and, 333
Ethanol, 195, 195f

Ethnic food traditions, 74
Ethnic and ancestral influences
    on diet
  African influences, 88
  Asian influences, 88–89
  Hispanic influences, 87–88
  Italian influences, 88
  Jewish influences, 90–91
  Native American influences,
      89–90
  Northwestern European
      influences, 87
  religious influences, 90, 90t
Evening primrose oil, 52t
Evidence based information, 33
Exchange System, 75–76
Exercise. See also Physical activity
  aerobic, 429
  benefits of regular, 426, 427f
  CVD and, 191
  defined, 425
  determining intensity level of
      physical activity, 426–428
  diabetes and, 149
  energy from ATP, 431, 431f
  energy metabolism for ATP
      formation, 429–432, 431f,
      431ff
  fat vs. carbohydrates for
      fueling, 436
  lactic acid energy system,
      433–434, 434f
  metabolic syndrome, 152
  osteoporosis and weight-
      bearing, 334
  oxygen energy system, 434–436
  PCr-ATP energy system,
      432–433, 433f
  physical activity pyramid,
      428–429, 428f
Exogenous source, 223
Experimental group, 38
Experimental (intervention)
    studies, 35
External anal sphincter, 117, 117f
Extracellular water, 318–319, 319f
Extra lean, legal definition, 82t
Extrusion reflex, 509

F

Fad diets, 404–405
  low-carbohydrate diet,
      405–406, 405t
  very-low-fat, 405t, 406
Farming. See Agriculture
Fat, body
  adipose cells, 373
  body composition of, 5f
  brown fat, 374
  cancer and, 304–305
  central-body obesity, 387–388
  consumption patterns of
      carbohydrates, 145

CVD and, 191–192
  diabetes and, 149
  distribution of, and effect on
      health, 387–388
  essential fat, 373
  fat-free mass, 372
  leptin and food intake, 389,
      390f
  liposuction, 403–404, 404f
  measuring, 374–375
  metabolic syndrome, 151–152
  as modifiable risk for
      cardiovascular disease, 186
  older adults, 525
  pear shape, 387, 387f
  subcutaneous fat, 373–374, 373f
  total body fat, 372
  upper-body obesity, 387f
  visceral, 374, 374f
  weight classifications based on,
      376, 377t
Fat, dietary, 165–208
  AMDR for, 64t
  ATP formation, 431, 431f
  average American intake of,
      142f
  benefits of, 165
  breast milk, 504, 508
  butter vs. margarine, 190–191
  cholesterol, 172
  Daily Value, A1
  Daily Values, 79
  dairy foods, 66
  dietary advice for athletes, 438
  dietary changes to reduce risk
      of atherosclerosis,
      188–194, 194t
  Dietary Guidelines, 68–69
  digestion of, 174–179
  Exchange System, 75
  fat compared to carbohydrate
      consumption, 145
  fat replacers, 192
  fats vs. oils, 167
  fatty acids, 166–169
  fatty acids, essential, 166–167
  food label, 180, 180f
  for fueling exercise, 436
  functions of, 165, 165t
  health claims and, 80
  increase in fat consumption,
      179
  insulin and metabolism, 141
  kcal in gram of, 12
  lipoproteins, 175–178
  as macronutrient, 12
  meats, 66
  monounsaturated fatty acids,
      166
  as nutrient, 5
  nutrient content claims, 82t
  Nutrition Facts panel, 180, 180f
  obesity and, 145

oils, 67
  phospholipids, 171–172
  polyunsaturated fatty acids, 167
  protein-rich food, 66
  recommended amount of, 179
  reducing by food selection and
      preparation, 191–192, 194t
  saturated fatty acids, 166–167
  solid fats, 67
  trans fats, 168–169
  triglycerides, 169–171, 178–179
  unsaturated fatty acids, 166
  very-low-fat diet, 405t, 406
  vitamin absorption, 262
Fat free, legal definition, 82t
Fat-free mass, 372
Fatigue, during pregnancy,
    496–497
Fat measurement, body
  air displacement, 375, 375f
  bioelectrical impedence, 376,
      376f
  dual-energy X-ray
      absorptiometry (DXA),
      375, 375f
  skinfold thickness, 376, 376f
Fat replacers, 192
Fat-soluble vitamins
  classifying vitamins, 259t
  classifying vitamins as, 259
  defined, 259
  MyPlate, 267f
  summary of, 266t
  toxicity and, 259
  vitamin A, 266–272
  vitamin D, 272–275
  vitamin E, 277–278
  vitamin K, 278–280
Fatty acids, 141, 166–169. See also
    Fatty acids, essential
  monounsaturated, 166
  omega end, 165, 166, 167f
  percentage of saturated in
      common fats/oils, 170f
  polyunsaturated, 166
  saturated, 166–167
  structure of, 167f
  trans fats, 168, 169
  unsaturated, 166
Fatty acids, essential, 166–167
  alpha-linolenic acid, 167, 168f
  linoleic acid, 167–168, 168f
  omega-3 fatty acid, 167, 168f
  omega-6 fatty acid, 167, 168f
Fatty liver, 202
Feces
  bacteria in, 118
  contents of, 117
Federal Food, Drug, and Cosmetic
    Act, 480
Federal Trade Commission (FTC)
  consumer protection on
      Internet, 47–48

role in food safety, 458
weight-loss supplements,
    407–408
Female athlete triad, 414, 446
Fermentation, 474
Fertility, vitamin A and, 268
Fetal alcohol syndrome (FAS),
    203, 203f, 501
Fetus, 494, 494f
Fiber, 136, 153–155
    Adequate Intakes for, 155
    average American consumption
        of, 140
    bowel movements and, 120
    cholesterol and, 154–155,
        193–194
    colorectal cancer and, 154
    Daily Value, A1
    defined, 136
    dietary advice for athletes, 439
    digestive tract and, 153–154
    fiber content of common
        foods, 138t
    fruits, 66
    heart health and, 154–155
    increasing, 155
    insoluble, 136, 137t
    metabolic syndrome, 152
    nutrient content claims, 82t
    nutritional value, 140
    Nutrition Facts panel, 144, 144f
    pregnancy, 497
    recommended intake for, 155
    satiety and, 155
    soluble, 136, 137t
    structure/function claim, 81, 82t
    viscous, 140
    weight control/loss, 155
Fibrin, 279
Fibrinogen, alcohol consumption,
    203
Fish
    Dietary Guidelines, 69
    as high-risk foods, 461t
    mercury in, 498–499
    omega-3 fatty acids, 189, 190,
        227
    pregnancy and, 69, 190, 498–499
    preventing food-borne illness,
        470–471
    reducing risk of CVD, 189
    as source of Vitamin D, 274,
        274t
    storage tips, 472, 472t
Fish oil supplements, 50, 52t, 190
Fitness plan, developing personal,
    449–451
    components of workout,
        450–451
    goals for, 449
    improvement and
        maintenance, 450
    initiation, 450

mixing it up, 451
    strength training, 451
Flavored drinks, 262
Flaxseed oil, 50, 52t
Flexibility exercise, in physical
    activity pyramid, 428–429,
    428f
Flies, 460, 460f
Flu, 462
Fluids
    dietary advice for athletes,
        443–445
    intake of, and breastfeeding,
        506
Fluoride, 356–357
    as essential element, 100t
    function of, 325f
    summary of, 346t
    in water, 327
Fluorosis, 357, 357f
Folate (folic acid), 259t, 287–290
    Alzheimer's disease, 298
    anemia, 289
    biological activity, 261
    CVD and, 298
    Daily Value, A1
    deficiency, 289–290
    defined, 287
    dietary adequacy, 288
    Dietary Guidelines, 69
    energy metabolism, A6
    enrichment, 262
    as essential nutrient, 7t
    food preparation and
        destruction of, 288
    food sources of, 287–288, 288t
    fruits, 66
    function of, 260f, 287
    health claim, 81t
    homocysteine and, 185
    neural tube defects, 290, 290f
    pregnancy and, 69, 290, 498
    RDA, 288
    red blood cell production,
        288–289, 289f
    summary of, 282t
    tetrahydrofolic acid
        (THFA), 287
    UL, 289
    vitamin B-12 and, 287, 288f, 289
    vitamin supplements, 298
Food additives. See Additives
Food Additives Amendment, 479
Food Allergen Labeling and
    Consumer Protection Act,
    239, 239f
Food allergy, 238–239
    anaphylaxis, 239
    food labels, 239, 239f
    genetics and, 239
    incidence of, 239
    mechanism of, 239
    most allergic foods, 239

signs and symptoms of, 239
    testing for, 239
    treatment for, 239
Food and Drug Administration
    (FDA)
    Daily Values (DVs), 64
    Delaney Clause, 480
    dietary supplement labels,
        82–83
    food additive safety, 479–480
    genetically engineered food
        and, 23
    health claims, 80
    irradiated food, 476
    label disclaimers, 47f
    Make Your Calories Count, 79
    nutrient content claims,
        81–82, 82t
    nutrition-and health-related
        claims on labels, 43
    regulation of bottled water, 362
    regulation of supplements,
        51, 54
    role in food safety, 458–459
    structure/function claims,
        81, 81f
    Supplement Facts label,
        82–83, ≈83f
    unintentional food additives,
        480
    website, 48t
Food and Nutrition Board (FNB),
    developing DRIs, 62
Food assistance programs, 21
Food-borne illnesses, 457
    defined, 457
    incidence of, 457–458
    incubation period, 462
    pathogens, 463–465
    preventing, 468–473
    signs and symptoms of, 462
Food-borne infections, 457
Food-cobalamin malabsorption,
    291
Food Distribution Program on
    Indian Reservations, 22t
Food dollars, stretching, 228–231,
    245–248
Food groups, major
    dairy foods, 65–66
    Dietary Guidelines, 68
    fruits, 66
    grains, 65
    oils, 67
    protein-rich foods, 66
    vegetables, 66
Food guidance system, 71
Food Guide Pyramid, 71
Food insecurity, 21
Food intoxication, 457
Food jags, in preschool children,
    513
Food labels

carbohydrates and fiber,
    143–144, 144f
country of origin, 76
Daily Values, 79
dietary supplements and, 51
disclaimers, 47–48, 47f
fat, 180, 180f
FDA and nutrition-and health-
    related claims on labels,
    43, 76–78
food allergies, 239, 239f
health claims, 80
ingredients listed on, 76–78,
    77f
light or lite food, 82
nutrient content claims, 81–82,
    82t
Nutrition Facts panel,
    76–78, 77f
organic, 85, 85f
% Daily Value, 79
protein content, 228, 228f
serving size, 79
structure/function claims, 81,
    81f
whole grains, 136, 137f
Food preparation and safety
    ground meats, poultry and fish,
        470–471
    hand washing, 468, 468f
    home-canned foods, 475
    maintaining proper
        temperature, 469–470
    preserving vitamin content in
        food, 264–265, 265f
    raw fish, 470
    to reduce dietary fat, 191–192,
        194t
    storing and reheating food,
        472–473
    summary of tips for, 467–469
    surfaces for, 468
Food preservation
    aseptic processing, 474
    fermentation, 474
    home-canned foods, 475
    irradiation, 476
    sterilization, 474
    summary of methods
        for, 475t
Food processing, nutrients and,
    17
Food Quality Protection
    Act, 480
Foods, energy and macronutrient
    contents of selected, 440t
Food safety, 457–488. See also
    Food-borne illnesses; Food
    preparation and safety
    alternative sweeteners,
        133–135
    benzene, 480
    federal agencies for, 458–459

Food safety, (continued)
  food additives, 479
  food preservation, 474–476
  hand washing, 460, 461f
  legislation, 479–480
  microbes in, 457, 459–460
  pesticides, 481–482
  preparing for disasters,
    476–478
  unintentional food additives,
    480
Food Safety and Inspection
  Service (FSIS), 458
Food storage, 472–473
Food waste, reducing, 24
Formula, infant. See Infant
  formula
Fortification, defined, 65, 262
Framingham Study, 38
Freezers/freezing
  preserving vitamin content in
    food, 265f
  storing food tips, 471–473, 472t
Freshman 15, 384
Fructooligosaccharides, sources/
  biological effect of, 8t
Fructose, 131f
  characteristics and sources
    of, 131
  high-fructose corn syrup, 130
  obesity and, 389
Fruitarian diet, 232t
Fruits
  American consumption of, 10
  cancer prevention and, 305
  Dietary Guidelines, 68–69
  eating to reduce refined sugar
    in diet, 142, 143
  fiber content in some, 138t
  as food group in MyPlate, 71, 71f
  fruit juice compared to soft
    drink, 142
  health claim, 81t
  hypertension, 40
  juice, 66
  as major food group, 66
  micronutrients in, 66
  preserving vitamin content in,
    264–265
  protein content, 230–231
  serving size, 66
  as vitamin C source, 295, 295f,
    296t
Functional foods, 18, 172
Fungi, as food-borne illness
  pathogen, 465
Fungicides, 481
Funk, Casimir, 257

G
Galactose, 131, 131f
Gallbladder, function in GI tract,
  111f, 115, 115f

Gallstones, 115, 115f
Gamma hydroxybutyric acid,
  448t
Garcinia cambogia, 407t
Gastroesophageal sphincter,
  113, 114f
Gastric banding procedure, 402
Gastric bypass surgery, 402, 403f
Gastric juice, 113
Gastroesophageal reflux disease,
  121–122
Gastrointestinal (GI) problems
  constipation, 120
  Crohn's disease, 118
  cystic fibrosis, 117
  diarrhea, 120–121
  heartburn, 121–122
  inflammatory bowel
    disease, 118
  irritable bowel syndrome, 123
  peptic ulcer, 122
  vomiting, 121
Gastrointestinal (GI) tract
  absorbing nutrients, 116–117
  adaptability of, 118
  alcohol's effect on, 200–201
  bioavailability, 111
  esophagus, 111f, 112–113, 113f
  fiber and, 153–154
  large intestines, 111f, 117–118
  liver, pancreas and gallbladder,
    111f, 115
  maintaining blood glucose
    level, 140–141, 140f
  microbes in, 118
  mouth, 111f, 113f
  organs of mouth, 111–112
  peristalsis, 113, 113f
  small intestines, 111f, 114,
    114f, 116f
  stomach, 111f, 113–114, 114f
  swallowing, 112–113
  tract, 111–119, 111f
Gastrointestinal ulcers, 113
Gelatin, 104
Gender differences
  alcohol metabolism, 197
  body composition, 5f, 317
  hereditary hemochromatosis,
    351
  iron intake, 347, 349
  metabolism, 379
  risk factor for cardiovascular
    disease, 185
  subcutaneous fat, 373f, 374
Generally Recognized as Safe
  (GRAS), 479
Genes, defined, 221
Genetically modified organisms
  (GMOs), concerns over, 23
Genetic disorders, PKU, 242
Genetic endowment, 437
Genetic expression, 242

Genetic factors
  atherosclerosis and cardiovascular
    disease, 185, 185t
  food allergy, 239
  obesity and overweight,
    389–391, 391f
Genetic modification, 22
Genetic obesity, 389–391, 391f
Genetic susceptibility, 38
Genetic testing kits, 244
Gestational diabetes, 148, 387,
  500
Ghee, 188
Ghrelin, 389, 390f, 402
Giardia, 465, 466f, 466t, 483
Gimmick diets, 405t
Ginger, 52t
Gingko biloba, 52t
Ginseng, 448t
  claims/benefits/risks, 53t
  in energy drinks, 443
GI tract. See Gastrointestinal (GI)
  tract
Glucagon, 215
Glucomannan, 407t
Glucosamine, 50, 53t, 448t
Glucose, 131f
  ATP formation, 431, 431f
  defined, 130
  for energy, 141
  as essential nutrient, 7t
  for fueling exercise, 436
  in glycogen, 136
  maintaining blood glucose,
    140–141, 140f
  as monosaccharride, 130
  stored as fat, 141
  stored in starch, 136
Glutamic acid, 217t, A5
Glutamine, 217t, A5
Gluten-free diet, 240, 240t
Glycated hemoglobin, 149
Glycemic index
  chronic diseases and, 157
  of common foods, 157t
  controlling diabetes and, 149
  criticism of, 157
  defined, 156
  weight control, 149
Glycemic load, 149
  of common foods, 157t
  defined, 156
Glycerol, 141
Glycine, 217t, A5
Glycogen, 136f
  carbohydrate loading, 439–441
  carbohydrates during event, 441
  characteristics and sources of,
    136
  dietary advice for athletes, 438
  maintaining blood glucose
    levels, 140–141
Glycogenolysis, 141

Glycolysis, 430, A2
Glycosides, sources/biological
  effect of, 8t
Goiters, 354, 354f
Goitrogens, 356
Goldberger, Joseph, 36
Good source of fiber, legal
  definition, 82t
Grains
  complamentary combinations,
    230t
  complementary combinations,
    230–231
  Dietary Guidelines, 68
  enrichment, 65, 262
  folate enriched, 288
  as food group in MyPlate, 71,
    71f
  fortification, 65
  as iron source, 347, 348t
  as major food group, 65
  micronutrients in, 65
  minerals and, 326
  protein consumption patterns,
    226–227, 227f
  riboflavin enriched, 284
  serving size, 65
  thiamin source, 281
  whole grains, 66, 136
Gram, 11
Green tea, 53t, 407t
Grocery shopping, 228–231,
  245–248
Guar gum, 407t
Guava, 295
Gums, 136, 137t

H
H. pylori, 122
Hair, 110
Hand washing, 460, 461f, 468,
  468f
Hazard Analysis and Critical
  Control Point (HACCP), 458
HDL (high-density lipoprotein)
  alcohol and raising, 193
  alcohol consumption, 203
  atherosclerosis and,
    183–184
  cholesterol, 184f
  defined, 183
  dietary changes to reduce
    risk of atherosclerosis,
    188–189
  healthy/unhealthy levels of,
    187–188, 187t
  metabolic syndrome, 151t
  percentages of lipid and
    protein, 183f
  role of, 183–184, 184f
Health claims
  on dietary supplement labels,
    82–83

on food labels, 80
weight-loss supplements, 407–408
Health on the Net symbol, 48t
Healthy Canada, 74
Healthy People 2020
  declining obesity goals of, 372
  objectives of, 10–11, 11t
Heart, structure and function of, 106f, 107
Heart attack, 182. *See also* Cardiovascular disease (CVD)
Heartburn
  causes and treatment for, 121
  defined, 113
  gastroesophageal reflux disease, 121–122
  during pregnancy, 497
  recommendations to reduce risk of, 122t
Heart disease. *See also* Cardiovascular disease (CVD)
  diet and chances of developing, 3
  health claim, 81t
  as leading cause of death in U.S., 4f, 9
  risk factors for, 9
Heart rate
  age-related maximum heart rate, 426–427
  radial artery, 428, 428f
  target heart rate zone, 426–427
Heat cramps, 443, 444t
Heat exhaustion, 443, 444t
Heat-related illness, 443
Heatstroke, 443, 444
Heme iron, 347
Hemicellulose, 136, 137t
Hemoglobin, 222, 222f
  defined, 347
  function of, 107
  monitoring diabetes and, 149
  Sickle cell anemia, 222, 223f
  vitamin B-6 and, 286
Hemoglobin A1c, 149
Hemorrhoids, 120, 154, 154f
Hepatic portal vein, 117
Hepatitis A, 463, 465t
Herbicides, 481
Hereditary hemochromatosis, 351
Hesperitin, sources/biological effect of, 8t
Heterocyclic amines, 304
HFCS (high fructose corn syrup), 130, 132, 132t
  obesity and, 145
  soft drinks and, 142
H⁺ (hydrogen ion), 101
High-birth-weight (HBW) infants, 495, 499
High blood pressure. *See* Hypertension

High-density lipoprotein cholesterol. *See* HDL (high-density lipoprotein)
High fiber, legal definition, 82t
High-fructose corn syrup, 130
High-protein bar, 442, 442f, 443t
High-protein diet, 236
High-quality protein, 219
High-sensitivity C-reactive protein (hs-CRP), 188
Hispanic influences on diet, 87–88
Histidine, 7t, 217t, A5
Home-canned foods, 475
Home-Delivered Meals, 22t
Homeostasis, 106
Homocysteine, 185, 286, 286f, 298
HONcode, 48t
Honey
  children and, 133
  compared to sugar, 131, 132t
  infants and, 510
  nutritional comparison of sweeteners, 132t
Hoodia, 407t
Hormones
  blood glucose levels and, 140–141
  defined, 109, 215–216
  in food, 99
  function of, 109, 215–216
  nitrogen balance and, 225
Household measurement units, 27
Human chorionic gonadotropin (hCG), 407t
Human growth hormone, 225, 448t
Human research. *See* Epidemiological studies
Hunger
  defined, 388
  ghrelin, 389, 390f
  hypothalamus and, 389, 390f
  taking action against, 24
Hydration
  defined, 318
  kidneys and, 321, 322f
  maintaining proper, 319f
Hydrocarbon, 167f
Hydrocarbon chain, 166, 167f
Hydrochloric acid
  sodium chloride formation, 103
  in stomach, 113
Hydrogen, as essential element, 100t
Hydrogenation, 169
Hydrogen ion, 101
Hydrolytic chemical reactions, 114
Hydrophilic, 171
Hydrophobic, 171
Hyperactivity, sugar and, 153
Hypercalcemia, 332
Hyperglycemia, 146

Hypertension, 336–340
  alcohol, 338
  arteriosclerosis, 183
  defined, 183, 336
  fruit, 40
  incidence of, 336
  lowering sodium intake, 338
  as modifiable risk for cardiovascular disease, 186
  obesity and, 338
  pregnancy-induced hypertension (PIH), 501
  prehypertension, 337
  real story of, 340
  reducing risk of, 339t
  risk factors for, 9, 338, 339t
Hyperthermia, 315
Hyperthyroidism, 378–379
Hypoglycemia, 150–151
Hyponatremia, 444
Hypothalamus, hunger and satiety, 389, 390f
Hypothesis
  defined, 33
  developing, in human experimentation, 40
Hypothyroidism, 378–379

I

Ileum, 114
Immune system
  food allergy, 238–239
  infants and breast feeding, 503
  normal aging changes, 523t
  vitamin A and, 268
Incomplete protein, 219
Indispensable amino acids, 217
Indoles, sources/biological effect of, 8t
Infant formula, 503, 507–508, 508t
  allergies and, 508
  baby bottle caries, 511
  undernutrition and, 20–21
  weaning, 509–510
Infants, 503–512. *See also* Breastfeeding
  allergies, 509
  baby bottle caries, 511
  cow's milk, 508–509
  high-birth-weight (HBW), 495
  infant formula, 503, 508, 508t
  introducing solid foods, 509–510
  iron deficiency anemia, 350
  monitoring growth of, 512
  nitrogen balance, 225, 225f
  nutrition for, 503–512
  premature infants and vitamin E, 278
  sudden infant death syndrome (SIDS), 502, 503
  undernutrition during, 20–21
  Vitamin D and exposure to sunlight, 506, 506f

vitamin K and, 280
  weaning, 509–510
  what not to feed, 510–511
Inflammation, 182
  atherosclerosis and, 182
  high-sensitivity C-reactive protein (hs-CRP), 188
  omega-6 and omega-3 fatty acids, 189–190
Inflammatory bowel disease (IBD)
  overview of, 118
  real story of, 119
  underweight and, 409
Influenza, 462
Insecticides, 481
Insensible perspiration, 321
Insoluble fiber, 136, 137t
Institute of Medicine
  athletes' protein consumption, 441–442
  television recommendation, 521
Insulin, 215
  chromium and, 358
  defined, 140
  diabetes and, 146
  fat and protein metabolism, 141
  maintaining blood glucose level, 140–141, 140f
  nitrogen balance and, 225
Insulin-resistant cells, 148
Integrated Pest Managment (IPM), 481
Integrative medicine, 51
Integumentary system, overview of, 107t, 110, 110f
Intensity, physical activity, determining, 426–428
Intentional additives, 478, 479t
Interesterified oils, 169
International Marathon Medical Directors Association (IMMDA)
  athletes' fluid consumption, 444
  sports drinks, 444
International Units (IUs), 258
Internet
  Health on the Net symbol, 48t
  nutrition information on, 47–48
  recipes on, 57
Intestine, large
  absorption, 117
  bacteria in, 118
  carbohydrate digestion, 139f, 140
  colorectal cancer and fiber, 154
  structure and function of, 111f, 117–118
Intestine, small
  absorbing nutrients, 116–117, 116f
  bacteria in, 118
  carbohydrate digestion, 139–140, 139f
  coenzymes and, 281

Intestine, small, *(continued)*
  duodenum, 114
  ileum, 114
  iron absorption, 347
  jejunum, 114
  lipid digestion, 175, 177f
  protein digestion and
      absorption, 222–223, 223f
  structure and function of, 111f,
      114, 114f, 116f
  vitamin absorption, 262
  vitamin B-12 absorption,
      291–293, 292f
  zinc absorption, 352
Intracellular water, 318–319, 319f
Intrinsic factor, 291, 293
in vitro experiments, 34
In vivo experiments, 34
Involuntary response, 113
Iodide, 325f
Iodine, 354–356
  Daily Value, A1
  deficiency, 356
  dietary adequacy, 356
  as essential nutrient, 7t, 100t
  food sources of, 355t, 356
  function of, 354–355
  goiters and, 354, 354f
  iodized salt, 355
  RDA, 355
  salt, iodized, 355
  summary of, 346t
  toxicity, 356
Ions, 100–101, 319t
Iron, 347–351
  adolescents, 518
  anemia, 349, 349f
  breastfeeding, 507
  Daily Value, A1
  deficiency, 349
  dietary adequacy, 347
  dietary advice for athletes, 445
  Dietary Guidelines, 69
  enriched grains and, 65
  as essential nutrient, 7t, 100t
  food sources of, 347, 348t, 349f
  function of, 325f, 347
  heme iron, 347
  hereditary hemochromatosis,
      351
  infant formula, 508
  meats, 66
  MyPlate, 348f
  nonheme iron, 347
  older adults, 527
  pregnancy and, 69, 498
  protein-rich foods, 66
  RDA, 347
  sports anemia, 445
  summary of, 346t
  toxicity, 351
  vegetarianism and, 233
  vitamin C and absorption of, 350
Iron deficiency, 349, 349t

Iron overload, 351
Irradiation, 476
Irritable bowel syndrome (IBS),
    123
Isoflavanoids, sources/biological
    effect of, 8t
Isoleucine, 7t, 217t, A5
Isothiocyanates, sources/
    biological effect of, 8t
Isotretinoin, 272
Italian influences on diet, 88

J
Jejunum, 114
Jewish influences on diet, 90–91
Journal of Nutrition, 41
*Journal of the American Medical
    Association,* 41, 41f
Junk food, empty-calorie vs.
    nutrient-dense foods, 15

K
Kava, 53t
Keratin, 215, 270
Ketoacidosis, 141
Ketone bodies, 141
Ketosis, 141
Kidneys
  antidiuretic hormone and
      aldosterone, 322, 322f
  in buffering system, 102
  deamination, 224, 225f
  function of, 108, 108f
  glucagon and, 141
  hydration and, 321, 322f
Kidney stones, 296, 321, 321f
Kilo, 12
Kilocalorie, 12
Kosher food, 90–91
Kwashiorkor, 237, 237f

L
Labels. *See* Food labels
Lactase, 139f, 140, 152
Lactate, 434, 434f
Lactation, 493
Lacteal lymph, 117
Lacteals, 175
Lactic acid, 433, 434f
Lactic acid energy system,
    433–434, 434f
Lactobacillus bifidus, 503
Lactoovovegetarian,
    232, 232t
Lactose, 131f
  characteristics and sources of,
    131
  galactose, 131
Lactose intolerance, 152
Lactovegetarian, 232, 232t
L-aginine, 53t
Large intestines. *See* Intestine,
    large

L-arginine claims/benefits/risks,
    53t
Larynx, 112, 113f
LDL (low-density lipoprotein)
  atherosclerosis and, 183–184
  butter vs. margarine, 190–191
  cholesterol, 183–184
  defined, 183
  dietary changes to reduce
      risk of atherosclerosis,
      188–189
  exercise and, 191
  healthy/unhealthy levels of,
      187–188, 187t
  niacin and, 298
  oxidized, 183–184, 184f
  percentages of lipid and
      protein, 183f
  role of, 183–184, 184f
  vitamin C, 299
Lead, 481
Lean, legal definition, 82t
Leavening agents, 479t
Lecithin, 171
Legumes, 219f
  complementary combinations,
      230–231, 230t
  defined, 219
  fiber content in some, 138t
  protein and fat in, 219
Le Leche League, 507
Leptin, 390, 391f
  food intake and, 389, 390f
  obesity, 389
Let-down reflex, 504, 505f
Let's Move, 521, 522
Leucine, 7t, 217t, A5
Levulose, 131
Life expectancy, 523, 523f
Life span
  defined, 524
  extending, 524, 529, 530
Life stages and nutritional needs,
    493–535
  adolescence, 517–518
  childhood, 512–514
  infants, 503–512
  older adults, 522–528
  pregnancy, 494–499
  prenatal period, 494–495
  school-age children, 515–516
Life stage/sex group, 62
Lifestyle, 9
Ligaments, 109
Light or lite food, 82
Lignans, sources/biological effect
    of, 8t
Lignin, 136, 137t
Limiting amino acids, 219
Lind, James, 257
Lingual lipase, 112
Linoleic acid, 167–168, 168f, 189
Lipase, 112, 174

Lipids. *See also* Fat, dietary
  benefits of, 165
  cholesterol, 172
  defined, 165
  dietary changes to reduce risk
      of CVD, 188–194, 194t
  digestion of, 174–179,
      175f–176f
  fatty acids, 166–169
  food label, 180, 180f
  functions of, 165, 165t
  lipoproteins, 175–178
  major functions of, 5t
  as nutrient, 5
  Nutrition Facts panel, 180, 180f
  phospholipids, 171–172
  triglycerides, 169–171, 178–179
Lipolysis, 141
Lipoprotein lipase, 175, 176
Lipoprotein profile, 187, 188
Lipoproteins, 175–178
  atherosclerosis and, 183–184,
      184f
  defined, 175
  elevated levels, as modifiable
      risk for cardiovascular
      disease, 186
  high-density lipoprotein,
      183–184, 184f
  low-density lipoprotein,
      183–184
  percentages of lipid and
      protein, 183f, 186
  very-low-density lipoproteins
      (VLDL), 184
Liposuction, 403–404, 404f
Listeria monocytogenes, 464t
Liter, 11
Lithium, 360t
Liver
  aflatoxin and, 465
  alcohol's effect on, 201–202
  cancer, 304
  carbohydrate digestion and
      absorption, 139–140, 139f
  cirrhosis, 202
  deamination, 224
  enterohepatic circulation, 178,
      178f
  function in GI tract, 111f, 115,
      115f
  glucagon and, 141
  hepatic portal vein, 117
  lipid digestion, 177, 177f
  metabolizing alcohol, 197
  protein digestion and
      absorption, 222–223, 223f
  recycling bile salts, 178, 178f
  saturated fat and, 188
  vitamin B-12 absorption, 291
Locusts, 19
Loperamide, 121, 485
Low-birth weight (LBW) infants,
    20, 495, 499

Low calorie, legal definition, 82t
Low-density lipoprotein cholesterol. *See* LDL (low-density lipoprotein)
Low fat, legal definition, 82t
Low-quality protein, 219, 221
Lumen, 114
Lungs
    in buffering system, 102
    structure and function of, 107, 108f
Lutein, 270
    age-related macular degeneration (AMD), 300
    sources/biological effect of, 8t
Lycopene, 8t, 270, 300
Lymph, 108, 117
Lymphatic system
    chylomicrons, 175, 177f
    normal aging changes, 523t
    overview of, 107t, 108, 108f
Lysine, 217, 217t, 230, 231f, A5
    as essential nutrient, 7t
    as limiting protein, 219

M
Macrobiotic diet, 232t
Macronutrients, 12
Macular degeneration, carotenoids, 300–301
Magnesium, 342–344
    Daily Value, A1
    deficiency, 343
    dietary adequacy, 343–344
    as essential nutrient, 7t, 100t
    food sources of, 342–343, 343t, 344f
    function of, 325f, 342
    MyPlate, 344f
    RDA, 343
    summary of, 328t
    toxicity, 344
Major minerals
    calcium, 328t, 329–332
    chloride, 328t
    magnesium, 328t, 342–344
    phosphorus, 328t
    potassium, 328t, 341–342
    sodium, 328t, 335–340
    sulfur, 328t
    summary of, 328t
Make Your Calories Count, 79
Malabsorption, 116
Malignant tumor, 303
Malnutrition
    defined, 19
    overnutrition, 19
    undernutrition, 19, 20–22
Maltase, 139, 139f
Maltodextrin, 136
Maltose, 131, 131f, 139, 139f
Manganese, 359
    Daily Value, A1
    as essential nutrient, 7t, 100t

function of, 325f
summary of, 346t
Mannitol, 133
Marasmus, 237f
Meals on Wheels, 528f
Measurements
    conversions, A0
    household, 27
Meat-and-potatoes diet, 87
Meats
    cancer and, 235, 304
    decreasing intake of, 228–229
    diabetes risk, 149
    Exchange System, 75
    fat content, 66
    as high-risk foods, 461, 461t
    as iron source, 347, 348t
    micronutrients in, 66
    MyPlate recommendations, 226–227
    nutrient content claims, 82t
    preventing food-borne illness, 469–471, 470t
    protein consumption patterns, 226–227, 227f
    serving size, 66
    storage tips, 472, 472t
    substitute protein-rich foods, 66f
    as vitamin B-6 source, 286
    as vitamin B-12 source, 291
Meat thermometers, 470
Mechanical digestion, 111
Medical treatment for weight loss
    bariatric surgical procedure, 402–403
    liposuction, 403–404
    weight-loss medication, 401
Mediterranean diet, 194
Mediterranean Diet Pyramid, 88, 88f
Megadoses, 298–299
    carotenoids, 300–301
    defined, 16
    disadvantages of, 16
    reasons people take, 296
    vitamin B-6, 298
    vitamin C, 296, 298–299
    vitamin E, 299
Megaloblastic anemia, 289
Melanin, 275
Melatonin, 53t
Men. *See also* Gender differences
    body composition, 5f, 317
    hereditary hemochromatosis, 351
Menaquinones, 279
Menu planning
    meatless menu planning, 234, 234t
    using MyPlate for, 72–73
    weight-loss plans and, 397
Messenger ribonucleic acid (mRNA), 221, 221f

Metabolic syndrome
    defined, 151
    signs of, 151t
Metabolic water, 320
Metabolism
    age and, 380
    basal, 378
    body composition and, 379
    body surface area, 379
    calculating energy need, 380
    calorie intake, 380
    defined, 5, 103
    energy, A2–A4, A6
    factors influencing, 379–380
    factors that increase, 380t
    gender and, 379
    genetics and thrifty metabolism, 389
    obesity and, 145
    resting metabolic rate, 378
    thyroid hormone, 378–379
Metastasized, 303
Meter, 11
Methionine, 217t, 230, 231f, A5
    as essential nutrient, 7t
    as limiting protein, 219
Metric system, 11–12
Mice, genetic obesity in, 391f
Micelle, 174
Micro, 12
Microbes
    in food, 457, 459–460
    in small and large intestine, 118
Micronutrients, 12
Microwave cooking
    preserving vitamin content in food, 264
    preventing food-borne illness, 469
Milk. *See also* Dairy foods
    allergies and infants, 509
    as calcium source, 330
    consumption of, 9
    as energy and nutrient source, 15, 15f
    fat content, 66
    fortification, 262
    as high-risk foods, 461, 461t
    infants, 508–509
    iron deficiency anemia and, 350
    lactose intolerance, 152–153
    micronutrients in, 66
    riboflavin and light, 284
    serving size, 66
    storage tips, 472, 472t
    Vitamin D fortification, 274
Milli, 12
Milo of Croton, 215
Minerals, 324–361. *See also* specific minerals
    bioavailability, 326
    body composition of, 5f
    calcium, 329–332
    defined, 100

as essential nutrient, 7t
    functions of, 5t, 324–325, 325f
    manganese, 359
    as micronutrient, 12
    molybdenum, 359
    narrow range of safety, 327, 327f
    as nutrient, 5
    with possible physiological roles, 360
    sources of, 326–327
    toxicity, 325, 327
    trace, 345–360
    water as source of, 327
Minerals, major
    calcium, 328t
    chloride, 328t
    magnesium, 328t, 342–344
    phosphorus, 328t
    potassium, 328t, 340–342
    sodium, 328t, 335–340
    sulfur, 328t
    summary of, 328t
Minerals, trace
    chromium, 358–359
    iodine, 354–356
    iron, 347–351
    selenium, 357–358
    summary of, 346t
    zinc, 352–354
Mineral water, 362t
Miso, 233
Mitochondria, 105, 105f, 431, 431f
Moderate-intensity physical activity, determining, 427
Moderation, 15
Modified starches, 136
Molds, food-borne illness and, 465
Molecules
    chemical reaction, 102–103
    defined, 100
Molybdenum, 359
    Daily Value, A1
    as essential nutrient, 7t
    summary of, 346t
Monoglycerides, 174, 175f
Monosaccharides, 130–131
Monosodium glutamate (MSG), 335
Monoterpenes, sources/biological effect of, 8t
Monounsaturated fatty acid
    defined, 166
    dietary changes to reduce risk of atherosclerosis, 188
    food label, 180, 180f
    percentage in common fats and oils, 170f
    recommended consumption of, 179
    structure of, 167f
Morning sickness, 496
Motivation, weight-loss plans and, 395

Mouth
  carbohydrate digestion, 139, 139f
  structure and function of, 111–112, 111f, 113f
mRNA, 221
Mucilages, 136, 137t
Mucus
  defined, 113
  small intestine, 114
  stomach walls, 113
  vitamin A and, 267–268
Multivitamin/multimineral (MVMM), 50, 262, 263
Muscle dysmorphia, 414
Muscle fatigue, 435
Muscles
  carbohydrate loading, 439–441
  dehydration and, 323
  energy sources for, 435t
  energy systems for, 432–435
  function of, 108, 108f
  older adults, 525
Muscular system
  normal aging changes, 523t
  overview of, 107t, 108, 108f
Mushrooms, toxic, 465
Myelin sheath, vitamin B-12, 291
Myocardial infarction, 182, 183
Myoglobin, 347
MyPlate, 71–72
  added sugars and, 142
  adolescents and, 518
  calcium, 326f, 331f
  for different calorie levels, 396
  empty calories and, 71, 142
  fat-soluble vitamins, 267f
  food groups of, 71, 71f
  iron, 348f
  for losing weight, 73
  magnesium, 344f
  oils and, 71
  for older adulthood, 524t
  overview of, 71
  physical activity and, 74, 392
  potassium, 344f
  preschool recommendations, 513, 513t
  protein intake, 226–227
  recommendations for average twenty-year old, 73t
  school-age children, 515–516, 515t
  tips for building a better plate, 72
  using for menu planning, 72–73
  water-soluble vitamins, 283f
  website for, 71
  zinc, 353f
MyPyramid Plan, 71

N
Nails, 110
Naringenin, sources/biological effect of, 8t

National Collegiate Athletic Association (NCAA)
  caffeine limits, 447
  rapid weight loss, 315
National Nutrient Database for Standard Reference, 86
National Osteoporosis Foundation, website, 48
National School Lunch Program, 22t
National Weight Control Registry, 401
Native American influences on diet, 89–90
Nausea, during pregnancy, 496
Negative energy balance, 384, 385f
Negative nitrogen balance, 225, 225f
Neotame, 134, 134t
Nerves, 109f
Nervous system
  normal aging changes, 523t
  overview of, 107t, 109, 109f
Neural tube defects, 290, 290f
Neurons, 109
Neurotransmitters, vitamin B-6, 286
New England Journal of Medicine, The, 41, 41f
Niacin, 259t, 285–286
  body's synthesis of, 262
  corn as source of, 285
  Daily Value, A1
  deficiency, 16, 286, 286f
  dietary adequacy, 285–286
  energy metabolism, A6
  enrichment, 262
  as essential nutrient, 7t
  food sources of, 285, 285t
  function of, 260f, 285
  LDL cholesterol, 298
  megadose of, 16
  pellagra, 36, 286, 286f
  summary of, 282t
  toxicity, 286
  tryptophan and, 259, 285
  vitamin supplements, 298
Nickel, 100t, 360t
Nicotinamide, 259t
Nicotinic acid, 259t
Night blindness, 268–269, 269f
Night eating syndrome (NES), 413–414
Nitrogen, as essential element, 100t
Nitrogen balance, 224–225, 225f
Nitrogen-containing group, 217
Nitrogen equilibrium, 225, 225f
Nitrosamines, 304, 305t
Nonchemical pest managment techniques, 481
Nonessential amino acids, 217, 217t

Nonexercise activity thermogenesis (NEAT), 382
Nonheme iron, 347
Nonnutrients, 6–7
Nonnutritive sweeteners, 133–135, 134t
  Acceptable Daily Intakes for, 135t
  safety of, 133–135
Norovirus, 465f, 465t, 469
Northwestern European influences on diet, 87
Nucleus, 99f, 105, 105f
Nutraceuticals, 50
NutraSweet, 134
Nutrient content claims, 81–82
Nutrient deficiency disease. See Deficiency and deficiency diseases
Nutrient-dense food, 15
Nutrient requirement, 34–35
Nutrients
  classes of, 5
  defined, 3
  essential, 6
  food as best source of, 17–18
  food as mixture of nutrients, 13
  macronutrients, 12
  major functions of, 5t
  megadose, 16
  micronutrients, 12
  physiological dose of, 16
Nutrient toxicity disorders, nutrient supplements and, 63
Nutrigenetics, 242, 244, 244t
Nutrigenomics, 242, 244, 244t
Nutrition, defined, 4
Nutritional genomics, 242, 244, 244f
Nutritional standards, 62–64
  Acceptable Macronutrient Distribution Ranges (AMDRs), 63
  Adequate Intakes (AIs), 63
  commercial applications, 64
  Daily Values, 64
  Estimated Average Requirement (EAR), 62
  Estimated Energy Requirement (EER), 62–63
  nutrition labeling purposes, 64
  Recommended Dietary Allowances (RDAs), 63
  Tolerable Upper Intake Level (UL), 63
  uses of, 64
Nutrition concepts, 13–19
  balance and variety of food, 13–14
  food as best source of nutrients and phytochemicals, 17–18
  food as mixture of nutrients, 13
  food in moderation, 15

food/nutrients not cure all, 18–19
  malnutrition as undernutrition and overnutrition, 19
  no "good" or "bad" foods, 14–15
  no "one-size fits all" diet, 18
  nutrition as dynamic science, 19
  safe intake of nutrients, 16
Nutrition Facts panel, 76, 78
  carbohydrates, 143, 144f
  Daily Values, 79
  fat, 180, 180f
  fiber, 143, 144, 144f
  fresh foods and, 78
  Make Your Calories Count, 79
  overview of, 76, 77f, 78
  % Daily Value, 79
  restaurants and vending machines, 79–80
  serving size, 76, 77f
  starch, 143, 144
  sugar, 143, 144, 144f
  trans fat and, 180
Nutrition information, 43–47
  ask questions about, 45–46
  pseudoscience, 44
  quackery, 46
  red flags for misinformation, 46–47
  registered dietitian as source for, 49
  skepticism of claims, 43–44
  testimonials, 43
  tips for using Internet wisely, 47–48
Nutrition labels. See also Food labels
  FDA using DVs for, 64
  nutritional standards and, 64
Nutritive sweetener, 132, 133
Nuts
  complementary combinations, 230–231, 230t
  as energy-dense food, 16
  food allergy to, 239
  as nutrient-dense food, 16
  protein and fat in, 219
  for protein consumption, 227

O
Oatrim, 192
Obesity. See also Childhood obesity; Overweight
  body mass index (BMI) classification, 386, 386t, 394, 394f
  central-body obesity, 387–388, 387f
  defined, 9, 371
  environmental influences, 391–392
  fructose, 389

genetic factors, 389–391
health effects of, 387–388, 387t
HFSC and, 145
hypertension and, 338
incidence of, 371–372
leptin, 389
medical treatment for, 401–404
percentage body fat
    classification, 376, 377t
physiological factors, 388–391
pregnancy and, 387
prevalence of, in U.S., 371,
    371f, 371t
psychological factors, 393
as risk factor, 9
set-point theory, 391
socioeconomic factors, 392
soft drink consumption and,
    39–40, 145–146
stigma of, 387
sugar and soft drinks, 145–146
weight-loss plans, medically
    sound, 395–401
weight-loss supplements, 407t
Observational studies, 35, 38
Oils
    fats vs. oils, 167
    hydrogenation, 169
    interesterified, 169
    as major food group, 67
    MyPlate and, 71, 71f
Older adults, 522–528
    aging process, 523–524, 523t
    anemia, 526
    calcium intake and, 332
    changes in body weight, 525
    community nutrition services
        for, 528
    constipation, 526
    daily food plan for, 527–528
    depression, 527
    dietary supplements and
        prescription drugs,
        526–527
    extending life span, 524, 529,
        530
    intestinal tract problems,
        526–527
    iron, 527
    life expectancy, 523
    pernicious anemia, 293
    physical inactivity, 525–526
    thirst and water intake, 323
    tooth loss, 526
    vitamin B-12, 526
    vitamin D and, 276
Olean, 192
Omega end, 166, 167f
Omega-3 fatty acid
    defined, 167
    dietary changes to reduce risk
        of atherosclerosis, 189–190
    in fish, 227
    fish oil supplements, 190

foods rich in, 189t
inflammation and, 189
supplements, 50
Omega-6 fatty acid
    blood clotting and
        inflammation, 167,
        189–190
    dietary changes to reduce risk
        of atherosclerosis, 189–190
    inflammation and, 189–190
Omnivore, 118
Opsin, 269
Organ
    accessory, 111
    defined, 107
    structure and function of, 106
Organelles, 105, 105f
Organic foods
    defined, 84
    increase in popularity of, 84
    labeling, 85, 85t
    as pesticide free, 481
Organosulfides, sources/biological
    effect of, 8t
Organ systems
    cardiovascular system, 107,
        107f, 107t
    defined, 107
    digestive system, 107t, 111,
        111f
    endocrine system, 107t, 109,
        109f
    function of, 106
    homeostasis and, 106
    integumentary system, 107t,
        110, 110f
    lymphatic system, 107t, 108,
        108f
    muscular system, 107t, 108,
        108f
    nervous system, 107t, 109, 109f
    overview of all, 107t
    reproductive system, 107t, 110,
        110f
    respiratory system, 107, 107t,
        108f
    skeletal system, 107t, 109, 109f
    urinary system, 107t, 108, 108f
Orlistat, 401–402
Osmosis, 318, 318f
Osteoblasts, 329
Osteocalcin, 279
Osteoclasts, 329
Osteomalacia, 276, 276f
Osteoporosis, 330f, 332
    adolescents, 518
    causes of, 333
    defined, 332
    estrogen and, 333
    high-protein diet, 235
    incidence of, 332
    reducing risk of, 333–335
    risk factors for, 333–335, 333t
    vitamin D and, 276

vitamin K and, 279
weight-bearing exercise, 334
Overnutrition, 19
Overweight. See also Childhood
    obesity; Obesity
    adolescents, 518
    body mass index (BMI)
        classification, 386, 386t,
        394, 394f
    carbohydrates and, 145
    defined, 371
    dietary fat and, 145
    environmental influences,
        391–392
    food composition factors, 389
    gallstones, 115
    genetic factors, 389–391
    health effects of, 387–388, 387t
    incidence of, 371–372, 519,
        519f
    medically sound weight-loss
        plans, 395–399
    percentage body fat
        classification, 376, 377t
    physiological factors, 388–391
    preschool, 514
    psychological factors, 393
    school-age children, 519–522,
        519f
    set-point theory, 391
    socioeconomic factors, 392
    stigma of, 387
    sugar and soft drinks, 145–146
    thrifty metabolism, 389
Ovovegetarian, 232, 232t
Oxalic acid, 330, 347, 350
Oxidant, 259
Oxidation, 430
    antioxidants, 169
    trans fats and, 169
Oxidative stress, 445
Oxidizing agent, 259
Oxygen, as essential element,
    100t
Oxygen energy system, 434–436
Oxytocin, 504, 505f

P
Paleo diet, 144
Pancreas
    alcoholic pancreatitis, 201
    function in GI tract, 111f, 115,
        115f
    lipase, 174
    lipid digestion, 174, 177f
    maintaining blood glucose
        level, 140–141, 140f
Pancreatic amylase, 139, 139f
Pancreatic cancer, 304
Pancreatic lipase, 174
Pantothenic acid, 259t, 294
    Daily Value, A1
    energy metabolism, A6
    as essential nutrient, 7t

function of, 260f
summary of, 282t
Parasite, as food-borne illness
    pathogen, 465, 466t
Parasitic worms, 465
Parathyroid, blood calcium levels,
    329, 329f
Parathyroid hormone (PTH)
    blood calcium levels, 329
    vitamin D and calcium levels,
        273, 274f, 331–332
Partial hydrogenation, 169
Pasteurization, 460
Pathogens
    bacteria, 463, 464t
    common routes for
        transmitting, 460
    defined, 457
    fungi, 465
    irradiated food and, 476
    parasite, 465, 466t
    virus, 463, 465t
Patient Protection and Affordable
    Care Act of 2010, 79
Pauling, Linus, 298
PCr-ATP energy system, 432–433,
    433f
Peanuts, food allergy, 239
Pear shape, 387, 387f
Pectin, 136, 137t
Peer review, 40
Pellagra, 16, 286, 286f
    medical research on, 36
    niacin and, 36
    signs and symptoms of, 286
Pepsin, protein digestion, 222,
    223f
Peptic ulcer
    causes and treatment for,
        122–123
    factors that increase risk of,
        122f, 122t
    H. pylori, 122
    stress, 122
Peptide bond, 220, 221f
Peptides, 221
Peptide YY, 389, 390f
% Daily Value, 79, 82
Peristalsis, 112, 113f
Pernicious anemia, 293, 526
Pesticides, 481–482
    defined, 481
    nonchemical pest managment
        techniques, 481
    pesticide residue, 481
    reducing exposure to, 85
    safety of, 481–482
pH
    of blood, 102, 102f
    defined, 101
    proteins and acid-base balance,
        216
    scale, 102, 102f
    water, 102, 102f

Pharmaceutical companies, using nutritional standards, 64
Pharynx, 112, 113f
Phenolics, sources/biological effect of, 8t
Phenylalanine, 134, 217t, A5
  as essential nutrient, 7t
  PKU and, 242
Phenylketunuria. *See* PKU (phenylketunuria)
Pheromones, 481
Phosphate, intracellular water, 319
Phosphocreatine (PCr), 432–433, 433f, 435t
Phospholipase, 174
Phospholipids
  body's use of, 171f
  deficiency, 171–172
  defined, 171
  digestion of, 174
  as emulsifier, 171–172
  lecithin, 171
  structure of, 171f
Phosphoric acid, 101
Phosphorus
  Daily Value, A1
  dairy foods, 65
  as essential nutrient, 7t, 100t
  function of, 325f
  summary of, 328t
  vitamin D and metabolism of, 272f, 273
Phylloquinone, 279
Physical activity, 425–453. *See also* Athletes
  adolescents, 518
  benefits of regular exercise, 426, 427f
  daily moderate-intensity physical activity, 392
  defined, 425
  determining intensity level of, 426–428
  developing personal physical fitness plan, 449–451
  diabetes and, 149
  Dietary Guidelines, 69
  energy expenditure for, 381–382, 381t
  energy metabolism for, 431–436, 432f, 433f
  as environmental influence in overweight, 392
  MyPlate and, 74
  MyPyramid Plan, 71
  older adults, 525–526
  osteoporosis and weight-bearing, 334
  physical activity pyramid, 428–429, 428f
  during pregnancy, 502
  school-age children and, 522

weight-loss plans, 396
Physical activity pyramid, 428–429, 428f
Physical fitness, defined, 425
Physical inactivity, as modifiable risk for cardiovascular disease, 186
Physician and Sportsmedicine, The, 437
Physiological anemia, 497
Physiological dose, 16
Physiological marker, 62
Physiology, 104–105
  cell, 105
  organ systems, 107
  tissues and organs, 104
Phytic acid, 330, 347, 350, 352
Phytochemicals
  defined, 6
  food sources vs. supplements, 17
  fruits, 66
  as nonnutrient, 6
  sources/biological effect of various, 8t
  vegetables, 66
Pica, 499
PKU (phenylketunuria), 242
  aspartame and, 134
  diagnosing, 242
  real story of, 243
  restrictive diet for, 242
Placebo
  defined, 35
  double-blind studies, 37
Placebo effect, 37
Placenta, 494f, 495
Plant sterols/stanols, 172
Plaque
  arteriosclerosis, 182
  atherosclerosis, 182
Plasma, 318
Plasma membrane, 105, 105f
Platelets
  alcohol consumption, 203
  vitamin K and, 279
Polychlorinated biphenols (PCBs), 480
Polycystic ovary disease, 386
Polypeptides, 220
Polysaccharides, 136
Polyunsaturated fatty acid
  defined, 167
  dietary changes to reduce risk of atherosclerosis, 188
  food label, 180, 180f
  percentage in common fats and oils, 170f
  recommended consumption of, 179
  structure of, 167f
Population control, 24
Portal vein, 223, 223f

Portion size
  estimating, 74f
  oversized restaurant, 391
Positive energy balance, 384, 385f
Positive nitrogen balance, 225, 225f
Potassium, 340–342
  AI, 341
  Daily Value, A1
  dietary adequacy, 341–342
  as electrolyte, 101
  as essential nutrient, 7t, 100t
  food sources of, 341, 342t
  fruits, 66
  function of, 325f, 340
  intracellular water, 319
  MyPlate, 344f
  summary of, 328t
Poverty, hunger and, 24
Prader-Willi syndrome, 391
Pre-diabetes, 146, 146f
Preeclampsia, 501
Pregnancy, 494–499. *See also* Breastfeeding
  alcohol consumption during, 203
  breast changes and, 496
  constipation during, 497
  Dietary Guidelines, 69
  digestive tract discomforts during, 497
  edema and, 497
  fatigue and, 496–497
  fetal alcohol syndrome, 203
  fish consumption during, 69, 190, 498–499
  folate, 290
  folic acid, 69
  general dietary recommendations, 497t, 498–499
  gestational diabetes, 148
  heartburn and, 497
  importance of good nutrition, 110
  iodine deficiency, 356
  iron, 69
  iron deficiency anemia, 349
  morning sickness during, 496
  neural tube defects, 290, 290f
  nitrogen balance, 225, 225f
  obesity and, 387
  PKU and, 242
  positive energy balance, 384
  pregnancy-induced hypertension (PIH), 501
  prenatal period of, 494–502, 494f
  preterm birth, 495–496
  vegetarianism, 233
  vitamin A, 271
  weight gain during, 500, 500t

Pregnancy-induced hypertension (PIH), 501
Prehypertension, 337
Premenstrual syndrome, vitamin B-6 and, 298
Prenatal care, 500–502
  defined, 500
  drug use, 501
  gestational diabetes, 500
  importance of, 500–502
  physical activity, 502
  pregnancy-induced hypertension (PIH), 501
Prenatal period
  defined, 493
  high-birth-weight infants, 499
  importance of prenatal care during, 500–502
  low-birth-weight (LBW) infants, 495, 499
  preterm birth, 495–496
  stages and development during, 494–495, 494f
Preschool children, 512–513
  allergies, 514
  daily food plan for, 513t
  dental caries, 514
  MyPlate daily food plan for, 513t
  overweight, 514
  snacks, 513, 513t
Preservatives, 479t
Preterm birth, 495–496
Probiotics, 51, 119
Produce, fresh, primary pathogens of, 461t
Prohormone vitamin D, 272, 276
Prolactin, 496, 504, 505f
Proline, 217t, A5
Prooxidant, 295
Prospective study, 38
Prostaglandins, 167
Prostate cancer, 304
Protein, 215–253
  acid-base balance, 216
  AMDR for, 64t
  amino acids, 216–217, 217t
  animal vs. plant sources, 218–219
  ATP formation, 431, 431f
  average American intake of, 142f
  blood pressure and blood proteins, 216, 216f
  body composition of, 5f
  body's synthesis of protein, 220–222, 221f
  complementary combinations, 230–231
  complete, 219
  consumption patterns, 226–227, 227f

daily recommendations, 442t
Daily Value, A1
dairy foods, 65
deamination, 224, 224f, 225f
decreasing intake of animal foods, 228–229
deficiency disease, 236–237, 237f
defined, 215
denaturation, 222, 222f
dietary advice for athletes, 441–442
diets with low-quality protein, 221
digestion and absorption of, 222–223, 223f
EAR for, 225
food allergy, 238–239
food labels, 228, 228f
in foods, 218–219, 218t
for fueling exercise, 436t
function of, 215–216, 215t
genetic defects and, 222
high-protein diet, 235
high-quality, 219
incomplete, 219
insulin and metabolism, 141
kcal in gram of, 12
low-quality, 219
as macronutrient, 12
major functions of, 5t
meatless menu planning, 234, 234t
meats, 66
MyPlate recommendations, 226–227
nitrogen balance, 225, 225f
as nutrient, 5
peptide bond, 220, 221f
protein-energy malnutrition, 236–237, 237f
protein-rich foods, 66
quality of, 219–220
RDA, 225
resistance training, 225f
shape of, 222, 222f
soy protein, 219
transamination, 224, 224f
triglycerides synthesis, 179
turnover, 224
vegetarianism, 232–234
Protein denaturation, 222, 222f
Protein-energy malnutrition, 236–237, 237f
kwashiorkor, 237, 237f
marasmus, 237–238, 237f
Protein Power diet, 236
Protein-rich foods
Dietary Guidelines, 68–69
fat content and, 66
as food group in MyPlate, 71, 71f
as major food group, 66
micronutrients in, 66

MyPlate recommendations, 226–227
serving size, 66
substitutes for meats, 66f
umami taste and, 112
Protein supplements, 441
Protein synthesis, 220–222, 221f
Protein turnover, 223–224
Prothrombin, 279
Protons, 99, 99f
Protozoans, 465
Provitamin, 259
Prudent diet, diabetes risk, 149–150
Pseudoscience, 44
Psyllium, 136
Puberty, 225, 225f, 517
Pulse, radial artery, 428, 428f
Purified water, 362t
Pyloric sphincter, 114
Pyridoxine, 259t
Pyruvate, 407t, 430

Q
Qsymia, 401
Quackery, 46
Quercetin, sources/biological effect of, 8t
Quinoa, 219, 219f, 251

R
Radial artery, 428, 428f
Radical
defined, 259
role of, 259, 261f
vitamin E and, 277, 277f
Radura symbol, 476, 476f
Rancidity, 261
Raspberry ketone, 407t
Reactive hypoglycemia, 151
Ready-to-use therapeutic food (RUTF), 22
Rebiana, 134t, 135
Recipes for healthy living
apricot quinoa, 251
bean and salsa dip, 419
chicken salad, 488
chicken soup, 57
egg salad, 125
food preparation basics, 27
low-fat applesauce oatmeal muffins, 28
mango lassi, 93
nutty energy bars, 453
oatmeal cereal with berries, 159
orange-strawberry smoothie, 366
salmon salad sandwiches, 207
stir-fried vegetables, 309
vegetable dip, 533
Recommended Dietary Allowances (RDAs), 64t
carbohydrate, 79

carbohydrates, 141
compared to Daily Values, 79
defined, 63
developing Daily Values (DVs), 64
establishing, 63, 63f
protein, 225
Rectum, 117, 117f, 223f
Red blood cells
anemia, 349, 349f
folate and production of, 288–289, 289f
vitamin B-12 and heme production, 289
Reduced or fewer calories, legal definition, 82t
Reduced or less fat, legal definition, 82t
Reduced sugar, legal definition, 82t
Refined grains, 65, 68
Refined sucrose, 131
Reflux, 113
Refrigeration, storing food tips, 471–473, 472t
Registered dietitian (R.D.), 49
clinical dietitians, 49
community nutritionists, 49
educational background, 49
finding one, 49
as sources of nutrition information, 49
types of work for, 49
work setting for, 49
Rehydration, 444
Reproductive system
normal aging changes, 523t
overview of, 107t, 110, 110f
Requirement, defined, 34
Research bias, 41
Resistance training
as component of fitness program, 451
nitrogen balance, 225, 225f
in physical activity pyramid, 428–429, 428f
Respiratory system
normal aging changes, 523t
overview of, 107, 107t, 108f
Restaurants
providing nutrition information, 79–80
weight loss and behavior modification, 396, 397
Resting metabolic rate (RMR), 378
Resveratrol, sources/biological effect of, 8t
Retinal, 259, 269
Retinoic acid, 259
Retinol (preformed vitamin A), 259, 259t
defined, 267
food sources of, 270

Retrospective study, defined, 38
R group, 217
Rhodopsin, 269
Riboflavin, 259t, 284
Daily Value, A1
dairy foods, 65
dietary adequacy, 284
energy metabolism, A6
enrichment, 262
as essential nutrient, 7t
food sources of, 284, 284t
function of, 260f, 284
RDA, 284
summary of, 282t
Ribosomes, 105, 105f
Rickets, 272, 272f, 276
Risk factors
cardiovascular disease, 184–185, 185t
compared to cause of disease, 186
defined, 9
diabetes mellitus, 147
Rodenticides, 481
Rods, 268, 269f
Rotavirus, 463, 465t
Roux-en-Y gastric bypass, 402, 403f

S
Saccharin, 134, 134t
Safe Drinking Water Act (SDWA), 362
Saliva, enzymes in, 112
Salivary amylase, 112, 139, 139f
Salivary glands, 111f
Salmonella, 461f, 464t, 476
Salt. See also Sodium
acid-base reaction, 103, 103f
iodized, 337, 355
Salty taste, benefit of, 112
Saponins, sources/biological effect of, 8t
Satiety
defined, 389
fiber and, 155
fructose and, 389
hypothalamus and, 389, 390f
Saturated fats
animal foods and cardiovascular disease, 67
Dietary Guidelines, 68–69
food label, 180, 180f
recommended consumption of, 179
reducing risk of atherosclerosis and, 188
Saturated fatty acid
Daily Value, A1
defined, 166
percentage in common fats and oils, 170f
structure of, 167f

Savory taste, benefit of, 112
School-age children, 515–516
  breakfast, 515t
  daily food plan
    recommendations, 513t,
    515–516
  MyPlate daily food plan for,
    515t
  overweight, 519–522, 519f
  physical activity, 522
  vegetarianism, 518
School Breakfast Program, 22t
School Lunch Program, 22t
Scientific method
  correlation, 39
  double-blind studies, 37
  epidemiological studies, 37–40
  follow-up research, 42
  historical perspective, 36
  human experimentation, 37–40
  peer review, 40
  pellagra, 36
  peptic ulcers, 33
  placebo effect, 37
  pseudoscience, 44
  research bias, 41
  steps in scientific investigation,
    33–34, 34f
Scurvy, 18, 296
  collagen synthesis, 295, 295f
  discovery of cure for, 257
  signs and symptoms of, 6
Secondhand smoke, 186
Seeds
  complementary combinations,
    230–231, 231f
  protein and fat in, 219
Segmentation, 114
Selectively permeable membrane,
    318, 318f
Selenium, A1
  cancer and, 357
  Daily Value, A1
  deficiency, 357
  dietary adequacy, 357
  as essential nutrient, 7t, 100t
  food sources of, 357, 358t
  function of, 325f, 357
  summary of, 346t
  toxicity, 357
  UL, 357
Selenoproteins, 357
Semivegetarian, 232, 232t
Senescence, 524
Serine, 217, 217t, A5
Serving size
  food labels, 79
  Nutrition Facts panel, 76, 77f
Set-point theory, 391
Shelf life, 474
Shigella, 464t
Shopping tips to save money,
    228–231, 245–248

Sickle cell anemia, 222, 222f
Silicon
  as essential nutrient, 100t
  summary of, 360t
Simple carbohydrates, 130–135
  disaccharides, 131
  monosaccharides, 130–131
  nutritive and non-nutritive
    sweeteners, 132–135
  sucrose, 131
Simple diffusion, 317–318, 317f
Simplesse, 192
Skeletal system, overview of,
    107t, 109, 109f
Skin
  function of, 110
  melanin and Vitamin D
    absorption, 275
  normal aging changes, 523t
  overview of integumentary
    system, 107t, 110, 110f
  tanning and cancer, 275, 275f
Skinfold thickness, 376f
Skinfold thickness measurements,
    376
Sleep apnea, 185, 386
Sleeve gastrectomy, 402, 403f
Small intestines. See Intestine,
    small
Smell, sense of, ability to taste,
    112
Snacks, preschool children, 513,
    513t
Socioeconomic factors, obesity
    and, 392
Sodium, 335–340
  AI, 335
  Daily Value, A1
  deficiency, 335
  dietary adequacy, 335
  Dietary Guidelines, 68–69
  as electrolyte, 101
  as essential nutrient, 7t, 100t
  extracellular water, 319
  function of, 325f, 335
  health claim, 81t
  health claims and, 80
  hypertension, 336–340
  intake assessment, 335, 337
  salty taste, 112
  sodium sentive people, 338
  sources of, 335, 336t
  summary of, 328t
  toxicity, 336
Sodium acetate, in acid-base
    reaction, 103, 103f
Sodium bicarbonate, 448t
Sodium chloride, 103, 335
Sodium citrate, 335
Sodium hydroxide, 101, 103
Sodium nitrate, 335
Soft drinks

added sugar in diet, 143
adolescents and calcium
    intake, 518
average American
    consumption, 143
consumption of, 14–15
energy and nutrient source of,
    15, 15f
fruit juice compared to, 142
HFCS in, 142
obesity and, 39–40, 145–146
Solid fats, 67f
Solid fats, characteristics of, 67
Solubility, 100, 100f
Soluble fiber, 136, 137t
  cholesterol and, 154–155
  health benefits of, 136, 137t
Solute, 100
Solution, 100
Solvent, 100
Sorbitol, 133, 511
Sour taste, benefit of, 112
Soy
  food allergy, 239
  as high-protein source, 219
  tips for using soybean foods,
    231
Sparkling bottled water, 362t
Spina bifida, 290
Spinal cord, 109f
Spirulina (blue-green algae), 407t
Splenda, 135
Sports anemia, 445
Sports bar, 442, 442f, 443t
Sports drinks, consuming during
    event, 441, 444–445
Sports nutrition, 437
Spring water, 362t
St. John's Wort, 53t
Stabilizers, 479t
Staphylococcus aureus, 464t
Starch
  characteristics and sources of,
    136
  digestion of, 139–140, 139f
  Nutrition Facts panel, 143, 144
Starvation
  kwashiorkor, 237f
  marasmus, 237–238, 237f
  muscle proteins for energy,
    141–142
  nitrogen balance, 225, 225f
Statins, 194
Steaming, as food preparation,
    264–265, 265f
Sterilization, 474
Steroids, anabolic, 448t
Sterols/stanols
  defined, 172
  reducing cholesterol
    absorption, 172
Stevia, 134, 134t, 135, 135t
Stomach

bariatric surgery, 402–403, 403f,
    404f
digestion and, 139f
in digestion process, 113
gastroesophageal sphincter, 113
hunger and satiety, 388–389, 390f
hydrochloric acid, 113
lipid digestion, 177f
mucus, 113
peptic ulcer, 122–123
protein digestion and
    absorption, 222, 223f
pyloric sphincter, 114
structure and function of, 111f,
    113–114, 114f
vitamin B-12 absorption, 291–
    293, 292f
Stress
  elevated levels, as modifiable
    risk for cardiovascular
    disease, 186
  peptic ulcer, 122
Stroke
  atherosclerosis and, 182
  as cause of death in U.S., 4f
  diet and chances of
    developing, 3
  incidence of, 181
  risk factors for, 9
Structure/function claims,
    81, 81f
  dietary supplement labels,
    82–83
Subcutaneous fat, gender
    differences, 373f, 374
Sucralose, 134, 134t, 135
Sucrase, 103, 104f, 139f, 140
Sucrose, 104f, 131f, 132
  added sugar, 68–69, 132t
  characteristics and sources of,
    131
  names for, 132t
  nutritional comparison of
    sweeteners, 132t
  nutritive and nonnutritive
    sweeteners, 132–135
  refined, 131
Sudden infant death syndrome
    (SIDS), 502, 503
Sugar
  added sugar, 15, 68–69, 132,
    132t, 143
  average American intake of,
    142f
  compared to honey, 131, 132t
  consumed by average
    American, 130
  disaccharides, 131
  fructose, 131
  galactose, 131
  glucose, 130
  hyperactivity and, 153
  lactose, 131

maltose, 131
monosaccharides, 130–131
names for, 132t
nutrient content claims, 82t
nutritional comparison of
sweeteners, 132t
Nutrition Facts panel, 143,
144, 144f
nutritive and nonnutritive
sweeteners, 132–135
obesity and, 145–146
reactive hypoglycemia and,
151
reducing consumption of, 143
refined, 131
soft drinks, 145–146
sucrose, 131
sugary foods, 67
tooth decay and, 152
Sugar alcohols, 133
Sugar beets, 131
Sugar cane, 131
Sugar free, legal definition, 82t
Sugar replacers, 133
Sugar substitutes, 133
Sulfites
as additive, 478
food allergy, 239
Sulfur, 345
as essential nutrient, 7t, 100t
summary of, 328t
Sunlight, vitamin D and, 272,
272f, 275
Sun protection factor (SPF), 275
Sunscreen, 275
Supplemental Nutrition
Assistance Program (SNAP),
22t
Supplement Facts label, 82–83,
83f
Supplements, weight loss,
407–408, 407t. See also
Dietary supplements; Vitamin
supplements
Surgery, for weight loss, 402–403,
403f, 404f
Sustainable agriculture,
23, 84
Swallowing, 112–113, 113f
Sweating, and sodium depletion,
335
Sweeteners, 479t
added sugar, 68–69, 132, 132t
alternative, 133–134, 134t
consumed by average
American, 130
nonnutritive, 133–134, 134t
nutritional comparison of
sweeteners, 132t
nutritive sweeteners, 132, 133
Sweet taste, benefit of, 112
Syndrome, 151
Systolic pressure, 336

T
Table salt. See Sodium
Tannins, 8t, 347
Target heart rate zone
age-related maximum heart
rate, 426–427
defined, 426
Taste
benefit of, 112
sense of smell and, 112
taste buds and, 112
Taste buds, 112
Taurine, 442
Teeth
baby bottle caries, 511
carbohydrate consumption and
tooth decay, 152
dental fluorosis, 357f
function in GI tract, 111f
infant's first teeth, 510, 511
preschoolers and dental
caries, 514
tooth loss in older adults, 526
Tendons, 109
Teratogen, 271
Testimonials, 43
Testosterone
nitrogen balance and, 225
osteoporosis and, 333
Tetrahydrofolic acid (THFA), 287
Therapeutic lifestyle changes (TLC)
defined, 149
diabetes, 149
metabolic syndrome, 152
Thermic effect of food (TEF), 381
Thiamin, 259t, 281–284
beriberi, 283, 284f
Daily Value, A1
deficiency, 202, 284
dietary adequacy of, 283
energy metabolism, A6
enrichment, 262
as essential nutrient, 7t
food sources of, 281, 285t
function of, 259, 260f, 281
RDA, 283
summary of, 282t
Wernicke-Korsakoff syndrome,
284
Thirst, as regulator of fluid
intake, 323
Threonine, 217t, 230, A5
as essential nutrient, 7t
as limiting protein, 219
Thrombus, 182, 182f
Thyroid
blood calcium levels, 329, 329f
iodine intake and, 355
Thyroid hormone, 355
hyperthyroidism, 378–379
hypothyroidism, 378–379
metabolism, 378–379

Thyroxin, vitamin C and, 295
Tin, as essential element, 100t
Tissue, 106, 107
Tobacco use
beta-carotene and, 300, 301
as modifiable risk for
cardiovascular disease, 186
during pregnancy, 501
vitamin C and, 296
Tofu, 66
Tolerable Upper Intake Level (UL),
63, 63f, 64t
Tomatillos, 66
Tomatoes, 270
Tongue
function of in GI tract, 111f
taste buds, 112
Total body fat, 372
Total water intake, 320
Toxicity and toxicity disorders
calcium, 332
carotenemia, 271–272
chromium, 359
fat-soluble vitamins, 259
hypercalcemia, 332
iodine, 356
iron, 351
magnesium, 344
minerals and, 325, 327
multiple vitamin, 263
risk of, 263
selenium, 357
sodium, 336
vitamin A, 271–272
vitamin B-6, 298
vitamin D, 276
vitamin E, 280
vitamin K, 280
water-soluble vitamins, 259
zinc, 353–354
Toxoplasma, 466t
Trace minerals
chromium, 358–359
iodine, 354–356
iron, 347–351
selenium, 357–358
summary of, 346t
zinc, 352–354
Transamination, 224, 224f
Transcription, 221, 221f
Trans fat, 168–169
butter vs. margarine, 190–191
defined, 168
Dietary Guidelines, 68
effect on body, 169
food label, 180, 180f
food labeled zero, 180
food storage and, 169
hydrogenation, 169
structure of, 168f
Transfer ribonucleic acid (tRNA),
221, 221f
Transition reaction, A3

Travelers' diarrhea, 483–485
Treatment group, 34, 35
Trichinella, 465, 466t
Triglycerides
atherosclerosis and, 183–184
defined, 169
digestion of, 174, 175f
exercise and, 191
healthy/unhealthy levels of,
187, 187t
storage of, in body, 178
structure of, 169f
using for energy, 178–179
tRNA, 221
Trypsin, protein digestion, 222,
223f
Tryptophan, 217t, 230, 231f, A5
as essential nutrient, 7t
as limiting protein, 219
niacin and, 285
as precursor to niacin, 259
2008 Physical Activity Guidelines
for Americans, 426
Type 1 diabetes, 146, 147–148
Type 2 diabetes, 146, 147–148
Tyrosine, 217t, A5

U
Ulcer
alcohol consumption and, 200
gastrointestinal, 113
peptic, 122
Ulcerative colitis, 118
Umami taste, 112
Umbilical cord, role of, 494f, 495
Undernutrition, 20
factors contributing to, 20
incidence of, 20
during infancy, 20–21
major U.S. food assistance
programs, 22t
during pregnancy, 20
during preschool years, 21
protein-energy malnutrition,
236–238, 237f
solutions to, 22
in United States, 21
Underwater weighing, 374–375,
374f
Underweight
classification as, body mass
index (BMI), 386t, 394,
394f
defined, 409–410
strategies for gaining weight,
409–410
UNICEF, 22
Unintentional food additives, 480
Unsaturated fatty acid
defined, 166
monounsaturated, 166, 167f
polyunsaturated, 167, 167f
structure of, 167f

Urea, 224, 224f, 321
Urinary system
    normal aging changes, 523t
    overview of, 108, 108f
Urine
    acidity of, 102
    daily output, 321
    as indicator of hydration status,
        322
U.S. Department of Agriculture
        (USDA)
    Basic Four, 71
    dietary analysis software, 85–86
    Dietary Guidelines, 67–69
    Food Guide Pyramid, 71
    Food Safety and Inspection
        Service (FSIS), 458
    MyPyramid Plan, 71–72
    organic food, 83–84
    role in food safety, 458
U.S. Department of Health and
        Human Services
    Dietary Guidelines, 67–69
    physical activity guidelines, 426
    role in food safety, 458
U.S. Food and Drug
        Administration. See Food and
        Drug Administration (FDA)
Uterus, 494, 494f

V
Valencia oranges, 86, 86f
Valine, 7t, 217t, A5
Vanadium, 100t, 360t
Variable, 34
Vegan, 232, 232t
Vegetables
    American consumption of, 10
    cancer prevention and, 305
    Dietary Guidelines, 68–69
    fiber content in some, 138t
    as food group in MyPlate, 71,
        71f
    health claim, 81t
    as magnesium source,
        342, 344t
    as major food group, 66
    micronutrients in, 66
    as potassium source, 341, 342t
    preserving vitamin content in,
        264–265
    protein content, 230–231
    serving size, 66
Vegetarianism, 232–234
    adolescents, 518
    breastfeeding and pregnancy,
        233, 507
    calcium deficiency, 332
    children and, 233
    complementary combinations,
        230–231
    defined, 232

health benefits of, 233–234, 233t
iron, 233, 445
iron deficiency anemia and,
    350–351
meatless menu planning, 234
school-age children, 518
teens and, 233–234
types of, 232, 232t
vitamin B-12, 293
vitamin D, 233
vitamins B-12, 233
zinc, 233, 352
Veins
    function of, 107
    hepatic portal, 117
    portal, 223
Vending machines, 79–80
Venter, J. Craig, 23
Vermin, 460
Very-low-calorie diets
    calorie restriction, 529
    metabolism and, 380
    regaining weight, 395
Very-low-density lipoproteins
        (VLDL), 184
    defined, 184
    percentages of lipid and
        protein, 183f
    role of, 184
Very-low-fat diet, success of, 405t,
    406
Vibrio vulnificus, 464t
Vigorous-intensity physical
        activity, determining,
        426–428
Villi, 116
Virus, as food-borne illness
        pathogen, 463, 465t
Visceral fat, 374, 374f
Viscous fiber, 140
Vision
    night blindness, 268–269, 269f
    vitamin A and, 268–269, 269f
    xerophthalmia, 271, 271f
Vitamin A, 259t, 266–272
    beta-carotene as precursor, 259
    chemical form, 259
    content of selected foods, 270t
    Daily Value, A1
    dairy foods, 65
    deficiency, 270–271
    dietary adequacy, 270–272
    epithelial cells and, 267, 267f
    as essential nutrient, 7t
    food sources of, 269–270, 270t
    function of, 260f, 267–268
    pregnancy and, 271
    RDA, 270
    retinol, 267
    summary of, 266t
    toxicity, 271–272
    vision and, 269, 269f, 270

Vitamin B
    energy metabolism, A6
    enriched grains and, 65
    as essential nutrient, 7t
    meats, 66
    protein-rich foods, 66
Vitamin B-1, 259t
Vitamin B-2, 259t
Vitamin B-3, 259t
Vitamin B-6, 259t, 286
    Alzheimer's disease, 298
    anemia, 287
    cardiovascular disease, 286
    CVD and, 298
    Daily Value, A1
    deficiency, 287
    dietary adequacy, 287
    energy metabolism, A6
    as essential nutrient, 7t
    food sources of, 286, 287t
    function of, 260f, 286
    homocysteine, 286, 286f
    homocysteine and, 185
    neurotransmitters, 286
    premenstrual syndrome, 298
    RDA, 287
    summary of, 282t
    toxicity, 287, 298
    vitamin supplements, 298
Vitamin B-12, 259t, 290–293
    absorption of, 291–293, 292f
    Alzheimer's disease, 298
    breastfeeding, 293, 507
    CVD and, 298
    Daily Value, A1
    deficiency, 292–293
    dietary adequacy, 291
    energy metabolism, A6
    as essential nutrient, 7t
    folate and, 287, 288f, 289
    food-cobalamin malabsorption,
        291
    food sources of, 291, 293t
    function of, 260f, 290–291
    myelin sheath, 291
    older adults, 526
    older adults and, 69
    pernicious anemia, 293
    RDA, 291
    summary of, 282t
    vegetarianism and, 233
    vegetarians, 293
Vitamin C, 259t, 294–296
    Alzheimer's disease, 299
    animal synthesis of, 294
    antioxidant activity, 295
    cancer and, 299
    collagen synthesis, 295
    common cold, 298–299
    Daily Value, A1
    deficiency, 6, 257, 258
    dietary adequacy, 296

    as essential nutrient, 7t
    food sources of, 295–296,
        296t
    fruits, 66
    function of, 259, 260f,
        294–295
    hormone production, 295
    iron absorption and, 350
    LDL cholesterol, 299
    megadose, 296
    in oranges vs. apples, 67f
    physiological marker for, 62
    preserving vitamin content in
        food, 264, 295
    RDA, 63, 296
    scurvy, 6, 257, 294f, 296
    smokers and, 63
    sour taste, 112
    summary of, 282t
    UL, 63, 296
    vitamin E and, 295
    vitamin supplements,
        298–299
Vitamin D, 259t, 272–275
    body's synthesis of, 262
    bone health and, 272–273
    bones health and,
        272f, 331
    breastfeeding, 507
    calcium supplements and,
        331–332
    cancer and, 275
    content of selected
        food, 274t
    Daily Value, A1
    dairy foods, 65
    deficiency, 273, 276
    dietary adequacy, 276
    as essential nutrient, 7t
    function of, 259, 260f, 272f,
        273
    as hormone, 272
    infants and exposure to
        sunlight, 506, 506f
    osteomalacia, 276
    osteoporosis and, 276
    RDA for, 276
    rickets, 272, 272f, 276
    sources of, 274–275, 274f
    summary of, 266t
    sunlight and, 272, 272f, 275,
        275f
    sunscreen and absorption of,
        275
    vegetarianism and, 233
Vitamin E, 259t, 277–278
    Alzheimer's disease, 299
    biological activity, 261
    cancer, 299
    content of selected
        food, 278t
    Daily Value, A1

deficiency, 278
dietary adequacy, 277–278
as essential nutrient, 7t
food sources of, 277, 278t
function of, 260f, 277–278
IU, 278
summary of, 266t
toxicity, 280
vitamin C and, 295
vitamin supplements, 299–300
Vitamin K, 259t, 278–280
body's production of, 262
content of selected food, 280t
Daily Value, A1
deficiency, 280
dietary adequacy, 280
as essential nutrient, 7t
food sources of, 279
function of, 260f, 279
summary of, 266t
toxicity, 280
Vitamins, 257–311. See also
specific vitamins
absorption of, 262–263
antioxidants, 260, 261f
basic concepts of, 258, 259,
260f
biological activity, 261
classifying, 259, 266t
daily multiple vitamin
supplement, 18, 262, 263
deficiency diseases, 263
defined, 258
discovery of, 257–258
enrichment and fortification,
262
estimate content in packaged
foods, 258, 258f
fat-soluble (See Fat-soluble
vitamins)
major functions of, 5t
megadose, 16
as micronutrient, 12
as nutrient, 5
physiological dose, 16
preserving vitamin content in
food, 264–265
sources of, 260–262
toxicity disorders, 263
vitamin D, 272–275
vitamin K, 278–280
water-soluble (See Water-
soluble vitamins)
Vitamin supplements, 297–301
carotenoids, 300–301
cure-all reputation, 297–298
folic acid, 298
incidence of using, 262
niacin, 298
nutrient toxicity disorders, 63
older adults, 526
pregnancy, 498

reasons people take, 297
toxicity and multiple
vitamin, 263
vitamin B-6, 298
vitamin C, 298–299
vitamin E, 299–300
VO$_{2\ max}$, 435
Vomiting
causes and treatment for, 121
danger signs, 121t
during pregnancy, 496

W
Waist circumference, obesity-
related disorder risk, 388,
388f
Warfarin, 279
Water, 316–324
absorption in small intestines,
117
adequate intake of, 320
antidiuretic hormone and
aldosterone, 322, 322f
body composition of,
5f, 317
body's conservation of,
321–323, 322f
boiling to sanitize, 484
bottled water vs. tap water,
361–362
characteristics of, 317
chemical contaminants, 480
chemical disinfection, 485
conservation of body water,
321–322
daily water balance, 320–323,
321f
dehydration, 323
dietary advice for athletes,
443–445
distribution of, in body,
318–319
diuretics, 322–323
EPA and regulation of drinking
water, 459
as essential nutrient, 7t
extracellular water, 318–319,
319f
filtration, 485
function of, in body, 317f
insensible perspiration, 321
intoxication, 323–324, 444
intracellular water, 318–319,
319f
kidneys and hydration,
321, 322f
major functions of, 5t
metabolic water, 320
as nutrient, 5
as nutrient in foods, 15
osmosis, 318, 318f

pH of, 102, 102f
preparing for disasters,
476–477
sanitizing drinking water to
prevent travelers' diarrhea,
484–485
in select food, 320t
simple diffusion, 317–318,
317f
as source of minerals, 327
sources of, 320, 320t
total water intake, 320
types of, 362, 362t
Water intoxication,
323–324, 444
Water-soluble vitamins
classifying vitamins as, 259,
259t
coenzyme action and,
281, 281f
defined, 259
folate, 287–290
MyPlate, 283f
niacin, 285–286
preserving vitamin content in
food, 264
riboflavin, 284
summary of, 282t
thiamin, 281–284
toxicity and, 259
vitamin B-6, 286
vitamin B-12, 290–293
vitamin C, 294–296
Weaning, 509–510
Weight
changes in older adults, 525
environmental influences on,
391–392
food composition factors, 389
genetic factors, 389–391
healthy, classification as, body
mass index (BMI), 386t,
394, 394f
physiological factors, 388–391
psychological factors, 393
set-point theory, 391
societal, 393
socioeconomic factors, 392
Weight classifications
based on body mass index
(BMI), 386, 386t
based on percentage body fat,
376, 377t
Weight control
body composition, 372–377
Dietary Guidelines, 68–69
energy balance, 383–385,
384f–385f
fiber, 155
gaining weight, 409–410
glycemic index, 149

Weight-control Information
Network (WIN), 396
Weight gain
energy balance, 383–385,
384f–385f
during pregnancy, 499–500,
500t
strategies for, 409–410
Weight loss and weight loss
procedures/plans, 393–401
advertising hype, analyzing,
407–408
bariatric surgical procedure,
402–403
behavior modification,
396–397
BMI and deciding if needed,
394
calorie reduction, 395–396
community-based programs,
399
dietary supplements, 407–408
energy balance, 383–385,
384f–385f
fad diets, 404–405
features of, 395, 395t
fiber and, 155
high-protein diet and, 236
liposuction, 403–404
low-carbohydrate diets, 144,
405–406, 405t
maintaining weight loss tips,
401
medication, 401–402
motivation, 395
MyPlate for, 73
older adults and, 525
rapid weight loss and
dehydration, 315, 323
real story of, 400
regular physical activity, 396
set-point theory, 391
Weight training. See Resistance
training
Weight Watchers, 399, 400
Wernicke-Korsakoff syndrome,
202, 284
Western diet, 87, 150, 235
What's in the Food You Eat, 86
Wheat
food allergy to, 239
food processing and, 17
White House Task Force on
Childhood Obesity, 521
Whole grains
defined, 65
enrichment vs., 262
fiber and, 136–137
food labeling guidelines and,
136, 137f
health claims and, 80
minerals and, 327

Widow's hump, 332, 333f
Women. *See also* Gender differences
　body composition, 6, 317
　iron intake, 347, 349
Women, Infants, and Children (WIC)
　iron deficiency anemia and, 350
　program, 22t
World Anti-Doping Agency (WADA), 447
World Health Organization (WHO), 236, 476

X

Xenical, 401–402
Xerophthalmia, 271, 271f
Xylitol, 133

Y

Yeast, alcohol production, 195
Yersinia enterocolitica, 464t
Yogurt, probiotics, 119

Z

Zeaxanthin, 270
　age-related macular degeneration (AMD), 300
　sources/biological effect of, 8t
Zinc, 352–354
　Daily Value, A1
　deficiency, 352–354
　dietary adequacy, 352–353
　as essential nutrient, 7t, 100t
　food sources of, 352, 353f, 353t
　function of, 325f, 352
　meats, 66
　MyPlate, 353f
　protein-rich foods, 66
　summary of, 346t
　toxicity, 353–354
　UL, 353
　vegetarianism and, 233

Dietary Reference Intakes (DRIs): Recommended Intakes for Individuals, Vitamins
Food and Nutrition Board, Institute of Medicine, National Academies

A

Life Stage Group	Vitamin A (µg/d)a	Vitamin C (mg/d)	Vitamin D (µg/d)b,c	Vitamin E (mg/d)d	Vitamin K (µg/d)	Thiamin (mg/d)	Riboflavin (mg/d)	Niacin (mg/d)e	Vitamin B–6 (mg/d)	Folate (µg/d)f	Vitamin B–12 (µg/d)	Pantothenic Acid (mg/d)	Biotin (µg/d)	Choline (mg/d)g
Infants														
0–6 mo	400*	40*	10	4*	2.0*	0.2*	0.3*	2*	0.1*	65*	0.4*	1.7*	5*	125*
7–12 mo	500*	50*	10	5*	2.5*	0.3*	0.4*	4*	0.3*	80*	0.5*	1.8*	6*	150*
Children														
1–3 y	300	15	15	6	30*	0.5	0.5	6	0.5	150	0.9	2*	8*	200*
4–8 y	400	25	15	7	55*	0.6	0.6	8	0.6	200	1.2	3*	12*	250*
Males														
9–13 y	600	45	15	11	60*	0.9	0.9	12	1.0	300	1.8	4*	20*	375*
14–18 y	900	75	15	15	75*	1.2	1.3	16	1.3	400	2.4	5*	25*	550*
19–30 y	900	90	15	15	120*	1.2	1.3	16	1.3	400	2.4	5*	30*	550*
31–50 y	900	90	15	15	120*	1.2	1.3	16	1.3	400	2.4	5*	30*	550*
51–70 y	900	90	15	15	120*	1.2	1.3	16	1.7	400	2.4h	5*	30*	550*
>70 y	900	90	20	15	120*	1.2	1.3	16	1.7	400	2.4h	5*	30*	550*
Females														
9–13 y	600	45	15	11	60*	0.9	0.9	12	1.0	300	1.8	4*	20*	375*
14–18 y	700	65	15	15	75*	1.0	1.0	14	1.2	400i	2.4	5*	25*	400*
19–30 y	700	75	15	15	90*	1.1	1.1	14	1.3	400i	2.4	5*	30*	425*
31–50 y	700	75	15	15	90*	1.1	1.1	14	1.3	400i	2.4	5*	30*	425*
51–70 y	700	75	15	15	90*	1.1	1.1	14	1.5	400	2.4h	5*	30*	425*
>70 y	700	75	20	15	90*	1.1	1.1	14	1.5	400	2.4h	5*	30*	425*
Pregnancy														
≤18 y	750	80	15	15	75*	1.4	1.4	18	1.9	600j	2.6	6*	30*	450*
19–30 y	770	85	15	15	90*	1.4	1.4	18	1.9	600j	2.6	6*	30*	450*
31–50 y	770	85	15	15	90*	1.4	1.4	18	1.9	600j	2.6	6*	30*	450*
Lactation														
≤18 y	1200	115	15	19	75*	1.4	1.6	17	2.0	500	2.8	7*	35*	550*
19–30 y	1300	120	15	19	90*	1.4	1.6	17	2.0	500	2.8	7*	35*	550*
31–50 y	1300	120	15	19	90*	1.4	1.6	17	2.0	500	2.8	7*	35*	550*

ng = milligram, µg = microgram

NOTE: This table (taken from the DRI reports; see www.nap.edu) presents Recommended Dietary Allowances (RDAs) in **bold type** and Adequate Intakes (AIs) in ordinary type followed by an asterisk (*). RDAs and AIs may both be used as goals for individual intake. RDAs are set to meet the needs of almost all (97 to 98%) individuals in a group. For healthy breastfed infants, the AI is the mean intake. The AI for other life stage and gender groups is believed to cover needs of all individuals in the group, but lack of data or uncertainty in the data prevents being able to specify with confidence the percentage of individuals covered by this intake.

[a] As retinol activity equivalents (RAEs). 1 RAE = 1 µg retinol, 12 µg β–carotene, 24 µg α–carotene, or 24 µg β–cryptoxanthin. To calculate RAEs from REs of provitamin A carotenoids in foods, divide the REs by 2. For preformed vitamin A in foods or supplements and for provitamin A carotenoids in supplements, 1 RE = 1 RAE.

[b] cholecalciferol. 1 µg cholecalciferol = 40 IU vitamin D.

[c] In the absence of adequate exposure to sunlight.

[d] As α–tocopherol. α–Tocopherol includes RRR–α–tocopherol, the only form of α–tocopherol that occurs naturally in foods, and the 2R–stereoisomeric forms of α–tocopherol (RRR–, RSR–, RRS–, and RSS–α–tocopherol) that occur in fortified foods and supplements. It does not include the 2S–stereoisomeric forms of α–tocopherol (SRR–, SSR–, SRS–, and SSS–α–tocopherol), also found in fortified foods and supplements.

[e] As niacin equivalents (NE). 1 mg of niacin = 60 mg of tryptophan; 0–6 months = preformed niacin (not NE).

[f] As dietary folate equivalents (DFE). 1 DFE = 1 µg food folate = 0.6 µg of folic acid from fortified food or as a supplement consumed with food = 0.5 µg of a supplement taken on an empty stomach.

[g] Although AIs have been set for choline, there are few data to assess whether a dietary supply of choline is needed at all stages of the life cycle, and it may be that the choline requirement can be met by endogenous synthesis at some of these stages.

[h] Because 10 to 30% of older people may malabsorb food–bound B–12, it is advisable for those older than 50 years to meet their RDA mainly by consuming foods fortified with B–12 or a supplement containing B–12.

[i] In view of evidence linking folate intake with neural tube defects in the fetus, it is recommended that all women capable of becoming pregnant consume 400 µg from supplements or fortified foods in addition to intake of food folate from a varied diet.

[j] It is assumed that women will continue consuming 400 µg from supplements or fortified food until their pregnancy is confirmed and they enter prenatal care, which ordinarily occurs after the end of the periconceptional period—the critical time for formation of the neural tube.

Adapted from the Dietary Reference Intakes series, National Academies Press. Copyright 1997, 1998, 2000, 2001, 2011, by the National Academy of Sciences. The full reports are available from the National Academies Press at www.nap.edu.

B

Dietary Reference Intakes (DRIs): Recommended Intakes for Individuals, Elements
Food and Nutrition Board, Institute of Medicine, National Academies

Life Stage Group	Calcium (mg/d)	Chromium (µg/d)	Copper (µg/d)	Fluoride (mg/d)	Iodine (µg/d)	Iron (mg/d)	Magnesium (mg/d)	Manganese (mg/d)	Molybdenum (µg/d)	Phosphorus (mg/d)	Selenium (µg/d)	Zinc (mg/d)
Infants												
0–6 mo	200*	0.2*	200*	0.01*	110*	0.27*	30*	0.003*	2*	100*	15*	2*
7–12 mo	260*	5.5*	220*	0.5*	130*	11	75*	0.6*	3*	275*	20*	3
Children												
1–3 y	700	11*	340	0.7*	90	7	80	1.2*	17	460	20	3
4–8 y	1000	15*	440	1*	90	10	130	1.5*	22	500	30	5
Males												
9–13 y	1300	25*	700	2*	120	8	240	1.9*	34	1250	40	8
14–18 y	1300	35*	890	3*	150	11	410	2.2*	43	1250	55	11
19–30 y	1000	35*	900	4*	150	8	400	2.3*	45	700	55	11
31–50 y	1000	35*	900	4*	150	8	420	2.3*	45	700	55	11
51–70 y	1000	30*	900	4*	150	8	420	2.3*	45	700	55	11
>70 y	1200	30*	900	4*	150	8	420	2.3*	45	700	55	11
Females												
9–13 y	1300	21*	700	2*	120	8	240	1.6*	34	1250	40	8
14–18 y	1300	24*	890	3*	150	15	360	1.6*	43	1250	55	9
19–30 y	1000	25*	900	3*	150	18	310	1.8*	45	700	55	8
31–50 y	1000	25*	900	3*	150	18	320	1.8*	45	700	55	8
51–70 y	1200	20*	900	3*	150	8	320	1.8*	45	700	55	8
>70 y	1200	20*	900	3*	150	8	320	1.8*	45	700	55	8
Pregnancy												
≤18 y	1300	29*	1000	3*	220	27	400	2.0*	50	1250	60	12
19–30 y	1000	30*	1000	3*	220	27	350	2.0*	50	700	60	11
31–50 y	1000	30*	1000	3*	220	27	360	2.0*	50	700	60	11
Lactation												
≤18 y	1300	44*	1300	3*	290	10	360	2.6*	50	1250	70	13
19–30 y	1000	45*	1300	3*	290	9	310	2.6*	50	700	70	12
31–50 y	1000	45*	1300	3*	290	9	320	2.6*	50	700	70	12

NOTE: This table presents Recommended Dietary Allowances (RDAs) in **bold type** and Adequate Intakes (AIs) in ordinary type followed by an asterisk (*). RDAs and AIs may both be used as goals for individual intake. RDAs are set to meet the needs of almost all (97 to 98%) individuals in a group. For healthy breastfed infants, the AI is the mean intake. The AI for other life stage and gender groups is believed to cover needs of all individuals in the group, but lack of data or uncertainty in the data prevents being able to specify with confidence the percentage of individuals covered by this intake.

Sources: Dietary Reference Intakes for Calcium, Phosphorus, Magnesium, Vitamin D, and Fluoride (1997); Dietary Reference Intakes for Thiamin, Riboflavin, Niacin, Vitamin B–6, Folate, Vitamin B–12, Pantothenic Acid, Biotin, and Choline (1998); Dietary Reference Intakes for Vitamin C, Vitamin E, Selenium, and Carotenoids (2000); Dietary Reference Intakes for Vitamin A, Vitamin K, Arsenic, Boron, Chromium, Copper, Iodine, Iron, Manganese, Molybdenum, Nickel, Silicon, Vanadium, and Zinc (2001); and Dietary Reference Intakes for Calcium and Vitamin D (2011). These reports may be accessed via www.nap.edu. Copyright 1997, 1998, 2000, 2001, and 2011 by the National Academy of Sciences. The full reports are available from the National Academies Press at www.nap.edu.

Adapted from the Dietary Reference Intake series, National Academies Press.

C

Dietary Reference Intakes (DRIs): Recommended Intakes for Individuals, Macronutrients
Food and Nutrition Board, Institute of Medicine, National Academies

Life Stage Group	Carbohydrate (g/d)	Total Fiber (g/d)	Fat (g/d)	Linoleic Acid (g/d)	α−Linolenic Acid (g/d)	Protein[a] (g/d)
Infants						
0–6 mo	60*	ND	31*	4.4*	0.5*	9.1*
7–12 mo	95*	ND	30*	4.6*	0.5*	**11.0**
Children						
1–3 y	**130**	19*	ND[b]	7*	0.7*	**13**
4–8 y	**130**	25*	ND	10*	0.9*	**19**
Males						
9–13 y	**130**	31*	ND	12*	1.2*	**34**
14–18 y	**130**	38*	ND	16*	1.6*	**52**
19–30 y	**130**	38*	ND	17*	1.6*	**56**
31–50 y	**130**	38*	ND	17*	1.6*	**56**
51–70 y	**130**	30*	ND	14*	1.6*	**56**
>70 y	**130**	30*	ND	14*	1.6*	**56**
Females						
9–13 y	**130**	26*	ND	10*	1.0*	**34**
14–18 y	**130**	26*	ND	11*	1.1*	**46**
19–30 y	**130**	25*	ND	12*	1.1*	**46**
31–50 y	**130**	25*	ND	12*	1.1*	**46**
51–70 y	**130**	21*	ND	11*	1.1*	**46**
>70 y	**130**	21*	ND	11*	1.1*	**46**
Pregnancy						
14–18 y	**175**	28*	ND	13*	1.4*	**71**
19–30 y	**175**	28*	ND	13*	1.4*	**71**
31–50 y	**175**	28*	ND	13*	1.4*	**71**
Lactation						
14–18 y	**210**	29*	ND	13*	1.3*	**71**
19–30 y	**210**	29*	ND	13*	1.3*	**71**
31–50 y	**210**	29*	ND	13*	1.3*	**71**

NOTE: This table presents Recommended Dietary Allowances (RDAs) in **bold type** and Adequate Intakes (AIs) in ordinary type followed by an asterisk (*). RDAs and AIs may both be used as goals for individual intake. RDAs are set to meet the needs of almost all (97 to 98%) individuals in a group. For healthy breastfed infants, the AI is the mean intake. The AI for other life stage and gender groups is believed to cover needs of all individuals in the group, but lack of data or uncertainty in the data prevents being able to specify with confidence the percentage of individuals covered by this intake.

[a]Based on 0.8g protein/kg body weight for reference body weight.

[b]ND = not determinable at this time.

Sources: Dietary Reference Intakes for Energy, Carbohydrate, Fiber, Fat, Fatty Acids, Cholesterol, Protein, and Amino Acids (2002). This report may be accessed via www.nap.edu.

Adapted from the Dietary Reference Intake series, National Academies Press. Copyright 1997, 1998, 2000, 2001, by the National Academy of Sciences. The full reports are available from the National Academies Press at www.nap.edu.

D

Dietary Reference Intakes (DRIs): Recommended Intakes for Individuals, Electrolytes and Water
Food and Nutrition Board, Institute of Medicine, National Academies

Life Stage Group	Sodium (mg/d)	Potassium (mg/d)	Chloride (mg/d)	Water (L/d)
Infants				
0–6 mo	120*	400*	180*	0.7*
7–12 mo	370*	700*	570*	0.8*
Children				
1–3 y	1000*	3000*	1500*	1.3*
4–8 y	1200*	3800*	1900*	1.7*
Males				
9–13 y	1500*	4500*	2300*	2.4*
14–18 y	1500*	4700*	2300*	3.3*
19–30 y	1500*	4700*	2300*	3.7*
31–50 y	1500*	4700*	2300*	3.7*
51–70 y	1300*	4700*	2000*	3.7*
> 70 y	1200*	4700*	1800*	3.7*
Females				
9–13 y	1500*	4500*	2300*	2.1*
14–18 y	1500*	4700*	2300*	2.3*
19–30 y	1500*	4700*	2300*	2.7*
31–50 y	1500*	4700*	2300*	2.7*
51–70 y	1300*	4700*	2000*	2.7*
> 70 y	1200*	4700*	1800*	2.7*
Pregnancy				
14–18 y	1500*	4700*	2300*	3.0*
19–50 y	1500*	4700*	2300*	3.0*
Lactation				
14–18 y	1500*	5100*	2300*	3.8*
19–50 y	1500*	5100*	2300*	3.8*

NOTE: The table is adapted from the DRI reports. See www.nap.edu. Adequate Intakes (AIs) are followed by an asterisk (*). These may be used as a goal for individual intake. For healthy breastfed infants, the AI is the average intake. The AI for other life stage and gender groups is believed to cover the needs of all individuals in the group, but lack of data prevent being able to specify with confidence the percentage of individuals covered by this intake; therefore, no Recommended Dietary Allowance (RDA) was set.

Source: *Dietary Reference Intakes for Water, Potassium, Sodium, Chloride, and Sulfate* (2005). This report may be accessed via www.nap.edu.

Acceptable Macronutrient Distribution Ranges

	Range (percent of energy)		
Macronutrient	**Children, 1–3 y**	**Children, 4–18 y**	**Adults**
Fat	30–40	25–35	20–35
omega–6 polyunsaturated fats (linoleic acid)	5–10	5–10	5–10
omega–3 polyunsaturated fats[a] (α–linolenic acid)	0.6–1.2	0.6–1.2	0.6–1.2
Carbohydrate	45–65	45–65	45–65
Protein	5–20	10–30	10–35

[a]Approximately 10% of the total can come from longer–chain n–3 fatty acids.

SOURCE: *Dietary Reference Intakes for Energy, Carbohydrate, Fiber, Fat, Fatty Acids, Cholesterol, Protein, and Amino Acids* (2002). The report may be accessed via www.nap.edu.

Adapted from the Dietary Reference Intakes series, National Academies Press. Copyright 1997, 1998, 2000, 2001, 2011, by the National Academy of Sciences. The full reports are available from the National Academies Press at www.nap.edu.

Dietary Reference Intakes (DRIs): Tolerable Upper Intake Levels (UL[a]), Vitamins
Food and Nutrition Board, Institute of Medicine, National Academies

Life Stage Group	Vitamin A (μg/d)[b]	Vitamin C (mg/d)	Vitamin D (μg/d)	Vitamin E (mg/d)[c,d]	Vitamin K	Thiamin	Riboflavin	Niacin (mg/d)[d]	Vitamin B-6 (mg/d)	Folate (μg/d)[d]	Vitamin B-12	Pantothenic Acid	Biotin	Choline (g/d)	Carotenoids[e]
Infants															
0–6 mo	600	ND	25	ND	ND	ND	ND	ND	ND	ND	ND	ND	ND	ND	ND
7–12 mo	600	ND	38	ND	ND	ND	ND	ND	ND	ND	ND	ND	ND	ND	ND
Children															
1–3 y	600	400	63	200	ND	ND	ND	10	30	300	ND	ND	ND	1.0	ND
4–8 y	900	650	75	300	ND	ND	ND	15	40	400	ND	ND	ND	1.0	ND
Males, Females															
9–13 y	1700	1200	100	600	ND	ND	ND	20	60	600	ND	ND	ND	2.0	ND
14–18 y	2800	1800	100	800	ND	ND	ND	30	80	800	ND	ND	ND	3.0	ND
19–70 y	3000	2000	100	1000	ND	ND	ND	35	100	1000	ND	ND	ND	3.5	ND
>70 y	3000	2000	100	1000	ND	ND	ND	35	100	1000	ND	ND	ND	3.5	ND
Pregnancy															
≤18 y	2800	1800	100	800	ND	ND	ND	30	80	800	ND	ND	ND	3.0	ND
19–50 y	3000	2000	100	1000	ND	ND	ND	35	100	1000	ND	ND	ND	3.5	ND
Lactation															
≤18 y	2800	1800	100	800	ND	ND	ND	30	80	800	ND	ND	ND	3.0	ND
19–50 y	3000	2000	100	1000	ND	ND	ND	35	100	1000	ND	ND	ND	3.5	ND

[a]UL = The maximum level of daily nutrient intake likely to pose no risk of adverse effects. Unless otherwise specified, the UL represents total intake from food, water, and supplements. Due to lack of suitable data, ULs could not be established for vitamin K, thiamin, riboflavin, vitamin B–12, pantothenic acid, biotin, or carotenoids. In the absence of ULs, extra caution may be warranted in consuming levels above recommended intakes.

[b]As preformed vitamin A only.

[c]As α–tocopherol; applies to any form of supplemental α–tocopherol.

[d]The ULs for vitamin E, niacin, and folate apply to synthetic forms obtained from supplements, fortified foods, or a combination of the two.

[β]β–Carotene supplements are advised only to serve as a provitamin A source for individuals at risk of vitamin A deficiency.

[f]ND = Not determinable due to lack of data of adverse effects in this age group and concern with regard to lack of ability to handle excess amounts. Source of intake should be from food only to prevent high levels of intake.

SOURCES: Dietary Reference Intakes for Calcium, Phosphorus, Magnesium, Vitamin D, and Fluoride (1997); Dietary Reference Intakes for Thiamin, Riboflavin, Niacin, Vitamin B–6, Folate, Vitamin B–12, Pantothenic Acid, Biotin, and Choline (1998); Dietary Reference Intakes for Vitamin C, Vitamin E, Selenium, and Carotenoids (2000); Dietary Reference Intakes for Vitamin A, Vitamin K, Arsenic, Boron, Chromium, Copper, Iodine, Iron, Manganese, Molybdenum, Nickel, Silicon, Vanadium, and Zinc (2001); and Dietary Reference Intakes for Calcium and Vitamin D (2011). These reports may be accessed via www.nap.edu.

Adapted from the Dietary Reference Intakes series, National Academies Press. Copyright 1997, 1998, 2000, 2001, 2011, by the National Academy of Sciences. The full reports are available from the National Academies Press at www.nap.edu.

E

Dietary Reference Intakes (DRIs): Tolerable Upper Intake Levels (UL[a]), Elements and Electrolytes[b,c]
Food and Nutrition Board, Institute of Medicine, National Academies

Life Stage Group	Arsenic[b]	Boron (mg/d)	Calcium (g/d)	Copper (μg/d)	Fluoride (mg/d)	Iodine (μg/d)	Iron (mg/d)	Magnesium (mg/d)[d]	Manganese (mg/d)	Molybdenum (μg/d)	Nickel (mg/d)	Phosphorus (g/d)	Selenium (μg/d)	Vanadium (mg/d)[e]	Zinc (mg/d)	Sodium (mg/d)	Chloride (mg/d)
Infants																	
0–6 mo	ND[f]	ND	1	ND	0.7	ND	40	ND	ND	ND	ND	ND	45	ND	4	ND	ND
7–12 mo	ND	ND	1.5	ND	0.9	ND	40	ND	ND	ND	ND	ND	60	ND	5	ND	ND
Children																	
1–3 y	ND	3	2.5	1000	1.3	200	40	65	2	300	0.2	3	90	ND	7	1500	2300
4–8 y	ND	6	2.5	3000	2.2	300	40	110	3	600	0.3	3	150	ND	12	1900	2900
Males, Females																	
9–13 y	ND	11	3	5000	10	600	40	350	6	1100	0.6	4	280	ND	23	2200	3400
14–18 y	ND	17	3	8000	10	900	45	350	9	1700	1.0	4	400	ND	34	2300	3600
19–70 y	ND	20	2.5[g]	10000	10	1100	45	350	11	2000	1.0	4	400	1.8	40	2300	3600
>70 y	ND	20	2	10000	10	1100	45	350	11	2000	1.0	3	400	1.8	40	2300	3600
Pregnancy																	
≤18 y	ND	17	3	8000	10	900	45	350	9	1700	1.0	3.5	400	ND	34	2300	3600
19–50 y	ND	20	2.5	10000	10	1100	45	350	11	2000	1.0	3.5	400	ND	40	2300	3600
Lactation																	
≤18 y	ND	17	3	8000	10	900	45	350	9	1700	1.0	4	400	ND	34	2300	3600
19–50 y	ND	20	2.5	10000	10	1100	45	350	11	2000	1.0	4	400	ND	40	2300	3600

[a]UL = The maximum level of daily nutrient intake that is likely to pose no risk of adverse effects. Unless otherwise specified, the UL represents total intake from food, water, and supplements. Due to lack of suitable data, ULs could not be established for arsenic, chromium, and silicon. In the absence of ULs, extra caution may be warranted in consuming levels above recommended intakes.

[b]Although a UL was not determined for arsenic, there is no justification for adding arsenic to food or supplements.

[c]Although silicon has not been shown to cause adverse effects in humans, there is no justification for adding silicon to supplements.

[d]The ULs for magnesium represent intake from a pharmacological agent only and do not include intake from food and water.

[e]Although vanadium in food has not been shown to cause adverse effects in humans, there is no justification for adding vanadium to food and vanadium supplements should be used with caution. The UL is based on adverse effects in laboratory animals and this data could be used to set a UL for adults but not children and adolescents.

[f]ND = Not determinable due to lack of data of adverse effects in this age group and concern with regard to lack of ability to handle excess amounts. Source of intake should be from food only to prevent high levels of intake.

[g]Upper Limit declines to 2 after age 50.

SOURCES: Dietary Reference Intakes for Calcium, Phosphorus, Magnesium, Vitamin D, and Fluoride (1997); Dietary Reference Intakes for Thiamin, Riboflavin, Niacin, Vitamin B–6, Folate, Vitamin B–12, Pantothenic Acid, Biotin, and Choline (1998); Dietary Reference Intakes for Vitamin C, Vitamin E, Selenium, and Carotenoids (2000); Dietary Reference Intakes for Vitamin A, Vitamin K, Arsenic, Boron, Chromium, Copper, Iodine, Iron, Manganese, Molybdenum, Nickel, Silicon, Vanadium, and Zinc (2001); and *Dietary Reference Intakes for Water, Potassium, Sodium, Chloride, and Sulfate* (2004). These reports may be accessed via www.nap.edu. The full reports are available from the National Academy of Sciences. Copyright 1997, 1998, 2000, 2001, 2011, by the National Academies Press.

Adapted from the Dietary Reference Intakes series, National Academies Press.

F